The Manual of Cytotechnology

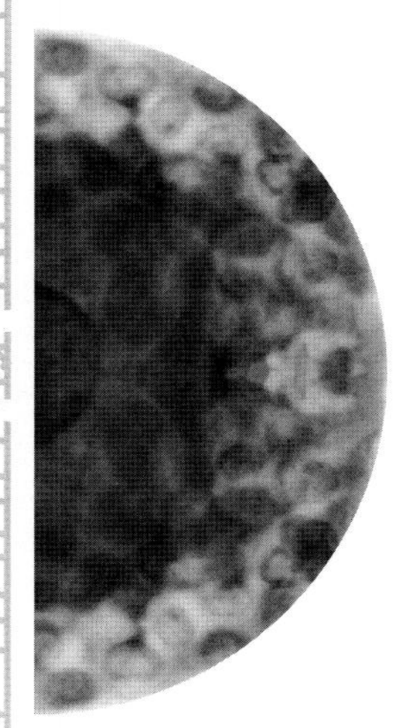

7th Edition

This publication was funded in part by grants from MetPath and Roche Biomedical Laboratories, Inc.

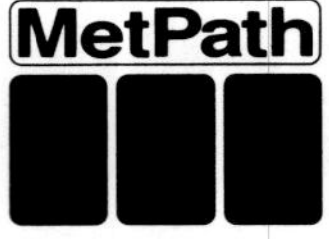

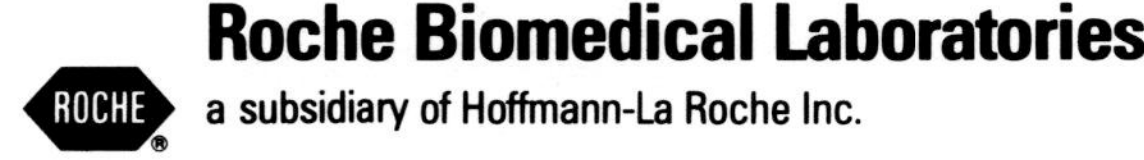

a **CORNING** Clinical Laboratory

Edited by

Catherine M. Keebler, CT(ASCP), CFIAC, ScD(hon)
Registrar, International Academy of Cytology
Chicago, Illinois

Theresa M. Somrak, JD, CT(ASCP), CFIAC
Director, Cytopathology Education Activities Consortium
Chicago, Illinois

The Manual of Cytotechnology

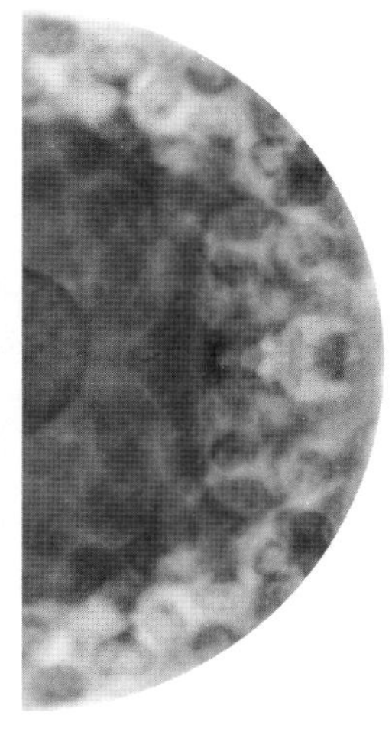

7th Edition

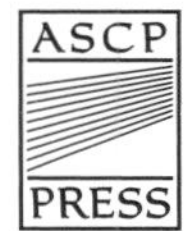

American Society of Clinical Pathologists
Chicago

Publishing Team

Jeffrey L. Carlson (design/production)
Shannon Hansford (marketing)
Andrea Meenahan (illustrations)
Philip Rogers (editorial)
Joshua Weikersheimer (acquisitions)

Notice:

Trade names for equipment and supplies described herein are included as suggestions only. In no way does their inclusion constitute an endorsement or preference by the American Society of Clinical Pathologists. The ASCP did not test the equipment, supplies, or procedures and, therefore, urges all readers to read and follow all manufacturers' instructions and package insert warnings concerning the proper and safe use of products.

Library of Congress Cataloging in Publication Data

The manual of cytotechnology/edited by Catherine M. Keebler, Theresa M. Somrak—7th ed.
p. 464
Includes bibliographical references and index.
ISBN 0-89189-352-0
1. Cytodiagnosis—Handbooks, manuals, etc.
I. Keebler, Catherine M. II. Somrak, Theresa M. III. American Society of Clinical Pathologists.
[DNLM: 1. Cytodiagnosis—laboratory manuals.
2. Neoplasms—diagnosis—laboratory manuals.
QZ 241 M294 1993]
RB43.M38 1993
616.07'582—dc20
DNLM/DLC 93-20250
for Library of Congress CIP

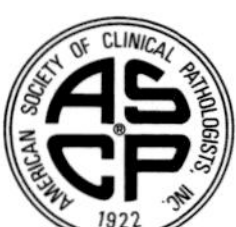

Printed in Hong Kong

97 96 95 94 93 5 4 3 2 1

Table of Contents

PART 3: NONGYNECOLOGIC CYTOLOGY

PART 4: FNA CYTOLOGY

PART 5: LABORATORY FUNCTION AND ADMINISTRATION

PART 6: TECHNICAL CONSIDERATIONS

Stanley F. Patten, Jr, MD, PhD, FIAC
Professor Emeritus and Senior Faculty Associate
Former Chairman and Director of Cytopathology
Department of Pathology and Laboratory Medicine
University of Rochester Medical Center
Rochester, New York

Stanley J. Radio, MD
Assistant Professor
Director, Cytopathology
Department of Pathology & Microbiology
University of Nebraska Medical Center
Omaha, Nebraska

Abraham E. Rakoff, MD, FIAC†
Professor Emeritus of Obstetrics and Gynecology
Medicine (Endocrinology)
Director, Division of Gynecologic Endocrinology
and Infertility
Jefferson Medical College
Thomas Jefferson University
Philadelphia, Pennsylvania

James W. Reagan, MD†
Professor of Pathology and Reproductive Biology
Director of Anatomic Pathology
Institute of Pathology
Case Western Reserve University
Cleveland, Ohio

Dorothy L. Rosenthal, MD, FIAC
Professor of Pathology
UCLA School of Medicine
Director, Section of Cytopathology
UCLA Medical Center
Los Angeles, California

Jan F. Silverman, MD
Professor and Director of Cytology
Department of Pathology and Laboratory Medicine
East Carolina University School of Medicine
Greenville, North Carolina

Diane Solomon, MD, MIAC
Chief, Cytopathology Section
National Cancer Institute
Bethesda, Maryland

Theresa M. Somrak, JD, CT(ASCP), CFIAC
Director, Cytopathology Education Consortium
Activities:
American Society of Cytology
American Society of Clinical Pathologists
American Society for Cytotechnology
Chicago, Illinois

George L. Wied, MD, FIAC
Former Professor and Chief, Section of Cytopathology
The University of Chicago
Chicago, Illinois

† Deceased.

Figures

Tables

Preface

The seventh edition of *The Manual of Cytotechnology* is dedicated to the memory of James W. Reagan, MD, internationally known surgical pathologist and cytopathologist, educator, and coeditor of previous editions of this book. Dr Reagan was instrumental in developing and refining what was once a simple method for detecting cancer and its precursors into a recognized, mature discipline in pathology. His meticulous, didactic approach to the teaching of cytotechnology is echoed in many of the chapters in this book written by friends and colleagues.

Since the first edition of *The Manual of Cytotechnology* in 1962, our knowledge and understanding of the cellular manifestation of various disease processes has increased exponentially. The seventh edition has been completely revised to include the most up-to-date information needed by cytotechnology students as well as cytopathology professionals. To provide this updated resource for individuals beginning their careers in cytotechnology as well as a reference for seasoned diagnosticians, 24 new authors were recruited to contribute chapters. In addition, 13 new chapters were added in the areas of fine needle aspiration cytology, human papillomavirus infection, gynecologic nomenclature, and laboratory function and administration. The editors hope this revision provides a current educational tool for all students in cytopathology.

The editors are indebted to many individuals who made this revised edition possible. We wish to express our appreciation to the authors who contributed their valuable time, expertise, and photomicrography. We are especially grateful to the ASCP Press staff for their support in the preparation of the manuscript: Jeffrey Carlson, design and production; Shannon Hansford, marketing; Andrea Meenahan, illustrations; Philip Rogers, editing; and Joshua Weikersheimer, coordinator of the project.

CHAPTER 1

Ethics and Liability

CATHERINE M. KEEBLER, CT(ASCP), CFIAC
THERESA M. SOMRAK, JD, CT(ASCP), CFIAC

CONTENTS

A CODE OF ETHICS FOR THE CYTOTECHNOLOGIST

Ethics is at the core of the health care profession, yet it is difficult to define. Ethics can be considered as the principles of conduct governing an individual or group. Ethics addresses conduct from a philosophical standpoint. It evokes a sense of moral and fundamentally correct behavior. Ethics in the health care profession transcends the law because the conduct of health care providers impacts directly on patients. Central to the health care profession is a responsibility and commitment to patients to prevent harm. Each time cytotechnologists review a cytologic specimen they must assure that their undivided attention and expertise is given to that patient. Ethics incorporates values above those that are minimally required by law. In other words, a code of ethics represents what we should do as cytotechnologists, not what we must do to fulfill government regulations.

The code of ethics outlined herein evolved from the authors' experience, as well as from concepts conveyed by cytotechnologists, cytopathologists, and clinicians; from examples set by supervisors and coworkers; and from knowledge of what the patient and medical community expect of an individual engaged in diagnostic cytology and cancer detection.

As cytotechnologists we have a duty:

- to patients to avoid endangering their welfare;
- to ourselves to uphold the high standards of our profession;
- to cytopathologists to assist them in preparing the final diagnostic assessment;
- to our employers to insure quality patient care;
- to clinicians to provide a reliable laboratory report; and
- to the community at large to provide the best possible cytologic service in detecting cancer as well as identifying premalignant and infectious conditions.

The following represent aspects of our profession that constitute an ethical practice of cytotechnology:

1. The cytotechnologist should practice in a clinical laboratory only under the supervision of a pathologist or other individual qualified to direct the laboratory.
2. The cytotechnologist should know the source of the cell sample, and should not render judgment on material for which this information is lacking, or on material from body sites of which the cytotechnologist has no experience.
3. The cytotechnologist should not perform assessments on clearly inadequate material and should report the reason for the inadequacy of the cellular sample.
4. The cytotechnologist should maintain a certain monthly (daily) minimum and maximum number of screened cellular samples. These numeric limits depend on the type of material received and the cytotechnologist's level of experience. The maximum number of cell samples evaluated should not exceed the current recommended number as designated by federal or state agencies or those suggested by the American Society of Cytology and other accrediting agencies.
5. The cytotechnologist should be expected to examine the entire representative cellular sample. Errors in inadequate screening of cell samples are more critical than errors in judgment.
6. The cytotechnologist is responsible to some extent for the internal quality control of the laboratory. The main responsibility for such control lies with the medical director; however, the cytotechnologist should participate in all phases of a laboratory quality assurance program.
7. The cytotechnologist should reevaluate previously interpreted specimens after their histologic verification, especially if there is a discrepancy between the histologic report and the original cytopathologic report.
8. The cytotechnologist should maintain patient confidentiality. Patients and their medical history should not be discussed outside of the laboratory setting. Laboratory reports should be issued only to authorized individuals.
9. The cytotechnologist should participate in continuing education programs. These may be internal programs within the laboratory, or programs provided by local, regional, national, or international organizations. Additionally, the cytotechnologist should keep up with current developments and/or writings concerning diagnostic cytology.

The practice of cytotechnology involves trust. The patient must be assured that the specimen is properly examined. The laboratory director must be assured that the cytotechnologist renders reliable judgments on the examined cell samples. The clinician must be assured that the service rendered is consistent with the highest standards and performed according to current concepts.

Individual cytotechnologists should realize that their behavior is representative of all cytotechnologists. The cytopathology laboratory is a focal point in contemporary medical practice. It is one of the major routes by which current concepts and diagnostic discoveries are transferred to patient care. Clinicians increasingly rely on the results of cytodiagnostic examinations to assist them in diagnosis and treatment. These forces create the continuing and growing need for highly motivated and competent cytotechnologists. Certifications, such as CT(ASCP), SCT(ASCP), and CT(IAC), attest to the qualifications of the individual at the time of issuance. Since the learning process does not stop with certification, continuing education and the desire to improve knowledge and skills are necessary to maintain high professional standards.

MEDICOLEGAL ISSUES IN THE CYTOPATHOLOGY LABORATORY

Specimens must be accurately evaluated and interpreted; misdiagnosis may result in inappropriate treatment of a patient. Recently, medicolegal concerns have been raised regarding the reliability of cytologic interpretation, especially in the gynecologic cytopathology field. Medicolegal implications are of particular concern to cytotechnologists, since they are responsible for the initial screening and interpretation of cytologic specimens.

This section discusses legal issues that may arise in the cytopathology laboratory. An overview of legal doctrines and theories as they apply to a laboratory, as well as technologist liability, is discussed. Approaches for reducing the risk of liability are then suggested.

Legal Doctrines Affecting the Cytopathology Laboratory

Legal doctrines affecting laboratory personnel include statutory law, administrative law, and common law. Statutory law is law enacted by either federal or state legislatures. The Clinical Laboratory Improvement Act of 1988 (CLIA '88) is an example of a statutory law that requires all laboratories and laboratory personnel to comply with its mandates. Administrative law is law created by an administrative government agency to implement statutory law via rules and regulations. The Health Care Financing Administration (HCFA) is such an administrative agency and is responsible for developing the regulations needed to implement CLIA '88.

Common law is distinguished from statutory law in that it derives authority from the courts rather than from the legislature. Common law is developed on a case-by-case basis through the judiciary system. Elements of the common law include judicial judgments and decrees, which establish precedent, as well as customary practices and common usages within society or a profession, as in the case of the laboratory. Common law imposes professional standards and corresponding liabilities on laboratory personnel if these standards are not met or if mistakes are made.

Legal Theories Affecting Laboratory Personnel

Negligence is a broad legal theory affecting laboratory personnel. It encompasses legal concepts such as professional responsibility and standard of care.

Negligence in its broad scope is best thought of in terms of the "reasonable person." The legal definition of negligence is either the omission to do something a reasonable person would do or the act of doing something a reasonable person would not do. Negligence is characterized by inadvertence, thoughtlessness, and inattention. The negligence theory is predicated on the duty of every person to exercise due care in his or her conduct toward others so that no harm results. For an act or an omission of an act to be found negligent the following elements must be satisfied: (1) A legal duty must exist. (2) A breach (violation or omission) of the duty must occur. (3) The breach of the duty must be the cause of the harm or injury. (4) Harm or injury must have occurred. (5) The person harmed or injured must have suffered actual damages. The following discussion focuses on professional responsibility and standard of care as they apply to laboratory personnel.

Laboratory professionals are responsible for proper evaluation of cytologic specimens. Professional responsibility and the standard of care have traditionally focused on the physician or pathologist in charge of a laboratory and are based on professional guidelines in the particular locale where the professional works. As the practice of medicine becomes more uniform, there is a trend in most states to expand this "locality rule" to a "similar locality rule" or a national standard. This wider focus has greater application to the cytopathology laboratory as procedures and protocols become standardized. With the passage of CLIA'88 and the implementation of HCFA regulations, courts will look to these documents for guidance to determine what is acceptable laboratory practice.

Another trend emerging is the implication of cytotechnologists along with pathologists when a laboratory mistake occurs that harms the patient. As was previously stated, cytotechnologists are responsible for the initial evaluation of the cytologic specimen. Cytotechnologists must accurately review specimens and bring abnormal findings to the attention of the pathologist. Legally this duty is applied not only to the person who performs the evaluation but also to those who employ or exercise direct control over the work of the technologist.

A legal theory called "respondeat superior," which means literally let the master answer, holds an employer responsible for the negligent acts of employees that occur within the scope of employment. An employee/employer relationship is established if the following criteria are met: (1) The employer hires the employee. (2) The employer pays the salary of the employee, deducting taxes and social security. (3) The employer has the power to control the employee. (4) The employer can fire the employee. Many cytotechnologists are employed by hospitals or private laboratories and therefore would be protected from liability under the theory of respondeat superior. However, self-employed cytotechnologists could be held liable for erroneous evaluation of a specimen. Thus, self-employed cytotechnologists should carry professional liability insurance.

Reducing the Risk of Liability

It is an accepted fact that liability risk cannot be eliminated. Human nature dictates that mistakes will occur.

However, the risk of liability can be reduced. This can be accomplished by adhering to the aforementioned code of ethics, participating in peer review accreditation programs, complying with government regulations, and establishing ongoing continuing quality improvement protocols. If a mistake occurs, a careful and truthful examination of the facts is the best reaction. If it is shown that there has been a cover-up, the situation can become greatly magnified and complicated.

Communication also plays an important role in managing risk liability. There should be effective communication between the laboratory and referring clinicians. The laboratory's findings should be correlated with the observations of the clinician who submits the specimen for interpretation. Laboratory personnel should report all cytologic findings using concise, descriptive, and unambiguous terminology. The primary purpose of diagnostic technology is to communicate to the referring clinician all information necessary to assure proper patient care.

CONCLUSION

The cytopathology laboratory and its personnel are an integral component of the health care team. Clinicians and their patients rely on an accurate evaluation of cytologic specimens. Liability in the laboratory cannot be eliminated but it can be reduced and effectively managed with the development of and the adherence to quality improvement procedures and ethical standards.

CHAPTER

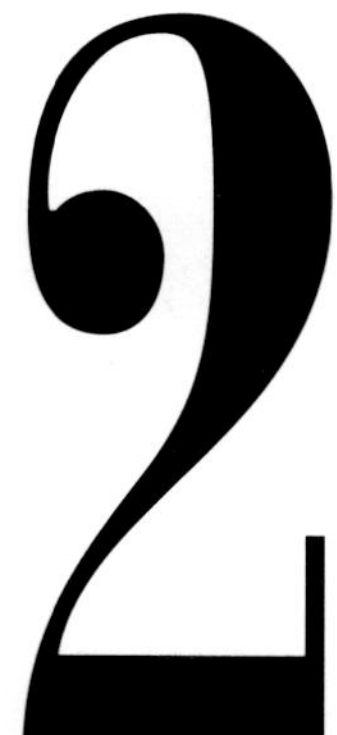

Clinical Cytology and Cytotechnology

SHIRLEY GREENING, MS, JD, CFIAC

CONTENTS

THE ORIGINS OF CLINICAL CYTOLOGY

Contemporary clinical cytology, also termed diagnostic cytology, reflects the culmination of centuries of trial, error, and discovery in traditional fields of anatomy, evolution, genetics, histology, pathology, and physiology, as well as the impact of more recent advances in biochemistry, computerization, and molecular biology. Modern cytology practice required the invention of the microscope, then the conception and development of cell theory, and breakthroughs in specimen fixation, staining, and processing methods, which allowed detailed visualization of cells and cell components. These philosophical and technical innovations are a mirror of their times, from the ancient, Greco-Roman, Medieval, and Renaissance eras, through the Industrial Revolution, the post-World War II period, and into the present.

Egyptians (circa 3000 BC) practiced embalming, although their exact method for preserving mummies is still not known. The Greek physician Hippocrates (circa 460-377 BC), the "father of medicine," theorized that disturbances in the balance of the four "humours" (blood, yellow bile, black bile, and phlegm) produced disease. The Roman Celsus (circa 30 BC-38 AD) described the four classical signs of inflammation: rubor (redness), tumor (swelling), calor (heat), and dolor (pain). The Renaissance (circa 1300-1600) produced the anatomists Beniveni, da Vinci, and Vesalius, each of whom performed human dissections and autopsies to determine anatomic structure and causes of illness and death. Between 1650 and 1700, scientists such as Malpighi, Hooke, Swammerdam, and Grew were among the first to study and describe the morphology of individual cells using rudimentary microscopes. The application of microscopy to advance understanding of cell structure and function earned this era the designation "golden age of microscopy."

The anatomist and pathologist Morgagni studied and reported the relationships between abnormal findings and patient symptoms from over 700 postmortem examinations during the "Age of Enlightenment" (circa 1700-1800). Textile manufacturing during the 19th century spurred development of synthetic (aniline) dyes, which were quickly applied to cellular study. The first half of the 20th century was marked by the introduction of electron microscopes, automated cell analyzers, computers, and emerging molecular biologic techniques, along with their earliest application to cellular diagnosis.

The acceptance of diagnostic cytology as a current and valid discipline in medicine is largely due to the work of Papanicolaou (1883-1962), the "father of modern cytology" [**F***2.1*]. In the 1920s Papanicolaou began to publish material on the cytologic method for hormonal evaluation and, in 1928, suggested that this method was of value in the diagnosis of cancer of the uterine cervix. Independently and earlier in the same year, Babes published material on the same subject. Recognition of cytology as a valuable diagnostic tool occurred following publication of monographs by Papanicolaou and Traut (*Diagnosis of Uterine Cancer by the Vaginal Smear* in 1943) and Papanicolaou et al (*The Epithelia of the Women's Reproductive Organs* in 1948). Since then the number of reports on cytologic techniques, results, and application to various body systems has been overwhelming in the United States and in many parts of the world. The cytologic method is now well recognized and accepted.

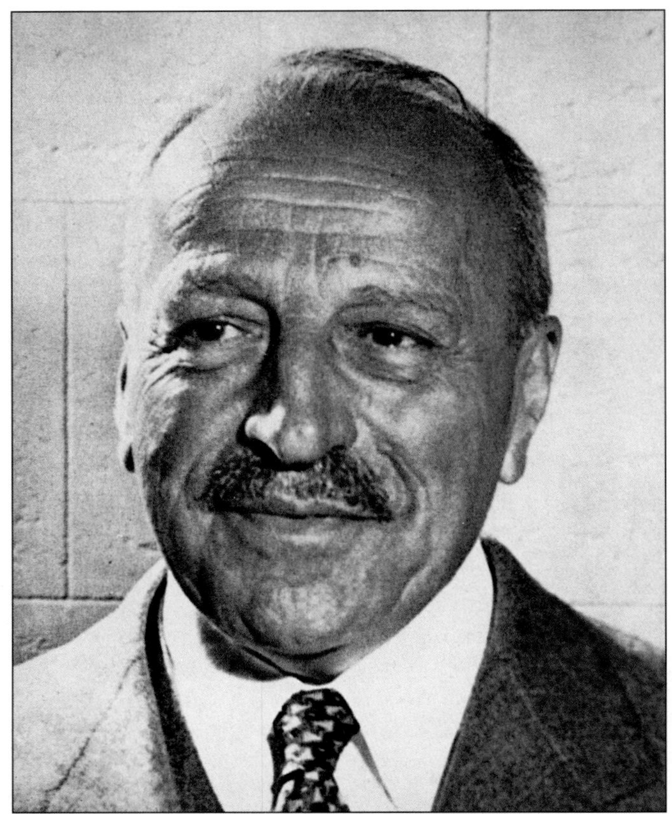

F*2.1*
George N. Papanicolaou, 1883-1962.

Papanicolaou also published the *Atlas of Exfoliative Cytology* in 1954 (with a supplement in 1956). The author of over 150 publications and the recipient of many honors and awards, Papanicolaou will long be remembered as the first to place cytology on firm ground.

Cytodiagnosis is currently applied to virtually every body site. The technique of applying a cell sample to a glass slide and staining the sample by various modifications of the staining method developed by Papanicolaou is sometimes referred to as a "Pap test." This technique, as well as endoscopic brushings, fine needle aspiration, and other collection methods, combined with sophisticated imaging techniques such as magnetic resonance and tomography, has placed the practice of clinical cytology in the forefront of preventive and diagnostic medicine.

DEVELOPMENT OF THE MICROSCOPE AND MICROSCOPIC CELL ANALYSIS

1590 Janssen builds the first compound microscope.
1624 Galileo builds microscopes patterned after his telescopes.
1625 Selluti publishes the first illustrations (of bees) made from microscopic observations.
1625 Faber first coins the word microscope (*microscopio*).
1653 Borel publishes *Historiarum et Observationum Medicophysicarum Centuria*, the first work linking microscopy with medicine.
1658 Kircher, with a microscope magnifying only x32, describes "worms" in plague victims (probably red and white blood cells) as a cause of disease.
1658 Swammerdam precisely describes red blood cells.
1665 Hooke publishes *Micrographia*, containing the first illustrations of cellular structures, and in doing so originates the word "cell."
1674 van Leeuwenhoek, using some of the over 200 microscopes and more than 400 lenses he constructed, reports his discovery of "animalcules" (protozoa) found in pond water.
1757 Dolland makes the first achromatic glass, thereby eliminating for future microscopists the shimmering, rainbow-like aberrations of objects placed under chromatic lenses.
1791 Beeldsnijder develops the first achromatic compound microscope.
1911 The fluorescence microscope is developed.
1926 Busch discovers that magnetic and electrostatic fields could be used as lenses to focus a beam to produce an ultramicroscopic image.
1931 Knoll and Ruska develop a prototype transmission electron microscope.
1934 Moldavan describes his attempts at photoelectric counting of cells flowing through a capillary tube, representing the first attempt at flow cytometry.
1935 Knoll outlines the principle of the scanning electron microscope.
1940 Videomicroscopy is developed for use as a diagnostic aid.
1941 Hillier and Vance construct an electron microscope capable of resolving power to 25 Å.
1947 Gucker describes an aerosol particle counter developed for the detection of airborne bacteria and spores, the principles of which are applied to flow cytometric analysis.
1950 Caspersson publishes his monograph *Cell Growth and Function*, describing microspectrophotometric measurements of normal and abnormal cell growth and metabolism.
1950 Friedman uses fluorescence microscopy for uterine cancer cell detection.
1951 Mellors and Silver develop a scanning microfluorometer to quantitatively measure DNA fluorescence in individual cells.
1952 Mellors, Keane, and Papanicolaou apply quantitative DNA measurement to squamous cancer cells.
1953 Coulter-type blood cell counters are developed.
1955 Tolles and Bostrom describe the automated optoelectronic "Cytoanalyzer," a system designed to detect malignant and premalignant cells based on size and density measurements.
1961 Hallerman describes a fluorochrome-based method for flow cytometric differential blood counts.
1967 Kamentsky uses a spectrophotometric cell sorter for cervical cytology classification.
1968 Finkel performs analysis of cervical cytology specimens using medium-resolution image analysis with ultraviolet absorption methods.
1968 Fulwyler describes experiments on cervical cell flow cytometric fluorescence using an argon ion laser.
1987 Computer-based digital image systems using neural network-emulating and algorithmic software are developed for use as automated cervical cancer screening devices.

DEVELOPMENT OF THE CELL THEORY AND THE FOUNDATIONS OF MOLECULAR CELL BIOLOGY

1656 Borel reports microscopic descriptions of what were probably red blood cells.
1661 Malpighi, founder of histology, refers to microscopic "utricles," "globules," and "saccules," all of which were probably cells.
1672 Grew publishes illustrations of the microscopic anatomy of plants, describing small "utricles" and "vesicles."
1759 Wolff, founder of embryology, describes "particles," which constitute all animal organs.
1802 de Mirbel observes that "plants appear to be entirely composed of cells and of tubes."
1824 Dutrochet writes that "all organic tissues are actually globular cells of exceeding smallness...united by adhesive forces."
1831 Brown reports his discovery of the cell nucleus.
1832 Dumortier reports his observation of cell division in algae.
1838 Schleiden publishes his treatise explaining the derivation of plant tissues from cells.
1839 Schwann applies Schleiden's cell theory to animal tissues. Schleiden's and Schwann's treatises establish the "cell theory" as a biologic concept.
1842 Nageli describes chromosomes during plant cell division.
1858 Virchow first applies cell theory to pathology, and is recognized as the founder of cellular pathology. In the same year Virchow, in his theory of cell lineage, postulates that present cells come from preexisting

cells in an unbroken line of descent, thus relating cytology to embryology, heredity, and evolution.

1859 Darwin postulates his evolution theory of natural selection.

1866 Mendel establishes the science of genetics with the publication of his preeminent work on inheritance in pea plants.

1869 Miescher separates "nuclein" (nucleic acid) from cell nuclei, presaging development of the field of biochemistry.

1875 Strasburger uses the terms "mitosis" and "karyokinesis" to describe cell division in plant cells. The stages of mitosis still bear the names he gave them.

1876 Flemming describes mitosis in animal cells and uses the term "chromatin" to describe nuclear material.

1888 von Waldeyer uses the term "chromosomes" to describe the fragmentation of nuclei during mitosis.

1897 Buchner shows that organic chemical transformations can be performed on yeast cell extracts by converting glucose into ethyl alcohol, one of the earliest experiments in the emerging field of biochemistry.

1898 Golgi first describes the cytoplasmic chemical and secretory apparatus (complex) that bears his name.

1900 Fischer demonstrates that peptide bonds form chemical links between amino acids.

1903 Sutton observes that each gamete receives only one set of chromosomes during germ cell division, and recognizes chromosomes as the carriers of Mendel's units of heredity.

1903 Levene discovers the chemical distinction between DNA and RNA

1904 Morgan, the founder of modern experimental genetics, begins his genetic studies of the fruit fly, *Drosophila melanogaster*

1909 Johannsen names Mendel's units of heredity "genes."

1909 Garrod recognizes the link between inherited recessive mutations and disease in his treatise *Inborn Errors of Metabolism*.

1931 McClintock correlates rearrangements of chromosome segments with redistribution of genetic traits in experiments with *Zea mays* (corn).

1938 Caspersson and Schultz show that nucleic acid content doubles during the mitotic cycle.

1941 Beadle and Tatum, in their experiments with the bread mold *Neurospora*, first demonstrate that genes control protein (enzyme) structure.

1944 Avery, MacLeod, and McCarty establish DNA as the carrier of genetic information.

1946 Lederberg first uses the bacterium *Escherichia coli* to study nutritional mutations and to demonstrate that genes could be transferred from one organism to another.

1951 Pauling suggests a helical arrangement for parts of protein chains.

1952 Hershey and Chase show that genetic information that causes new viral production resides in DNA.

1953 Watson and Crick demonstrate the double-helical structure of DNA.

1959 Kendrew determines the spatial position of each atom in myoglobin using x-ray crystallography.

1961 Jacob and Monod introduce the principle that protein products of certain genes regulate activity of other genes, thus unifying the biochemical, electron microscopic, and genetic study of cell function under one unifying field, molecular cell biology.

1962 Eagle perfects the first defined cell growth medium and successfully cultures mammalian cells in vitro.

1962 Puck pioneers culturing of single mammalian cells.

1962 Dulbecco introduces animal virology as a quantitative science.

1978 Gene cloning and recombinant DNA technology emerge.

DEVELOPMENT OF STAINS, FIXATIVES, AND CYTOHISTOLOGIC TECHNIQUES

1660 Hooke uses natural dyestuffs (logwood and cochineal) to stain wool and hair.

1665 Hooke first uses "thin sectioning" to study the architecture of a piece of cork.

1714 van Leeuwenhoek uses saffron to improve microscopic visibility of muscle fibers.

1735 Belchier introduces intravital staining for bovine bone specimens.

1770 Hill uses carmine to show plant vascular systems.

1807 Link uses an iron salt to microscopically identify tannin cells in plants.

1825 Raspail uses iodine to demonstrate starch granules.

1849 Goppert and Cohn first use carmine as a histologic stain.

1850 Hartig uses the dark purple juice from pokeweed berries as a nuclear stain (phytolacca).

1852 Babo introduces centrifugation as a cell separation technique.

1856 Perkins produces first aniline purple dyes.

1858 Gerlach introduces staining as routine laboratory procedure.

1861 Grohe uses ferrocyanide staining for tissue iron.

1865 Bohmer first uses hematoxylin.

1869 Bottcher introduces alcohol differentiation as a staining technique.

1869 Klebs introduces paraffin embedding of tissues.

1875 Ranvier uses synthetic dyes for histologic sections, including quinoline blue for fat droplets.

1877 Ehrlich uses aniline dyes to stain specific granules in white blood cells, thus introducing the field of hematology.

1893 Blum first uses formalin as a tissue fixative.

1896 Daddi introduces Sudan III as a lysochrome stain.
1897 Macallum adds the hematoxylin reaction to ferrocyanide staining.
1899 Fischer publishes his monograph on the fixation of tissues.
1900 Widal introduces ether-alcohol as a cellular fixative.
1910 Harrison introduces in vitro tissue culture technique.
1917 Papanicolaou develops trichrome stain to demonstrate hormonal changes in vaginal epithelial cells in guinea pigs.
1953 Porter and Blum introduce the first widely adopted ultramicrotome.
1959 Lehrer and Ornstein introduce enzyme localization using organic enzyme histochemical stains.
1961 Caro demonstrates the use of autoradiography in electron microscopy.
1963 Sabatini introduces gluteraldehyde as a fixative for electron microscopy.
1966 Nakane uses an enzyme-tagged antibody for electron microscopic localization of antigen.

THE FOUNDATIONS OF CLINICAL DIAGNOSTIC CYTOLOGY

1845 Lebert studies malignant cells in effusions.
1847 Pouchet publishes a monograph on ovulation.
1860 Beale examines exfoliated cancer cells in sputum.
1864 Sanders describes malignant cells found in urine specimens.
1869 Dickenson examines discharges from women with uterine cancer but fails to find diagnostic cells.
1891 Quincke and Wynter introduce lumbar puncture, enabling cytologic examination of cerebrospinal fluid.
1895 Lucatello performs aspiration biopsy of liver for cellular diagnosis.
1896 Bahrenberg reports the usefulness of cytology in diagnosing peritoneal carcinomatosis.
1896 Daiber publishes his atlas on urine sediment.
1901 Ewing publishes *Clinical Pathology of the Blood*.
1904 Dufour reports his findings of malignant cells in cerebrospinal fluids.
1909 Marissi employs gastric lavage to study esophageal and gastric cancers.
1920 Papanicolaou publishes materials on the cytologic method for hormonal evaluation.
1924 Cowdry publishes his edition of *General Cytology*.
1928 Papanicolaou presents his finding that cytology is of value in diagnosing cancer of the uterine cervix.
1928 Babes publishes *Diagnosis of Cancer of the Uterine Cervix by Smears*.
1943 Papanicolaou and Traut publish *Diagnosis of Uterine Cancer by the Vaginal Smear*.
1947 Ayre documents that a cell sample obtained directly from the uterine cervix by a wooden spatula is more efficient and easier to examine than a vaginal smear.
1948 Papanicolaou et al publish *The Epithelia of Women's Reproductive Organs*.
1954 Papanicolaou publishes *Atlas of Exfoliative Cytology*.

CYTOTECHNOLOGY

Some of the first cytotechnologists were not identified by that name—they were called laboratory technicians in the 1930s and cytologic technicians or technologists in the 1940s. By the 1950s, however, the professional designation "cytotechnologist" was firmly established.

Cytotechnologists initially received their training "on the job," which consisted of intensive microscopic study and review of available cytologic specimens as they were received in the few established cytology laboratories of the late 1930s and early 1940s. Formal lectures were rare, since knowledge of cytodiagnostic criteria for each organ system was still developing. The first formal cytology training programs, ranging in length from 1 week to 1 year, were set up as fellowships to support physicians in their study of cytology. However, as the concept and availability of cervical cytology mass screening programs became commonplace, the need for additional technical assistance to handle the increasing specimen volume became critical. By 1947, several structured programs offered lectures and microscopy to both prospective cytotechnologists and physicians. Uniform national standards (called *Essentials*) for cytotechnology training programs were approved in 1962, and have been revised and updated four times since then.

THE PROFESSIONAL ROLE OF THE CYTOTECHNOLOGIST

Cytotechnologists are employed in hospital and private laboratories, and in research, education, managerial, or other health care industry positions. As valued members of health care diagnostic teams that include pathologists, clinicians, and other specialists, cytotechnologists are proficient in:

- determining and implementing the appropriate procedures for collecting and processing biological specimens for cytologic analysis.
- detecting, differentiating, and diagnosing presence or absence of disease in gynecologic and nongynecologic samples.
- selecting and clearly marking the cells most representative of the nature of any pathological process present.
- evaluating gynecologic material with sufficient competency to meet the entry-level responsibility

of issuing the final report for gynecologic specimens within normal limits.
- integrating and relating data generated by the various clinical departments while making judgments regarding possible discrepancies; confirming cytologic results; verifying quality control procedures; and developing solutions to problems concerning the generation of laboratory data.
- using contemporary and uniform diagnostic terminology in reporting laboratory results.
- making judgments concerning the results of quality assurance measures and instituting proper procedures to maintain accuracy and precision.
- evaluating current and new techniques, instruments, and procedures in terms of their clinical and diagnostic usefulness and practicality, including consideration of a given facility's personnel, equipment, space, and budgetary resources.
- demonstrating professional conduct and interpersonal communication skills with patients, laboratory personnel, other health care professionals, and the public.
- recognizing, encouraging, and acting on an individual's need for continuing education as a function of growth and maintenance of professional competence.
- applying sound principles of management and supervision.
- understanding and/or applying sound principles of scientific research and educational methodology.

EDUCATION PROGRAMS

Contemporary cytotechnology programs are sponsored by universities, hospitals, medical schools, or laboratories, or combinations of these facilities. Program length may vary from 1 to 4 years, depending on whether cytotechnology training is continuous or integrated into undergraduate programs that culminate in a baccalaureate degree. One-year programs may constitute the fourth year of college ("3+1" programs), or postbaccalaureate certificate or graduate-level programs. Some programs are interspersed through the 4 years of college, while others are termed upper division ("2+2" programs), where cytotechnology training takes place in the third and fourth years of college.

All cytotechnology programs in the United States, regardless of length and structure, are collaboratively reviewed for approval and accreditation by the Cytotechnology Programs Review Committee of the American Society of Cytology. The accreditation process assures that programs meet standards of quality in areas of administration, educational resources, curriculum content, and preparation of students for entry-level competencies in cytotechnology. Cytotechnology program faculty design courses, microscopic sessions, and clinical experiences so that students will meet these competencies on completion of their training.

CYTOTECHNOLOGY COMPETENCIES

1. On presentation of a cytologic specimen to the laboratory, the cytotechnologist will be able to
   - accept or reject the specimen.
   - select and perform the most advantageous preparation technique.
   - select and perform the most advantageous staining procedure.
   - coverslip and label the specimen.
   - apply principles of quality control.
   - solve problems in staining and preparation procedures.
   - evaluate and implement new preparation procedures.
2. When given cervicovaginal cellular samples, the cytotechnologist will be able to microscopically identify and discriminate among the following entities:
   - Specimen adequacy
   - Cellular constituents within normal limits
   - Cellular changes associated with infections
   - Reactive and reparative cellular changes, including inflammation, effects of therapy, effects of mechanical devices, and effects of diethylstilbestrol exposure
   - Epithelial squamous cell abnormalities, including atypical squamous cells of undetermined significance, low-grade and high-grade squamous intraepithelial lesions, and squamous cell carcinoma
   - Glandular cell abnormalities, including presence of endometrial cells, atypical glandular cells of undetermined significance, and adenocarcinoma
   - Nonepithelial malignant neoplasms
   - Extrauterine malignant neoplasms
   - Hormonal evaluation
3. The cytotechnologist will be able to evaluate gynecologic material with sufficient competence to meet the entry-level responsibility of issuing the final report for gynecologic specimens within normal limits.
4. When given cellular samples from any nongynecologic cytology specimen, including fine needle aspirations, the cytotechnologist will be able to microscopically identify and discriminate among the following entities:
   - Specimen adequacy
   - Cellular constituents within normal limits
   - Inflammatory cells
   - Microbiologic entities and associated cytomorphology
   - Manifestations of cellular degeneration
   - Atypical cellular manifestations related to benign conditions

- Cellular manifestations of various premalignant processes
- Cellular manifestations of benign neoplasms
- Squamous cell carcinoma, adenocarcinoma, and other malignant neoplasms
- Cellular effects of radiation and chemotherapy
- Altered cellular morphology due to collection methods

5. When given a cellular preparation, the cytotechnologist will be able to detect with a high level of accuracy, select, and clearly mark the cells most representative of the nature of any pathologic process present.
6. On detection of cellular manifestations of disease, the cytotechnologist will be able to develop a differential diagnosis based on the cellular evidence in conjunction with
   - current histologic and cell block specimens.
   - pertinent cognitive knowledge and clinical data.
   - knowledge of the significance of symptoms.
   - knowledge of the various modes of treatment.
   - review of previous patient material.
7. The cytotechnologist will be able to prepare a report using a contemporary and uniform system of diagnostic terminology for gynecologic specimens (such as the Bethesda System or its equivalent) and nongynecologic specimens.
8. The cytotechnologist will demonstrate ability to review histologic tissue sections and pertinent clinical data to build cognitive correlation between tissue patterns of disease and the cellular manifestations of disease, and for the purposes of quality control and quality assurance.
9. The cytotechnologist will demonstrate ability to read and evaluate published professional literature for its pertinence and reliability and use this information in the preparation and evaluation of specimens.
10. The cytotechnologist will demonstrate understanding of basic principles and potential uses of adjunct diagnostic technologies (eg, immunologic stains, flow cytometry, image analysis).
11. The cytotechnologist will apply knowledge of the following practical components of laboratory organization and management:
    - Quality assurance methodology
    - Supply and inventory methods
    - Interpersonal communication skills
    - Annual reports and statistics
    - Budget preparation
    - Reporting methods
    - Policy and procedure manual preparation
12. The cytotechnologist will be able to incorporate quality control and assurance measures in the preparation and microscopic evaluation of specimens as required by appropriate accrediting agencies and regulatory programs.
13. The cytotechnologist will comply with laboratory safety measures and regulations.
14. The cytotechnologist will demonstrate understanding of the principles of preparing and the importance of participating in continuing education sessions.
15. The cytotechnologist will demonstrate understanding of the basic principles of scientific research.
16. The cytotechnologist will demonstrate knowledge of the consequences of specimen evaluation on patient management.
17. The cytotechnologist will demonstrate knowledge of the ethical role and responsibilities of the cytotechnologist by practicing
    - discretion and confidentiality in regard to laboratory and patient reports.
    - honesty and integrity in professional duties.
    - the principles of good personal relationships with peers, staff, and faculty.

SUGGESTED CURRICULUM FOR A CYTOTECHNOLOGY PROGRAM

Cytology is a cumulative learning process; more advanced diagnostic, technical, and clinical course work and practice by their nature require retention and application of basic and fundamental knowledge and concepts. A cytotechnology curriculum should reflect a systematic and progressive sequence of classroom and practical laboratory experiences, including frequent evaluation to assess students' understanding of the principles of diagnostic cytology.

Diagnostic cytology instruction forms the "core curriculum" of a cytotechnology program. Courses and instruction in basic cytomorphology, gynecologic and nongynecologic cytology, fine needle aspiration, cytopreparation techniques, and microscopic study are common to all programs. Study of histology, pathology, management and supervision, research and education methods, and professional issues are also required components of cytotechnology curricula. In addition, students should be exposed to emerging diagnostic technologies and understand basic concepts and operation of laboratory information systems.

The following curriculum illustrates a progressive sequence of courses in a cytotechnology program, the schedule and course credits of which may be modified to conform to 1-year or multiyear integrated programs.

Term/Phase 1

Morphologic Cytology

Two credits (equivalent to 2 hours lecture and 3 hours microscopy per week for 15 weeks). Basic cellular structure and function, methods of examining the cell sample, and general cytomorphology in normalcy, inflammation, infection, reaction to injury, atypia, neoplasia (benign and malignant), and cellular changes due to therapy (lecture and microscopy sessions).

Functional Histology

Two credits (equivalent to 2 hours lecture and 3 hours microscopy per week for 15 weeks). Microscopic study of the human body, including normal structure and function and relationships to life processes (lecture and microscopy sessions).

Cytopreparatory Techniques

Two credits (equivalent to 4 hours of laboratory practice per week for 15 weeks). Study and practice in the techniques used for preparation and staining of specimens for cytologic study, including compliance with laboratory safety and biohazard precautions.

Gynecologic Cytopathology

Four credits (equivalent to 5 hours lecture per week for 15 weeks). Study of normal anatomy, physiology, and benign and malignant pathophysiology of the female genital tract and corresponding cytomorphologic features, and value of cytologic diagnosis in patient management.

Gynecologic Cytopathology Laboratory

Four credits (equivalent to 10 hours microscopy per week for 15 weeks). Application of cytodiagnostic criteria to develop practical expertise in microscopic analysis prior to clinical practice.

Term/Phase 2

Nongynecologic Cytopathology

Five credits (equivalent to 6 hours lecture per week for 15 weeks). Study of normal anatomy, physiology, benign and malignant pathophysiology, and corresponding cytomorphologic features of the respiratory, gastrointestinal, urinary, breast, and central nervous systems, and effusions, and value of cytologic diagnosis in patient management.

Nongynecologic Cytopathology Laboratory

Five credits (equivalent to 12 hours microscopy per week for 15 weeks). Application of cytodiagnostic criteria to develop practical expertise in microscopic analysis of respiratory, gastrointestinal, urinary, breast, and central nervous system, and effusion cytology specimens prior to clinical practice.

Diagnostic Laboratory

Two credits (equivalent to 2 hours lecture and 3 hours microscopy per week for 15 weeks). Review and discussion of selected cases in gynecologic and nongynecologic cytology, including clinical correlations, using microscopy, literature review, and patient simulations.

Term/Phase 3

Pathology Lecture

Two credits (equivalent to 2 hours lecture per week for 15 weeks). Study of basic disease processes of the body, including inflammation, repair, fluid and hemodynamic disorders, and neoplasia; and specific disease processes affecting the major body systems.

Pathology Laboratory

One credit (equivalent to 2 hours microscopy per week for 15 weeks). Laboratory instruction in the microscopic presentation of general pathologic processes.

Advanced Diagnostic Cytology

Two credits (equivalent to 1 hour lecture and 3 hours microscopy per week for 15 weeks). Discussion and microscopic examination of challenging cases in diagnostic cytology from all body sites, emphasizing fine needle aspiration cytology, with histologic and clinical correlation.

Clinical Practicum I

Eight credits (equivalent to 24 hours clinical laboratory experience per week for 15 weeks). Clinical internship in a cytopathology laboratory. Students participate in all phases of diagnostic service work and laboratory functions, including experience in continuing education activities and diagnostic seminars.

Term/Phase 4

Clinical Practicum II

Eight credits (equivalent to 24 hours clinical laboratory experience per week for 15 weeks). Continuation of the clinical internship in a cytopathology laboratory.

Laboratory Management

Three credits (equivalent to 3 hours lecture per week for 15 weeks). Management functions (planning, organizing, directing, coordinating, and controlling) as applied to laboratories in the health care delivery system, including quality control and assurance, inventory methods, reporting methods, budgeting, and information systems.

Biochemical and Imaging Technology

Two credits (equivalent to 2 hours per week for 15 weeks). Discussion, technical demonstrations, and practical experience in emerging diagnostic and treatment methods involving laboratory diagnosis, including immunochemistry, flow cytometry, molecular diagnostic techniques, biotechnology, and digital image analysis.

Seminar

Two credits (equivalent to 2 hours per week for 15 weeks). Problem-solving strategies and case studies encompassing management, supervision, education, professional ethics and responsibility, government regulation, and medicolegal issues as they relate to medical testing laboratories, technologists, the health care system, health services research, and policy formulation.

Health Services Research

Two credits (equivalent to 2 hours per week plus research time for 15 weeks). Guided study and/or research in cytopathology or a related discipline, under faculty supervision. Oral and written presentation of results of study/research is required. Prerequisite: Completion of advanced laboratory science course work.

The following laboratory experiences or courses may be incorporated into cytotechnology programs to augment the study of diagnostic cytology, or to expand students' learning and experiences:

Histopreparatory Techniques

Two credits (equivalent to 4 hours laboratory practice per week for 15 weeks). Introduction to histologic preparatory techniques and special stains.

Histopathology

Two credits (equivalent to 4 hours laboratory practice per week for 15 weeks). Technical preparation of tissue specimens for microscopic examination, including gross dissection of tissues, paraffin processing, sectioning, routine and special staining, and preparation of a histopathologic report.

Electron Microscopy

Two credits (equivalent to 4 hours laboratory practice per week for 15 weeks). Preparation techniques, principles of operation, and diagnosis for electron microscopic study.

Other courses could be conducted in statistics and research methodology, microcomputer software program analysis, biochemistry and/or introduction to molecular cell biology, and interpersonal communications.

CERTIFICATION OF CYTOTECHNOLOGISTS

The Board of Registry of the American Society of Clinical Pathologists (ASCP) offers national certification examinations in cytotechnology to students and experienced cytotechnologists who fulfill the eligibility requirements. The written and visual examinations consist of approximately 200 questions. The examinations are also available in computer interactive format. Certification conveys recognition that an individual has met the competencies and qualifications for the profession of cytotechnology.

The Cytotechnologist, CT(ASCP), examination, offered in August each year, requires:

1. Baccalaureate degree from a regionally accredited college/university with 20 semester hours (30 quarter hours) of biologic science (eg, general biology, microbiology, parasitology, cell biology, physiology, anatomy, zoology, histology, embryology, or genetics), 8 semester hours (12 quarter hours) of chemistry, and 3 semester hours (4 quarter hours) of mathematics, AND successful completion of a cytotechnology program accredited by the Committee on Allied Health Education and Accreditation, OR
2. Baccalaureate degree from a regionally accredited college/university with 20 semester hours (30 quarter hours) of biologic science (eg, general biology, microbiology, parasitology, cell biology, physiology, anatomy, zoology, histology, embryology, or genetics), 8 semester hours (12 quarter hours) of chemistry, and 3 semester hours (4 quarter hours) of mathematics, AND 5 years full-time acceptable clinical laboratory experience, including cytopreparatory techniques, microscopic analysis, and evaluation of the body systems, within the last 10 years. At least 2 of these years must be subsequent to the completion of the academic component, and at least 2 years must be under the supervision of a licensed physician who is a pathologist certified, or eligible for certification, by the American Board of Pathology in Anatomic Pathology or has other suitable qualifications acceptable to the Board of Registry.

The Specialist in Cytotechnology, SCT(ASCP), examination is offered yearly and requires:

1. CT(ASCP) certification AND a baccalaureate degree from a regionally accredited college/university AND 5 years of full-time acceptable experience in cytology within the last 10 years. These 5 years of experience must be obtained following CT(ASCP) certification and under the supervision of a licensed physician who is a pathologist certified, or eligible for certification, by the American Board of Pathology in Anatomic Pathology or has other suitable qualifications acceptable to the Board of Registry, OR
2. CT(ASCP) certification AND a master's degree from a regionally accredited college/university AND 4 years of full-time acceptable experience in cytology within the last 10 years. These 4 years of experience must be obtained following CT(ASCP) certification and under the supervision of a licensed physician who is a pathologist certified, or eligible for certification, by the American Board of Pathology in Anatomic Pathology or has other suitable qualifications acceptable to the Board of Registry, OR
3. CT(ASCP) certification AND a doctorate from a regionally accredited college/university AND 3 years of full-time acceptable experience in cytology within the last 10 years. These 3 years of experience must be obtained following CT(ASCP) certification and under the supervision of a licensed physician who is a pathologist certified, or eligible for certifica-

tion, by the American Board of Pathology in Anatomic Pathology or has other suitable qualifications acceptable to the Board of Registry.

For general information and to receive an application for these examinations, write to the Board of Registry, PO Box 12270, Chicago, IL 60612.

PROFESSIONAL SOCIETIES

Membership and involvement in societies and organizations on the local, state, or national level present an excellent means to maintain competence in diagnostic cytology, continue education in general or specialized areas of cytology, and stay updated on professional, legislative, and regulatory issues affecting the practice of cytopathology. Attendance at society meetings provides the opportunity to meet other cytology professionals to talk about relevant issues, and to renew acquaintances with colleagues from other laboratories and institutions.

American Society for Cytotechnology (ASCT)

Established in 1979 by cytotechnologists for cytotechnologists, the ASCT is a nationally recognized peer group organization in which all full members have voting privileges and are eligible to hold office. Membership is also open to physicians, dentists, veterinarians, students, and other professionals interested in cytology. The ASCT represents the professional, legislative, legal, and educational interests of cytotechnologists, and promotes quality practice and professional standards in cytology. At its annual meeting, and in conjunction with state and regional cytology organizations, the society conducts workshops and seminars covering timely issues of interest to the cytology community. The ASCT sponsors National Cytotechnology Day (May 13, Papanicolaou's birthday) each year, and annually recognizes cytotechnologists with its Cytotechnologist Achievement Award, and outstanding students with the Warren R. Lang Memorial Scholarship Award.

The *ASCT News* is the monthly publication of the society, and is sent free of charge to all members. Information about membership, publications, and programs may be obtained from the ASCT National Office, 920 Paverstone Dr, Suite D, Raleigh, NC 27615.

American Society of Cytology (ASC)

The ASC is the field's national medical cytology society and was founded in 1951 as the Inter-Society Cytology Council. The society's aim is to foster the cytologic method in clinical practice through education and research. Cytotechnologists may first become nonvoting associate members, and after 5 years may apply for voting cytotechnology membership. Student membership is also welcome. Cytotechnologists participate on ASC committees and may be nominated and elected by their peers to serve on the Cytotechnology Advisory Committee, which acts as an advisory board to the Executive Committee. Associate and cytotechnologist members contribute to and receive the society's bimonthly publication, the *ASC Bulletin*.

Two cytotechnology awards are presented at the annual ASC scientific meeting. The Cytotechnologist of the Year Award is presented to a cytotechnologist for meritorious service or achievement in the field of cytology. The Cytotechnologist Award of the ASC is presented to the cytotechnologist who gives the best presentation of a scientific paper at the meeting.

The ASC's annual scientific meeting and the interim meeting include poster sessions, platform presentations, panel discussions, guest lectures, workshops, and diagnostic seminars. The ASC also conducts its voluntary laboratory inspection program, which enables qualified laboratories to become accredited, and actively participates in accreditation of schools of cytotechnology through its Cytotechnology Programs Review Committee. Information on membership, and listings and information about accredited laboratories and schools of cytotechnology may be obtained from the ASC, 1015 Chestnut St, Suite 1518, Philadelphia, PA 19107.

American Society of Clinical Pathologists (ASCP)

Associate membership in the ASCP is contingent on certification and current registration with the Board of Registry. Cytotechnologists receive a free subscription to *Laboratory Medicine* with their membership and receive discounts on all education programs and products. Associate members serve on a variety of committees, including the Associate Member Section (AMS), the Council on Cytopathology, and the Cytotechnology Examination Committee of the Board of Registry.

The ASCP conducts a wide range of clinical and anatomic pathology workshops, seminars, and teleconferences throughout the year. The society also publishes textbooks, manuals, videotapes, and other audiovisual teaching aids and reference materials. For information about the ASCP, write to ASCP, 2100 W Harrison St, Chicago, IL 60612.

International Academy of Cytology (IAC)

Academy membership is open to cytotechnologists after successful completion of the IAC Registry Examination in Cytotechnology. CT(IAC) registration offers the only worldwide recognition of cytotechnology performance, therefore candidates from countries in which there is a national certification examination must first pass that country's examination before applying for CT(IAC) certification. Cytotechnologist members (CMIAC) and cytotechnologist fellows (CFIAC) serve as chairs and members of educational and scientific committees of the Academy.

The IAC cosponsors week-long Tutorials of Cytology in the United States and around the world, and international conferences on cytology computerization and cell image analysis. Every 3 years the International Congress of Cytology is held. The journal of clinical cytology, *Acta Cytologica*, is the official periodical of the IAC (as well as of the ASC and numerous national cytology societies). The Tutorials of Cytology publishes teaching slide sets in cytology and the *Compendium on Diagnostic Cytology*. Write to the registrar for information about the registry examination, or the Committee on Continuing Education for information about education programs, both located at the IAC, 1640 E 50th St, Suite 20B, Chicago, IL 60615-3161, USA.

REVIEW EXERCISES

1. The person who first described the four classical signs of inflammation was
   a) Hippocrates.
   b) Vesalius.
   c) Malpighi.
   d) Celsus.
   e) Galen.

2. Knoll and Ruska are (were)
   a) anatomists of the 16th century.
   b) developers of the electron microscope.
   c) responsible for the cell theory.
   d) makers of microscopes in the 17th century.
   e) the first to describe red blood cells.

3. Fundamental cell discoveries made possible with microscopes from 1650 to 1700 earned this period the designation
   a) the Age of Enlightenment.
   b) the Renaissance.
   c) the Golden Age of Microscopy.
   d) the Scientific Revolution.
   e) the Modern Cytology Era.

4. The two scientists credited with early development of the cell theory were
   a) Schleiden and Schwann.
   b) Mendel and Darwin.
   c) Beadle and Tatum.
   d) Brown and Flemming.
   e) Watson and Crick.

5. Morgan, the founder of modern experimental genetics, conducted his research on inheritance with
   a) *Zea mays*.
   b) pea plants.
   c) *Escherichia coli*.
   d) *Drosophila melanogaster*.
   e) utricles and saccules.

6. The scientist credited with introducing the field of hematology, by being the first to use aniline dyes to stain and differentiate white blood cells, was
   a) Hooke.
   b) van Leeuwenhoek.
   c) Perkins.
   d) Klebs.
   e) Ehrlich.

7. Papanicolaou's earliest work in human cancer cytodiagnosis concentrated on cancer of the
   a) respiratory system.
   b) nervous system.
   c) female reproductive tract.
   d) gastrointestinal tract.
   e) urinary tract.

8. The uniform national education standards under which accredited cytotechnology training programs operate are called
   a) competencies.
   b) essentials.
   c) health care teams.
   d) licenses.
   e) certificates.

9. Cytotechnologist competencies are entry-level education and diagnostic standards that cytotechnologists are expected to possess
   a) by the time they retire from the profession.
   b) after 5 years in the field of cytotechnology.
   c) prior to admission to a cytotechnology program.
   d) at the completion of their cytotechnology training program.
   e) before introductory cytology course work is completed.

10. Certification in cytotechnology recognizes that individuals
    a) are ready to begin a cytotechnology training program.
    b) have worked in a hospital laboratory before admission to a training program.
    c) have met the competencies and qualifications for the profession of cytotechnology.
    d) are members in professional societies.
    e) have been cytotechnologists for 25 or more years.

SELECTED READINGS

American Medical Association Committee on Allied Health Education and Accreditation. *Essentials and Guidelines of an Accredited Educational Program for the Cytotechnologist.* Chicago, Ill: American Medical Association; 1992.

Bender GA, Thom RA. *Great Moments in Medicine.* Detroit, Mich: Parke-Davis; 1961.

Carmichael DE. *The Pap Smear: Life of George N. Papanicolaou.* Springfield, Ill: Charles C Thomas Publisher; 1973.

Darnell J, Lodish H, Baltimore D. *Molecular Cell Biology.* 2nd ed. New York, NY: Scientific American Books; 1990.

Gelehrter TD, Collins FS. *Principles of Medical Genetics.* Baltimore, Md: Williams & Wilkins Co; 1990.

Hajdu SI. Cytology from antiquity to Papanicolaou. *Acta Cytol.* 1977;21:668-676.

Koprowska I. George N. Papanicolaou: living memories, monuments, and archives. *Diagn Cytopathol.* 1985;1:68-72.

Koss LG. Analytical and quantitative cytology: a historical perspective. *Anal Quant Cytol.* 1982;4:251-256.

Koss LG. A quarter of a century of cytology. *Acta Cytol.* 1977;21:639-642.

Lillie RD, ed. *H. J. Conn's Biological Stains.* 9th ed. Baltimore, Md: Williams & Wilkins Co; 1977.

MacLeod AG. *Cytology: The Cell and Its Nucleus.* Kalamazoo, Mich: The Upjohn Company; 1973.

Report of a National Study of Cytotechnologists: Education and Performance Relationships. Bethesda, Md: National Council on Medical Technology Education; 1968.

Shapiro HM. *Practical Flow Cytometry.* 2nd ed. New York, NY: Alan R Liss Inc; 1988.

Wischnitzer S. *Introduction to Electron Microscopy.* 2nd ed. Elmsford, NY: Pergamon Press Inc; 1970.

C H A P T E R

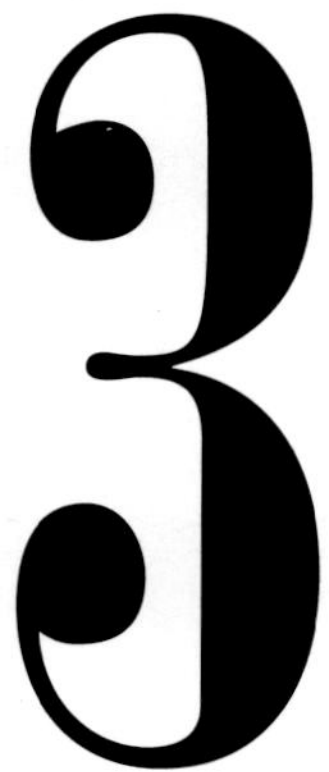

Basic Cellular Structure and Function

GUNTER F. BAHR, MD, FIAC

CONTENTS

There are two principal types of cells: primitive ones without a distinct nucleus, called prokaryotic cells; and those with a nucleus, called eukaryotic cells. It is believed that nucleated cells derived from the more primitive forms some 2 billion years ago. Bacteria are prokaryotes, while eukaryotes, the nucleated cells, are the building blocks of such divergent species as molds, trees, and animals. The body of a nucleated cell is called its cytoplasm.

The following sections describe a typical nucleated cell and the functions of its organelles as a principal example of the cells of the human body (somatic cells) seen in cytologic preparations.

NUCLEUS

Nuclear Envelope

In a nondividing cell, the nucleus can be clearly distinguished because it is enclosed by a thin membranous structure, the nuclear envelope [**F**3.1]. The term "envelope" is used by cell biologists today in recognition of the complexity of this structure, the meaning of which is not adequately conveyed by the term "membrane." (Since the two membranes of the envelope cannot be seen under the light microscope, continued use of the term "nuclear membrane" is practical for light microscopists.) The nuclear envelope consists not only of two membranes, but also of doughnut-like structures (tori) on the inside of the envelope, where the two membranes closely approach each other. The inner nuclear membrane is slightly thicker than the outer one and encloses the nuclear content in a taut fashion. This impression of tautness is produced partly because the chromatin, some of the fibrous content of the nucleus, is anchored in many places to the inner nuclear membrane.

In many vertebrate and invertebrate cells, and in some cancer cells, an additional structure has been described. It is called the fibrous lamina and is usually a uniform, dense layer—100 to 200 Å (0.01-0.02 µm) thick (1 Å = about the distance of -C-C-, or two carbon atoms in a molecule)—tightly applied to the inside of the inner nuclear membrane. Its function is not known, but it may contribute to the prominence of the nuclear envelope under the light microscope, especially in cancer cells.

The outer nuclear membrane is often wavy. It is part of the endoplasmic reticulum, which will be discussed later. Sometimes ribosomes are found attached to the outer nuclear membrane. Space between the outer and inner nuclear membranes, the perinuclear cisterna, is variable and may increase considerably, eg, after radiation injury to the cell; it may become visible as a vacuole or a space adjacent to the nucleus. The perinuclear halo seen in

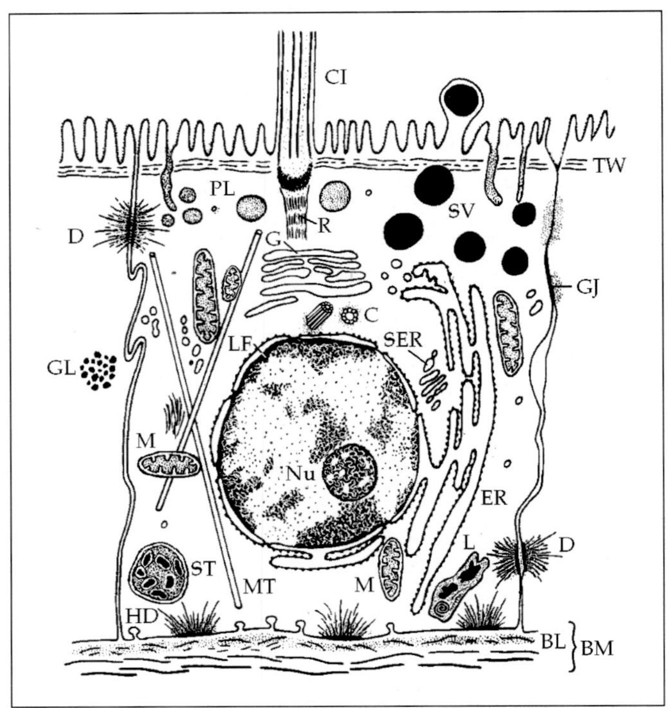

F3.1
This cell in a one-layered epithelium illustrates a number of nuclear and cytoplasmic features not seen in one single cell. Toward the lumen of the body cavity, the apical portion of the cell, thick microvilli are covered with the mucopolysaccharide fuzz of the glycocalyx. Between microvilli, the cell takes up small molecules in fluid and packages them in small vesicles. A cilium (CI) is inserted into the plasma membrane and rootlets (R) anchor the cilium to the apical cytoplasm. A secretion vesicle (SV) leaves the cell with an outpouching of the plasma membrane. Fibers of the terminal web (TW) underlay the apical cell membrane and assist not only in anchoring the cilium (see [F3.4]) but the proteins of the cell membrane as well. Between the nucleus and apical cell surface, the Golgi apparatus (G) is situated. There are also primary lysosomes (PL) fusing with food vacuoles taken up between microvilli. Mitochondria (M) and microtubules (MT) are found throughout the cytoplasm. The nucleus is surrounded by the nuclear envelope, inside of which the lamina fibrosa (LF) is depicted. Within the nucleus is the nucleolus (Nu). Two centrioles (C) are shown, one longitudinally, the other in cross section. On the right side of the nucleus and around it is depicted the endoplasmic reticulum (ER). The endoplasmic reticulum is connected with the perinuclear cisterna and by pinched-off vesicles with the Golgi apparatus. It is studded with attached ribosomes. Other vesicles in the cytoplasm belong to the smooth endoplasmic reticulum (SER) without ribosomes. A group of glycosomes (GL) represents the cell's storage of energy in the form of glycogen in an adjacent cell. Material not digestible by lysosomes is stored in storage vesicles (ST) or as pigments, eg, lipofuscin (L). Cell-to-cell connections and contacts are found in desmosomes (D), the gap junction (GJ), and hemidesmosomes (HD). The cell sits on the basement membrane (BM), a component of which is the basement lamina (BL). (Adapted from Compendium on Diagnostic Cytology. *Chicago, Ill: Tutorials of Cytology; 1983.)*

inflammation has a different origin and will be part of the discussion below on tonofilaments.

Both the inner and outer membranes are pierced by the regular but complex structure of the nuclear pores. Some nuclear material is believed to pass through them on its way to the cytoplasm, but these pores are not truly open holes because the nucleus behaves as a closed compartment and may change its size with the osmotic conditions and ionic composition of its surrounding milieu. When chromatin fibers contract toward the nuclear envelope, as will be discussed, they tend not to cover the sites of the nuclear pores. Nuclear chromatin, therefore, may appear under the light microscope partitioned into segments or lumps along the nuclear envelope. The nuclear envelope consists chiefly of lipids and protein.

Chromatin

Chromatin is the major constituent of the nuclear content. It occupies on the average 25% to 28% of the volume of the nucleus. Chromatin consists almost entirely of thin, 150- to 250-Å (0.015- to 0.025-μm) fibers of considerable but unknown length. In electron micrographs, these fibers are uneven, kinky, curving, and bending. Chromatin fibers are composed of 14% to 17% DNA; the remainder is protein and a very small amount of RNA. DNA consists of two matching, very long molecular chains twisted around each other (double helix). The DNA double helix is rolled up into a seemingly endless coiled structure inside the chromatin fiber and is protected by protein. Within every 1 μm of fiber there may be 28 lengths of DNA coiled up.

There is a considerable tendency for chromatin to change its state of distribution, ie, to expand and to contract. The expanded state in the nuclear space is the normal state. Contraction occurs with even minor changes in the intranuclear ionic milieu. Chromatin has been shown to be most sensitive to changes in the concentration of calcium (Ca^{++}) and magnesium (Mg^{++}) ions. When chromatin contracts, part of it always contracts onto the nuclear membrane, on which it is somehow anchored at numerous places. This state of contraction is called nuclear margination; a lesser degree of contraction creates the chromatinic membrane. The coarseness of chromatin is seen in the "salt-and-pepper" distribution of carcinoma in situ nuclei or more coarsely still in some malignant nuclei, and is a consequence of chromatin contraction. Many states of disease bring about a change in the ionic balance between nucleus and cytoplasm, and some, therefore, cause nuclear margination, and/or chromatin clumping. This is not true clumping, however, since the chromatin fibers maintain their individuality.

Dehydrating alcohols or other dehydrating fixatives produce only minor changes in chromatin, such as the slight coarsening of the fine chromatin meshwork. The aldehydic fixatives formaldehyde and glutaraldehyde invariably produce some degree of margination, while the acid fixatives, such as Carnoy's, produce considerable swelling of chromatin fibers and a dissolution of structure, because most of the proteins are separated from the DNA. Chromatin changes to a gel on acid fixation.

DNA is the carrier of genetic information in the cell. DNA determines a cell's properties and abilities. It is believed that all body cells normally contain the same set of genetic instructions that are established when the egg (ovum) and the sperm cell (spermatozoon) fuse in the process of fertilization. Recent investigations reveal that throughout life pieces of genes (transposons) change place and that therefore the location of genetic functions in the nucleus of an adult tissue cell clearly differs from the location of functions in the fertilized ovum.

DNA is often compared with a book of instructions, according to which not only each cell but also the whole organism is constructed—determining how it will function and even how it will age. Cells with different functions use different portions of this instructional text. A cell in the pancreas makes enzymes for the digestion of food, while a muscle cell makes the proteins for muscle contraction. The unused portions of the book of instructions, or DNA, are tightly "repressed" by protein. Only under the pressure of disease and injury can a cell open other portions of the book and thus perform other functions.

This vital activation and deactivation of genetic expansion is accomplished by proteins, which guard the structural integrity of DNA. Some proteins (enzymes) can repair damaged DNA, while others can remove damaged pieces. Two major categories of nuclear proteins, histone and nonhistone proteins, are recognized. The five major histones that have all been chemically analyzed in great detail are basic (in contrast to acidic). Histones are considered responsible for supercoiling of the DNA molecule. They neutralize most of the acidic groups of DNA. Nonhistone proteins are a heterogeneous group of proteins among which the many regulators, initiators, and controllers of the complex machinery of the nucleus are gradually being discovered.

In cancer cells, an enrichment in acidic nonhistone nuclear proteins may take place, leading to an increased uptake of basic dyes. This increase in acidic nonhistone nuclear proteins is one of three reasons for the occurrence of nuclear hyperchromasia. A second reason is that a cancer cell may double its chromatin as if preparing for division, but it may never divide. This will not be so apparent from its microscopic profile because a sphere or ovoid having doubled the volume looks only about 25% to 30% larger; in other words, the difference is between 10 and 13 μm in diameter.

A third reason for the occurrence of nuclear hyperchromasia is that because of Beer's law of light absorption in the bright-field microscope, ie, the absorption (loss) of light increases exponentially with linear increase in dye concentration, there is a tendency to confuse human visual judgment. Thus, for a nucleus of doubled volume, approximately a 30% increase in diameter, light will have to pass through roughly 30% more chromatin. Its visible density will almost have doubled! On the other hand, a swollen nucleus appears much paler than its normal neighbor, even when both have exactly the same content of chromatin and stain.

It is generally true that the repressed or inactive portion of the chromatin aggregates more easily and is then recognized as heterochromatin. Heterochromatin stains more heavily (because of chromatin concentration) than the intervening areas, the euchromatin. Euchromatin is the active, sparse, often clear appearing portion of chromatin. The fluid between the fibers contains a wide variety of organic and inorganic molecules in water and is called the nuclear "sap."

A normal nucleus contains a number of chromosomes that result from the fusion of spermatozoon and ovum. In humans this number is 46 and is called normoploid or euploid. This state of the nucleus is also called diploid, because each characteristic (except sex) of an individual is represented twofold, namely, by a pair of homologous chromosomes. Half this number has been contributed by sperm cell and half by ovum; therefore, these germ cells are called haploid. Any deviation from the normal number of chromosomes, and therefore from the normal amount of DNA, is called aneuploid or heteroploid. The latter term is frequently used also to describe great variation in aneuploidy of a population of cells, such as is seen in cancer. Older cells especially tend to delay mitosis but increase DNA, resulting in multiples of diploid. They are tetraploid with an exact doubling of the diploid amount of DNA, octoploid with an exact quadrupling of the diploid amount of DNA, etc. Triploidy, ie, a diploid plus a haploid amount of DNA, in humans is abnormal.

Several observations point to an ordered arrangement of chromosomes in the nucleus ("everything has its place") [**F***3.2*]. A normal cell seen in exfoliative cytology has a round to ovoid nuclear shape. If the genetic machinery is activated at an abnormal or unusual site, eg, inside the nucleus, the nuclear envelope will be deformed presumably to bring this newly activated site (or sites) closer to the cytoplasm, the effector site. Nuclear shape will change when chromosomes are lost or multiplied. For this reason, heteroploid nuclei are likely to possess odd shapes.

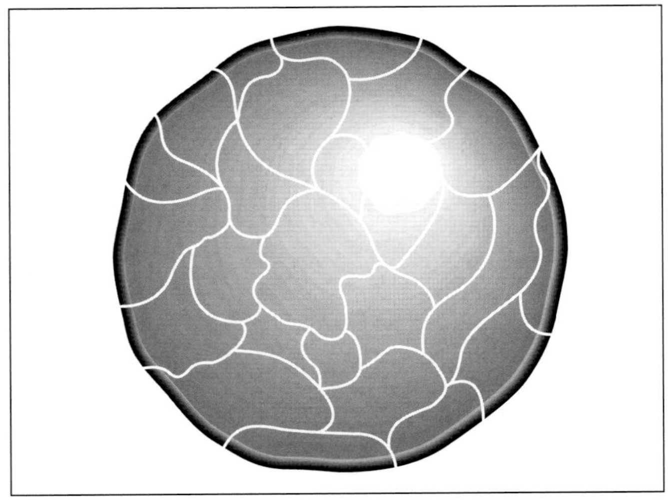

F*3.2*
Representation of the distribution of chromosomes into defined spaces of a normal nucleus. Extra chromosomes (heteroploidy) and the loss of chromosomes disturb this order, a fact recognizable in altered shapes of the nucleus. Genetic reactivation of repressed chromosomal sites is likely to have the same morphologic consequences. (Adapted from Compendium on Diagnostic Cytology. *Chicago, Ill: Tutorials of Cytology; 1983.)*

Flow of Instructions From Nucleus to Cytoplasm

A process by which the genetic instructions are read in the nucleus has been discovered [**F***3.3*]. The key mechanism is the making of an exact copy (transcription) of a portion of the instructional text, DNA, or genetic code. This copy is RNA. Ribonucleic acid is a single-stranded, usually long molecule with the sugar molecule and one nucleotide different from those of DNA. The strandedness of a nucleic acid influences its staining property. Double-stranded DNA fluoresces green with acridine dyes, but single-stranded RNA fluoresces orange-red. With other types of dyes, the accompanying proteins may determine

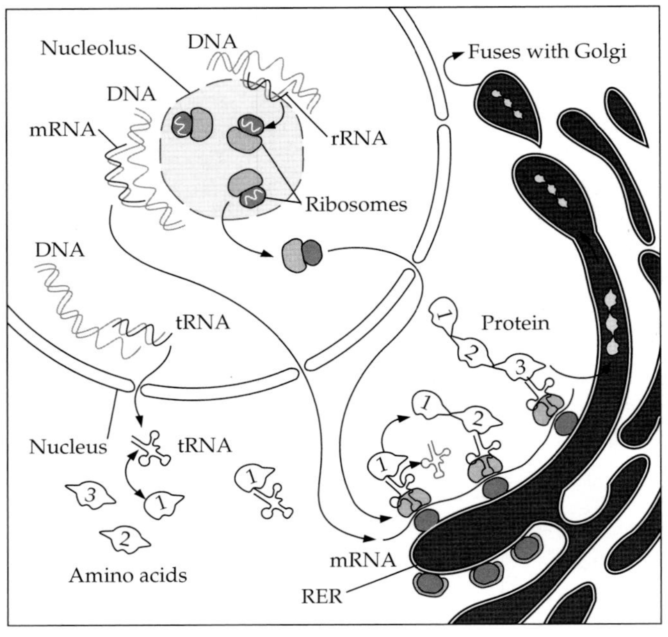

F*3.3*
Flow of instructions from nucleus to cytoplasm to direct protein synthesis. RER is the rough, ribosome-studded vesicular structure into which protein molecules are synthesized and transported to the Golgi apparatus.

the color and degree of intensity. In chromatin acidic groups of DNA and nonhistone proteins dominate, while basic proteins predominate in the nucleolus, much as in the cytoplasm. The nature of dye binding decides what color will be seen under the light microscope.

While RNA is composed of the nucleotides adenine, guanine, cytosine, and *uridine*, DNA contains adenine, guanine, cytosine, and *thymine*. The sugar in RNA is ribose; in DNA it is deoxyribose. There are three major types of RNA: messenger (mRNA), ribosomal (rRNA), and transfer (tRNA). Imagine the following: DNA, ie, the book of genetic instructions, is read in the nucleus. One chapter specifies what protein should currently be made. A copy of this instruction, mRNA, is sent to the cytoplasm. Previously, another chapter has been read, and instructions for the machinery to make proteins have been copied. rRNA is made at the site of the nucleolus by intranucleolar chromatin. The rRNA is packaged together with protein and dispatched to the cytoplasm in the form of ribosomes. Relatively short pieces of tRNA are sent to the cytoplasm to find specific building blocks (amino acids) needed for the protein specified by the messenger. Eventually the three RNAs meet and hook the amino acids together in the precise sequence translated from the messenger. This is how a protein is synthesized.

One can now understand that actively growing and synthesizing cells have large nucleoli because many ribosomes are needed for protein synthesis. Furthermore, one can now understand that cytoplasm stains in the manner of the nucleolus because there is much RNA-associated basic protein in both for the same purpose. There is speculation also that the tinctorial properties of the nucleolus are influenced by its high sulfhydryl content. The nucleolus derives largely from the stalk of 12 satellited chromosomes, so-called nucleolar organizers, which in normal cells collaborate in forming one nucleolus. In a disturbed state, especially in cancer, nucleolar organizers are separated from each other and form multiple nucleoli.

Many generations of cells and, for that matter, many generations of individuals produce some of the same proteins over and over. This is because the primary instructions lodged in the nucleus remain unchanged and have been faithfully reproduced and carefully protected over millions of years.

CYTOPLASM

Cell Membrane

Cell biologists prefer the terms "plasma membrane" or "plasmalemma" to distinguish the cell membrane from other cellular membranes. A single membrane separates the cell from its environment. There is an extraneous coat of glycoproteins—a combination of polysaccharides and protein—on almost all cell membranes [**F***3.1*]. This coat is called glycocalyx and is thickest on cells lining body cavities or intercellular spaces. On protrusions of the cell membrane such as microvilli, this coat may be furry and thick.

While discussing the cell membrane, there is good reason to look a little closer at the nature of all cellular membranes [**F***3.4*]. Each membrane is actually composed of two layers of lipid molecules [**F***3.5*]. These molecules are stacked in such a way that their hydrophilic (water-loving) portions face outward from the cell membrane, while the hydrophobic (water-fleeing) portions point inward. Embedded in this lipid double layer are protein molecules. They may face the cytoplasm in an outward direction, or they may face in both an outward and inward direction. These protein molecules accomplish their role in cell

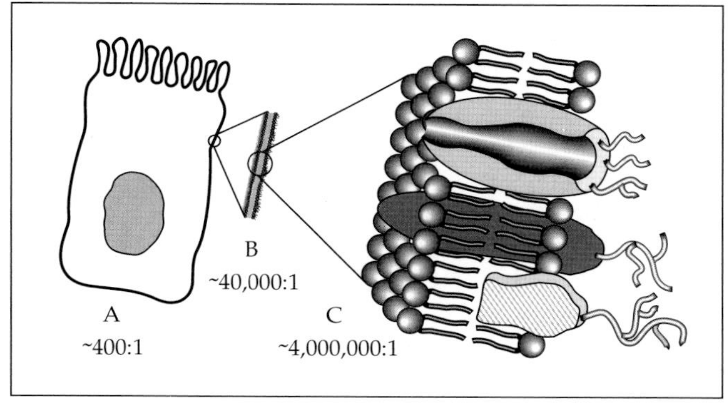

F*3.4*

A columnar cell is shown with its limiting membrane at light microscopic magnification (A). A portion of the membrane is enlarged in the electron microscope (B), and again in a hypothetical model (C). The fuzz on the outside of the cell in B, glycocalyx, consists of the carbohydrate extensions of glycoproteins embedded in the lipid bilayer of the membrane. There are fine fibers of the cytoskeleton immediately under the lipid bilayer.

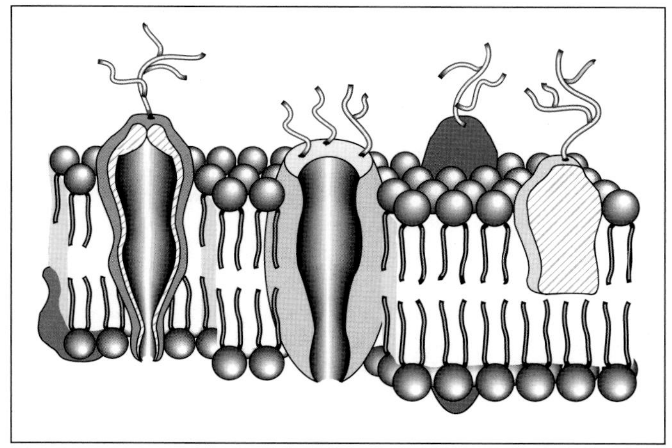

F*3.5*

The model C of F3.4 is shown in greater detail. Two protein molecules of the ion-pumping mechanism are cut in half to show the concept of an open and a closed channel.

metabolism in intake and release of molecules. Last, but not least, these protein molecules in the cell membrane account for the immunologic properties of the cell surface. One function is the recognition of one cell from another.

Urothelial cells possess a specialized membrane on the cell surface facing the urine. The inner lipid layer of this membrane is thicker than the outer layer, which is why this membrane is called an asymmetric membrane. Vesicles under the luminal cell membrane constitute a reserve for the considerable extension of the epithelium in a filled bladder.

Membrane Specializations

There are few cells in the human body that do not possess specializations of the cell membrane [**F***3.1*]. Even the free-floating white blood cells have microvilli, ie, irregularly arranged finger-like protrusions of the cell membrane 0.1 to 0.5 µm in length, as well as ruffles. Microvilli can be prominently seen under the light microscope as the brush border on the luminal side of columnar cells of the small intestine. No instrument has revealed cell surfaces better than the scanning electron microscope. It shows that the ruffles are extended cytoplasmic flaps or folds assuming a wavy or crenated configuration.

Microvilli and ruffles are often responsible for an indistinct cell border seen by light microscopy. Liquid-filled outpouchings of the cell membrane, frequently seen in degenerating and dying cells, are called blebs. In cancer cells, especially those derived from solid tumors, one may find broad or thin cytoplasmic extensions; conversely, deep infoldings of the cell membrane into the cytoplasm may also be seen. Normal tissue cells have a tendency to fill "their place" only. They are inhibited by contact with other cells. Malignant cells lose this contact inhibition and tend to extend their cytoplasm for considerable distances and to abandon their place. The majority of cells of the human body normally do not grow beyond the organ size of the adult, except as replacement for worn-out and dying cells. Replacement is, however, an essential, limited, and specified function of epithelia and bone marrow.

Of interest to cytologists is another modification of the cell surface, cilia. In contrast to microvilli of irregular position, thickness, and length, and unlike the brush border of absorptive cells, cilia contain microtubules (discussed in the section below on the cytoskeleton) believed to be responsible for the beating motion. Microtubules are anchored below the cell surface to the basal body (also called the kinetosome when cilia are actively beating) and are covered by cell membrane. The anchoring mechanism is reinforced by rootlets of striated fibers extending like a plant's roots from the basal body into the cytoplasm. In fact, this anchoring structure imparts much density to the uppermost cell layer, giving it a solid appearance easily recognized by light microscopy. Individual cilia 0.2 µm thick can actually be observed by light microscopy. They are motile structures moving with a lashing stroke. The cilia of the columnar epithelia of oviduct, uterus, and trachea beat in small groups because the impulses are locally propagated.

Cell-to-Cell Contacts

Columnar or cuboidal epithelial cells are held together by a series of surface modifications. At the apical portion of the intercellular contact, close to the lumen or body cavity, the two outermost layers of the plasma membrane [**F***3.5*] of each cell are fused so that three layers result: the inner layer of one cell, the fused layers, and the inner layer of the other cell. This is called the tight junction (zonula occludens). Directly beneath and away from the lumen follows another structure, the intermediate junction (zonula adherens), where, as the term implies, the intact membranes adhere closely to each other. Both junctions are associated with dense material on either cytoplasmic side that tends to stain in light and electron microscopy. Since these junctions form a girdle-like structure around the cell, a narrow, dense stripe is seen under the free cell surface, which is called the terminal bar. The prominent staining of terminal bars is due to the combination of properties of the junctions and the meshwork of rootlets and basal bodies in ciliated cells, or of the junctions and the terminal web, a meshwork of fine fibrils in cells with a brush border. The impression of density is enhanced by a network of intermediate fibers that is found directly under the cell membrane. This network is believed to aid in fixing the location of intramembrane proteins and assist in the anchoring of ciliary basal bodies. The intercellular junctions constitute a seal between the lumen, toward which the cell faces, and the intercellular and tissue spaces, while its tight junction permits the passage of electrical signals from cell to cell (eg, coordination of ciliary activity).

It is not unusual to find wide liquid-filled intercellular spaces basal to or adjacent to the terminal bar. However, another surface specialization, the desmosome (macula adherens) [**F***3.1*], prevents epithelial cells from separating too far. The desmosome is a round structure on each of two adjacent cells with some dense material in between the two cell membranes. Desmosomes constitute "intercellular bridges" but do not provide true cytoplasmic continuity between cells. Desmosomes are points at which two cells appear "welded" together and to which cytoplasmic filaments (tonofilaments) from deep within the cell radiate, with the result that not only the membranes but the bodies of cells are held together. Tonofilaments are not directly attached to desmosomes but are held with loops of intermediate fibers. Furthermore, desmosomes help cells to recognize each other in mixed cell populations so that enduring contact can be established among cells of the same type. Desmosomes are nevertheless known to disappear in short intervals of time. They are lost in the uppermost, mature layer of the nonkeratinizing and keratinizing squamous epithelium.

Many times, two neighboring cell membranes are extensively folded or interdigitated, perhaps to increase cell surface and thus transmembrane exchange, but mostly to provide a certain "give" under mechanical stress. The deeply convoluted membranes of neighboring cells in the transitional epithelium of an empty bladder are good examples of this function. They disappear when the bladder is distended and the urothelial cells are stretched. Interdigitation of membranes provides cell-to-cell adherence in the superficial epithelial layers when desmosomes are gone.

Basement Membrane

All epithelia rest on a membranous structure, the periodic acid-Schiff–positive basement membrane. Two structurally discrete components can be discerned [**F***3.1*]. First, the basal lamina, a rather homogeneous layer of neutral mucopolysaccharides containing thin 30- to 40-Å collagen fibers, is situated closest to the basal portion of the cell membrane. Second, there is a layer of fine collagen fibers in ground substance of mucoproteins and neutral mucopolysaccharides. The greater the mechanical stress to which an epithelium is exposed, the thicker the collagenous portion of the basement membrane. The more intense a filtering function assigned to the basement membrane, the thicker the basal lamina. Where there is no mechanical stress, only the basal lamina will be found, as in the glomerulus of the kidney. Light microscopic methods cannot distinguish the two components of the basement membrane. There is evidence that epithelial cells secrete the unstructured portion of the constituents of this membrane. Collagen is contributed by fibroblasts in the connective tissue under the basement membrane.

Normally, capillaries and lymphatic vessels do not reach the epithelium proper but remain under the basement membrane. Desmosomes also attach epithelial cells to the basement membrane. Since there is no other cell partner to attach to, however, a row of half-desmosomes (hemidesmosomes) is formed to anchor the cellular mass of the epithelium [**F***3.1*].

Mitochondria

It has often been said that mitochondria [**F***3.1*] are the powerhouses of the cell because one of the major energy carriers, adenosine triphosphate (ATP), is synthesized and regenerated there. In this process, the sugar glucose is oxidized to carbon dioxide, and water and oxygen are consumed (glycolysis). In green plants, the reverse takes place. By means of energy from the sun, carbon dioxide is converted to glucose (photosynthesis). Mitochondria in animal cells and the green chloroplasts in plant cells contain an independent genetic system based on a short piece of DNA quite similar to the DNA in bacteria. Some believe these two organelles were bacteria that invaded the cell at the dawn of cellular development and remained symbionts ever since.

To the light microscopist, mitochondria appear as round or rod-shaped cytoplasmic particles that can fuse and divide. Mitochondria propagate by growth and division; their own DNA, however, is insufficient to render instructions for all the proteins necessary to make a mitochondrion and is therefore assisted by the nucleus. In nondividing cells, when actively synthesizing a product, eg, mucus or protein, mitochondria are large and numerous. Rapidly dividing cells have few, small mitochondria functioning only for the cell's own energy needs. Masses of tightly packed mitochondria are found in muscle cells in which large amounts of energy are required.

Rough Endoplasmic Reticulum

Among the compartments in the cytoplasm, the endoplasmic reticulum is the most extensive system of membrane-enclosed cisternal space. Two major types of endoplasmic reticulum have come to be distinguished by the presence or absence of ribosomes on the cytoplasmic surfaces of the endoplasmic reticulum. Numerous chains of ribosomes are found attached to one type, rough-surfaced endoplasmic reticulum, giving it its name. As stated before, ribosomes are synthesized and rRNA is incorporated in the nucleolus, and they migrate as two parts to the cytoplasm to be assembled at the site of protein synthesis for internal cellular use. Some attach to the endoplasmic reticulum to join with mRNA and tRNA in the synthesis of proteins for export or secretion. The newly synthesized protein is directly discharged into the cisternal space. Mitochondria are close by to provide the energy for this demanding process. The products for export now move in membrane-enclosed spaces to the Golgi apparatus [**F***3.4*].

Golgi Apparatus

The Golgi apparatus [**F***3.1*], first described in 1898 by the Italian microanatomist Camillo Golgi, is a characteristic stack of connected, flat, smooth membranous vesicles typically located close to the nucleus, and is connected with the rough endoplasmic reticulum either by smooth-surfaced channels or by a flow of small vesicles. In epithelial cells, it is situated between the nucleus and the apical portion of the cell facing the lumen. The raw products from the rough endoplasmic reticulum enter the stack of Golgi vesicles from one side, molecules are added, and portions are eliminated. Finally, the finished, packaged product appears at the other side of the polar stack to be released into special vesicles wherein it may be stored or transported to the cell membrane for discharge.

The hormones of the thyroid are stored as thyroglobulin in follicles. Thyroglobulin is synthesized in the rough endoplasmic reticulum and transported to the Golgi apparatus where galactose (a sugar) is added to the molecule. Then it is packed in vesicles and excreted into the follicle when the vesicles reach the luminal cell membrane. This process illustrates well the cooperation of rough endoplasmic reticulum, Golgi apparatus, and cell membrane in the synthesis and export of an important protein. It can now be understood why the Golgi apparatus is large in secretory cells and small in cells with predominantly mechanical functions, such as muscle and squamous epithelial cells. It has been shown that in some cells lysosomes are formed at the Golgi apparatus in conjunction with portions of the smooth endoplasmic reticulum.

Smooth Endoplasmic Reticulum

The second type of endoplasmic reticulum is the smooth-surfaced endoplasmic reticulum [**F**3.1]. It is found in many places scattered throughout the cytoplasm. As the name implies, the membranes of this organelle are smooth. No ribosomes are attached, although this organelle may be found connected to the rough endoplasmic reticulum. Smooth-surfaced endoplasmic reticulum differs also from the rough endoplasmic reticulum because the smooth type consists mostly of rather small, sometimes connected tubules and vesicles. Perhaps its most clearly understood function is detoxification, the elimination of substances harmful to the cell or the organism. Many drugs, eg, barbiturates, are metabolized in the smooth endoplasmic reticulum of liver cells. Steroid hormone-producing cells, eg, of the adrenal gland, ovary, testis, and hypophysis, contain large amounts of smooth endoplasmic reticulum, whereas cells of exocrine glands contain little or none. It has been proposed that smooth endoplasmic reticulum, the structural substrate on which the great variety of enzymes are anchored, is needed to accomplish the diverse metabolic functions of the cell. Smooth endoplasmic reticulum is known to be active in glycogen metabolism of liver cells and in transport of lipids and fat from the intestine into the hepatic vein.

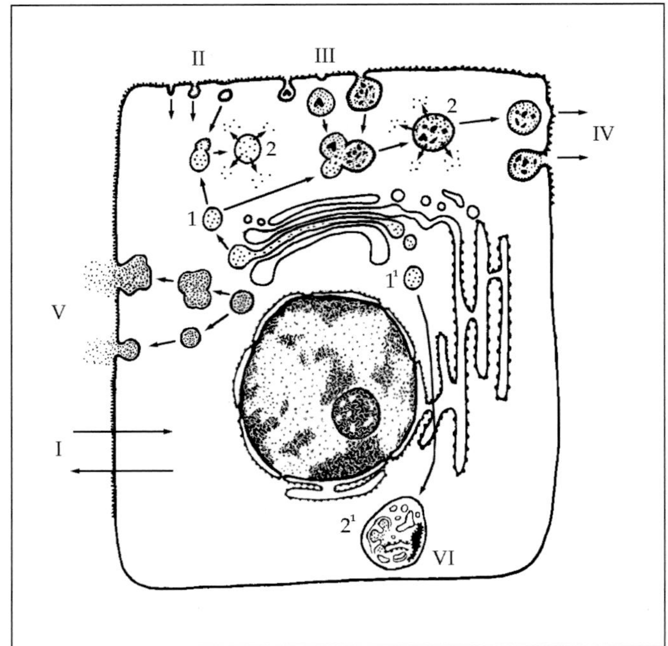

F3.6

Demonstration of uptake and discharge (I) across cell membrane. Uptake—or release of small molecules, salts, and water—does not noticeably change appearance of cell membrane. Cell can actively pump both in and out or use concentration gradients. Pinocytosis ("cell-drinking," as was formerly believed to be the way cells fed) concerns transport of large molecules (II), essentially a variant of phagocytosis (III), or "cell-eating." Illustrated here is uptake of chunks of material. Roth vesicles from phagocytosis at II and III fuse with primary lysosomes (1) for digestion of ingested substances and materials. Small molecules produced this way then pass through a wall of secondary lysosome (2) into cytoplasm as nutrients, which is suggested by short arrows. Indigestible portions and debris from cellular activities are defecated when secondary lysosomes fuse with cell membrane (IV, V). Lysosomal enzymes (which are proteins) are produced in the rough endoplasmic reticulum and flow to the Golgi apparatus, where they are activated and move as membrane-enclosed digestion bags, primary lysosomes (1^1), to cytoplasm. Here they meet phagocytized material and fuse and digest what they can (2^1). Other material is stored in storage vesicles (VI).

Lysosomes

So far the synthetic activities of the cell and the flow of information and products have been discussed. All nucleated cells contain in various quantities a group of organelles summarily called lysosomes [**F**3.1, **F**3.6], which belong to the intracellular digestive system. They were first identified as organelles of common function by the presence of acid phosphatase, an acid hydrolase, which is a digestive enzyme. Today about 70 different enzymes have been reported to occur in lysosomes, which can digest almost everything made in the cell, from nucleic acids to proteins, carbohydrates, and lipids. Most substances introduced from the outside are also digested; some, however, as we have seen before, are broken down by the smooth endoplasmic reticulum.

Consider the following dynamic scene [**F**3.6]. Digestive enzymes, proteins made by the ribosomes, are released directly into the cisternae of the rough endoplasmic reticulum; transported to the Golgi apparatus, where they are modified; and activated. They are then packaged in thick-walled vesicles—the primary lysosomes—and moved into the cytoplasmic space. Here they meet other thick-walled vesicles that have just been released from the cell membrane, where they have picked up material from outside the cell. The cell "eats" in two ways, namely, in big chunks (phagocytosis, III) or in minute bites (pinocytosis, II). Pinocytosis originally implied cell-drinking, but water uptake and release are largely regulated by osmosis. Phagocytosis and pinocytosis result in the formation of vesicles at the cell membrane; these vesicles do not contain digestive enzymes yet. When a phagocytic vesicle meets a primary lysosome, fusion results. The enzymes of the primary lysosome act on the contents of the vesicle. A newly formed body, called a secondary lysosome results. Although most cells can phagocytize, the macrophage is the most active of all cells in this respect. Not only is material beneficial to the cell taken up, but also deleterious material from the cell's environment, such as dust and coal particles, is transitionally stored in the cytoplasm.

Organelles of the cell itself age, wear out, and break down and must be eliminated or, rather, recycled. Thus, mitochondria and pieces of rough and smooth endoplasmic reticulum enclosed by a membrane (autophagic vacuole) are eventually joined by a primary lysosome, and digestion starts (secondary lysosome). Many of the dark granules seen in the squamous cells of cytologic preparations are inactivated lysosomes containing remnants of the remodeling process occurring on the way from basal to superficial cell (residual body). Such granules are also seen when a high dose of estrogen has been recently administered. Material that cannot be digested is often brought to the cell membrane and excreted (exocytosis or defecation). Autophagy reduces organ size during involution. Examples are the reduction in the size of the breast after lactation or of the uterus after a pregnancy. Macrophages remove the debris.

Glycogen, Lipids, Pigments, and Crystalloids

Cells have the capacity to store products, most often their own. One can demonstrate that certain stored products are kept as a reserve of energy and building material. Glycogen and fat belong in this category.

In spite of the effective ways in which cells can handle waste, as will be seen, cells may retain some cellular waste in the cytoplasm, apparently for lack of another way of handling it. Many nonfunctional pigments belong in this category.

The following inclusions will be briefly discussed in this order: hemosiderin, hematoidin, bilirubin, hematin, anthracotic pigment, lipofuscin, melanin, other inclusions, and Reinke crystalloids. Hemosiderin is a yellow or brown intracellular pigment. It is the product of phagocytosis and digestion of red cell hemoglobin. It contains easily demonstrable iron and is soluble only in strong alkali. After formalin fixation, even dilute acids can dissolve it. Ferritin is the major component of hemosiderin, and enough polysaccharide is present in this pigment to render a strong periodic acid–Schiff reaction.

Hematoidin and bilirubin are closely related, if not identical, intracellular pigments. Like hemosiderin, these two pigments derive from the digestion of erythrocytes. They are bright orange-yellow to brown and do not remain in the cytoplasm but are eliminated by exocytosis. Hematoidin occurs as crystals, bilirubin as amorphous masses. Both are soluble only in chloroform and are insoluble after formalin fixation.

Hematin is a precipitation of dark brown or black pigment caused by acid formalin fixation of blood-rich tissue areas. It should be considered an artifact; its formation can be prevented by buffering formalin to neutral pH.

Anthracotic pigment is a black, amorphous substance, insoluble in all solvents. It occurs frequently in macrophages. Anthracotic pigment is carbonaceous dust derived from our environment. Coal dust, soot, incompletely burned organic compounds, and automotive tire carbon are some of the sources of this pigment.

"Lipofuscin" is a term describing autochthonous pigments of varying composition and reactivity. The color of lipofuscin is often brown. It is the product of intracellular oxidation of lipids, chiefly phospholipids and unsaturated fats. Lipofuscin is considered the result of the wear and tear of cellular membranes. The gradual process of oxidation entails changing histochemical reactivity, so that fat reactions as well as the periodic acid–Schiff reaction are positive. Some of the myeloid bodies or storage bodies familiar to the electron microscopist contain lipofuscin at the light microscopic level.

The melanins occur as normal cytoplasmic substances in pigmented skin and hair. Melanins are actually a group of pigments, of which eumelanin ranges in color from yellow, brown, and black to violet, and phaeomelanin from yellow, brown, and black to red. Eumelanin is responsible for the scale of brown colorations in humans and animals, while phaeomelanin contributes the red color, eg, that of hair and freckles. Both melanins are complex, high-molecular-weight polymers, insoluble in almost all solvents. Melanosomes average in size from 150 to 700 nm and vary in degree of melanin polymerization and cross-linking. Most often melanosomes are grain-shaped. Melanosomes are synthesized in melanocytes and are subsequently moved to cells of the malpighian layer of the epidermis. Melanocytes may then appear empty. The malignant state of melanocytes is melanoma.

Cell inclusions in the form of crystalloid bodies are rare occurrences. Both proteins and polysaccharides may crystallize, but viruses are also known to form crystalloids in heavily infected cells. Sometimes the inclusion turns out to be a myelin body (a defense mechanism) and can be recognized with crossed polarizer and analyzer as a brightly birefringent body. The birefringence of other inclusions is usually weak. Reinke crystalloids are said to occur extracellularly in virilizing ovarian tumors, in hilus cells of adrenal tumors, and in Leydig cells of testis. Their nature is not well understood except for the fact that Reinke crystalloids consist only of protein.

Microbodies (Peroxisomes and Glyoxisomes)

Cell biologists recognize a family of small, 0.1 to 1.5 μm in diameter organelles in the cytoplasm, collectively called microbodies. Two main subgroups have become known. Peroxisomes have been recognized as separate organelles for some time. They contain enzymes capable of destroying toxic peroxide compounds, the significance of which in the life of the cell is not clear. Glyoxisomes contain some of the enzymes of the glyoxylate cycle, which is a modification of the Krebs cycle, providing energy through cellular respiration (oxidation).

CELL SHAPE

Forces From Inside

Most undifferentiated cells will assume a spherical shape when released from the context of tissue structure, reflecting the same physiochemical principle that makes a drop of oil round in water. The cell membrane is an elastic structure that foreshortens or stretches as the need arises. In this instance, it will contract and surround the cytoplasm in tight fashion. Small and large molecules in the cell water seek constantly to dilute themselves. To accomplish this, they try to get out of the cell and push against the cell membrane, producing osmotic pressure. Molecules on the outside are driven by the same force, and thus these forces are in balance. A medium for cells designed to maintain this balance is called an isotonic medium. When imbalance occurs through uptake of metabolites and salts, the cell either takes up water or releases it to keep the balance. The cell also has the option of taking in or putting out more salt. The proper balance of ions is actively maintained through proteinaceous pumps in the cell membrane [**F**3.5]. Energy is required for this process, which means that the process stops when the cell is fatally injured. The cell swells or, seldomly, shrinks.

Forces From Outside

In tissue, cells arrange themselves according to instructions from their nucleus. They align themselves into rows forming the carpet of an epithelium and are arranged in one or more layers. Erythrocytes at the edge of a drop of blood align under the phase microscope. The "voluntary" alignment of the cells into a "cuboidal epithelium" may become apparent. In three-dimensional tissue, neighboring cells soon hold onto each other by desmosomes and form a coherent layer. At the same time, tight and intermediate junctions form. Then the cells secrete the basal lamina and attach themselves to it by half-desmosomes.

Maintenance of Shape: The Cytoskeleton

The cytoskeleton consists of the following components:

- Microtubules (250 Å)
- Intermediate filaments (70-110 Å)
  - Keratin filaments (80 Å)
  - Neurofilaments (70 Å)
  - Glial filaments, glial fibrillary acidic protein
  - Filaments containing vimentin, desmin, synemin, and pectin
- Actin filaments, also called stress fibers (60 Å)
- Microtrabecular meshwork (15 Å)

In recent years, much progress has been made in clarifying what is generally called the cytoskeleton. Specific fluorescent labels for isolated and purified proteins of the cytoskeleton have helped in localizing fiber types.

Microtubules

Microtubules are among the best-studied components of the cytoskeleton. They are long, slender tubes assembled from subunits. They originate from microtubule-organizing centers distributed throughout the cytoplasm but particularly around centrioles [**F**3.1]. From here the mitotic spindle forms, consisting of microtubules. Microtubules are considered the chief structural element through which the shape of the cell is maintained. This function is exemplified in cytology by the columnar cell not rounding up when it leaves its epithelial space. Microtubules are found in beating cilia of respiratory, endocervical, and uterine fallopian epithelium, in sperm tails, and last but not least, in the flagella of *Trichomonas*. Microtubules are assembled in the moving front of migratory cells and disassembled in the trailing cytoplasm.

Intermediate Filaments

Intermediate filaments are an enlarging family of filaments, so-called because their diameters are intermediate between microtubules and actin filaments. However, they occur in all cells in varying relative proportions, and they may even occur as composite filaments. Because of the apparent cell-specific combinations, they are assumed to have a cell type-specific function. One of the most ubiquitous of intermediate fibers is the tonofilament (80 Å in diameter), occurring without exception in all ectodermal or epithelial cells. Tonofilaments are a member of the keratin family of epidermis (hair, nails, silk, feathers) and are found in greatest abundance in keratinizing cells. It has been found that all structures based on keratin have the same basic keratin molecule as a structural element. This molecule occurs with different degrees of polymerization and different extents of phosphorylation. Thus, many of the tonofilaments of the superficial cell of squamous cervical epithelium are already present in the basal cell. Tonofilaments serve to preserve the coherence of the cytoplasm; they provide the cell relative toughness against stretching. A multitude of antibodies are available to demonstrate by fluorescence the types and location of human keratin.

Neurofilaments can be found in nerve axons. Filaments containing glial fibrillary acidic protein may occur along with neurofilaments. Against the protein of glial filaments, an antibody has been developed so that it can be recognized in glia (astrocytes).

Filaments containing the polypeptides vimentin, desmin, pectin, synemin, and others await clarification of composition and function.

Actin Filaments

Cells with contractile properties, such as the myoepithelial cells around mammary gland acini, are endowed with contractile fibers, the actin filaments (60 Å). Bundles of actin filaments are called stress fibers. Almost all cells possess to a varying degree contractile actin filaments; blood platelets, which contract during clot formation, are included. They share the contractile property with muscle. In some cells, as in muscle, both actin and myosin have been demonstrated, although the latter is found in cells in much smaller concentration.

Microtrabecular Meshwork

A cytoplasmic structure was found that is believed to be the smallest structural entity of the cytoskeleton. It is called the microtrabecular meshwork, its highly labile and variable elements being 10 to 15 Å in diameter. The meshwork gives the cytoplasm its gel-like property, ie, a cell does not "run out" when injured as an egg would.

All cells studied carefully up to this point have been found to contain microtubules in varying quantities and arrangements. All epithelial cells contain, in addition, tonofilaments. In malignant tumor cells, large quantities of diffuse or aggregated filaments, comparable but not identical with tonofilaments, are often observed. In a normal squamous cell, one finds tonofilaments fairly evenly intermixed with mitochondria, endoplasmic reticulum, and other cell organelles throughout the cytoplasm. When cells are injured by irradiation, or when cells react to a marked change in their environment, one finds tonofilaments aggregated to bundles, and a dense meshwork may occupy a broad area between nuclear envelope and cell membrane. As a consequence, a zone of varying width around the nucleus is relatively free of tonofilaments. Endoplasmic reticulum and mitochondria in low concentration occupy this zone, easily recognized under the light microscope as a perinuclear halo. A comparable halo effect is produced when a filament-free zone arises at the cell border.

Differences in concentration of organic material between the peripheral cytoplasm (sometimes called exoplasm) and the filament-rich region result in a difference in optical refraction. With an almost closed aperture diaphragm of the substage condenser or with phase-contrast microscopy, this difference in refraction can be clearly seen. Prominent concentration of tonofilaments in wavy bundles at the border of these zones is sometimes called the spiral of Eberth. Among the factors in the environment likely to produce cytoplasmic patterns of filament aggregation is inflammation, with its attendant changes in pH, in concentration of salts, and notably in the release of lytic enzymes from leukocytes.

Cancer cells often display long cytoplasmic extensions, a consequence of weak or failing contact inhibition. In differentiating squamous cancer cells, a fair quantity of tonofilaments may be located in these extensions. When such a cell is subject to the process of filament aggregation described earlier, a prominent bundle of filaments may become apparent under the light microscope. Moreover, when these filaments are wavy, which they often are, the bundle in the cytoplasmic extension appears as a Herxheimer spiral.

CELL DIVISION

One of the basic tenets of life is the statement that "all cells derive from cells," paraphrasing Virchow's statement, "*Omnis cellulae e cellulae*." For a new cell to originate, a cell has to grow until it reaches a size (mass) that triggers cell division [**F***3.7*, **F***3.8*], resulting in two equivalent daughter cells. It is sometimes difficult to realize how effective this process is; after only 10 successive divisions, 1024 cells result, and after 10 further divisions, the population will have swollen to over 10 million cells, provided that each daughter cell divides again.

The first preparatory step for cell division is the meticulous replication of nuclear DNA in a so-called synthetic phase (S) of the cell cycle [**F***3.7*]. The two resulting sets of genetic instructions are then packaged into the form of chromosomes (prophase) at the end of a brief phase of reorganization, G_2, after termination of S. G_2 and G_1 were once called gaps in the division cycle. The designating letter (G) is retained.

In the meantime, a small cytoplasmic double-structure, the diplosome or pair of centrioles, replicates itself; it is barely visible with the light microscope [**F***3.1*, **F***3.8*]. The two centrioles migrate to opposite ends of the cell to form the anchoring points for two sets of microtubules. One set spans from one pair of centrioles to the other; the other set connects one half of each chromosome to opposite centrioles. The mitotic spindle has been formed. By this time, most of the nuclear envelope and the nucleolus have disappeared at light microscopic resolution, while the chromosomes have assembled during metaphase in a plate-like formation [**F***3.8*] in the middle of the cell. Each chromosome is now split into two equal parts, each chromosome half carrying one strand of the original DNA double helix plus the newly synthesized complementary strand. These chromosome halves are "pulled" by the connecting microtubules (spindle fibers) to the respective centrioles, perhaps by using the centriole-to-centriole microtubules as a brace. These microtubules also elongate and thus appear to help in the separation of the two sets

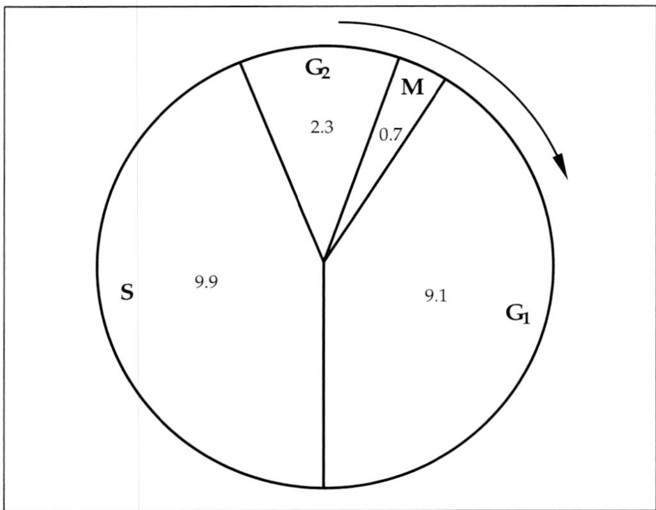

F3.7

When a cell grows and divides, its stages of DNA synthesis can be described by a circle. Mitosis (M lasts for 0.7 hour and is followed by a gap period (G_1) before synthesis of DNA. Duplication of the genome starts in the synthetic period (S). Another gap period (G_2) follows when synthesis has been completed before another mitosis (M) and the division of the cell starts a new cell cycle.

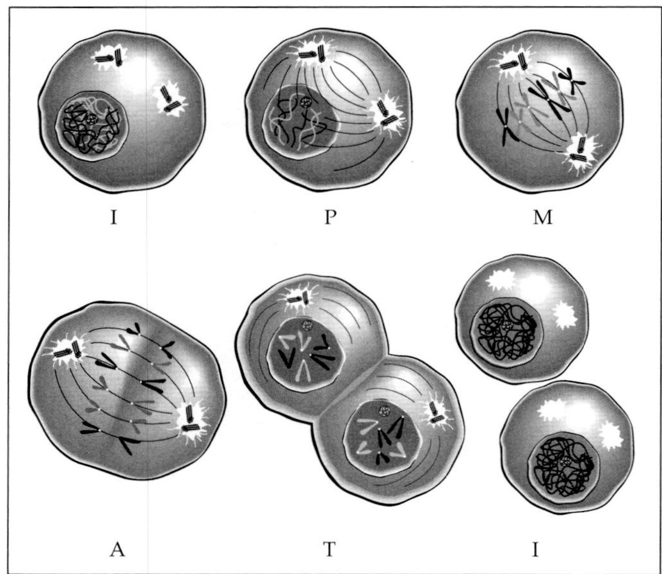

F3.8

Sequence of events of cell division. At interphase (I), nuclear division has progressed to the G_1 phase. A pair of centrioles (diplosome) is close to a shallow indentation of the nuclear envelope. In prophase (P), chromosomes form out of the mass of chromatin fibers. The diplosome has divided and the two resulting pairs move to opposite sites of the nucleus. The envelope dissolves, a spindle is formed, and chromosomes gather in the mitotic plate during metaphase (M). In anaphase (A), the chromatids part in opposite directions; when they collect at the centrioles, it is called telophase (T). At this time, cytokinesis, the division of the cytoplasm, takes place by pinching off at a waistline (T).

of chromosomes and ultimately of the daughter cells. This phase of chromosome movement is called anaphase.

When the chromosomes are eventually assembled at opposite poles (telophase), they are unraveled, and their chromatin assumes the distribution it had before prophase. A new nuclear envelope and nucleolus are formed for each set. At this time, also, the cytoplasm divides without much precision (cytokinesis). Cell division is over, and the new cells have entered G_1, in which they remain for the rest of their lives, perhaps undergoing differentiation as they do in epithelia, or perhaps growing and preparing for the next division as basal cells do in the same tissue.

The G_1, S, G_2, and mitotic phases of the cell cycle have different lengths for different kinds of cells and tissues. Division is the most intricate and complex process the cell performs. On consideration of this complicated task , it is not difficult to see why dividing cells, of all cells in the body, are the ones most susceptible to injury from the outside, such as from chemicals, radiation, or viral infection. A majority of malignant tumors occur in rapidly proliferating tissues, ie, in tissues with many cell divisions.

Disturbances in the regular movement and replication of the pair of centrioles can cause havoc, because with only one centriole no mitosis occurs; with three of four centriolar pairs, multipolar mitosis results, in which the chromosomes are pulled in three or four directions without achieving mitosis or complete cell division. Sometimes one or a few chromosomes do not move in mitosis (nondisjunction) and are caught in the middle between the separating daughter cells. All these abnormalities are seen in cancer and after irradiation with x-rays.

CELL DIFFERENTIATION

One of the most intriguing aspects of cells is their ability to differentiate. Different functions are often reflected morphologically in different shapes and appendices and in different cytoplasmic organelles mirroring differences in biochemical equipment.

As the basal cell of cervical epithelium differentiates, bundles of tonofilaments increase in quantity, while other cellular functions decrease, as is evident in the disappearance of most mitochondria, the endoplasmic reticulum, and the Golgi apparatus. Also, the nucleus ceases most of its activities. This becomes first evident with the disappearance of its nucleolus. While the nucleus shrinks, it compresses its chromatin into the dense pyknotic pattern. By this time, the cell has attained its characteristic squamous shape, and many tonofilaments coalesce with the remaining cellular proteins to form solid intracellular masses. Chemically, a process of progressive cross-linking of molecules is involved. The conversion of cellular sulfhydryl-SH to disulfide-S-S- is a prominent feature of this process. Only the desmosomes continue to function as connecting elements. Metabolic processes have ceased; the cell is dead. Its attachments to neighboring cells gradually loosen under the influence of mechanical forces and the influence of chemical factors in the vaginal fluid, leading ultimately to the cell's exfoliation, the total separation of the cell from its connections with the epithelium, and the passive transport into the lumen of the anatomic structure. Its shape and surface structure are rigidly maintained.

We have already touched on the fact that proteins control whatever portions of chromatin remain active. Heterochromatin is considered to be the repressed portion of the general genetic code embodied in DNA. Early in the development of an embryo, cells are omnipotent, ie, they can adapt themselves functionally to any place in the embryo. Later on, one finds the daughter cells locked to specific functions; they are developmentally determined and will remain so even if transplanted. Only selected chapters of the code of instruction remain open and the remainder is firmly closed. Many more chapters are open in the embryo than in the adult. Maturation is the process of continued differentiation associated with an ever more limited access to the genetic code (the genome).

Finally, a limited set of instructions resides in a basal cell of cervical epithelium, to use an example befitting the specific group of readers of this manual. This set specifies within narrow limits the sequence of events leading to the formation of squamous epithelial cells, including the approximate turn-on and turn-off sequence for such chemical events as the synthesis and assembly, or both, of more tonofilaments. Superimposed on the effect of genetic instructions are environmental influences. These become apparent when a basal cell divides and one of the daughter cells, namely, the one receiving most of the cytoplasm, further differentiates, while the other commences collecting material for the next division, always mindful of the given instructions. Cells also have a series of options as to how much and what to produce. An example of this flexibility, admittedly limited, is seen in the consequences of varying the hormonal output to a cell. It is known that hormones enter the cell and bind to a receptor protein and that both the hormones and the protein then enter the nucleus. Here they act as a message to the nucleus, inducing it to order the production of more, less, or different proteins.

Can closed chapters of the genetic code be opened again? Depending on the cell type and degree of maturation, the answer is a qualified yes. Usually, reopening (derepression) leads to abnormal cells, such as those in a malignant transformation, and to regression to less differentiated states, with disturbances in the mechanism of cell division and loss of harmonic collaboration among cellular components. An example of disproportionate activity is a large nucleolus in a cell with little cytoplasm or the replication of nuclear DNA without subsequent mitosis or cell division. How these events are regulated at the molecular level is still a matter of speculation; it appears certain, however, that a cell cannot change its assignment. It can only move forward (to a point) in the direction of determined differentiation or move back (with considerable difficulty) the same way. Cells can be turned off for a time but some can be reactivated.

REVIEW EXERCISES

1. The cellular nucleus is separated from the cytoplasm by a specific structure. Name this structure and three of its components.

2. Chromatin constitutes the major portion of the nucleus. What does chromatin consist of?
   a) Name three chemical categories of molecules and their functions.
   b) Describe the major structure of chromatin.

3. Explain terms associated with ploidy (heteroploidy, etc).

4. What are the three major types of RNA produced for protein synthesis?

5. What are the principal functions of
   a) rough endoplasmic reticulum?
   b) smooth endoplasmic reticulum?
   c) the Golgi apparatus?

6. What is the function of mitochondria?

7. Name at least three components of the cytoskeleton.

8. How do epithelial cells adhere to each other? Name two mechanisms by which cells attach themselves to each other and the individual function of each mechanism.

9. Cells take in substances from their surroundings and release rejected substances from the cell interior to their surroundings. What are these two opposite processes called, and how do they take place?

10. Interphase chromatin tends to change its pattern of distribution. What makes chromatin contract? What leads to hyperchromasia?

SELECTED READINGS

Alberts B, Bray D, Lewis J, et al. *Molecular Biology of the Cell.* New York, NY: Garland Publishing; 1983.

Bloom W, Fawcett DW. *A Textbook of Histology.* Philadelphia, Pa: WB Saunders Co; 1975.

CHAPTER

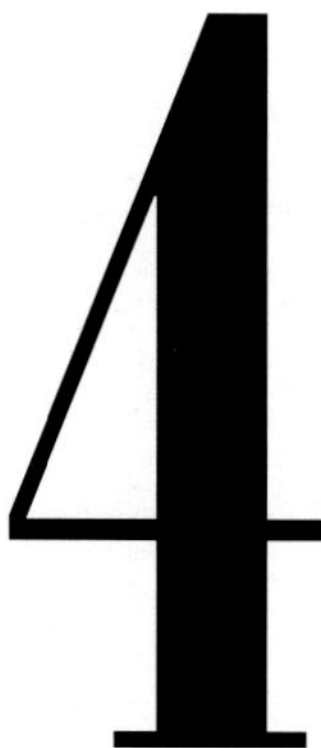

Evaluation of the Cell Sample

James W. Reagan, MD†
Theresa M. Somrak, JD, CT(ASCP), CFIAC

CONTENTS

† Deceased.

A meaningful evaluation of the cellular sample requires much more skill than is needed to merely detect the presence of abnormality. The microscopist must initially acquire a detailed knowledge of normal cellular morphology. This is an important first step because the ability to appreciate the abnormal is directly related to an understanding of the normal.

To evaluate cellular alterations it is helpful to use a systematic approach that provides for the assessment of all abnormal manifestations in the cellular sample. For optimal cellular evaluation, the source of the sample and the method of collection must be known. Pertinent patient history must be provided if the evaluation is to be precise, especially in the evaluation of samples from many different anatomic sites. Without this information the accuracy of the cellular sample is reduced.

When evaluating the cellular sample there are a number of questions the cytotechnologist must answer, including: Is the specimen adequate? Are there an appropriate number of cells? What is the origin of the cells? Is the cellular sample within normal limits? If not, what is the cellular abnormality? To answer these questions the cytotechnologist must assess the background, the cellular features, and the nuclear features of the cytologic specimen. With experience the thought process that takes place occurs subconsciously and simultaneously as the slide is screened.

A checklist to aid in evaluating the cellular sample is shown [**T**4.1]; a detailed discussion of each component follows.

Milieu/Background

Cellular Features
- Number of cells
- Distribution
  - Isolated
  - Aggregates
- Surface modifications
- Size
- Shape
- Cytoplasmic appearance
- Cytoplasmic staining
- Products of functional adaptation
- Inclusions
- (Organelles)

Nuclear Features
- Size
- Size variation
- Position
- Number
- Chromatin pattern
- Hyperchromasia
- Chromatinic membrane
- Chromocenters
- Nucleolar size
- Nucleolar shape
- Nucleolar number
- Mitoses
- Degeneration

T4.1
Checklist for Evaluating the Cellular Sample

MILIEU/BACKGROUND

The milieu/background of the cellular sample is important to evaluate, because it is an indication of the host response to the disease process. Erythrocytes, lymphocytes, plasma cells, and neutrophils reflect a host response to inflammation, which may be accompanied by transudate in some inflammatory reactions and by the causative agent. When the aforementioned findings are accompanied by fibrin, recent hemorrhage, and detritus (the breakdown products of cells), a destructive process must be considered. In and of itself the milieu is not pathognomonic of cancer; however, when considered in relation to other cellular evidence it adds significantly to an understanding of the disease process.

CELLULAR FEATURES

Number of Cells

The cellular sample is usually composed of a variety of cells. The number of cells contained in a cellular sample depends on many factors, including the anatomic location, the sampling method, the procedure used to prepare the sample, and the lesion in the underlying epithelium. Cellular samples from the female reproductive tract should have numerous epithelial cells. A cellular sample from the respiratory tract should contain macrophages if the specimen is a sputum or a bronchial lavage, and abundant bronchial cells if the specimen is collected by a bronchial brush or wash. In samples from the pleural or peritoneal cavities the lining cells of the cavity are common; however, a minimal amount of cellular material from a cerebrospinal sample could be within normal limits. Fine needle aspiration cytologic specimens vary dramatically from site to site as to the number and types of cells present (see chapters on fine needle aspiration cytology).

In the presence of an altered epithelium the desquamation of cells is related to the differentiation of the epithelium. Generally, carcinomas (malignant tumors of epithelial origin) that are poorly differentiated (bearing little resemblance to normal tissue of origin) have a higher rate of desquamation than those that are well differentiated (resembling normal tissue of origin). These factors also influence the distribution of cells.

Distribution

Cells may occur isolated or in aggregates. It is important to assess the relative frequency of isolated abnormal cells, which may reflect the decreased mutual adhesiveness of the cells in the parent tissue. In samples from sarcomas (malignant tumors arising in connective tissue), the cells are often isolated, while in carcinomas some abnormal cells are isolated while others occur in aggregates. Many different types of aggregates may occur [**F***4.1*]. Cells that are regularly arranged in relationship to one another and have discernible cell boundaries are said to occur in a sheet-like arrangement. This is usually associated with a normal cellular polarity in the parent epithelium. In a syncytial arrangement the cells are irregularly arranged in relationship to one another and have poorly defined cell boundaries. This three-dimensional mass of cells reflects an altered polarity in the parent epithelium.

Syncytial arrangements of cells from the uterine cervix may be observed in the presence of high-grade squamous intraepithelial lesions, carcinoma in situ, microinvasive carcinoma, or squamous cell carcinoma. During "exodus" (days 6-10 of a normal menstrual cycle), aggregates made up of an inner core of small compact cells and an outer rim of larger cells are often encountered. Other three-dimensional aggregates may be sufficiently characteristic to suggest the nature of the pathologic process. Cell balls, rosette-like arrangements, and loosely cohesive groups in a side-by-side arrangement of cells may suggest the presence of adenocarcinoma (a malignant tumor arising in glandular epithelium). Epithelial pearls may be shed from normal squamous epithelium as well as from carcinomas. Papillary growths are often associated with branching aggregations of cells.

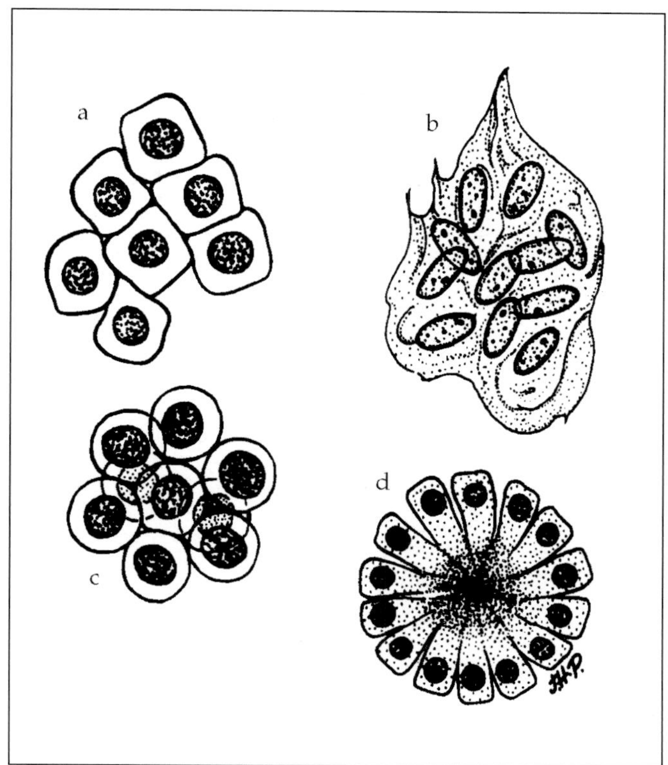

F*4.1*

Examples of common cellular arrangement. (a) This is a sheet-like arrangement of abnormal cells regularly situated in relationship to one another and having distinct cell boundaries. This arrangement is usually associated with altered epithelium having relatively normal cellular polarity in surface layers. (b) This is a syncytial arrangement of abnormal cells, irregularly arranged in relationship to one another. The cell boundaries are poorly defined. Haphazard arrangement of cells is appreciated by drawing a line through the long axis of each nucleus and comparing nuclear polarity of one cell with another. Arrangements of this type are usually observed in the presence of altered epithelium having abnormal or inconstant cellularity polarity. (c) This schematic drawing of cell balls shows a compact, three-dimensional mass of cells. Glandular cells will often occur in this type of arrangement. In fluid media there is a tendency for some cells to grow in spherical aggregates of cell balls. (d) This is an example of altered cell balls. Cells are usually tall columnar forms with basally placed nuclei (ie, endocervical adenocarcinoma).

Size and Shape

The volume of a normal cell is related to its origin and function. The volume is relatively constant for any type of normal epithelial cell. In disease the cell may be larger or smaller than its normal counterpart. There may be significant cell enlargement in folic acid deficiency and after ionizing radiation. Conversely, in cancer the cells may be smaller than their normal counterpart. Variation in cell size characterizes the cells of some malignant tumors, while other neoplasms are composed of uniform cells.

The cytoplasm provides information about the origin of the cell, its function, and its degree of differentiation. Most epithelial cells have a relatively constant form. While all cells are three-dimensional, a polygonal form is often related to epithelial cells. The cells derived from the upper layers of a stratified squamous epithelium are polygonal and wafer-like. This configuration is ideally suited for cells that serve a protective function.

Depending on the perspective from which they are viewed, other cells have a cuboidal, columnar, spherical, or prismatic form. When viewed "on end" cuboidal cells (cells that are of comparable height and thickness) or columnar cells (cells that are taller than they are wide) have a polygonal form. Columnar and cuboidal forms are often associated with absorption or secretion usually of exocrine type. Some but not all spherical cells are related to endocrine secretion. Abnormal cells may either retain their shape or assume a form unlike their tissue of origin. Some abnormal processes are characterized by a predominance of isodiametric cells (ie, spherical cells), while others are associated with nonisodiametric cells (elongate, caudate, or otherwise irregular in form).

Cells that are forcibly removed from an epithelial surface often have morphologic features that are quite different from those observed in cells shed spontaneously from the same epithelium. When cells are forcibly removed from an epithelium, their configuration usually resembles that of component cells of the epithelium. In contrast, cells spontaneously shed into a fluid medium tend to obey certain laws of surface tension and assume a spherical form. This explains the columnar shape of endometrial cells in samples obtained by abrading the endometrium and the spherical form of desquamated endometrial cells. Similarly, columnar cells shed from the lining of the pleural or abdominal cavities tend to have a spherical form when observed in fluid withdrawn from these sites. The appearance of cells may be affected by their metabolic state at the time of shedding, by the environment into which they are desquamated, and by the time interval between exfoliation and sampling of the cellular material.

Cytoplasmic Appearance

There are factors other than cell function that are believed to be related to the shape of the cell within the tissue. The action of the microtubules, the "rigidity" of the cell membrane, the viscosity of the cytoplasm, the surface tension, and the pressure exerted by the contiguous cells are believed to be important. Neoplastic cells that are ovoid when observed in the cellular sample are often associated with neoplasms having a high rate of cell division. The pressure exerted on cells in the tissue may contribute to their form, which indirectly reflects a high rate of cell division (mitosis).

Although invisible by light microscopy, a structural barrier exists between the cell and its environment. Over this membrane is a coating of mucopolysaccharide secreted by the cell. The external coating is conspicuous in plant cells and lacking in human epithelial cells. Cell function is reflected to some extent in the modifications of the cell surface. Numerous folds representing the microvilli observed by ultramicroscopy increase the surface area and augment the transfer of materials across the cell membrane. When observed over a free margin of columnar epithelium this has been designated as a brush border, and is observed in intestinal and renal epithelium. Other cells have more discrete filamentous processes over their free margins. When multiple and short they are referred to as cilia. Ciliation is observed in cells of the respiratory tract and female reproductive tract. When the processes are long and few in number they are considered flagella. Flagella are observed in spermatozoa and *Trichomonas hominis* (an organism of the genital area). Cells that have a complex infolding of the surface membrane are provided with a reserve of surface area to permit the epithelium to adapt to a rapid change in the size of a distensible cavity.

Although the limiting membrane of the cell cannot be visualized by light microscopy, some cells have a well-defined boundary when observed in an isolated state and other cells have an ill-defined outline. The preservation of the cell as well as the methods used in fixation and staining may influence the definition of the cytoplasmic boundary and may reflect cellular differentiation. Well-differentiated cells are more likely to have well-defined cytoplasmic boundaries that are less apparent in poorly differentiated cells. There is a condensation of the cytoplasmic matrix at the periphery of some cells (ie, metaplastic cells). As a result there is a dense peripheral ectoplasmic zone and a more lightly stained central endoplasm. In some metaplastic cells there is an irregular fibril encircling the cell at the junction of the ectoplasm and endoplasm, referred to as the fibril of Eberth. It is evident that the cell has the capacity to undergo keratinization.

Cytoplasmic Staining

Factors that influence the color of the cytoplasm include the metabolic state of the cell, the method of fixation, and the staining technique. With Papanicolaou staining techniques the cytoplasm may appear eosinophilic (pink), indeterminate (gray-blue), or cyanophilic (blue-green). Metabolically active cells and cells derived from tissues known to be associated with RNA synthesis are characterized by cyanophilic cytoplasm. Intense cytoplasmic eosinophilia is often observed in cells undergoing degeneration. An orangeophilic staining reaction is seen in anucleate squamous cells and cells that have the potential to undergo keratinization. Cells derived from keratinizing squamous cell carcinoma have orange-staining cytoplasm.

The appearance of the cytoplasmic matrix is also important. A granular cytoplasm is observed in some secretory cells while others have delicate cytoplasmic vacuolization. Squamous epithelial cells have a delicate homogenous staining cytoplasm. In some cells the cytoplasm has a fibrillar quality. The appearance of the cytoplasm may be related to the method for fixation and the staining technique used.

Products of Functional Adaptation

Within the cytoplasm of some cells there are specific structures that relate to the function of the cell. They have been referred to as the products of functional adaptation. These are best demonstrated by selective staining but may be observed with Papanicolaou staining techniques. Represented are the tonofibrils, myofibrils, and neurofibrils. The tonofibrils are known to be related to the process of keratinization. The elongate or caudate cells observed in keratinizing squamous cell cancer sometimes have a delicate fibril running through the cell, which probably accounts for the bizarre configuration of cells seen in keratinizing processes. Myofibrils and neurofibrils similarly reflect specific functions in muscle cells and nerve cells, respectively.

Inclusions of fat, carbohydrate, protein, and mucus may be contained within the cytoplasm. The identification of these inclusions requires special staining methods. Secretory granules and intracytoplasmic pigment may be identified in the cytoplasm. Hemosiderin, hematoidin, or anthracotic pigment (carbon) may be observed in the cytoplasm of histiocytes. Melanin pigment may occur in both epithelial and connective tissue cells. The lipofuscins, sometimes termed "wear-and-tear" pigments, occur in many tissues. Crystalloids as well as cytoplasmic granules observed in most cells and eosinophilic leukocytes reflect specific cell functions. Cytoplasmic inclusions are inconstant in their occurrence and are not observed in all cells. Organelles or organoids, in contrast, occur in all cells and are best studied by selective staining or by ultramicroscopy.

NUCLEAR FEATURES

While the cytoplasm provides information about the origin of the cell, its function, and its differentiation, the nucleus reflects the reproductive potential of the cell. Except for the mature erythrocyte and the squames derived from the surface of stratified squamous epithelium all human cells contain a nucleus, which is a three-dimensional mass that is visualized in two dimensions by the microscopist. The size of the nucleus is a critical factor in the evaluation of the cell. This may be assessed directly or by considering the nuclear size in relation to the cell size. The latter may be expressed as a nucleocytoplasmic index, a nuclear/cytoplasmic ratio, or a relative nuclear area. Minor changes in the nuclear area are associated with significant changes in nuclear volume. In a spherical nucleus a 50% increase in area reflects a 100% increase in volume. For this reason slight changes in nuclear area must be appreciated in cellular evaluation.

When dealing with small nuclei, minor differences in size are difficult to appreciate. Generally, cells originating from a mature or differentiated epithelium tend to have small nuclei while those arising from an immature or poorly differentiated epithelium have large nuclei. Cancer cells tend to have larger nuclei than their normal counterparts, although as the result of degeneration their nuclei may be reduced in size. Variations in nuclear size may be conspicuous in some cancer cells. In neoplasms having a homogenous cellular content, this variation is often related to an alteration in the nuclear DNA content. To some extent this may occur in neoplasms derived from two or more types of tissue. These tumors are characterized by a heterogeneous cellular population. The position of the nucleus is also important. When a cell is in equilibrium the nucleus is centrally placed. The nucleus can be displaced by secretions or any of the cytoplasmic inclusions. A single nucleus exists in most epithelial cells.

Cells from liver and cartilage are more often binucleated. Osteoclasts and syncytiotrophoblasts are characteristically polynucleate. Multinucleated cells occur in certain disease states [**F**4.2]. They are also observed in viral infections. The Reed-Sternberg cell observed in Hodgkin's disease is usually binucleate. The nuclear configuration

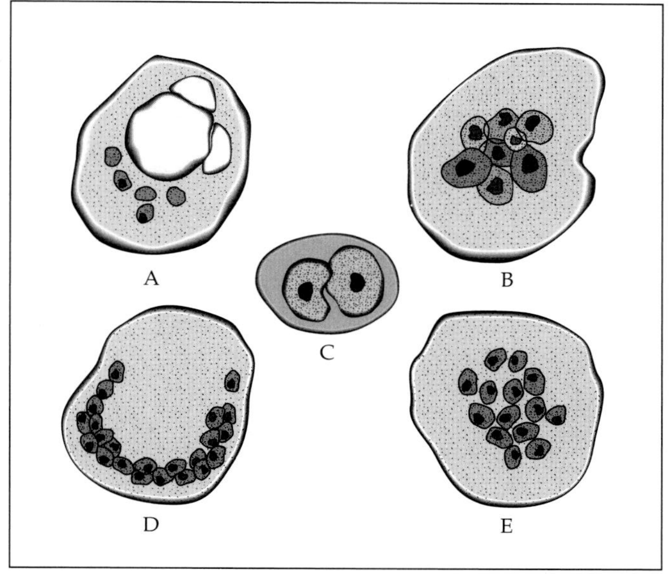

F4.2

Different types of multinucleated giant cells. (a) Touton giant cell is characterized by vacuolated cytoplasm and 5 to 25 irregularly arranged nuclei. Cytoplasmic vacuoles reflect lipid that has been dissolved out of cytoplasm in fixation and staining. (b) Malignant tumor giant cell is large compared with other malignant tumor cells. Multiple and inconstantly arranged nuclei have features observed in malignancy: they are enlarged, varied in size and shape, and hyperchromatic with altered chromatin and macronuclei. (c) Reed-Sternberg cell, a giant cell observed in Hodgkin's disease. The cell is large with poorly stained cytoplasm. Nuclei are enlarged and may appear to overlap one another. The number of nuclei observed are fewer than in other types of giant cells. One or more nuclei may be reniform (kidney-shaped). Nuclear chromatin is clumped and nucleoli may be prominent. (d) Langhans' giant cell, usually associated with tuberculosis. The cell is large with finely granular cytoplasm, and may have an irregular outline. Nuclei are oval, uniform in appearance, and arranged at the periphery of the cell. Long nuclear axis may be radially or inconstantly arranged. With special stains the tubercle bacilli may be observed in the cytoplasm. (e) Foreign body giant cell. The cell is the result of fusion of individual cells, observed in tissues around foreign material introduced into the body, eg, suture material or talc. Cells are large with multiple nuclei and are irregularly arranged in relationship to one another, often near the center of the cell. Nuclei are small and uniform.

may be related to the shape of the cell. In spherical cells the nuclei are usually spherical, while in cylindrical or fusiform cells the nuclei are usually ovoid or compressed. In other cells the nuclear shape is unrelated to the shape of the cells.

Nucleus

The nucleus is surrounded by the nuclear envelope, which is not visible by light microscopy. The nuclear chromatin may be deposited beneath the nuclear envelope, constituting the chromatinic membrane. In the presence of a chromatinic membrane the nuclear envelope appears to be thickened but this is not the case.

The nucleus contains chromatin, which has an affinity for the basic dyes. It stains a deep blue with hematoxylin when using the Papanicolaou technique. The euchromatin stains lightly and has no well-defined masses. In this type of chromatin the DNA strands are unwound or only loosely twisted and are metabolically active. The heterochromatin stains deeply and is arranged in sharply defined clumps. In this form of chromatin the DNA is tightly twisted, folded together, and in an inactive state.

By light microscopy most normal nuclei appear to have a finely granular and uniformly distributed chromatinic material that does not have a great affinity for the nuclear dyes. Hyperchromasia implies an increased nuclear cyanophilia, which may be related to an increase in nuclear DNA. Alterations in the size and distribution of the chromatin aggregates must be considered. Viewed by light microscopy the chromatin pattern may be uniformly finely granular, finely granular and irregularly distributed, uniformly coarsely granular, or coarsely granular and irregularly distributed. With degeneration the nucleus may be transformed into a translucent or opaque mass indicating pyknosis. In cancer cells the chromatin clumps are often separated by clear interchromatinic spaces. Some nuclei contain one or more large discrete masses of chromatin, which stain cyanophilic (blue). These have been termed "chromocenters" or "false nucleoli". Round, well-defined intranuclear masses staining eosinophilic (red) with the Papanicolaou stain are sometimes called true nucleoli. The nucleolus may be surrounded by a rim of DNA referred to as the nucleolus-associated chromatin [**F**4.3].

Unless the nucleus is carefully evaluated the nucleolus-associated chromatin may mask the nucleolus. One or more nucleoli may be observed. They are small in normal cells. Large nucleoli (macronucleoli) are observed in some cancer cells. Macronucleoli may also be seen in benign conditions such as a reparative process. Irregular nucleolar configurations are sometimes observed in cells from poorly differentiated cancers. Ultrastructural changes have been demonstrated in nucleoli observed in cells from some cervical cancers; however, this is not associated with recognizable changes by light microscopy.

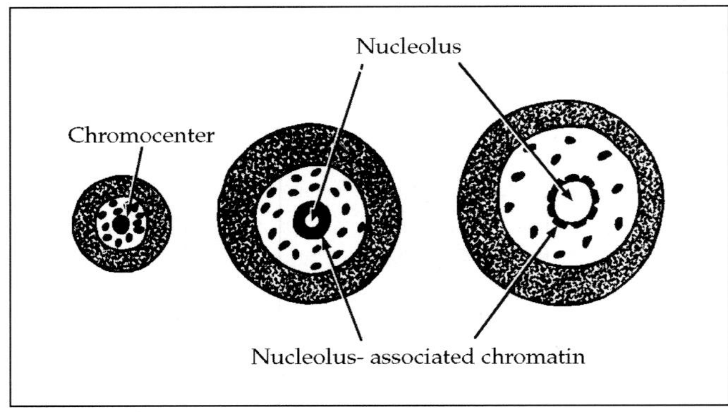

F4.3
Nucleolus surrounded by a rim of DNA (nucleolus-associated chromatin). Modified from Casperson TO. Cell Growth and Cell Function. *New York, NY: WW Norton Co; 1950:104. Figure 48.*

Mitosis

During cell division the appearance of the chromatinic material reflects the stage of mitosis. Prophase, metaphase, and anaphase are associated with characteristic arrangements of the chromatin. The nucleus is reconstituted in telophase. Abnormal form of mitosis also occurs. Mitoses are infrequently observed in cellular samples and are more frequently encountered in histiocytes rather than in epithelial cells. Characteristic changes in the nuclear chromatin occur in degeneration and necrosis. This may be manifested as pyknosis, chromatolysis, or karyorrhexis.

EVALUATION OF THE CERVICOVAGINAL SAMPLE

The evaluation of the cervicovaginal sample has been the subject of much controversy. There is considerable debate as to what constitutes an optimal sample. The utility of the Pap test as well as any laboratory test depends on the quality of the specimen provided and its accurate interpretation. Care must be taken to report to the clinician any unsatisfactory or suboptimal specimen so the clinician can repeat the cellular examination. A specimen may be reported as unsatisfactory for a number of reasons, including paucity of cellular material, obscuring or dilution by excessive blood, obscuring by inflammatory cells, and drying artifact or poor fixation of cellular material. It is recommended that an additional specimen be taken immediately in the event of an unsatisfactory specimen. These criteria and recommendations are not in dispute. The controversy centers around what constitutes an optimal cervicovaginal sample.

The crux of the dispute is whether an endocervical component (material from the transformation zone) must be present for a cervicovaginal sample to be optimal. The presence of endocervical cells and/or metaplastic cells traditionally has indicated that the transformation zone has been sampled. The laboratory should report the presence of an endocervical component to the clinician. The decision as to whether a specimen should be repeated because of the lack of an endocervical component should be made by clinicians based on patient information. The importance of proper sampling methods, including a discussion on the importance of the presence of an endocervical component, is addressed elsewhere (Chapters 6 and 9).

CONCLUSION

This chapter covers the basic features to be considered in a comprehensive cellular evaluation. When these features are taken into consideration a meaningful examination is provided. The evaluation of the cells provides information about the underlying nature of disease. This is cellular pathology in the true sense of the term, a new parameter in the study of disease. However, cellular pathology is not a substitute for biopsy; instead, its use facilitates biopsy findings, and the nature of the underlying disease process is more readily documented.

REVIEW QUESTIONS

1. What are the characteristics of the milieu in a normal sample as compared with a sample from a patient with advanced cancer?
2. What are the features to be assessed in examining the cell?
3. What features provide information about the origin and differentiation of the cell?
4. What features provide information about the reproductive capacity of the cell?
5. Define the difference between "true" and "false" nucleolus.

SELECTED READINGS

Bloom W, Fawcett DW. *A Textbook of Histology.* 10th ed. Philadelphia, Pa: WB Saunders Co; 1975.

Casperson TO. *Cell Growth and Cell Function.* New York, NY: WW Norton Co; 1950.

Cowdry EV. *Cancer Cells.* Philadelphia, Pa: WB Saunders Co; 1955.

Crick FHC, Watson JD. The complementary structures of dioxyribonucleic acid. *Proc R Soc.* 1954;223:80-96.

Goellner JR. Evaluation of the cellular sample. In: Bibbo M, ed. *Comprehensive Cytopathology.* Philadelphia, Pa: WB Saunders Co; 1991.

CHAPTER 5

Anatomy and Histology

STANLEY F. PATTEN, JR, MD, PHD, FIAC

CONTENTS

To fully appreciate the cellular changes associated with disease of the female genital tract organs, an understanding of normal anatomy and histology of these structures is essential. The organs of the female genital tract constitute an internal group within the body and an external group on the surface of the body.

EXTERNAL GENITALIA

The external genitalia, commonly referred to collectively as the vulva, include a number of structures [**F**5.1]. The mons pubis is a diffuse midline elevation overlying the junction of the pelvic bones anteriorly (toward the front of the body). It is formed by a pad of subcutaneous fat. At puberty, this area becomes covered with pubic hair. The labial folds are two longitudinal folds of skin on each side of the midline, beginning inferiorly (toward the feet) and posteriorly (toward the back of the body) to the mons pubis. The larger and more lateral (toward the sides of the body) folds are called the labia majora and the medial (toward the center of the body) and smaller folds are called the labia minora.

The labia majora are the counterparts of the two halves of the male scrotum and contain a large amount of fibrous fatty tissue. Their external aspects are covered by pubic hair. They begin anteriorly at the mons pubis, where their medial borders are in continuity. They pass backward, becoming less prominent, to again meet in the midline anterior to the anus. The area of skin between the posterior junction of the labia majora and the anus is called the obstetrical perineum. This is often the site of injury or tearing during childbirth. To prevent such an injury, an incision, or episiotomy, is made shortly before delivery. This is repaired immediately following delivery.

The labia minora are more slender and contain no fat, appearing as redundant folds of skin. They bound the vestibule of the vagina. Anteriorly, they split to enclose a small, erectile organ called the clitoris, which is homologous with the male penis. It is relatively small, measuring approximately 2.5 cm in length, and is composed of highly vascular tissue. Posteriorly, the labia minora are joined by a fold called the fourchette.

The vestibule of the vagina is a cleft between the labia minora. Within the vestibule, about 1 to 2 cm posterior to the clitoris, is a slightly elevated opening. This is the external opening of the urinary tract, or urethral orifice (external urethral meatus). Below or posterior to the urethral opening is the vaginal orifice, or introitus, which is the external opening of the female genital tract. Immediately within is a thin, incomplete membranous fold called the hymen. The remnants of the hymen persist as small tags or elevations. Opening into the vestibule are numerous small, mucous-secreting glands. At the lower border of the vaginal orifice are the ducts from two relatively large mucous glands called Bartholin's glands.

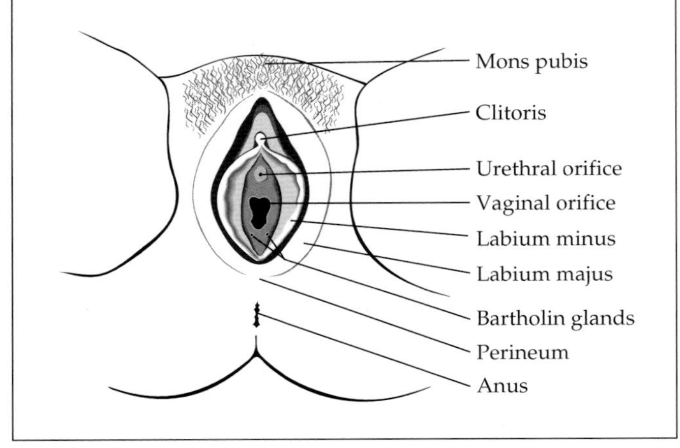

F5.1
External genitalia of the female genital tract.

The microscopic structure of the external genitalia is quite variable from one site to another. The labia majora are covered by skin, or epidermis, similar to that observed elsewhere on the surface of the body. The epidermis is composed of a keratinized, stratified squamous epithelium. Beneath this epithelium, the connective tissue stroma, or dermis, contains the usual skin appendages, such as hair follicles and sebaceous glands. In addition, special apocrine or sudoriferous glands similar to those present in the axilla and breast may be identified. The labia minora and vestibule of the vagina are usually covered by a nonkeratinizing stratified squamous epithelium, and the underlying connective tissue stroma usually lacks hair follicles.

INTERNAL GENITAL ORGANS

The portions of the female genital tract that lie within the body include the vagina, uterus, uterine tubes, and ovaries [**F**5.2]. These structures occupy the lower portion of the abdominal, or peritoneal, cavity referred to as the pelvic cavity. The abdominal and pelvic cavities are lined by a smooth glistening membrane called the peritoneum. Its surface is composed of a single layer of flat, pavement-like cells frequently termed mesothelial cells. This layer of peritoneum is reflected onto the surfaces of various organs present in the abdominal and pelvic cavities, providing a so-called serosal coat or layer.

In addition to the organs of the female genital tract, portions of the urinary and gastrointestinal systems also occupy areas of the pelvic cavity. The female genital tract is suspended in the pelvic cavity by a series of supports called ligaments. These are reflections of the peritoneum passing between the organs and the body wall. The broad ligament envelops the uterus and passes from its lateral margins to

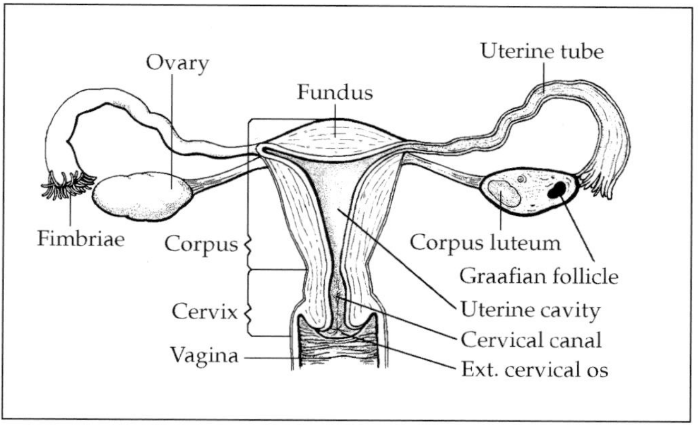

F5.2
Internal organs of the female genital tract.

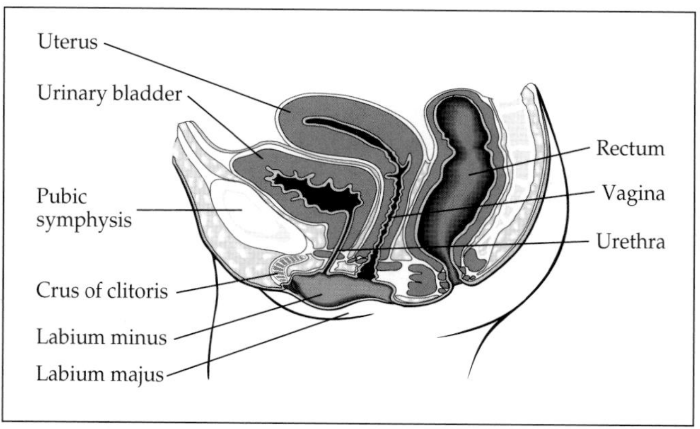

F5.3
Sagittal view of internal organs of the female genital tract in relation to other organ systems.

the lateral wall of the pelvis. It is triangular in shape and its upper border is occupied by the uterine tubes. The round ligaments are true ligamentous fibromuscular cords. They pass from the superior portions of the uterus to the inferior portions of the pelvic wall. The function of the round ligaments is to draw the uterus forward after it has been displaced backward by pregnancy or a distended urinary bladder. Should they fail to function, intra-abdominal pressure forces the uterus downward, putting strain on ligamentous supports, resulting in descensus, or prolapse, of the uterus into the vagina. Other ligaments aid in the suspension of the ovaries, cervix, and vagina.

Vagina

The vagina is a flattened, but distensible, musculomembranous canal measuring about 7 cm in length. It extends from the vestibule to the lower end of the uterus, passing posteriorly and upward into the pelvis. It is situated posterior to the urinary bladder and urethra and anterior to the rectum and anal canal [**F**5.3]. The upper end of the vagina invests the lower portion of the uterus or cervix. The latter projects into the vagina through the upper portion of the anterior wall at an oblique angle. The recesses of the vagina around the cervix are termed fornices. The posterior vaginal fornix is the deepest, and a "pool" of secretions, cells, and cellular debris may accumulate at this site. Papanicolaou utilized the vaginal pool sample to prepare his cell films for examination. Because cells accumulating at this site had exfoliated, the study of these cells was called "exfoliative cytology."

The vagina has four layers or coats. The outer coat is composed of fat containing many small veins. Inside this is a layer of smooth or nonstriated muscle. Next to the layer of muscle is a submucous coat of elastic fatty tissue containing a dense complex of veins. The innermost layer is the mucosa, which is composed of a multilayered epithelium made up of flattened, pavement-like cells. This type of epithelium is referred to as stratified squamous. Unlike the skin (epidermis), the vaginal mucosa (epithelium) is nonkeratinized; however, like the skin, its main function is protection. The thickness (number of cell layers) comprising the epithelium of the vagina varies during different periods of life, since it is affected by hormones. In the child, except in the immediate postpartum period, the cell layers are few in number. At the onset of menstruation, when the hormone estrogen is formed by the ovaries, the epithelium grows, matures, and becomes highly stratified. At this time, the squamous cells composing the epithelium contain a large amount of glycogen. When menstruation ceases in later years, the vaginal epithelium, lacking stimulation by estrogen, becomes thin, undergoing a process known as atrophy. Thus, the stratified squamous epithelium of the vagina is a relatively sensitive indicator of the hormonal status of the female. This is examined in greater detail in Chapter 7, "Hormonal Cytology."

Uterus

The uterus, a pear-shaped, hollow, muscular organ lying behind the urinary bladder and in front of the rectum [**F**5.3], measures about 7 x 5 x 2.5 cm. The uterine tubes and broad ligaments are attached to its lateral margins. The uterus is divided into three parts: a base, or fundus; a main portion, the body; and the lower prolongation known as the neck, or cervix, which projects into the vagina. The fundus and corpus form the upper 5 cm and the cervix forms the lower 2 cm.

The interior of the uterine corpus, or uterine cavity, is a small, triangular space that communicates laterally with the uterine tubes and the cervix below. The cavity (channel) through the cervix is called the cervical or endocervical canal. Its upper, or proximal, junction with the uterine cavity is called the internal os, or opening. The lower, or distal, opening into the vagina is the external os. The uterine cervix, constituting the lower third of the uterus, may be divided into two portions. The lower portion, lying within the vaginal canal, is called the portio vaginalis (ectocervix). The portion lying above the vaginal attachment and in continuity with the uterine corpus is referred to as the portio supravaginalis (endocervix). During a pelvic examination by a physician, the ectocervix may be viewed by dilating the vaginal canal with an instrument called a vaginal speculum. From this perspective, the cervix appears as a thick, circular ring, with the external os in the center. Viewed in this position, the ectocervix is commonly described as having an anterior and posterior lip. Before childbirth (nulliparous), the external cervical os is usually smooth and circular, but following childbirth (parous) is transverse or stellate in appearance.

Microscopic Structure of the Uterine Corpus

The uterine corpus has three layers: an outer serosa, which represents the reflection of the peritoneum over the uterus; an intermediate, thick (about 1.5 cm) muscular layer composed of interlacing bundles, the myometrium; and an inner mucosal coat, the endometrium. The endometrium undergoes regular cyclic changes during the reproductive years as a result of hormonal influences. The uterine cavity and the glands that open into this cavity are lined by a simple columnar or cuboidal epithelium. In the region of the internal cervical os, this epithelium merges with the epithelium lining the cervical canal. This epithelium is composed principally of columnar, secretory forms. Occasionally, ciliated columnar cells may also be identified. In general, the cells are not as tall as those lining the endocervical canal and their secretory product is glycogen. In addition to the cells lining the surface of the uterine cavity and the underlying endometrial glands, the endometrium includes a peculiar type of connective tissue, known as endometrial stroma, in which the endometrial glands are embedded. Both the epithelial and connective tissue components of the endometrium undergo definite cyclic changes in response to ovarian hormones.

The cyclic changes observed in the endometrium may be divided into three phases: menstrual or bleeding phase; proliferative, preovulatory, or luteal phase; and secretory, postovulatory, or follicular phase. In general, the menstrual cycle is set as a 28-day period. The first day of the cycle is designated as day 1 and is characterized by the onset of menstrual flow. During the next 3 to 4 days, bleeding continues and the bulk of the endometrium is desquamated, leaving a thin layer of endometrial stroma and glandular stumps over the myometrium. Following the cessation of menstrual flow, from day 5 to day 14, the endometrium is stimulated by the ovarian hormone estrogen. During this period, the stromal and epithelial cells that remain after desquamation of the endometrium during the menstrual phase, proliferate in number and increase in size. The thickness of the endometrium increases rapidly with the formation of new endometrial glands and stroma. At the beginning of the proliferative phase, the surface and glandular epithelium is composed of relatively small, cuboidal cells. Toward the end of the proliferative phase, the cells assume a definite columnar form. Thus, in the early proliferative phase, the glands are straight and narrow with low, cuboidal lining epithelium. Later, the glands increase in size, appear tortuous, and are lined by a distinctly columnar epithelium [❚*5.1*].

Ovulation usually occurs in the middle of a 28-day cycle. Following this event, the ovaries begin to produce a new hormone, progesterone, which exerts its influence on the endometrium. Under the influence of progesterone, the endometrium enters the secretory phase. The first evidence of secretory activity is characterized by the presence of glycogen secretion in the base of the epithelial cells beneath the nuclei. As glycogen accumulates, it moves around the nuclei and comes to lie in the apical portion of the cells. As the secretory phase proceeds, the endometrial glands become plumper and more tortuous, and the lining epithelial cells appear pale and frayed as their secretions are released into the lumens of the glands [❚*5.2*]. Toward the end of the secretory phase, the stromal cells begin to enlarge and assume an epithelial-like appearance in the upper portions of the endometrium (predecidual reaction). If pregnancy occurs, this process continues with the formation of the decidua. A similar decidual reaction may occur within the stroma of the uterine cervix in a small percentage of women during pregnancy. If pregnancy does not occur, with the cessation of progesterone formation by the ovaries, the secretory phase of the cycle ends with the onset of menstrual flow and the eventual desquamation of the endometrium, marking the beginning of a new cycle.

Microscopic Structure of the Uterine Cervix

The uterine cervix is composed chiefly of fibromuscular tissue often referred to as the cervical stroma. Covering the canal surfaces of the cervix is a mucosal coat (epithelium). Like the vaginal canal into which it projects, the ectocervix is covered by a nonkeratinizing stratified squamous epithelium. This is similar to that lining the vaginal canal, except that the glycogen content of the cells is lower. Like the vaginal epithelium, the thickness and appearance of the ectocervical epithelium varies with the age of the individual, and it undergoes minor changes during the menstrual cycle. In the approximate region of the external cervical os, there is an abrupt transition of the lining epithelium from stratified squamous to a simple or one-layered type called columnar, as the cells composing the epithelium are taller than they are wide. This transition zone, variable in its anatomic location between the epithelium covering the ectocervix and that lining the endocervix, is referred to as the squamocolumnar junction [❚*5.3*].

From the perspectives of clinical examination and sample collection for cytologic examination, it is important to recognize that the anatomic site of the squamocolumnar junction and the configuration of the external cervical os varies with age and that their locations can be artificially

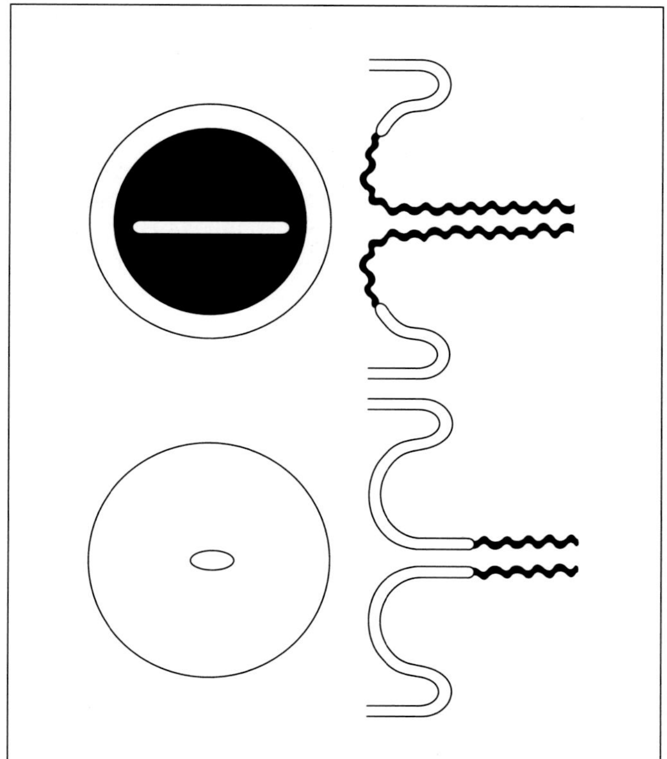

F5.4

Variations in the site of the squamocolumnar junction and shape of the external cervical os in relation to age: before the age of 30 years (top); after the menopause (bottom). Reproduced with permission from Practical Colposcopy *(Figures 8a and 8b, p 18).*

modified by clinical examination and pathologic study. In the parous woman under 30 years of age, the external cervical os is horizontal and broad with the squamocolumnar junction lying outside the cervical canal [**F**5.4, top]. After the menopause, the external cervical os is small and narrower, with the squamocolumnar junction lying well within the cervical canal [**F**5.4, bottom] as a result of cervical fibrosis and stenosis. Under these circumstances, the clinical external os and the anatomic cervical os coincide. Therefore, it is important to note that the squamocolumnar junction is not always synonymous with the external os. Similarly, from a clinical standpoint, ectocervix is not synonymous with squamous epithelium nor is the endocervix necessarily synonymous with columnar epithelium. As previously indicated, the anatomic location of the squamocolumnar junction can be artificially modified by clinical and pathologic examination. The normal location of the squamocolumnar junction of a parous cervix from the perspectives of frontal and sagittal views is shown [**F**5.5, left]. Note that only a small area of glandular (endocervical) mucosa is visible around the external os (dark zone). However, during clinical examination, the valves of the vaginal speculum exert traction on the anterior and posterior fornices in opposite directions, which separates the lips of the cervix and tends to pull out the lower or distal portions of the endocervical canal [**F**5.5, right]. When the valves of the vaginal speculum are closed, the distal portion of the endocervical epithelium retracts into the canal and can no longer be viewed.

In contrast with the above, when the squamocolumnar junction is visible on the ectocervix by clinical examination with a vaginal speculum in place [**F**5.5, right], a cone biopsy specimen of the same cervix after fixation may reveal a squamocolumnar junction 10 to 15 mm within the cervical canal [**F**5.6].

The squamocolumnar junction is not a static junction between two types of epithelia, squamous and columnar. Rather, during a woman's life, this junction undergoes a dynamic transformation. It is on this basis that it is called the "transformation zone." Not only does this zone undergo epithelial-type transformation but it is also the most common site of neoplastic transformation.

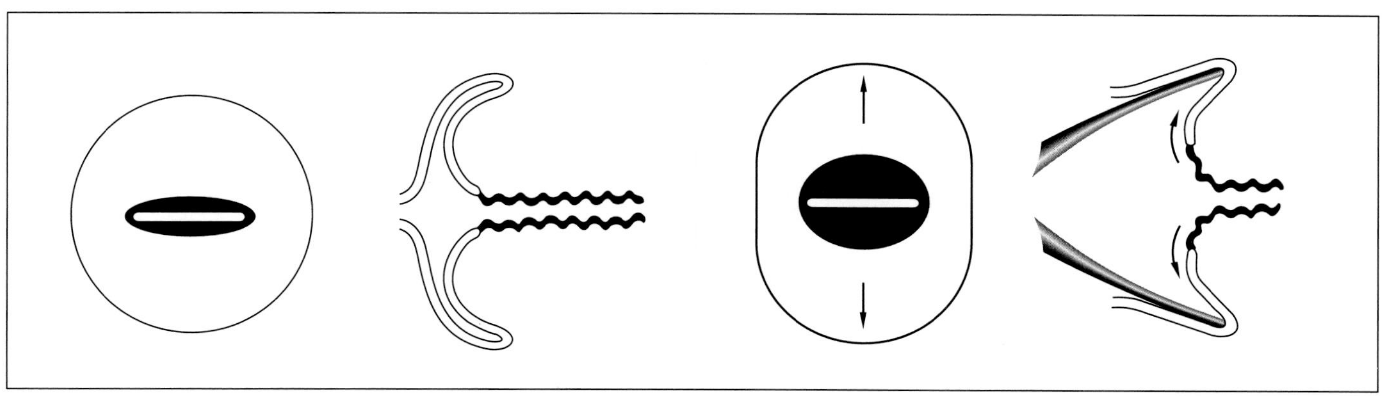

F5.5

Site of the squamocolumnar junction. With vagina in normal collapsed state, a small amount of glandular (endocervical) mucosa may be visible as depicted by the dark zone surrounding the external cervical os on frontal and sagittal views (left). With vaginal speculum in place with valves expanded, the external cervical os is opened with a wide zone of glandular (endocervical) mucosa, becoming visible in frontal and sagittal views (right). Reproduced with permission from Practical Colposcopy *(Figures 9a and 9b, p 18).*

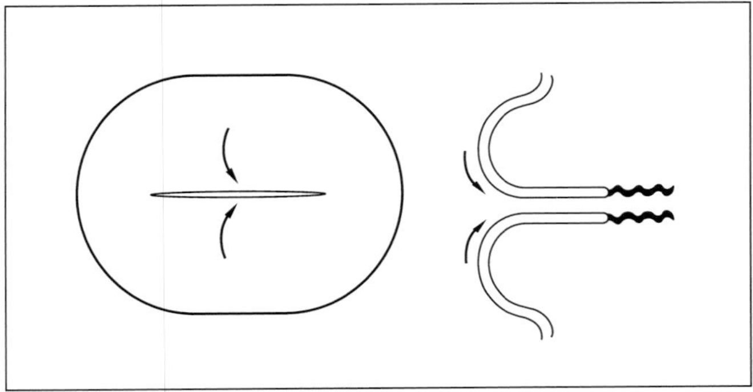

F5.6

Position of the squamocolumnar junction in a fixed cone biopsy specimen. The external cervical os pushes the glandular (endocervical) mucosa far into the canal. Reproduced with permission from Practical Colposcopy *(Figure 9c, p 18).*

Simple Columnar Epithelium

The columnar epithelium lining the cervical canal contains at least two cell types. One is a secreting columnar cell and the other is a ciliated columnar cell, although each may represent various stages in the complete life cycle of the cell. In the premenstrual and postmenopausal years, the cells are not tall and lack the secretory activity present during the reproductive years. There is some evidence to suggest that they undergo cyclic changes under hormonal influence during the menstrual cycle, becoming taller and plumper during the latter half of the cycle. The simple columnar epithelium lining the canal extends into and lines the so-called endocervical "glands," crypts or folds that lie beneath the surface in the cervical stroma. The columnar cells lining these crypts or gland-like spaces are chiefly of a secreting type. They produce mucus, in contrast with the glands of the endometrium, which produce glycogen.

Located within the stroma at the extreme lateral margins of the uterine cervix may be seen small tubular structures lined by a single layer of low, columnar cells. These structures represent the embryologic remnants of a portion of a primitive urinary tract. In the female, they are called Gartner's ducts. Portions of this system may be identified in the wall of the uterine corpus and/or in the broad ligament.

Stratified Squamous Epithelium

The epithelium that lines the vagina and covers the outer portion of the uterine cervix, or for practical purposes, the ectocervix, is classified as nonkeratinizing stratified squamous epithelium. The designation stratified is used to indicate that the epithelium is made up of many cell layers. The epithelium is characterized as squamous because the superficial cells at the surface are flat and scale-like, resembling squames. The primary function of this epithelium is the protection of the underlying tissues, although it has been suggested that its production of glycogen is concerned with the nourishment of spermatozoa when they enter the female genital tract.

The cells making up the stratified squamous epithelium have a relatively short life span. They are cast off from the surface, ie, exfoliated, and new cells must be formed constantly in the deeper layers of the epithelium to replenish those that are shed. The life cycle of the squamous cell begins in the deep layers of the epithelium where new cells are formed by division of preexisting cells. At this level, the cells are characterized as immature because they have not as yet attained the features of adult squamous cells. As the cells are pushed upward in the epithelium, they acquire the physical and chemical characteristics of adult, or mature, squamous cells. Having acquired these features, the cells are said to be differentiated. As the cells are pushed closer to the surface of the epithelium, away from their main source of nourishment, evidence of aging becomes apparent in the cells. They undergo senescence, but even in this state will continue to provide a protective function. Once aging develops, the cells have completed their life cycle and will soon be shed, only to be replaced by new cells. Since mature and senescent cells are incapable of cell division, any replacements for the exfoliated cells must come from the immature cells lying deep in the epithelium.

Under the microscope, several different layers can be identified in the stratified squamous epithelium of the uterine cervix and vagina [**I**5.3]. From the epithelial-stromal junction to the surface, these are the basal cell layer, or stratum cylindricum or germinativum; the parabasal zone, or deep spinous layer; the intermediate zone, or superficial spinous layer; the so-called intraepithelial layer; and the superficial zone, or stratum corneum. The stratified squamous epithelium of the uterine cervix and vagina retains the potential for further differentiation, and a modification of the foregoing arrangement may be observed under presumably normal conditions. Typically this occurs in the region of the intraepithelial layer, where the cells may become specialized with the formation of keratohyalin granules in the cytoplasm. This zone of squamous cell specialization is termed the granular cell layer. The function of this layer is to produce a surface zone of keratin or keratinized squames, resulting in a stratified epithelium that affords greater protection like the skin or epidermis.

When viewed on cross section under the microscope, the basal cell or germinal layer is made up of a single thickness of cells, which are referred to as columnar cells. The nucleus appears to be relatively large and is round or oval. Overlying the basal layer are several layers of round or small polygonal cells, which are referred to as parabasal cells because they lie near the basal cells. They are sometimes called spinous cells because, with special stains, delicate fibrils may be observed within their cytoplasm. These are the tonofibrils that give the cell a spinous appearance. On cross section, these cells appear to be larger than the basal cells. The nucleus is centrally placed and appears to be relatively large in relation to the amount of visible cytoplasm. These cells may contain glycogen, which is apparent with special stains. The number of cell layers in the parabasal or deep spinous layer and the shape of the cells are related to the amount of estrogen present.

There are several layers of cells in the intermediate or superficial spinous zone that appear to be elliptical or navicular in form. Their configuration suggests that of a flattened polygonal cell. These cells have tonofibrils in their cytoplasm, giving them a spinous appearance. They also contain glycogen. The nuclei appear to be smaller than those in the deeper-lying cells. Although some cells have a central nucleus, other cells possess an eccentric nucleus whose displacement is probably related to the presence of glycogen. In some cells, the nucleus is round on cross section, while in other cells it is flattened. The intermediate zone is variable in its thickness, being better developed when the entire epithelium is thick and under the influence of estrogen stimulation.

The intraepithelial layer, made up of flattened cells with small, dense nuclei, may be present above the intermediate zone. The significance of this layer is not well understood and is not always present in the human. Overlying this layer, in the stratum corneum, are several thicknesses of flat cells. On cross section, these cells are so thin that their nuclei appear thicker than the cells themselves. The nucleus is quite small and dense.

As alluded to previously, under certain conditions, in place of the intraepithelial layer, there may be a layer composed of flattened cells with numerous small cytoplasmic granules. This constitutes the granular cell layer, which is usually observed in conjunction with surface keratinization. The latter is characterized by the presence of flat cells that do not possess nuclei, although the position usually occupied by the nucleus may be represented by a small clear area. These anucleated cells often degenerate. Although a thin layer of anucleated squames may be observed on the surface of an otherwise normal epithelium, a thick layer of so-called keratinized cells constitutes an abnormal reaction in the uterine cervix or vagina.

A microscopic description of the cross section of a stratified squamous epithelium provides information about two cell dimensions. It must be kept in mind, however, that all cells have three dimensions. The surface cells are thin, wafer-like forms on cross section but are large, polygonal forms when viewed in a plane parallel to the surface. The cells of the intermediate layer, which are ellipsoidal on cross section, are also polygonal in form when viewed on a plane parallel to the surface. When viewed from above, they appear smaller than the surface cells, largely because much of their volume is not appreciated in this perspective. Cells of the parabasal zone are polygonal, round, or oval in form, regardless of the plane in which they are viewed. They appear smaller than the cells from the overlying layers, largely because much of their total mass is not appreciated in two-dimensional studies.

When viewed from above, the cells of the basal layer are polygonal in shape, although they are columnar in configuration when viewed on cross section.

Atrophy may occur in the stratified squamous epithelium of the uterine cervix and vagina as a result of estrogen deficiency. Atrophy constitutes a reduction in the size of an organ or tissue that formally was mature. When it occurs during the reproductive years of life, it represents an abnormal change. After menopause, however, atrophy is a normal physiologic process. The appearance of an atrophic stratified squamous epithelium depends to some extent on the relative degree of estrogen deficiency that exists. Usually, an atrophic epithelium is reduced in thickness and lacks a surface maturation characteristic of a normal mucosa. The component of cells may be reduced in size and, because of the absence of maturation, there are immature-appearing cells lying at superficial levels in the epithelium.

Squamous Metaplasia

Within the transformation zone of the uterine cervix, a sharp demarcation between stratified squamous and simple columnar epithelia at the squamocolumnar junction [▮*5.3*] is replaced by an immature stratified squamous epithelium representing a gradual transition between the two principal types of epithelium [▮*5.4*]. The term metaplasia denotes the substitution of one adult cell type for another. In the uterine cervix, the process represents a squamous metaplasia, as there is a replacement of a columnar epithelium by a stratified squamous epithelium. This change may involve both the surface epithelium and the gland-like crypts of the endocervical canal. With advancing age, the size of the transformation zone and linear progression up the cervical canal increases. In the premenopausal woman, the squamous metaplastic-columnar junction may lie near the region of the internal cervical os. A three-dimensional drawing of the normal squamocolumnar junction is shown [**F***5.7*].

The concept of squamous metaplasia is extremely important for an understanding of the process of carcinogenesis in the uterine cervix and, therefore, is equally important in diagnostic cytopathology. The term metaplasia implies that there is a transformation of the endocervical columnar cell into another type of adult cell type, the squamous cell. This, of course, is not true. For purposes of classification, squamous metaplasia can be arbitrarily subdivided into the stages of reserve cell hyperplasia, immature squamous metaplasia, and mature squamous metaplasia. The microscopic structure of reserve cell hyperplasia may be defined as the appearance or development of one or more layers of primitive, germinal-type cells beneath the columnar epithelium. These so-called reserve cells closely resemble the cells normally observed in the basal cell layer of stratified squamous epithelium but lack well-defined boundaries, thus giving the appearance of nuclei residing in a syncytium of cytoplasm. Immature squamous metaplasia spans the morphologic spectrum from the development of well-defined cell boundaries in the reserve cells to a stratified squamous epithelium composed of three of the four classical layers observed in a completely mature nonkeratinizing stratified squamous epithelium. When the newly

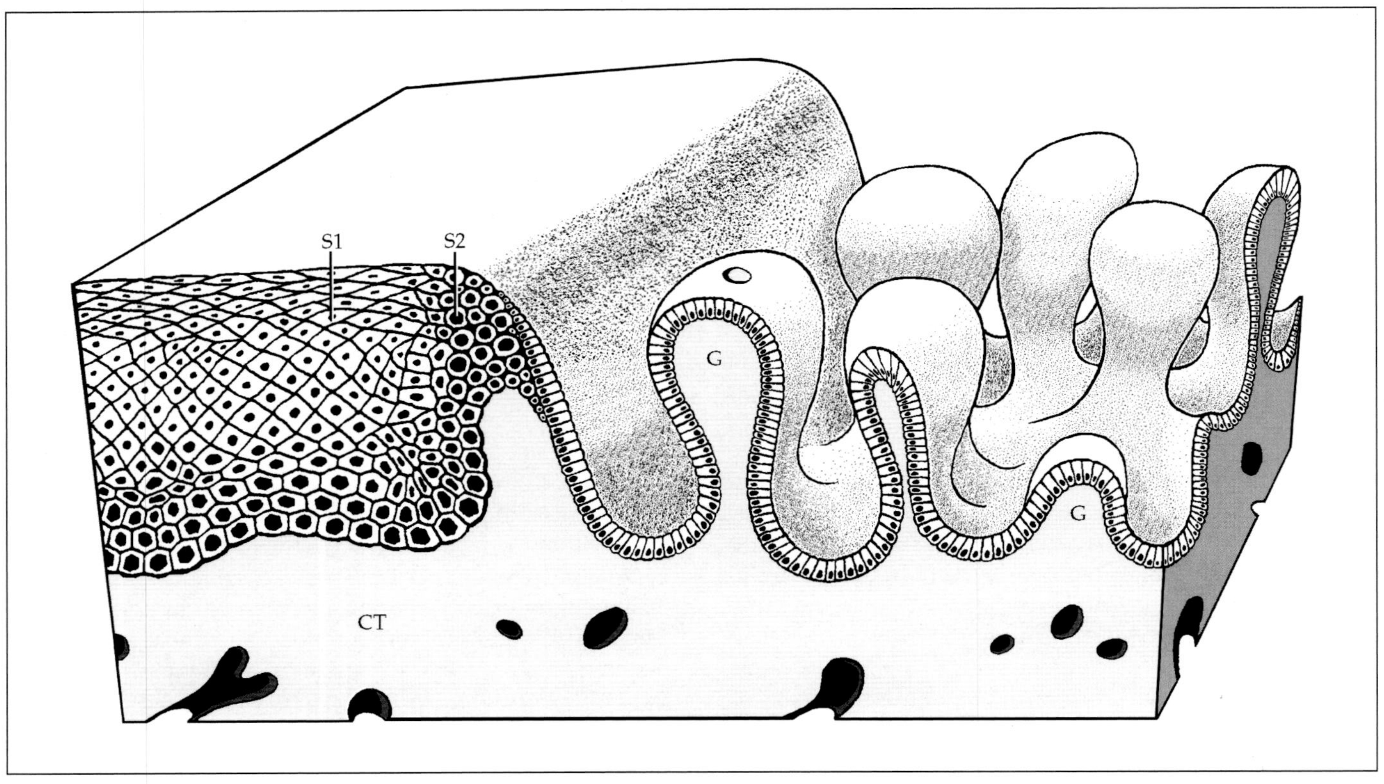

F5.7

Original squamocolumnar junction. S1, normal squamous epithelium laden with glycogen; S2, small area of squamous epithelium lacking glycogen, representing a white margin; G, papillae of glandular mucosa; CT, connective tissue. Reproduced with permission from Practical Colposcopy *(Figure 2b, p 24).*

formed epithelium is morphologically indistinguishable from adult stratified squamous epithelium, it constitutes mature squamous metaplasia. It is not uncommon to observe columnar epithelial-lined gland-like spaces beneath zones of squamous metaplasia, with or without extension of the squamous metaplastic process into these spaces.

While the process of squamous metaplasia is considered to be a normal physiologic protective response to a variety of stimuli, this process may be replicated in an abnormal fashion during cervical carcinogenesis, with the various stages of squamous metaplasia being composed of abnormal cell populations.

Uterine Tubes

The uterine tubes (fallopian tubes or salpinges) are the paired oviducts that convey the ovum from the ovary to the uterus. Each is about 10 cm long and 0.8 cm in diameter, with a sometimes tortuous appearance. They emerge from the lateral uterine wall at the junction of the corpus and fundic portions. Four subdivisions of the uterine tubes are recognized: an interstitial portion, represented by a very short segment passing through the uterine wall, or cornu; a narrow isthmus lying adjacent to the uterus; the ampulla, which is the longest, widest section and is slightly convoluted; and the infundibulum, which is funnel-shaped and is the lateral opening of the uterine tubes. The margins of the infundibulum are broken into numerous finger-like processes called fimbria, which give the free margins a fringed or ragged appearance. This portion of the uterine tube curves over, but is not attached to, the superior pole of each ovary.

The uterine tubes are composed of three coats or layers: an outer serosa, representing the peritoneal envelope; a middle muscular layer; and an inner mucosa, or endosalpinx. The endosalpinx is thrust forward into three or four longitudinal folds, or rugae. It is composed of an inner connective tissue layer and a lining epithelium. The epithelium is of a simple columnar type. Three distinct cell types may be identified in the lining epithelium: ciliated columnar cells, nonciliated or secretory columnar cells, and the so-called intercalated or peg cells, which represent another phase in the life cycle of the secretory cell. Like the epithelial cells in other portions of the female genital tract, the ciliated and secretory cells of the uterine tubes appear to undergo cyclic changes during the menstrual cycle, reaching their greatest height during the midportion and secretory portion of the cycle. During pregnancy, the epithelium becomes low and may even appear flat in many places. Evidence of secretory activity is not seen at this time. In addition to presence or absence of cilia, the ciliated and secretory cells may be distinguished on the basis of nuclear staining qualities. The nucleus of the ciliated cell is relatively pale, whereas the secretory cell nucleus may appear quite hyperchromatic.

Ovaries

The two ovaries, resembling large almonds in both size and shape, are situated on each side of the uterus in close relationship to the free ends of the uterine tubes. They are suspended from the posterior surface of the broad ligament of the uterus by a short peritoneal fold, the mesovarium. Before puberty, their surfaces are smooth, but as a result of ovulation and especially pregnancy, the surfaces become scarred. In elderly, multiparous women, the surfaces are very uneven and puckered.

Structurally, the ovary is composed of two zones: a central medulla, containing numerous blood vessels and connective tissue; and an outer cortex. The cortical layer consists of a distinctive, fibromuscular tissue or stroma enclosing the follicular elements of the ovary in various stages of development. The cortex comprises about two thirds of the depth of the ovary during reproductive life. Surrounding the cortex is a fibrous capsule. Scattered through the cortical zone are the graafian follicles. In the ovaries of children and younger women, there are numerous primordial follicles, consisting of a central germ cell or ovum encircled by a flattened or low cuboidal layer of epithelium called the follicle epithelium, or granulosa. In the later phases of reproductive life their number becomes progressively less, and after menopause they are almost entirely absent.

During reproductive life, follicles in various stages of development are seen. The features of these various stages can be best described by tracing the life history of the follicle from the primordial stage to full maturation, ovulation, and involution. As the follicle grows, the granulosa proliferates, forming several layers of cells. At this time, the follicle begins to show a central cavity or antrum, the ovum being located at one pole in an accumulation of granulosa cells called the cumulus oophorus. The stroma surrounding the developing follicle gives rise to a layer of modified connective tissue called the theca. The developing follicle is responsible for the production of the ovarian hormone, estrogen, which exerts its influence on the endometrium, reaching its highest level during the proliferative phase of a cycle.

The mature follicle is of considerable size and may reach a diameter of 0.8 cm. At ovulation, the ovum, with a varying number of granulosa cells, is extruded from the ovary, passing into the uterine tube. Immediately following ovulation, the follicle collapses, and subsequent involution or alteration depends on whether implantation (pregnancy) takes place.

The granulosa cells become modified by the accumulation of fatty material, and the entire structure is called the corpus luteum. The corpus luteum produces the ovarian hormone, progesterone, along with diminishing amounts of estrogen. The former stimulates the secretory activity of the endometrium during the second half of the menstrual cycle. In the late portion of the cycle, progesterone initiates the predecidual reaction and also a decidual reaction of pregnancy if implantation occurs. The mature corpus luteum measures 1.0 to 1.5 cm in diameter. If pregnancy has not occurred, the corpus luteum enters a retrogressive phase, resulting in diminution of progesterone formation and eventual onset of menstruation. Complete involution transforms the corpus luteum into a scarred structure called the corpus albicans. In the event of pregnancy, the mature corpus luteum does not involute, but becomes larger and forms the corpus luteum of pregnancy.

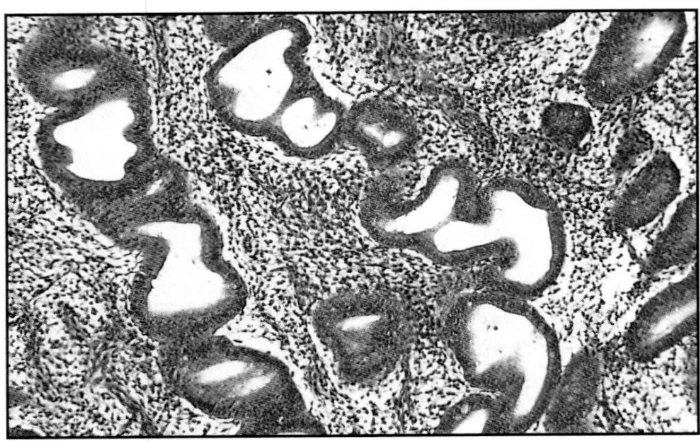

▮5.1
Endometrium in late proliferative phase (x130).

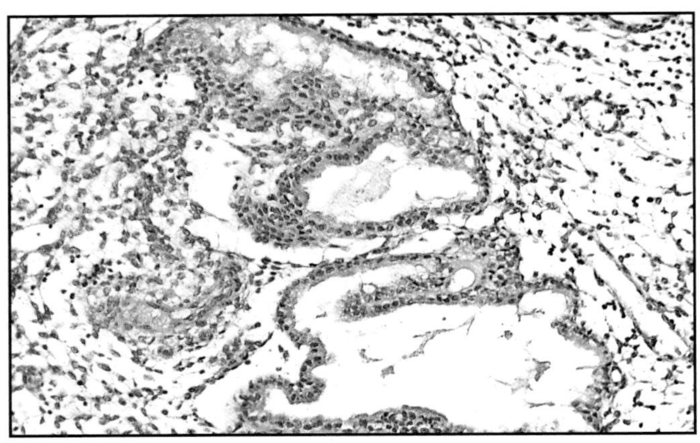

▮5.2
Endometrium in late secretory phase (x130).

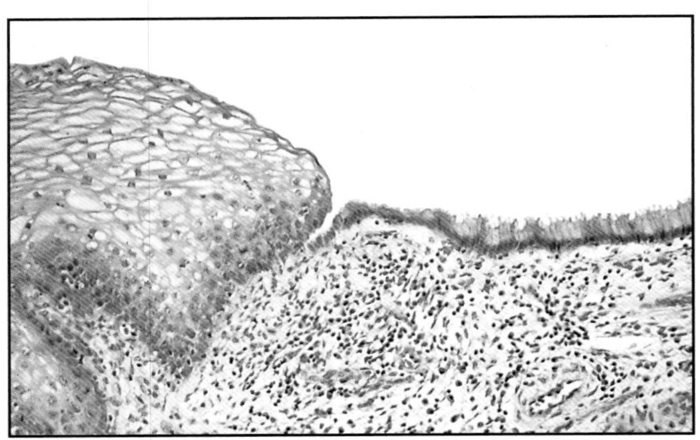

▮5.3
Squamocolumnar junction in uterine cervix (x128).

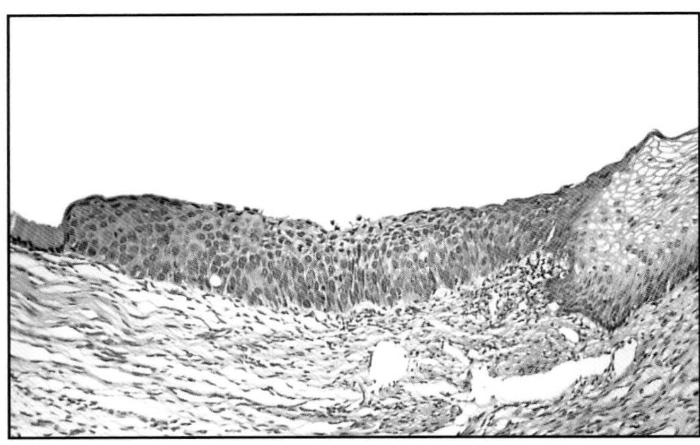

▮5.4
Early transformation zone in the uterine cervix. Note zone of immature squamous metaplasia between original (native) stratified squamous epithelium and simple columnar epithelium (x85).

REVIEW EXERCISES

1. Draw and label a line diagram of the female internal genital tract organs.

2. Draw and label a cross-sectional diagram of each internal female genital tract organ, including the major layers or coats and the type of epithelium covering or lining each organ as appropriate.

3. Briefly define the following terms:
   a) Decidual reaction
   b) Estrogen
   c) Salpinges
   d) Round ligament
   e) Squamous metaplasia
   f) Deep spinous layer
   g) Internal cervical os
   h) Luteal phase
   i) Progesterone
   j) Granular cell layer
   k) Uterine prolapse
   l) Transformation zone
   m) Ectocervix
   n) Posterior vaginal fornix
   o) Posterior cul-de-sac (pouch of Douglas)

4. Draw and label a diagram of nonkeratinizing stratified squamous epithelium. Opposite this diagram, draw an individual cell that would be representative of each principal layer.

SELECTED READINGS

Cartier R, Cartier I. *Practical Colposcopy*. 3rd ed. Paris, France: Laboratoire Cartier; 1993.

Clement PB. Anatomy and histology of the ovary. In: Kurman RJ, ed. *Blaustein's Pathology of the Female Genital Tract.* 3rd ed. New York, NY: Springer-Verlag NY Inc; 1987:438-470.

Ferenczy A. Anatomy and histology of the uterine corpus. In: Kurman RJ, ed. *Blaustein's Pathology of the Female Genital Tract.* 3rd ed. New York, NY: Springer-Verlag NY Inc; 1987:257-291.

Ferenczy A, Winkler B. Anatomy and histology of the uterine cervix. In: Kurman RJ, ed. *Blaustein's Pathology of the Female Genital Tract.* 3rd ed. New York, NY: Springer-Verlag NY Inc; 1987:141-157.

Parmley T. Embryology of the female genital tract. In: Kurman RJ, ed. *Blaustein's Pathology of the Female Genital Tract.* 3rd ed. New York, NY: Springer-Verlag NY Inc; 1987:1-14.

Sedlis A, Robboy SJ. Diseases of the vagina. In: Kurman RJ, ed. *Blaustein's Pathology of the Female Genital Tract.* 3rd ed. New York, NY: Springer-Verlag NY Inc; 1987:97-104.

Wheeler JE. Diseases of the fallopian tube. In: Kurman RJ, ed. *Blaustein's Pathology of the Female Genital Tract.* 3rd ed. New York, NY: Springer-Verlag NY Inc; 1987:409-413.

CHAPTER

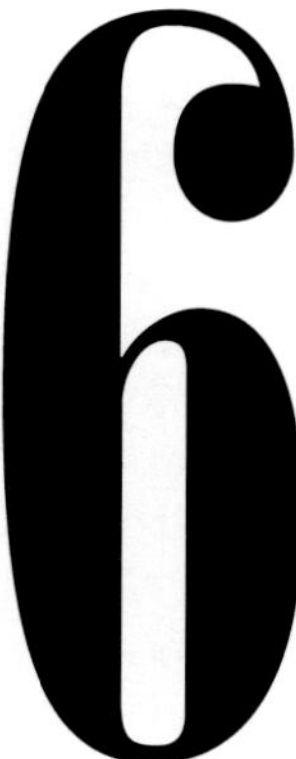

Normal Epithelial Cells

Stanley F. Patten, Jr, MD, PhD, FIAC
Alan B. P. Ng, MD, FIAC

CONTENTS

SQUAMOUS CELLS

Cells originating from the upper levels of nonkeratinizing stratified squamous epithelium constitute the most common cell types in scrape specimens from the uterine cervix and vagina. These arise from the upper levels of the intermediate or superficial spinous zone and the superficial layer (stratum corneum).

Classically, four cell types corresponding to the histologic layers of the cervicovaginal epithelium are described. These include basal cells, parabasal cells, intermediate cells, and superficial cells. However, in samples collected from intact, mature stratified squamous epithelia, so-called basal and parabasal cells probably do not originate from the deep layers of the epithelium. These cells have been related to the deeper layers of a squamous epithelium because of their resemblance to cells normally occupying these layers in histologic material. Except in those instances where partial degeneration or destruction of the mature stratified squamous epithelium has occurred, the presence of basal or parabasal-like cells in the cellular sample usually implies that immature cells lie at the surface of the epithelium of origin. Such a situation is observed before puberty and in the postmenopausal period. The identification of basal or parabasal-like cells in a cell sample obtained during a women's reproductive period of life would be suggestive of an estrogen deficiency or, more often, a benign proliferative epithelial reaction composed of relatively immature cells, such as occurs in the presence of reserve cell hyperplasia or immature squamous metaplasia. Cells derived from the latter are most often identified in samples obtained directly from the transition or transformation zone.

Superficial Squamous Cells

These cells, derived from the upper layers of the epithelium, are abundant in cell samples from the ectocervix [▮*6.1*]. In the past, they have also been referred to as cornified or karyopyknotic cells. They are senescent cells ready to be shed, are relatively large and polygonal in shape, and have a small, dense nucleus that lacks any discernible structure. Cell boundaries are usually sharply defined. The cytoplasm is thin and relatively transparent, staining eosinophilic or cyanophilic with common polychrome techniques. Because of the relative thinness of the cytoplasm, folding or rolling up of the cell is not uncommon. In addition to their size and configuration, the most significant characteristic of superficial squamous cells is the small, opaque, or translucent nucleus that is a manifestation of senescence and degeneration (pyknosis). In most cellular samples derived from the uterine cervix and/or vagina, the superficial squamous cells appear in an isolated fashion, although clumping of the cells may suggest a sheet-like arrangement.

Intermediate Squamous Cells

The cells depicted [▮*6.2*] are polygonal but vary somewhat in size, ranging between the most mature superficial cells to cells approximately half that size. The cytoplasm of the smaller polygonal cells may be relatively transparent, but is often somewhat more dense than the more mature squamous cells. The cytoplasm usually stains cyanophilic, but may be eosinophilic. Except for differences in size and staining reaction, the major distinction between the intermediate, or precornified, cell and the superficial cell is the nucleus. The nucleus is approximately two to three times the size of the superficial squamous cell nucleus and is often characterized as vesicular. The chromatin pattern is uniformly finely granular except for the presence of occasional small chromocenters and a sex chromatin mass. Particularly prominent during pregnancy are those intermediate squamous cells that have an angulated or ellipsoidal shape. Such forms are sometimes termed navicular cells because their configuration resembles that of a boat. These angulated forms are more likely to have flattened nuclei that may be displaced from the more commonly observed central position in the cell.

The relative proportion of superficial and intermediate squamous cells varies, being dependent on the phase of the menstrual cycle. Intermediate cells are present in greatest numbers during the midfollicular to late follicular phase. Superficial squamous cells are most numerous at the time of ovulation.

As a group, the superficial and intermediate squamous cells constitute the largest cells observed in routine cellular specimens from the uterine cervix. The mean cell area of normal squamous cells has been reported to be $1604 \pm 312\ \mu m^2$. The normal cell diameter would then be in the range of 40 to 50 µm. The nuclear diameter is approximately 5 to 6 µm or, in terms of nuclear area, $36 \pm 13\ \mu m^2$. The relative nuclear area of the superficial squamous cell is 2% to 3 %, whereas that for the intermediate cell is 3% to 5%.

Anucleate Squamous Cells (Squames)

These are squamous cells without nuclei [▮*6.3*]. While approximating the size and configuration of superficial and intermediate squamous cells, anucleated squames are often shrunken or wrinkled. The area formerly occupied by a nucleus may appear as a pale zone or "nuclear ghost." In addition to staining eosinophilic, the cytoplasm may stain orange, yellow, or red. Although a few isolated cells or sheets may be observed in the presence of an otherwise normal epithelium, when present in large numbers they are indicative of an excessive formation of keratin over the surface of the stratified squamous epithelium. In the absence of other epithelial abnormality, anucleated squames are most often observed in the presence of uterine descensus or prolapse. Often associated with the presence of anucleated squames are superficial squamous cells containing numerous, small discrete granules in the cytoplasm. These are keratohyaline granules, and these specialized superficial cells presumably arise from the granular cell layer of the ectocervical epithelium, possessing evidence of keratin formation.

Cells of Squamous Metaplasia

Cells referred to as parabasal, basal, or deep cells are also observed in many cell samples from the uterine cervix. As previously noted, when observed in cell specimens collected from an intact epithelium, they probably do not originate from the deep layers of the epithelium. True basal or parabasal cells may be identified in the presence of epithelial destruction or ulceration.

Cells derived from various stages of reserve cell hyperplasia and squamous metaplasia are commonly observed in cellular samples from the uterine cervix. However, their number depends on the extent of the epithelial alteration in the transformation zone and the method used to collect the sample. Because of a relatively low rate of exfoliation, in combination with their anatomic site of origin in the uterine cervix, samples collected from the posterior vaginal fornix (pool) will contain relatively few cells from squamous metaplasia.

The cytologic manifestations of reserve cell hyperplasia [▮*6.4*] are best observed in specimens obtained directly from the endocervical canal or the transformation zone. In spite of the frequency of reserve cell hyperplasia in histologic material, the cells are infrequently observed and/or recognized in routine cell samples. The so-called reserve cell in isolated form is often difficult to differentiate from a small histiocyte or stromal cell. Cells from reserve cell hyperplasia are usually observed in groups with a sheet-like arrangement. Often, sheets of reserve cells resemble a syncytium because of poorly defined cell boundaries. Cells derived from reserve cell hyperplasia are irregular or polygonal in form and are relatively small. The mean cellular area is approximately 200 μm^2. The cytoplasm is usually cyanophilic and finely vacuolated. The nuclei are small, round, or oval, and in some instances, reniform in configuration, with longitudinal grooves or folds. The mean nuclear area is 50 μm^2 with a relative nuclear area of about 25%. The chromatin pattern is usually finely granular with scattered, small chromocenters. No nucleoli are present.

Cells derived from squamous metaplasia are relatively more common in all types of cellular specimens compared with cells from reserve cell hyperplasia. Any difficulty in their recognition can be ascribed to the fact that squamous metaplasia is represented by a spectrum of histologic patterns resulting in an admixture of cells of varying maturity in the cell sample. In contrast to reserve cell hyperplasia, cells originating from squamous metaplasia tend to be isolated, only rarely occurring in small, loose sheets with well-defined cell borders. The number of squamous metaplastic cells in any particular sample will vary depending on the location and extent of the reaction in the transformation zone as well as the method of obtaining the sample.

The shape of the squamous metaplastic cell will vary from round or oval to polygonal. Those cells originating from immature squamous metaplasia [▮*6.5*] tend to be round or oval, whereas those from a more mature process assume a polygonal configuration. The mean cell area of those cells classified as immature squamous metaplasia is 318 ± 47 μm^2. Those cells derived from a mature squamous metaplasia have a mean cell area of 642 ± 54 μm^2 [▮*6.6*]. The cytoplasm of immature squamous metaplastic cells is homogeneous, frequently dense, and predominantly cyanophilic in its staining reaction. The cytoplasm of cells derived from mature squamous metaplasia may be similar to that described above. Some, however, appear to have cytoplasm divided into an outer dense zone (ectoplasm) and a relatively pale perinuclear zone (endoplasm). As the squamous metaplastic cell approaches the size and configuration of the normal intermediate squamous cell, the only distinguishing feature may be that the cell derived from a metaplastic process possesses a denser cytoplasm. Histologic foci of complete mature squamous metaplasia will give rise to cells that are indistinguishable from normal intermediate and superficial squamous cells.

When cells are forcibly removed from a focus of squamous metaplasia, cytoplasmic processes may be a prominent feature [▮*6.6*]. This configuration has no diagnostic significance except to suggest to the observer that the cells were removed from their natural setting rather than exfoliated.

Nuclei of cells originating from squamous metaplasia are generally centrally located and have a round or oval configuration. The mean nuclear area of those cells derived from immature squamous metaplasia is 51 ± 12 μm^2 compared with 51 ± 9 μm^2 for those derived from mature squamous metaplasia. However, the relative nuclear area of cells originating in immature squamous metaplasia is approximately 16% compared with 8% for those cells derived from mature squamous metaplasia. The range for the relative nuclear area of cells from squamous metaplasia has been reported as being from 4.5% to 19.5 % compared with a range of 1.5% to 7.5 % for normal superficial and intermediate squamous cells.

Like the nuclei of intermediate squamous cells, the nuclei of cells derived from squamous metaplasia possess a uniformly finely granular chromatin pattern with rare, small chromocenters. Nucleoli are not normally identified in the nuclei of these cells. Their identification may suggest their proper origin as true parabasal cells.

Atrophic Squamous Cells

Cells originating from an atrophic stratified squamous epithelium are reminiscent of those derived from immature squamous metaplasia. Because of their round or oval configuration and relatively small size, an origin from the deep or parabasal levels of the squamous mucosa is suggested. However, atrophic squamous cells are not true parabasal cells, as they originate from the surface of the atrophic epithelium. A morphologic distinction between the atrophic squamous cell and cells originating from immature squamous metaplasia may be impossible. However, in contrast with cells of squamous metaplasia, which generally present in an isolated fashion, the atrophic squamous mucosa is extremely fragile and sheets of cells may be dislodged by sampling techniques employing physical force.

ENDOCERVICAL COLUMNAR CELLS

Within the simple columnar epithelium of the endocervical canal, three cell types can be identified: the secretory cell [▮*6.7*], the ciliated cell (some consider the presence of cilia as a tubal metaplastic transformation), and the intercalated cell. The secretory cells are most frequently observed. Ciliated cells are less numerous and inconstant in their occurrence. While less commonly observed in the uterine cervix compared with the endometrium, the intercalated cells are believed to represent compressed or exhausted secretory cells. The columnar cells of the endocervical canal may be found in the fluid of the posterior vaginal fornix. However, they are more abundant in samples collected directly from the uterine cervix. Their frequency in ectocervical scrapings in part depends on the size of the transformation zone, site of the squamocolumnar junction, and shape of the cervix as well as configuration of the scraping device. When the squamocolumnar junction occurs on the ectocervix (as in the young, nulliparous woman), ectocervical scrapings may contain numerous endocervical columnar cells. When the squamocolumnar junction occurs higher in the endocervical canal (as in the older, multiparous woman), the ectocervical scraping may contain few or no endocervical columnar cells. Endocervical columnar cells are less apt to be observed in the presence of atrophic ectocervical epithelium or in association with certain benign proliferative reactions (reserve cell hyperplasia and squamous metaplasia) or abnormal proliferative reactions (squamous intraepithelial lesions, cervical intraepithelial neoplasia, dysplasia, and/or carcinoma in situ). The increasing utilization of endocervical brushing devices has had a significant effect on the numbers of endocervical columnar epithelial cells in routine cervical cell samples.

In cellular specimens, the endocervical columnar cells occur singly, in strips, in rosettes, and in sheets. The appearance and size of the cells are variable, related in part to the type of cellular sampling, the perspective from which the cell is viewed, and the configuration of the cell. The cells have a mean area of 188 ± 40 μm^2. When viewed on end, the cells appear small and polygonal in form and the sheet has a honeycomb arrangement [▮*6.8*]. When viewed from the lateral aspect, the cells possess a columnar or prismatic configuration [▮*6.7*]. These forms are more common in cells forcibly removed from their mucosal position. When spontaneously desquamated, some cells tend to assume the shape of a soap bubble. Depending on the metabolic state of the cell, the cytoplasm may be diffusely vacuolated, granular, or dominated by a single secretion vacuole. The cytoplasmic staining reaction is usually eosinophilic with the EA-65 modification of the Papanicolaou stain, but under other conditions it may be cyanophilic or indeterminate. Ciliated columnar cells have fine, delicate fibrils or cilia arranged parallel to one another and extending from what represents the free margins of the cells. The cilia are usually eosinophilic. Beneath the free margin of the cell, there may be a more intensely stained zone. In some instances, a row of tiny granules can be identified in this site. These are basal granules that serve to anchor the cilia. The presence of ciliated endocervical cells has recently been considered to be evidence of "tubal metaplasia."

Depending on the nature of the cell sample, the mean nuclear area of the endocervical columnar cell ranges from 54 ± 8 to 82 ± 12 μm^2. The nuclei are approximately one and a half to two times the nuclear size of an intermediate squamous cell. The round or oval nucleus is often indented or possesses a protrusion of the nuclear contents at one pole, referred to as the nuclear nipple. The cells are usually mononuclear. However, binucleation or multinucleation is not uncommon. The nuclear chromatin is delicately finely granular and evenly dispersed. Within the nucleus, there are usually several small chromocenters and/or eosinophilic nucleoli. The nucleus tends to appear more complex than the structure of the nucleus of the normal endometrial cell.

It may not be possible to always distinguish endocervical columnar cells from the region of the internal cervical os from endometrial cells. This is a more frequent problem with the increasing routine use of endocervical brushing devices. In the atrophic, postmenopausal woman, the cytoplasm of endocervical columnar cells tends to undergo lysis more frequently, resulting in isolated stripped or bare nuclei.

NORMAL CELLS OF THE ENDOMETRIUM

The cavity of the uterus and the glands opening into this cavity are lined by a columnar or cuboidal epithelium. This epithelium merges almost imperceptibly with the epithelium lining the cervical canal in the vicinity of the internal os. The columnar epithelium lining the uterine cavity differs from that lining the cervical canal in that it is lower and has different chemical characteristics. The mucosa of the uterine cavity, referred to as the endometrium, undergoes definite cyclic changes in response to the ovarian hormones, and is in large part desquamated at the time of menstruation. The cells shed from the endometrium include both epithelial cells [▮*6.9*, ▮*6.10*] and cells forming supportive tissue, referred to as stromal cells [▮*6.11*, ▮*6.12*]. The appearance of the normal endometrial cells is related to many factors, most important of which are the site of origin of the several different cell types of the endometrium, the stage of the menstrual cycle, the perspective from which the cells are viewed, the method used to collect the sample, and the processing technique.

Endometrial cells are observed at any time in the menstrual cycle and may be identified during the postmenopausal period. There are three types of epithelial cells: the secretory cell, the ciliated cell, and the intercalated cell. In addition, there are superficial [▮*6.11*] and deep stromal [▮*6.12*] cells. Many of these cell types respond to hormonal stimuli. The relative frequency of these cells is related to the stage of the menstrual cycle and the functional state of the epithelium. The cells are usually observed in strips or sheets. Openings may be observed in sheets of epithelial cells that correspond to the stomas of the glands. They are more closely approximated in the proliferative phase and more widely separated in the secretory phase. Depending on the perspective from which the cells are viewed, they may appear columnar, round, or oval.

The secretory, or nonciliated, cell is the most common of the cells found. During endometrial growth, this cell increases in size. The cellular outlines are often ill defined. As a result, it is difficult to accurately measure the cell size. The scanty cytoplasm is cyanophilic and finely vacuolated. The nucleus, which is round or oval, has a mean area of 41 ± 6 μm^2 when the uterine cavity is sampled directly. There is a uniformly distributed finely granular chromatin with usually one or two small chromocenters. Subnuclear vacuolization may be seen during the early secretory phase. Later, vacuolization becomes more diffuse. Cytoplasmic cyanophilia is less pronounced as secretion accumulates, and an indeterminate or slightly eosinophilic cytoplasm is observed. With accumulating secretion, the nucleus is displaced to the base of the cell and may be indented. The discharge of secretion from the cell is followed by a reduction in cell size, with associated shrinkage of the nucleus and variable evidence of degeneration.

The intercalated cells are believed to be compressed secretory cells. They are long, thin, prismatic forms, some of which have a bulbous dilatation in the vicinity of the centrally placed nucleus.

Ciliated cells are prismatic in form and may be truncated. When viewed in the proper perspective, cilia may be identified. A distinct row of anchoring granules may be present beneath the free border of the cell, occurring alone or with cilia.

The endometrial stromal cells vary in size. During early endometrial growth the cells have a mean area of 45 μm^2. There is progressive enlargement until the late secretory phase, at which time they have a mean area of 72 μm^2. This growth is more characteristic of the superficial stromal cells. They are round or irregular in form, with ill-defined cytoplasmic outlines and poorly stained indeterminate cytoplasm. Cells originating in the deep stroma are small, spindle shaped, and sometimes stellate in form. Cytoplasmic vacuolization is conspicuous in the stromal cells. The nucleus has a mean area of 46 ± 8 μm^2 and undergoes cyclic changes similar to those described for cell size. The nucleus is round, oval, or reniform. The nuclear chromatin is finely granular, becoming more coarsely granular as the proliferative phase progresses. Mitoses may occur in the stromal cells. During the secretory phase there is a peripheral condensation of the cytoplasmic matrix associated with the increased glycogen content. As a result, the cell acquires some features of an epithelial cell. These changes are characteristic of the decidual cell. With the cell block techniques, small fragments of endometrium are represented in the sample, and both epithelium and stroma can be studied. The presence of tissue fragments enables the microscopist to interpret and date the endometrium, as is done in histologic specimens.

The cells spontaneously desquamated from the endometrium into the cervical or vaginal secretion are quite different in appearance from those forcibly removed from the endometrium. As is characteristic of other cells shed into a fluid medium, the desquamated endometrial cells tend to obey the laws governing surface tension, and approach a spherical form in many instances. As a result, cells with columnar configurations are inconspicuous in the cervical or vaginal aspirates. The cervical mucus usually provides a more favorable environment for the preservation of desquamated endometrial cells than the contents of the posterior vaginal fornix. For this reason, samples obtained from the cervical canal are more apt to be satisfactory for cell evaluation than those obtained from the vagina.

Spontaneously desquamated endometrial cells may be of epithelial or stromal origin. They occur in isolated form or in aggregates. In aggregates, the cells and nuclei have a comparable size. Isolated cells are small, with a round or oval configuration. The cytoplasm is scanty and ill defined. One or more minute vacuoles may be seen in the cytoplasm, which usually stains cyanophilic or indeterminate and less often eosinophilic. The nucleus has a mean area of 37 ± 4 μm^2. The nucleus is round or oval and usually eccentric in location. Within the nucleus, the chromatinic material is finely granular and evenly distributed. One or sometimes two distinct chromocenters are observed. The chromatin may be deposited beneath the nuclear membrane. This constitutes the "chromatinic membrane" and is probably a manifestation of degeneration.

While it is usually possible to identify stromal cells, under some conditions they resemble epithelial cells. The cytoplasm of superficial stromal cells appears poorly stained, finely vacuolated, and ill defined. The nuclei are round, oval, or uniform in shape, and often eccentric. Variation in cell size may be observed. In contrast, the deep stromal cells are usually spindle shaped, and infolding of the nuclear envelope produces a longitudinal nuclear groove. The deep stromal cells are prone to be desquamated on days 6 to 10 in the normal cycle. During this period, referred to as exodus, stromal cells are frequently desquamated from the endometrium. Double-contoured masses made up of an inner core of stromal cells and an outer rim of epithelial-like cells are also observed. The latter may be superficial stromal cells or epithelial cells, which are often accompanied by neutrophils. Under normal conditions, endometrial cells are more frequently desquamated in samples collected in the first half of the menstrual cycle. For practical purposes, the desquamation of the endometrial cells during the second half of the cycle in the premenopausal woman and at any time in the postmenopausal woman should be regarded as abnormal and should be explained.

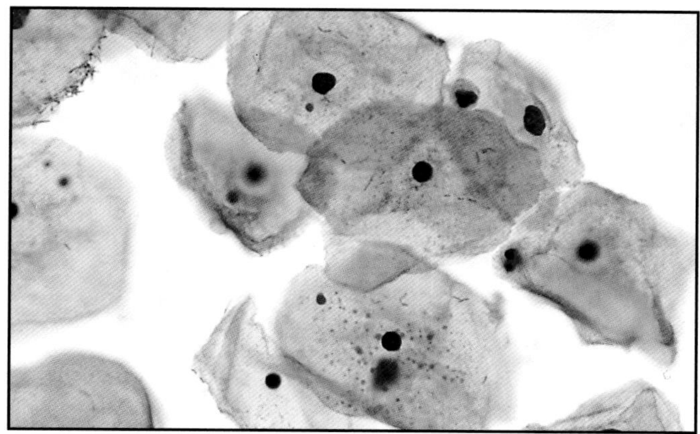

6.1
Normal superficial squamous cells. Note pyknotic nuclei (x400).

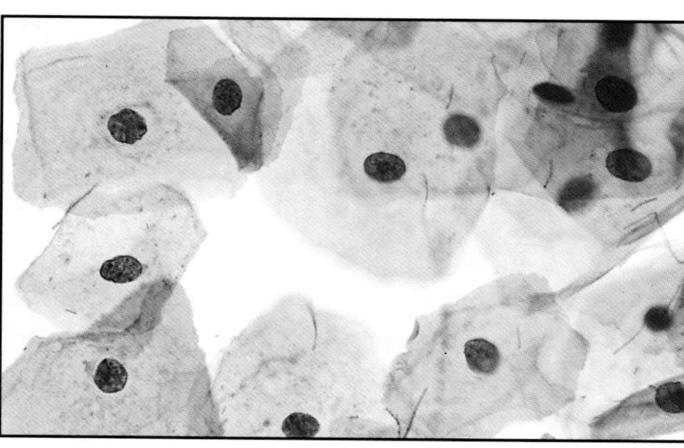

6.2
Normal intermediate squamous cells. Note vesicular nuclei (x400).

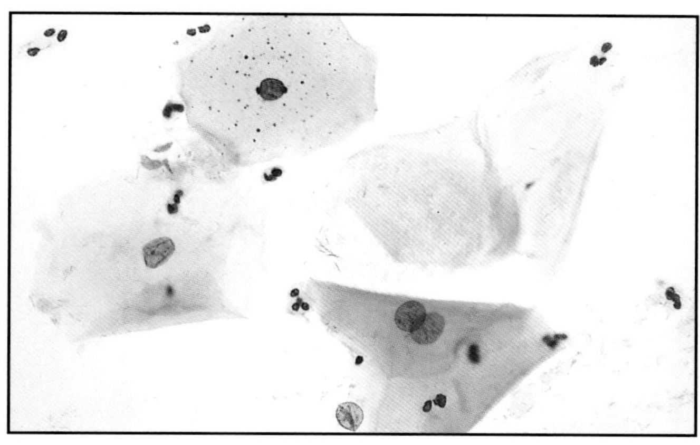

6.3
Anucleate squamous cells. Note nuclear "ghosts" (x400).

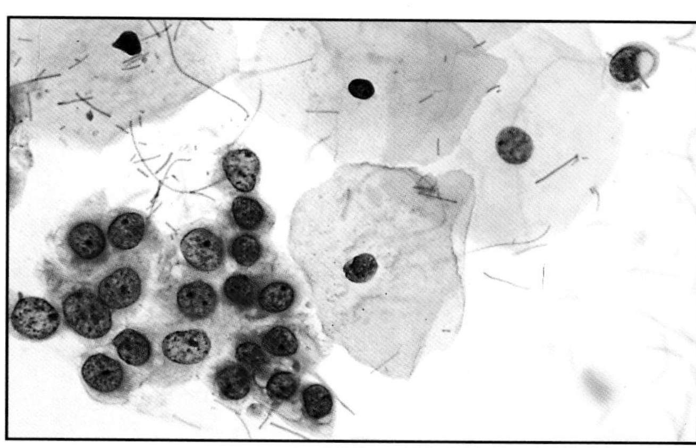

6.4
Normal superficial and intermediate squamous cells with immature (primitive) cells derived from reserve cell hyperplasia (x400).

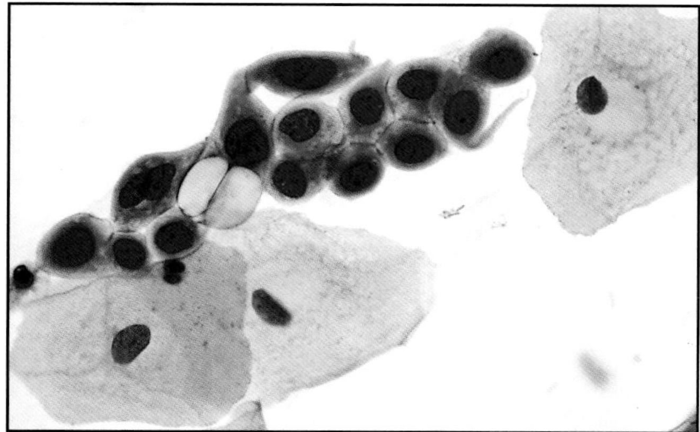

6.5
Normal intermediate squamous cells with cells derived from immature squamous metaplasia (x400).

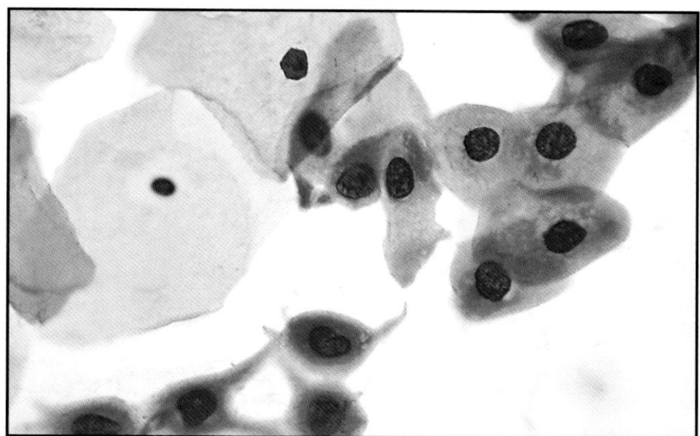

6.6
Normal superficial and intermediate squamous cells with immature cells derived from squamous metaplasia. Note cytoplasmic pseudopods (x400).

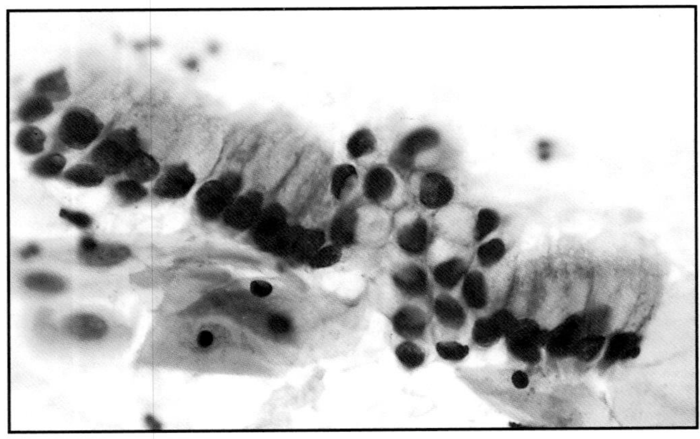

6.7
Normal glandular epithelial cells of endocervical origin in "picket fence" or side-by-side arrangement (x400).

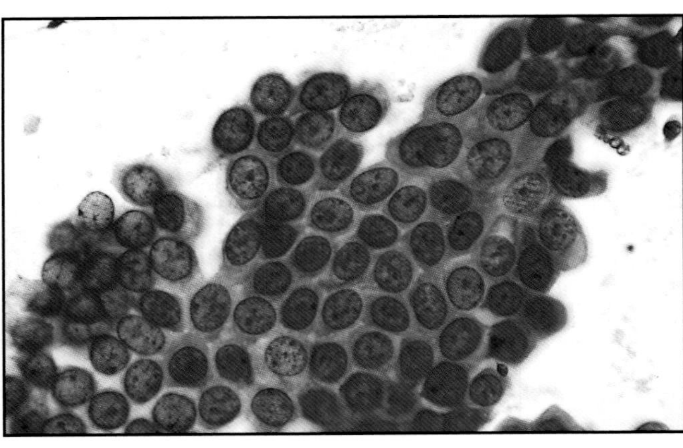

6.8
Normal glandular epithelial cells of endocervical origin in "honeycomb" pattern (x400).

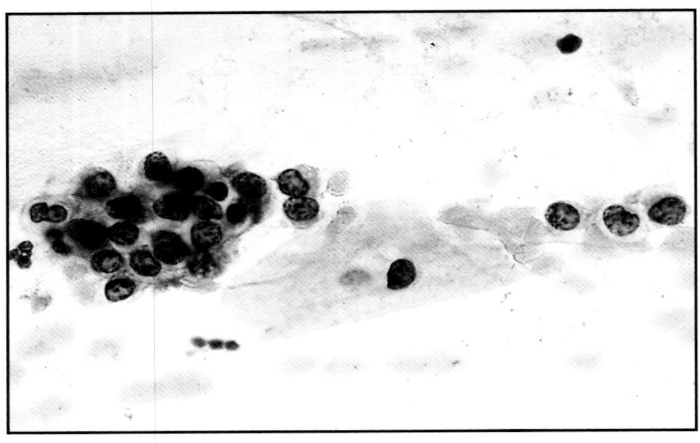

6.9
Normal glandular epithelial cells of endometrial origin, day 3 (x400).

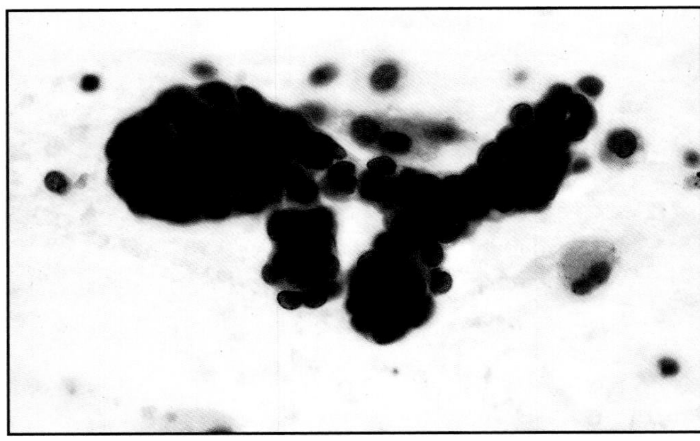

6.10
Normal glandular epithelial cells of endometrial origin arranged in a three-dimensional papillary cluster, day 6 (x400).

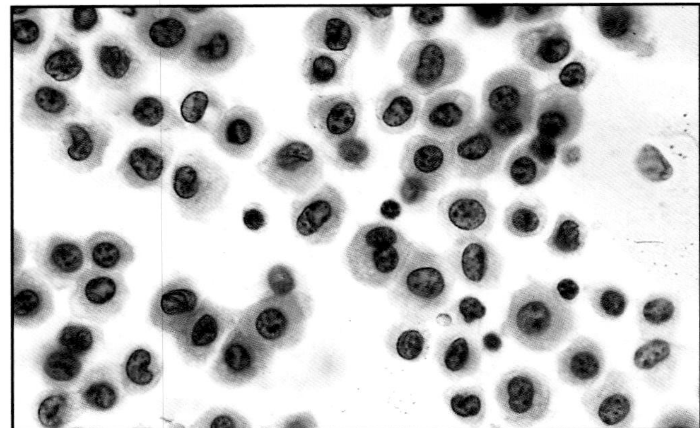

6.11
Normal superficial stromal cells of endometrial origin (x400).

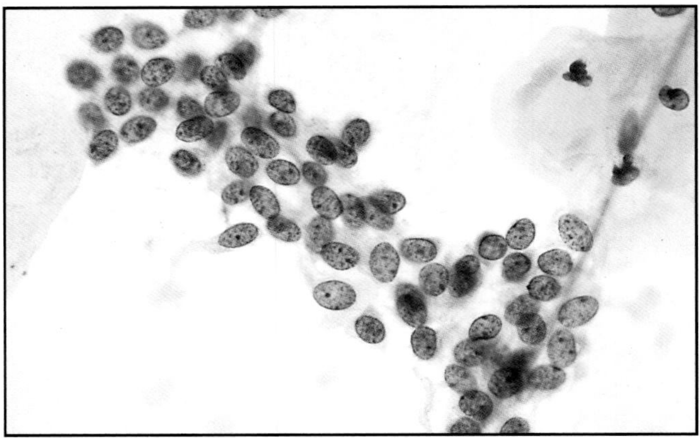

6.12
Normal deep stromal cells of endometrial origin (x400).

REVIEW EXERCISES

1. Briefly define the following terms:
   a) Relative nuclear area
   b) Parabasal cell
   c) Sheet of cells
   d) Atrophic cell
   e) Transformation zone
   f) Squamous metaplastic cell
   g) Intercalated cell
   h) Squame
   i) Cilia
   j) Luteal phase

2. List and briefly describe the cells that may arise from the normal epithelium lining the endocervical canal.

3. Define the approximate relative cytoplasmic and nuclear areas of the following cells:
   a) Superficial squamous cell
   b) Intermediate squamous cell
   c) Immature squamous metaplastic cell
   d) Mature squamous metaplastic cell
   e) Endocervical cell
   f) Endometrial cell

4. List and briefly describe the cells that may arise from the normal endometrium.

SELECTED READINGS

Koss LG. *Diagnostic Cytology.* 4th ed. Philadelphia, Pa: JB Lippincott Co; 1992:256-272.

Naib ZM. *Exfoliative Cytopathology.* 3rd ed. Boston, Mass: Little, Brown & Co; 1985:21-39.

Ng ABP. Endometrial hyperplasia and carcinoma and extrauterine cancer. In: Bibbo M, ed. *Comprehensive Cytopathology.* Philadelphia, Pa: WB Saunders Co; 1991:259-265.

Patten SF Jr. *Diagnostic Cytopathology of the Uterine Cervix.* 2nd ed. Basel, Switzerland: S Karger; 1978;3. Wied GL, ed. Monographs in Clinical Cytology.

Reagan JW, Ng ABP. *The Cells of Uterine Adenocarcinoma.* 2nd ed. Basel, Switzerland: S Karger; 1973;1. Wied GL, ed. Monographs in Clinical Cytology.

Vooijs GP. Benign proliferative reactions, intraepithelial neoplasia and invasive cancer of the uterine cervix. In: Bibbo M, ed. *Comprehensive Cytopathology.* Philadelphia, Pa: WB Saunders Co; 1991:153-167.

CHAPTER

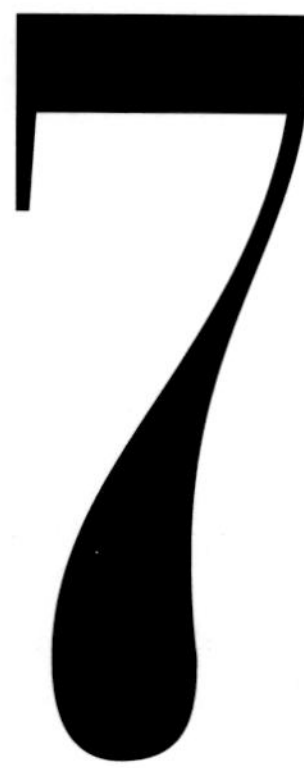

Hormonal Cytology

GEORGE L. WIED, MD, FIAC

CONTENTS

PHYSIOLOGY

The endocrinologic function of the female reproductive tract is essentially controlled by estrogens and progestogens, although other hormones such as androgens and cortisone-like hormones are also produced and influence endocrine function. These hormones are steroid hormones, as contrasted with proteohormones (such as follicle-stimulating hormone, luteinizing hormone, and several others). Steroid hormones, which can be synthesized, possess the steroid ring (cyclopentenophenanthrene-ring system) in their molecules. In the human they are produced in such glands as in the gonads and adrenals. Proteohormones are hormones produced by the anterior lobe of the pituitary, the chemical structures of which are based on protein molecules. They influence the growth and activity of the gonads and the function of other endocrines.

The proteohormones control the growth of the graafian follicles and their transformation into a corpus luteum, which produces the progestational hormone. In the human female only one graafian follicle ripens in the ovary each month and discharges its egg. There are two ovaries, but through a coordinative system of the body that is not fully understood, only one ovulation occurs each month. The process of ovulation, its contributing and resulting changes in the pituitary cycle, the urinary excretion of hormonal metabolites, and the endometrial response are demonstrated [**F** *7.1*].

During the time an egg is maturing in the graafian follicle of the ovary, the endometrium becomes thick and richly vascularized. This proliferation of the endometrium is induced largely by estrogens produced in the ovary. This portion of the cycle is usually called the proliferative or estrogenic phase of the menstrual cycle. After the egg is discharged (ie, after ovulation has occurred), the ruptured follicle changes its appearance and develops into the corpus luteum. The hormone produced in the corpus luteum is referred to as the corpus luteum hormone, and chemically is progesterone. The influence of this hormone contributes to the final maturation of the endometrium, which is then ready for implantation of the fertilized egg. The name progesterone comes from the stem word gestation (ie, carrying the embryo), since it is essential for implantation. Stimulated by the corpus luteum hormone, the endometrial glands develop secretion during this phase of the menstrual cycle, which is called the secretory or luteal phase. Usually, the corpus luteum functions for about 14 days after ovulation, generally fixing this time from the occurrence of ovulation to menstruation. The duration of the proliferative estrogenic phase of the menstrual cycle is often rather variable. Menstruation occurs normally at the end of the functional life of the corpus luteum. Menstruation-like bleeding may, however, also occur if ovulation has not taken place, such as in the case of a persisting follicle. Bleeding in such cases is the result of estrogen withdrawal related to the degenerating follicle.

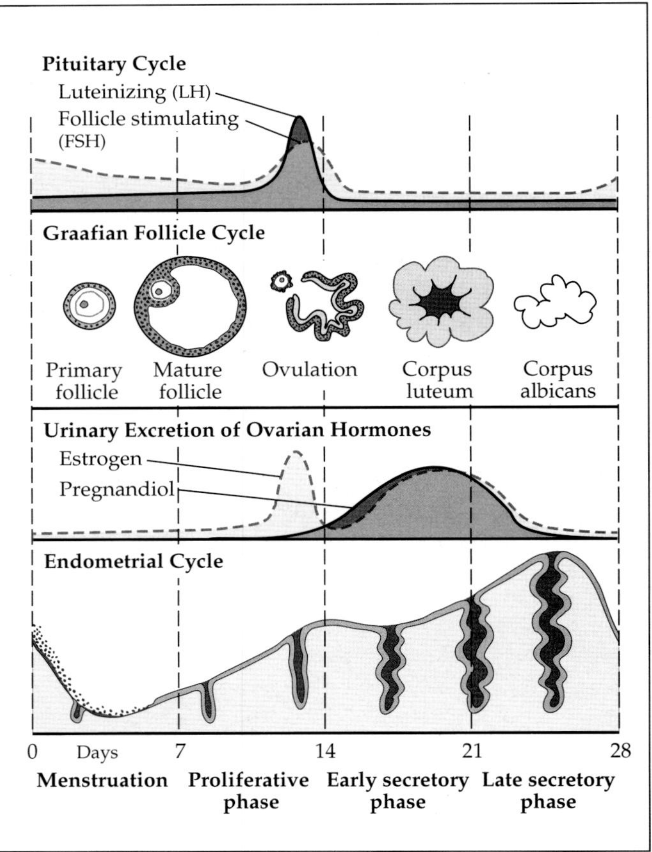

F *7.1*

The female reproductive endocrine cycle.

If implantation (pregnancy) does not occur, the cycle is repeated. If conception takes place, the corpus luteum persists (now called the corpus luteum of pregnancy) and produces estrogens and progestogens in relatively large quantities. The developing placenta takes over hormone production early in pregnancy, particularly after the third month of gestation. The sex steroids and hormones continue to be produced until a few hours or days after delivery of the child. After delivery, there is a dramatic decrease in estrogenic and progestational hormones, since the ovaries are inactive at that time and the placental production has ceased.

At this time lactation is induced by a proteohormone of the pituitary gland (prolactin). The estrogen and progestational titers usually remain low throughout the period of lactation. This occurrence of lactation can be inhibited by administering a steroid hormone (such as estrogen) that acts on the pituitary gland and prevents it from producing prolactin (which stimulates the secretion of milk in the breasts).

At the end of the reproductive years in the human female there is a reversal of the development that took place from infancy and childhood to puberty. In late childhood the ovaries (which are so far inactive) start to produce estrogens in nonovulatory cycles. At the end of the reproductive years, ovulation usually ceases first whereas some menstrual-like uterine bleeding may continue for some time as a result of nonovulatory cycles. The onset of menopause depends on racial and socioeconomic factors. Some women cease menstruating as early as their late thirties or as late as their middle or even late fifties. While atrophy of the vaginal epithelium occurs almost instantly following removal of the ovaries in laboratory animals, menopausal atrophy of the ovaries, or castration, in women does not have the same result. This leads to the assumption that steroid hormonal substances, produced namely in the adrenals, continue to stimulate epithelial growth for a certain time.

Androgens are also produced in small amounts in the ovaries, and corticosteriods (ie, cortisone-like hormones) as well as androgens are produced in the adrenal glands, which may have minor, but in some instances, clearly discernible effects on the vaginal epithelium.

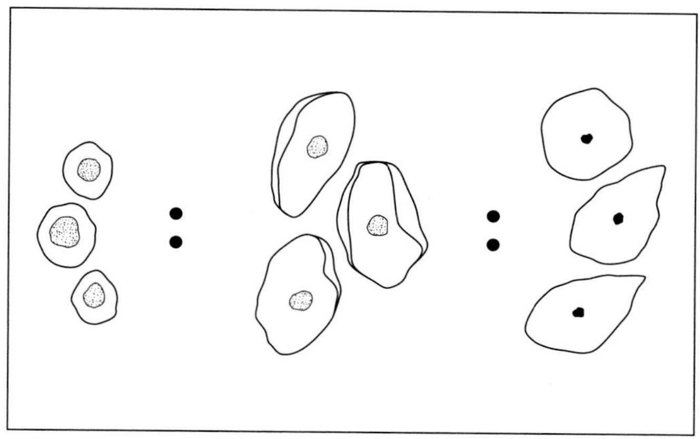

F *7.2*

The Maturation Index expresses the relationship of parabasal to intermediate to superficial squamous cells.

BASIC CYTOPHYSIOLOGIC PATTERNS IN THE VAGINAL SMEAR

There are basically three major cell types: superficial squamous cells, ie, mature squamous usually polygonal cells containing a pyknotic nucleus, regardless of the staining reaction of the cytoplasm; intermediate squamous cells, ie, mature squamous usually polygonal cells containing a clearly structured vesicular nucleus that may be either well preserved or peptolytically changed as a result of bacterial cytolysis; and parabasal cells, ie, immature squamous cells that are usually round or oval, and contain one, and rarely more than one, relatively large nucleus [**F** *7.2*]. These cells occur either well preserved or in proteolytic clusters as a result of degeneration or necrosis. (Note that previously used terms, such as cornified, precornified, navicular, or keratinized cells, have been discontinued since 1957 when the terminology was revised with the assistance of Papanicolaou.)

Squamous cells without nuclei (anucleated squames) do not normally occur in the proximal two thirds of the human vagina. If they appear in the cytologic sample, they may be due to preparation of the sample on the vulvar area or distal one third of the vagina, or due to cervical hyperkeratosis (leukoplakia).

How should cytohormonal samples be handled and reported? The first prerequisite is a vaginal sample, not a cervical or endocervical sample. The ectocervix differs in its response to hormonal stimuli from that of the vaginal epithelium, and is usually involved in transformation (eg, squamous metaplasia [**I** *7.1*], ectopias) and in inflammation, rendering hormonal evaluation impossible. A vaginal smear from the upper (ie, proximal) portion of the vagina must be examined for its usefulness to hormonal assessments. As a general rule, hormonal assessments should not be made on the following types of samples: on cell samples that were air-dried prior to fixation, on cell samples that show definite evidence of marked inflammation, and on specimens that exhibit an unusual or significant bacterial content not normally observed in this site.

After receiving a vaginal sample and determining that the sample is cytomorphologically useful for hormonal readings, the clinical information received from the gynecologist should be reviewed to obtain essential data about the patient (ie, age, menstrual history, possible medication with sex steroids, contraceptive medication, and history of any gynecologic surgery, such as hysterectomy, oophorectomy, or castration by irradiation). If these pertinent data are not available, one may safely assume that the clinician does not care for a proper cytohormonal assessment, and the cytology laboratory should not render a hormonal evaluation. An appropriate statement should be appended to the report indicating that the laboratory cannot provide a diagnostic assessment without appropriate clinical information.

The clinician should be informed as to what constitutes an adequate sample and proper clinical information. In many instances, this may be circumvented for the sake of expediency and for the reason that some cytologists may not be aware of the cytophysiology of the vagina and its endocrinologic bases. By issuing cell counts rather than hormonal readings, the responsibility for diagnostic assessment is transferred to the recipient of the report rather than to the issuer of the diagnostic findings. The recipient, in this case the gynecologist, is then expected to know what these indices mean. The clinician merely receives a "number," such as the Maturation Index, the Karyopyknotic Index, the Eosinophilic Index, the Folded Cell Index, and/or the Crowded Cell Index. Some clinicians believe that maturation equals estrogenic effect, thus disregarding the basic endocrinologic knowledge that the vaginal epithelium is practically always stimulated by multihormonal substances (ie, estrogens, androgens, progestogens, and cortisone-like agents). Nothing can be further from the truth than to believe that a Karyopyknotic Index of 50 necessarily indicates an absolutely higher estrogenic titer than a Karyopyknotic Index of 25. This misconception may go so far as to result in requests for an "estrogenic index." The most commonly used indices are shown [**F***7.2*-**F***7.6*].

It is necessary to count more than one index to properly describe the cellular pattern in the form of numbered reports. For example, a Karyopyknotic Index of 50 indicates a much more marked effect by estrogens if it is accompanied by an Eosinophilic Index of 45 (instead of an index of, say, 10), a Folded Cell Index of 10 (instead of an index of 75), and a Crowded Cell Index of 10 (instead of an index of 50). In another example, if a given degree of nuclear maturity occurs in flat, reddish, and single-lying cells, it indicates more meaningfully the probable presence of a marked estrogenic effect than if the same Karyopyknotic Index occurs in predominantly bluish, folded, and crowded cells. Either all the important cellular parameters are assessed by cell counts or the reading on a single slide is incomplete at best, senseless at worst.

How should an expert cytotechnologist report a given endocrinologic condition if indices are not the appropriate manner of diagnostic response? The optimal diagnostic reply, especially for cases that are not submitted as serial hormonal evaluations, follows: "The cytohormonal pattern *is* (*not*) compatible with the age and menstrual history of the patient because...(insert reason)."

Such a reply is diagnostically useful for the gynecologist and represents an appropriate communication between

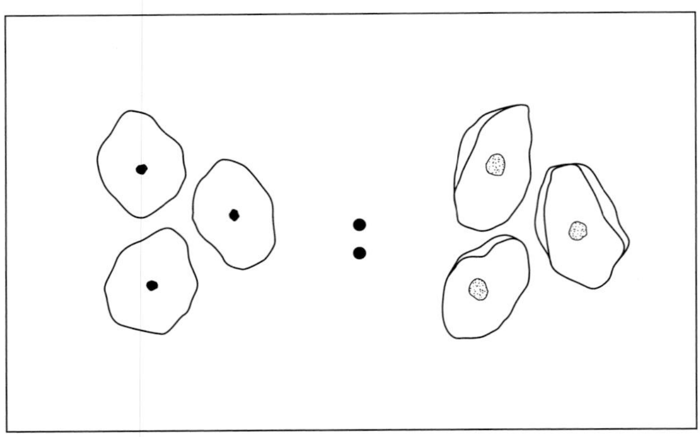

F*7.3*
The Karyopyknotic Index expresses the relationship of superficial squamous cells to mature intermediate cells.

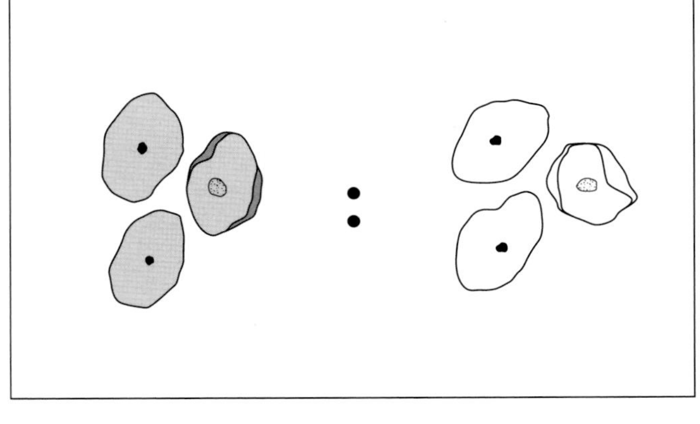

F*7.4*
The Eosinophilic Index expresses the relationship of eosinophilic mature cells to cyanophilic mature squamous cells.

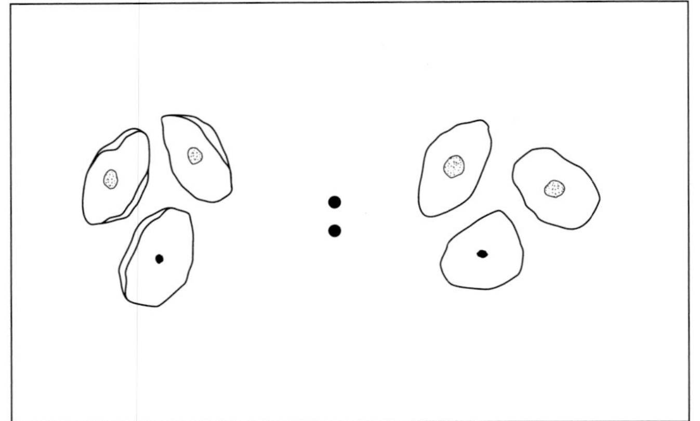

F*7.5*
The Folded Cell Index expresses the relationship of mature squamous cells with folded cellular borders to all mature squamous cells without cytoplasmic folding.

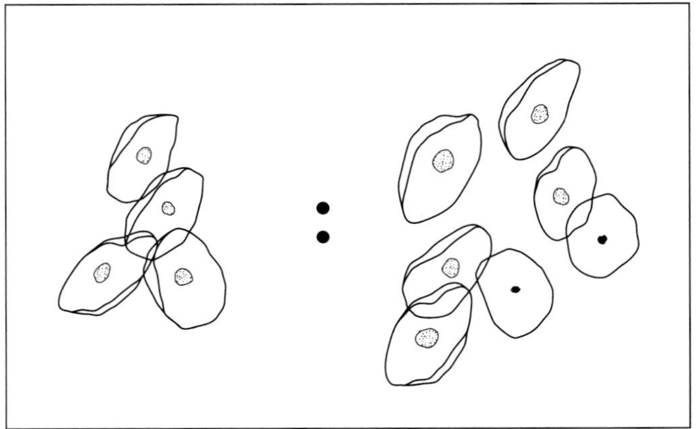

F*7.6*
The Crowded Cell Index expresses the relationship of mature cells occurring in cell clusters of four or more to mature squamous cells lying singly, as twins, or as triplets.

the laboratory and the recipient of the report. Gynecologists who routinely request cellular indices (especially those who request only one index) on primary screenings are generally unaware of the potential and limitations of cytohormonal evaluations. They usually believe that "ovulation occurs at a certain index level," or "normal pregnancy exists only up to a certain index level," or "height of maturity equals amount of estrogens as a titer," and so on. The expert cytotechnologist knows that this is nonsense and would perpetuate the practice of "magic cytology" if he or she leaves the gynecologist with this misconception.

CYTOPHYSIOLOGIC PATTERNS

Newborn

The vaginal epithelium of the newborn female usually exhibits the same pattern shown in the mother at the time of delivery. The exfoliated cells are overwhelmingly of intermediate type, some cells may be superficial squamous cells, and there are no parabasal cells. The smears are free of leukocytes and practically sterile.

Early Childhood

During the first few weeks (up to 10 weeks) of childhood, the pattern usually changes. The cells are less mature, with a significant increase in parabasal cells. An increasing number of coccoid bacteria are observed, leukocytes are more numerous, and mature squamous cells gradually disappear.

Premenarche

The cellular pattern of early childhood (namely, epithelial atrophy) may exist for several years, depending on ovarian maturation. Up to 3 or 4 years prior to the onset of menstruation the parabasal cells are gradually replaced by mature mostly intermediate squamous cells. One year prior to menarche certain cyclic changes may be observed (apparently due to nonovulatory ripening and degeneration of follicles). These premenarche phases often consist of two consecutive patterns that closely resemble the future menstrual changes, with the exception that crowding and folding of the intermediate squamous cells in the second portion of these nonovulatory phases are not as pronounced as those seen during menstrual phases.

Menstrual Cycle

The phases of the menstrual cycle (proliferative, ovulatory, secretory, and menstrual) are well documented. Essentially, they consist of increased maturation of the vaginal epithelium up to the time of ovulation (ie, about 14 days prior to the onset of the menstrual period), followed by a decrease in maturation after ovulation. The latter is demonstrated by increased numbers of intermediate squamous cells with tendency toward increased cyanophilia, folding, and cellular crowding. Bacterial cytolysis due to lactobacilli (*Bacillus vaginalis*) [▮*7.2*] may often be found in the late luteal phases of the cycle.

Pregnancy

After conception occurs there is a gradual cellular change similar to that seen in the luteal phases of the normal menstrual cycle, with the exception that the decrease in maturity takes weeks rather than days. The "ideal" luteal pattern of pregnancy (ie, exclusively cyanophilic intermediate squamous cells with marked tendency toward folding and crowding) occurs sometimes as late as the third month of pregnancy. It should be emphasized that in some instances the "classic luteal pattern" may never occur and pregnancies have been observed to go normally to term with a consistent Karyopyknotic Index of 20 or more. The important feature in these rare cases is that the cellular patterns unfluctuatingly have a rather high degree of maturity and do not change from a cell type consisting only of intermediate squamous cells to a more mature cell type. As in all cytophysiologic conditions in which there are intermediate squamous cells, bacterial cytolysis [▮*7.2*] often occurs as a result of the enzymes of Döderlein's bacillus (*B vaginalis*). The appearance of parabasal cells in vaginal smears of pregnant patients is usually a poor prognostic sign, often indicating that the fetus is either dead in utero or has been expelled.

Postpartum

The postpartum pattern is often characterized by the presence of many parabasal cells in the vaginal smear. These are related to the sudden drop in hormonal production after the placenta is expelled. The postpartum type of smear may persist for as long as lactation lasts.

Climacterium, Menopause, and Senium

The decreasing ovarian function at the end of the reproductive age of the woman expresses itself in a manner similar to the changes occurring prior to menarche, only in reverse order. In some patients, senile atrophy [▮*7.3*] occurs rather rapidly; in others, it never appears and an intermediate cell pattern may persist for the duration of the woman's life. The latter may occur in patients who underwent hysterectomy and oophorectomy during their reproductive years. One theory, which was advanced to explain the two major types of cellular patterns in the older woman, is that the subepithelial vascularization is deficient in women who exhibit senile atrophy, whereas the vascularization of the connective tissue is better maintained in those who show intermediate cell patterns. This is supported by the fact that women with epithelial atrophy who undergo estrogen therapy for a few weeks (which results in revascularization of the connective tissue) may not exhibit epithelial atrophy for months or years after cessation of the medication. This suggests that the rather weak adrenal substances that are active in every woman now have a chance to act on the stratum germinativum of the epithelium and to stimulate intermediate cell maturation.

EFFECT OF EXOGENOUS SEX STEROIDS ON THE VAGINAL EPITHELIUM

The effects of administered estrogens, androgens, and progestogens may vary greatly in accordance with the basic hormonal condition of the patient (as demonstrated by the cell sample) prior to the time of the hormonal medication.

Theoretically, the administration of estrogens will induce cellular maturity, and the administration of androgens or especially progestogens will induce increased desquamation and thus decreased maturity.

These general expectations hold true if only one hormone is involved, or under controlled laboratory conditions. These, however, are improbable situations. Because of the polyhormonal influence on the vaginal epithelium and the individual differences in end-organ response from one patient to another, no two women receiving identical amounts of exogenous sex steroids will exhibit identical cell patterns. These findings of variability of epithelial response have resulted in an overestimation by some observers of the significance of minor cell alterations seen in the cell sample, while others regard hormonal cytology in patients receiving exogenous hormonal substances as having little or no clinical value. The truth lies somewhere between these extreme views. The prior cell pattern must be known to assess the effect of the administered steroid hormones.

The effect of exogenous sex steroids depends greatly on the maturity of the epithelium at the time of administration of the hormone. The administered substance may induce cellular maturation, inhibit cellular maturation, and induce increased desquamation. Sex steroids may act synergistically or antagonistically, depending to a great extent on the endocrinologic state of the patient and the dosage and chemical structure of the substance.

Effects of Administered Estrogens

During pregnancy oral and parenteral administration of estrogen will not induce increased cellular maturity unless a hormonal imbalance exists. In the postmenopausal patient the intermediate cell type as well as the completely atrophic (parabasal) cell type will be replaced by mature cells, when the administration is of relatively short duration, eg, 3 to 6 months [▮*7.4*]. However, long-term administration will result in the occurrence of intermediate cells that may be peptolytically cytolyzed by Döderlein's bacilli [▮*7.2*]. In the event that the postmenopausal patient has exhibited a cytolytic cell pattern prior to the administration of estrogen, there may often be no increase in cellular maturity. The surface epithelium may be cytolyzed before attaining sufficient maturity to resist the cytolytogenic effect of Döderlein's bacilli (*B vaginalis*).

Effects of Administered Progestogens

During normal pregnancy, the administration of progestogens in almost any dosage will not induce cytomorphologic alterations of the "normal" intermediate cell pattern. However, if the cell pattern during pregnancy is more mature than expected, eg, a Karyopyknotic Index of 25 or more, progestogen administration may induce decreased maturity to the intermediate levels, usually a good prognostic criterion.

The administration of progestogens during the postmenopausal years induces no effect in patients for whom an intermediate cell pattern already existed. In patients whose initial cell pattern reflected senile atrophy (parabasal cell type), about 50% will demonstrate an intermediate cell pattern and the other 50% will show no reaction, probably depending on the status of the vascularization of the subepithelial tissue.

Effects of Administered Androgens

In most postmenopausal patients with an intermediate cell type, the administration of androgen causes no change in the cytomorphology. In a minority of cases there are regressive cell changes to a mixed pattern containing parabasal and intermediate squamous cells. The estrogen-stimulated epithelium is usually reduced in its degree of maturity.

In postmenopausal patients in whom epithelial atrophy (parabasal cells) exists prior to androgen administration, an admixture of intermediate squamous cells and parabasal cells results in about 40% and a uniform intermediate cell pattern occurs in another 40%. In a minority of cases (about 20%) there is no response.

CYTOLOGIC EFFECT OF CONTRACEPTIVE DRUGS

Contraceptive drugs that have cytologic effects on the squamous epithelium of the female genital tract may be considered as follows: combined (estrogen-progestogen) agents, sequential substances, long-acting oral agents, long-acting parenteral substances, continuous progestogen administration, and postcoital administration of steroid agents.

The cytologic response depends on the type of steroid administered, its absolute and relative dosage, and the variable responsiveness of the squamous epithelium to these two steroids. It is possible to find cell patterns resembling those observed at the height of cellular maturity, ie, at the time of ovulation in the untreated woman, or more closely resembling those of the late luteal phase in the untreated woman.

In addition to these two major responses, inflammatory cell patterns or, in rare cases, admixtures of parabasal cells are sometimes encountered. In the ectocervical epithelium of untreated women there may be a relative increase of metaplastic cells at the time of ovulation. The occurrence of parabasal cells in women treated with combined estrogen-progestogen drugs could be the result of a similar effect, at least in those individuals in whom the basic cell pattern is predominantly estrogenic.

The epithelial response after administration of combined estrogen-progestogen substances is varied. Observation of daily smears in several women taking the same type of medication shows a rather wide variation in epithelial response. The cytomorphologic assessment of women taking combined agents is therefore of rather limited value.

TEST ADMINISTRATION OF ESTROGENS TO RESOLVE DIFFERENTIAL DIAGNOSTIC PROBLEMS

Papanicolaou first suggested administering estrogens to patients whose vaginal smears exhibited equivocal cellular criteria. Short-term estrogen therapy was administered to induce maturation of the normal squamous epithelium without essentially affecting malignant tumor cells.

Occasionally, interpretative difficulties may be due to the inexperience of the individual evaluating the cell sample. However, there are certain cell patterns that may, even in retrospect, present diagnostic problems for the experienced interpreter [▮*7.5*-▮*7.7*]. Vaginal parabasal cells in the patient with epithelial atrophy tend to degenerate proteolytically, and the resulting autolytic cell pattern may bear certain similarities to highly degenerated tumor cells from the necrotic surface of squamous cancers. Cells exhibiting benign changes in patients with epithelial atrophy accompanied by inflammation may be misinterpreted as malignant because of certain similarities between cells deriving from reparative and inflammatory processes and those deriving from malignant lesions.

The best results can be achieved using one of the following methods:

1. Oral administration of 1 mg of diethylstilbestrol daily for 5 days with repeat smears 2 days after cessation of test therapy
2. Oral administration of 3.75 mg of conjugated estrogens (Premarin) daily in divided dosages for 5 days with repeat smears 2 days after cessation of therapy
3. Intramuscular injection of an estrogenic substance with repeat smears taken on the fourth day after the parenteral administration

A proliferation test may be requested for one of the following reasons:

1. When it is questionable whether there are merely benign, immature cells or those from a potentially malignant condition of squamous origin
2. When there is an inadequate cell sample in the postmenopausal patient, and a repeat smear would most likely yield a similar cell sample
3. When there are apparent malignant cells, the exact type and extent of which cannot be determined from the provided cell sample

Short-term administration of estrogens in patients with epithelial atrophy induces the following changes in the cell sample:

1. The background becomes "clean."
2. Superficial and intermediate squamous cells become the predominant cell types in the vaginal and ectocervical cell samples.
3. Cells apparently deriving from squamous metaplasias are often increased in number, especially in endocervical samples but also in some ectocervical samples.
4. Previously observed parabasal cells usually are not seen in repeat smears or, if present, are few in number.

After cessation of this short-term oral administration of estrogen, there is a gradual return to the atrophic cell pattern, occurring as early as 15 days and as late as 6 months.

Although the epithelial response varies from patient to patient as a result of the administration of test dosages of estrogen, there is an absence of parabasal cells and an increase in maturation of the epithelial cells in all three cell spreads (ie, vaginal, ectocervical, and endocervical samples).

There is an apparent "hormonal deafness" of malignant tumor cells to the administration of estrogenic substances. Thus, if malignant tumor cells are present, the repeat cell sample will reveal clearly defined malignant tumor cells amid abundant mature squamous epithelial cells [▮*7.8*].

After estrogen administration, the repeat cell sample may appear deceptively normal at first glance because of the abundance of normal squamous epithelial cells and the decrease in the tumor diathesis. On occasion, the malignant tumor cells may be few. It is important, therefore, to have information that this is a repeat specimen after estrogen test administration. These cell samples require diligent screening on the part of the cytotechnologist. While the estrogen test is not considered useful in the presence of lesions derived from glandular epithelium, it is helpful in ruling out the presence of a squamous cell carcinoma or dysplasia of the uterine cervix or vagina.

CONCLUSIONS

Hormonal evaluation of the female by means of exfoliative cytology should be performed only on vaginal smears taken from the lateral vaginal wall (or from the vaginal fornix). Smears prepared from the surface of the ectocervix or from the endocervix cannot be used for hormonal evaluation, since metaplasia, cervicitis, ectopia, and other conditions preclude the evaluation.

The cytologic specimens should be accompanied by pertinent clinical information, including the age of the patient, dates of last and previous menstrual periods, previous hormonal or surgical therapy, and past treatment using ionizing radiation.

Although a variety of staining techniques are useful for specific applications, the most practical and efficient staining technique for hormonal evaluation is the one designed by Papanicolaou, requiring that the specimen be fixed immediately (while still wet) in 95% ethanol or spray fixed with a commercially available cytologic fixative.

Reporting the cytohormonal interpretation should be a meaningful communication between the cytopathologist and the gynecologist. The cytopathologist should relate the cytomorphologic findings to the given clinical data and make a hormonal assessment on the basis of the received data, rather than routinely or exclusively providing the clinician with an index that is in most cases meaningless. Indices may be useful for follow-up in some cases during hormonal therapy or pregnancy, but generally a verbal communication would be more meaningful than the mere presentation of an index.

Characteristic physiologic cellular changes exist from the time of birth through the postmenopausal years. The deviations from the physiologic cell patterns may indicate the presence of pathologic conditions within the various limitations of the technique.

Cytology may also be used for assessing the efficacy of administered steroid hormones, although estrogens, androgens, and progestogens may act synergistically or antagonistically under certain conditions.

There are a number of conditions, mostly infections, metaplasias, faulty preparation of the specimens, and lack of or deficient clinical information, that render cytohormonal evaluation inaccurate. However, if these conditions are met or taken into account, and if the cytohormonal assessment is being interpreted by an experienced individual, the technique is very useful, diagnostically accurate, and an inexpensive method for the evaluation of the endocrinologic condition of the female patient.

The following are some facts concerning hormonal cytology that are often misunderstood and may render the hormonal interpretation useless unless taken into consideration:

1. The vaginal epithelium is influenced by estrogens, progestogens, and adrenal substances. It is impossible to express the degree of maturity of the epithelium in degrees of estrogenic effects or estrogen deficiencies, since more than one hormonal stimulus is involved.
2. Different patients react differently to the same dosage of steroids, whether it is estrogen, androgen, or progestogen. It is therefore impossible to tell whether a certain degree of cellular maturity found in a patient indicates the same hormonal condition as observed in another patient.
3. Surgical removal of the ovaries and uterus does not necessarily result in epithelial atrophy. In a large percentage of patients intermediate squamous cells persist. It is therefore impossible to tell whether the ovaries are inactive or whether there is a multihormonal condition associated with functioning ovaries.
4. Cell samples prepared from the lower third of the vagina and from the ectocervix or endocervix are useless for hormonal assessment. Contamination with cervical material renders specimens inadequate for hormonal assessment. Only specimens prepared from the lateral vaginal wall or from the vaginal fornix may be used.
5. There are only two cell types that can be identified with some degree of accuracy without knowing the age and menstrual history of the patient. One type is found in the specimen containing abundant flat, single-lying superficial squamous cells (indicating unequivocal estrogenic effect), and the other in the specimen containing only parabasal cells (indicating lack of maturation of the vaginal epithelium, due to a lack of steroid hormone stimulation of the stratum germinativum).
6. The gynecologist who requests an "estrogenic index" is apparently unaware of the limitations of cytology regarding hormonal assessment of the patient, because the height of maturation is not a titer of the estrogens present.
7. It is impossible to predict from an individual cell specimen whether a patient will ovulate or has recently ovulated. Similarly, it is impossible to predict the stage of the menstrual cycle from an individual specimen. This is only possible by examining serial specimens from the same patient.

8. An intermediate cell type is an intermediate cell type regardless of its size, folding, or clustering (ie, one cannot distinguish an intermediate cell of pregnancy from that observed in the late luteal phase, in secondary amenorrhea, in a surgical castrate, in a patient receiving long-term low estrogen administration, in a postmenopausal patient, or in the premenarche).
9. The laboratory that indiscriminately and routinely issues epithelial indices (such as the Karyopyknotic and the Maturation Indices) on every patient usually issues "estimograms" rather than counted indices. Few of us have the time to count 300 cells in various random selected sites on the glass slide for every cell sample.
10. A cell pattern containing superficial, intermediate, and parabasal cells usually indicates the presence of infection, metaplasia, or other factors unrelated to the hormonal condition. Therefore, a hormonal assessment should not be done on cell spreads containing all three cell types.
11. No hormonal assessment should be made without knowing the age of the patient, her menstrual history, and whether she has received exogenous hormones. Requests for hormonal assessment should be rejected if there is inadequate information, or if the sample was obtained by scraping the ectocervix.

Hormonal cytology is valuable in the assessment of the endocrinologic condition of the patient in the following cases:

1. Assessment of ovarian function in a woman who has undergone hysterectomy
2. Assessment of ovarian function in patients with menstrual disorders
3. Assessment of ovarian function in early childhood and premenarche
4. Assessment of the prognosis and guidance of therapy for pregnant women with possible hormonally imbalanced conditions and for habitual aborters
5. Determination of impending onset of the menstrual cycle in the postpartum patient
6. Diagnosis of follicular persistency
7. Assessment of the ovarian function in climacteric and postmenopausal women
8. Guidance of hormonal therapy as to duration of effect and efficiency of hormonal substances
9. Assessment of proper admixture of administered multihormonal agents
10. Diagnosis of hormone-producing tumors in children and postmenopausal women
11. Ruling out the presence of squamous cancer in the equivocal atrophic cell pattern

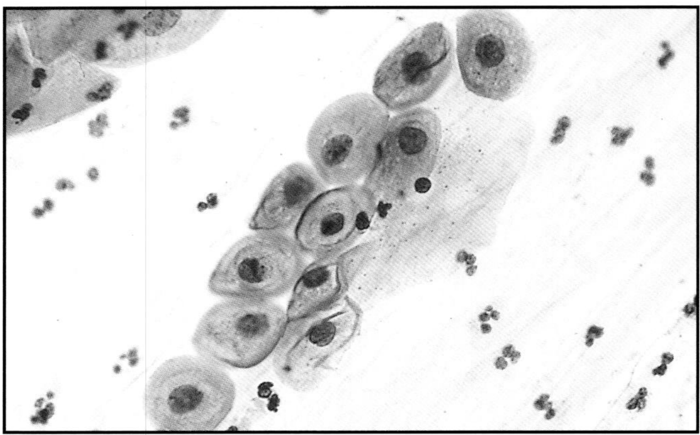

7.1
Cells deriving from a squamous metaplasia in a cervical scraping (x400).

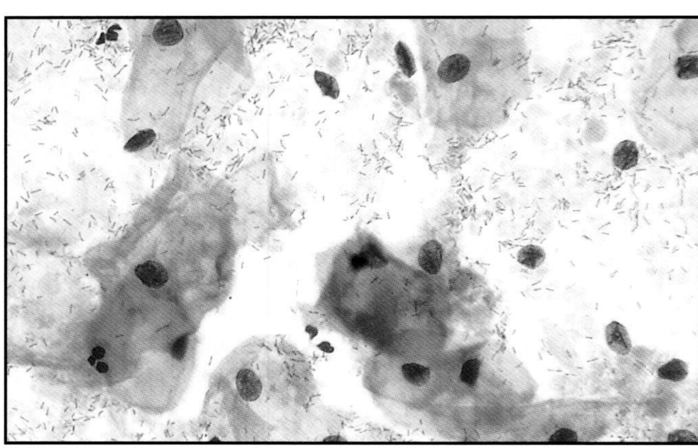

7.2
Bacterial cytolysis and intermediate cells in a smear taken from the lateral vaginal wall (x400).

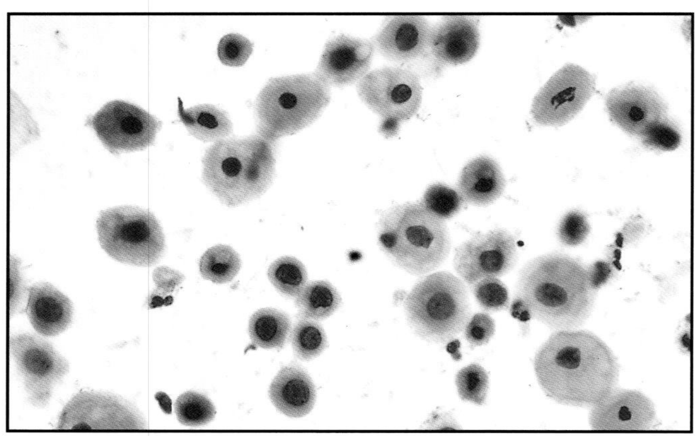

7.3
Atrophic cell pattern in a smear taken from the lateral vaginal wall (x400).

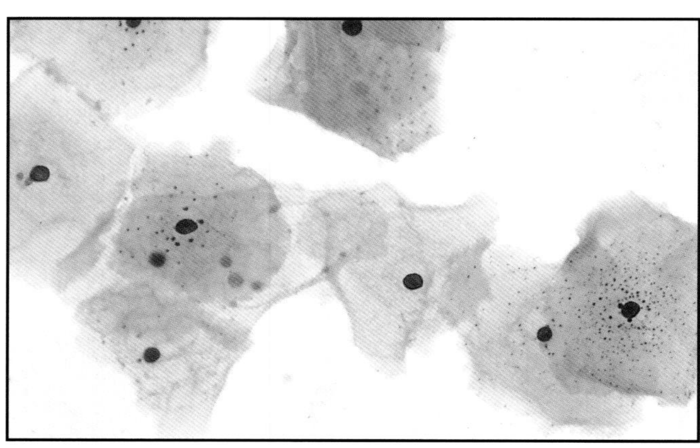

7.4
Superficial cells (estrogenic effect) in a smear taken from the lateral vaginal wall (x400).

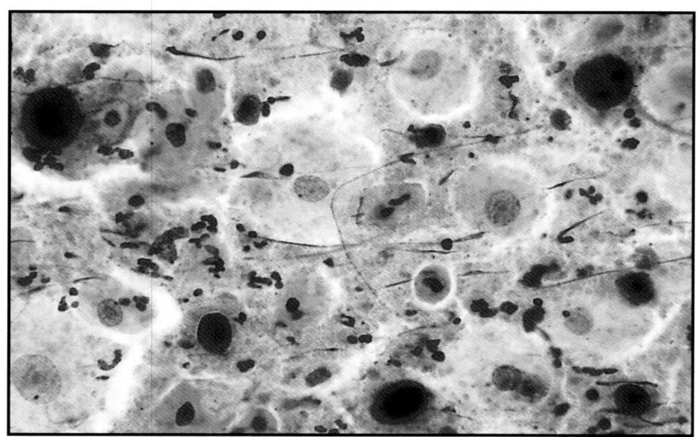

7.5
Atrophic cell pattern exhibiting inspissated mucous—so-called blue blobs—in a smear taken from the lateral vaginal wall (x400).

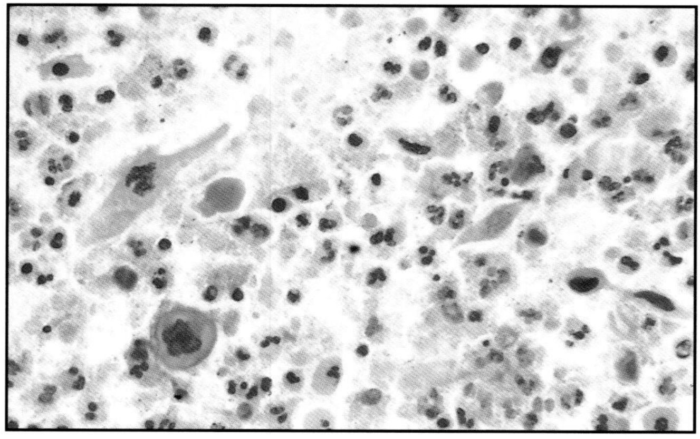

7.6
Atrophic cell pattern containing malignant tumor cells from a keratinizing squamous cancer in a smear taken from the lateral vaginal wall (x400).

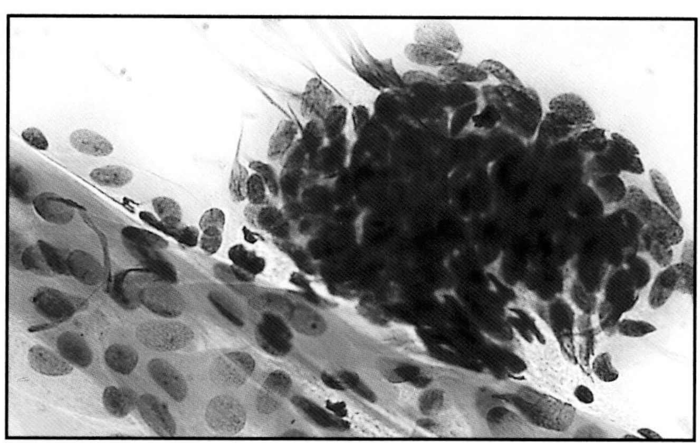

I7.7
Atrophic cell pattern containing autolyzed malignant tumor cells in a smear taken from the lateral vaginal wall (x400).

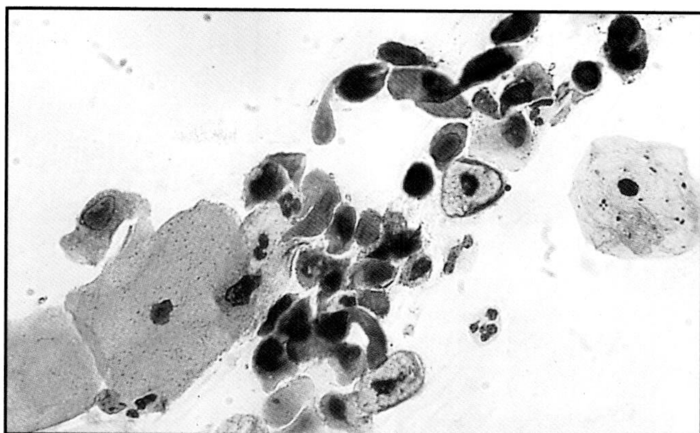

I7.8
Cell sample after proliferation test in same patient as depicted in I7.7. Biopsy revealed carcinoma in situ (x400).

REVIEW EXERCISES

1. Does the same index in two different patients indicate the same hormonal status?

2. Does surgical removal of the ovaries always result in epithelial atrophy?

3. List six conditions in which a patient may normally exhibit an intermediate cell pattern. Can one distinguish these cell patterns from one another without knowing the age and clinical history of the patient?

4. The vaginal epithelium responds to exogenous estrogen therapy in all but which physiologic condition?

5. Long-term administration of estrogens in postmenopausal years will most likely result in the occurrence of what type of cell pattern?

SELECTED READINGS

Keebler CM, Wied GL. The estrogen test: an aid in differential cytodiagnosis. *Acta Cytol.* 1974;18:482.

Papanicolaou GN, Traut HF. *Diagnosis of Uterine Cervix by the Vaginal Smear.* Cambridge, Mass: Harvard University Press; 1943.

Papanicolaou GN. Is the term "cornified cell" scientifically correct as applied to exfoliated cells from vagina and uterine cervix? *Acta Cytol.* 1958;2:28.

Soost HJ. Comparative studies on the degree of proliferation of the vaginal and ectocervical epithelium in the hormonal evaluation of a patient by means of exfoliative cytology. *Acta Cytol.* 1960;4:199.

Wied GL, Bibbo M. Evaluation of endocrinologic condition by means of exfoliative cytology. In: Gold JJ, ed. *Gynecologic Endocrinology.* New York, NY: Paul B. Hoeber; 1975.

Wied GL, Bibbo M. Evaluation of the endocrinologic condition of the patients by means of vaginal cytology. In: Wied GL, Koss LG, Reagan JW, eds. *Compendium on Diagnostic Cytology.* 3rd ed. Chicago, Ill: Tutorials of Cytology; 1974.

Wied GL, Davis ME. *Cytologic screening during pregnancy.* In: *Clinical Obstetrics and Gynecology.* New York, NY: Paul B. Hoeber; 1963:45-74.

CHAPTER

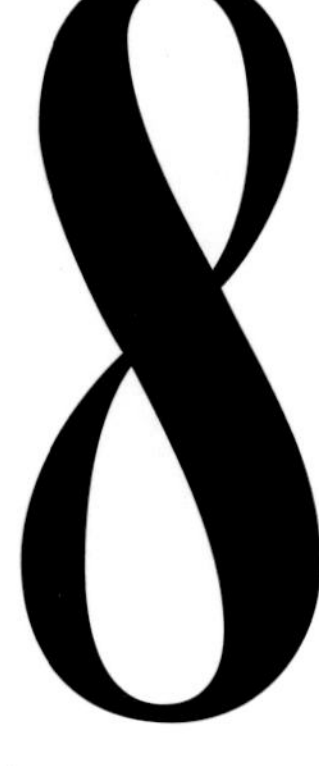

Endocrinopathies

Abraham E. Rakoff, MD, FIAC†

CONTENTS

† Deceased.

Many disorders of the endocrine glands cause alterations in the hormonal patterns seen in vaginal smears [**T**8.1]. Such changes result from the effect of endocrine disturbances on the secretion of steroid hormones that can influence the proliferation, maturation, and desquamation of the vaginal epithelium, namely, estrogens, progestins, androgens, and, to a lesser degree, the corticosteroids.

In women, these hormones are normally secreted by the ovary and the adrenal cortex. It is therefore apparent that endocrine dysfunctions arising in either of these glands will be reflected in the vaginal smear. Furthermore, since the endocrine functions of the ovary and the adrenal are controlled by the pituitary and the hypothalamus, and to some degree by the thyroid, disorders arising in these structures may also indirectly cause an alteration in the vaginal hormonal picture. In addition, since certain genetic defects of the gonads are associated with aberrations of the sex chromosomes, the sex chromatin pattern as seen in the exfoliated cells of the vaginal and buccal epithelium may also show deviations from the normal. Exfoliative hormonal cytology is therefore a simple and useful adjunctive tool in the evaluation of various gynecologic endocrinopathies.

To use this modality effectively it is essential to collect the smears from the correct sites, then properly prepare them. They must then be interpreted by a cytologist who is familiar not only with the various normal hormonal patterns, but also with the variations that may be encountered in patients with different endocrine abnormalities. In addition, the cytologist should be provided with essential clinical information about the patient, including age, date of last menstrual period, and suspected clinical diagnosis. Indeed, the method is used most effectively when the clinician and the cytologist interpret the smear together. For this

Condition	Usual Smear Types
Adrenal hyperplasia, congenital	Atrophic to atypical intermediate proliferation
Adrenogenital syndrome (hyperplasia)	Atrophic to atypical intermediate proliferation
Adrenal tumor (masculinizing)	Usually atrophic; sometimes "multihormonal" with cells from all layers
Chiari-Frommel syndrome	Markedly atrophic
Cushing's syndrome	Intermediate proliferation or atypical regressive types
Eunuchoidism, ovarian	Atrophic
Feminizing testicular syndrome	Proliferative; nuclear sex chromatin negative
Follicular cytosis	Persistently high Eosinophilic Index and Karyopyknotic Index
Gonadal dysgenesis	Atrophic; nuclear sex chromatin negative in 80%
Hirsutism, genetic	Normal cycling
Hypothalamic (psychogenic) amenorrhea	Most often atrophic to slight proliferation, but great variation from atrophic to highly proliferative
Menopausal syndrome	At first highly proliferative, some with cycling; later intermediate proliferation or atrophic
Ovarian tumors, feminizing	Proliferative, some with high Eosinophilic Index and Karyopyknotic Index, occasionally regressive
Ovarian tumors, masculinizing	Variation, many atrophic, some with atypical proliferation or multihormonal
Precocious puberty, constitutional	Proliferative, some with high Eosinophilic Index and Karyopyknotic Index, some with cycling
Pituitary hypogonadism	Atrophic to slight proliferation
Pseudocyesis	"Progestational" types, with varying regression
Stein-Leventhal syndrome	Variation; most with intermediate proliferation, occasionally highly proliferative
Uterine defect (congenital absence or irresponsiveness)	Normal cycling

T*8.1*
Vaginal Cytologic Smear Findings in Gynecologic and Related Endocrinopathies. Reprinted with permission from Clin Obstet Gynecol *(1961;4:1045), Copyright ©1961, JB Lippincott Co.*

reason many gynecologists have developed expertise in hormonal cytology and, with the help of rapid staining methods, do their own vaginal hormonal cytology in the office or clinic while the patient is still present.

DETERMINATION OF CELLULAR PATTERNS

In examining the smear for hormonal effect, the cytologist should first carefully scan the entire slide to gain an impression of the general cellular pattern. As a rule there is no need to count individual cells for a maturation or other index, except when requested or required for special purposes. If the patient is suspected of having a chromosomal aberration, a sex chromatin count is also made, using the Papanicolaou-stained preparation. If the vaginal smear is not satisfactory for this purpose, a buccal smear may be requested.

The various hormonal patterns that may be found in normal women have been described in the chapter on hormonal cytology (Chapter 7). Unusual patterns are described below in conjunction with the various endocrinopathies with which they may be associated.

It is the role of the cytopathologist and cytotechnologist to describe the pattern noted on the smear and to determine whether it is consistent with the clinical data presented. If findings suggestive of a specific endocrinopathy are noted, this possibility can be suggested to the clinician by the cytopathologist.

HORMONAL CYTOLOGIC PATTERNS IN VARIOUS ENDOCRINOPATHIES

Syndromes of Primary Amenorrhea

Primary amenorrhea is a term used to indicate that menstrual function has not started by the age of 18 years. In a high percentage of cases this condition may be due to a serious genetic defect involving the ovaries or uterus. In other instances it may result from dysfunctions or lesions involving the pituitary gland, the hypothalamus, the adrenal cortex, or the thyroid gland; or it may be the result of a systemic disease, metabolic disorder, or a psychogenic disturbance that has secondarily affected the endocrine system.

Gonadal Dysgenesis: Turner's Syndrome and Variants

In the typical Turner's syndrome the ovaries are genetically defective and are represented by streaks of connective tissue that do not contain ovarian follicles. Clinically, the condition is characterized by shortness of stature, failure of sexual maturation, and a variety of somatic defects.

The vaginal smear is of the markedly atrophic type and, in approximately 80% of the cases, the sex chromatin pattern is negative (XO karyotype). For this reason, a sex chromatin determination should be done on all smears from patients with primary amenorrhea. In cases that are sex chromatin positive the karyotypes may show mosaicism, with two or more stem lines (such as XO/XX, XO/XX/XXX). The finding of two sex chromatin, or Barr, bodies in some cells may provide a clue to mosaicism. Sex chromatin determinations may be done on vaginal as well as buccal smears. The finding of unusually large or small Barr bodies suggests the possibility of a structural abnormality, such as an isochromosome, for the large or small arms of the X, respectively. It is also important to note that in some of the sex chromatin–positive cases the karyotype may show a normal XX pattern. In such instances it is probable that one of the X or autosomal chromosomes is genetically defective.

In some patients with atypical gonadal dysgenesis, described as variants of Turner's syndrome, slight proliferation may be noted on the vaginal smear as evidenced by the presence of small intermediate type cells; these patients are usually sex chromatin positive and often exhibit mosaicism. In some instances, however, they may be sex chromatin negative with an XY or XO/XY karyotype.

Testicular Feminization Syndrome

In this condition the subject is a well-developed phenotypic female, who is really a genetic male (XY) and has testes. "She" has failed to develop as a male because of a genetic defect, in which the male-directed tissues are insensitive to androgens but responsive to the effects of estrogens, so that the breasts undergo development. There is a congenital absence of the uterus.

The smear shows a proliferative pattern consisting of large, flat intermediate and superficial type cells. It is sex chromatin negative. This type of smear is diagnostic for this condition, as this combination (good estrogen effect, sex chromatin negative) occurs in no other condition in an untreated patient. It should be noted, however, that a similar smear can be produced by estrogen therapy in a patient with gonadal dysgenesis of the XO or XY types.

Male Pseudohermaphroditism

The external genitalia of a genetic male have failed to develop properly, and because of the ambiguous genitalia the individual may be raised as a female.

The smear collected from the urogenital sinus is of the atrophic type and is sex chromatin negative.

Ovarian Eunuchoidism

The ovaries have undergone premature failure prior to puberty as a result of some destructive cause, such as infection, excessive radiation, or immune antibodies.

Pituitary Infantilism

In this condition there is failure of sexual maturation because of a deficiency of the pituitary gonadotropic hormones, which may result from a lesion in or near the pituitary or hypothalamus, or from a genetic defect in these structures.

The vaginal smear is atrophic or shows only slight proliferation. It is sex chromatin positive.

Simple Congenital Absence of Uterus

The individual is a normally developed woman in every respect except with regard to the uterus and sometimes also the vagina. These organs have failed to develop because of an embryologic defect, and therefore the individual does not menstruate even though she may ovulate.

The smear shows good proliferation and is sex chromatin positive. On smears taken at daily or nearly daily intervals a normal cyclic pattern is evident.

Congenital Adrenal Hyperplasia

This condition is due to a genetic defect of the adrenal cortex in which an excessive amount of androgen is secreted, beginning in utero. The woman is born with ambiguous external genitalia and undergoes progressive virilization.

Smears taken from the urogenital sinus show an atrophic pattern. Buccal smears, as well as the vaginal smears, are sex chromatin positive—an important fact in establishing the true sex of the infant. Smears taken later in childhood may show some degree of proliferation. If the initial smears are sex chromatin negative, they should be taken again several days later.

Syndromes of Secondary Amenorrhea

The cessation of menstrual function after a normal pattern has been established is referred to as secondary amenorrhea. This may result from a large variety of causes, some of which are physiologic, such as pregnancy or the menopause, and others, which can be attributed to interference with the normal hypothalamic-pituitary-ovarian endocrine mechanism. The latter may be due to an organic lesion in one of these structures or a functional disorder of the controlling endocrine mechanism. Functional disorders are particularly common as a cause of secondary amenorrhea during the reproductive years.

Hypothalamic Amenorrheas

This category includes amenorrheas attributable to psychogenic disturbances, physical stress, environmental changes, dieting, and obesity. These factors generally act at the hypothalamic level, inhibiting the secretion of gonadotropins with resulting anovulation and varying degrees of ovarian hypofunction.

The vaginal smears in these patients may vary widely, and are of value chiefly in indicating the degree of ovarian inhibition. In the more severe psychogenic amenorrheas the pattern may be of the atrophic type, while in the milder cases there may be a persistently good estrogenic effect; on serial smears there may be no evidence of progesteronic effect, indicating that the cycles are anovulatory. The type of pattern noted is of prognostic significance and is also helpful to the clinician in selecting the type of hormonal therapy.

For patients in whom both psychogenic and nutritional factors are involved, eg, in the syndrome of anorexia nervosa, the atrophic pattern may be particularly severe with the presence of only very small parabasal cells.

Also included in the category of hypothalamic amenorrheas are the cases of "postpill" amenorrhea. About 2% of the women who stop taking contraceptive pills may develop amenorrhea of some months' duration due to persistent partial inhibition of the gonadotropic hormones. The vaginal smear in patients with postpill amenorrhea usually shows intermediate proliferation, with small intermediate cells predominating.

When no obvious clinical cause for an atrophic smear is apparent, and the gonadotropins measured in the blood and urine are low, it becomes necessary for the clinician to rule out an organic lesion involving the pituitary or hypothalamus, such as a pituitary tumor or a craniopharyngioma.

Syndromes of Oligomenorrhea and Hirsutism

The combination of infrequent menstruation (oligomenorrhea) and excessive hair growth on face and body (hirsutism) may occur in women who are secreting increased amounts of androgen. Normally, the androgens in a woman are secreted by the adrenal cortex, but small amounts are also secreted by the ovaries. The chief androgens secreted by these glands are dehydroepiandrosterone, androstenedione, and testosterone, the last being the most potent of the androgens. In females with certain dysfunctions or tumors of the ovary or adrenal cortex these androgenic hormones may be secreted in excess. This results in inhibition of the pituitary gonadotropins, causing anovulation and oligomenorrhea, and also varying degrees of virilization, which may be evidenced by acne, hirsutism, and, in more severe cases, deepening of the voice and enlargement of the clitoris. The vaginal hormonal pattern is disturbed in all these conditions, but the pattern may vary considerably depending on the amount of androgen secreted and the ratio of androgen to estrogen. The more common syndromes of this type are discussed below.

In the Stein-Leventhal syndrome, also known as the polycystic ovary syndrome, the ovaries are enlarged, contain multiple small cysts, and secrete a moderately increased amount of androgen, as well as varying amounts of estrogen. Ovulation does not occur and thus progesterone is not secreted.

The vaginal hormonal pattern generally shows some degree of intermediate proliferation, but may vary considerably in degree. In many instances, atypical intermediate cells of the navicular type are present. Occasionally large, so-called hypertrophic parabasal cells may also be noted, while in other cases a considerable number of superficial cells can be seen. When cells from all three layers are noted in the same field, the picture is often described as a "mixed" hormonal effect.

Masculinizing tumors of the ovary occur in women with androgen-secreting ovarian tumors, such as an arrhenoblastoma, hilar cell tumor, or adrenal rest cell tumor. The vaginal smear is usually of the atrophic type.

The term adrenogenital syndrome is applied to amenorrhea and virilization of adrenal origin; it may be associated with hyperplasia of the adrenal (virilizing adrenal hyperplasia) or with a tumor of the adrenal cortex.

The vaginal hormonal cytologic pattern varies widely, depending on the amount and type of androgen secreted. In cases of mild adrenal hyperplasia a mixed hormonal pattern is often encountered. Atypical intermediate cells of the navicular type are often present as well as large parabasal cells, some of which contain considerable glycogen while others are aglycogenic. In the more severe cases, particularly those associated with adrenal tumors, the smear tends to consist chiefly of parabasal cells.

Cushing's syndrome results from increased secretion of cortisol by the adrenal cortex, either because of tumor or hyperplasia. These patients show a "buffalo" type of obesity, moon-shaped face, purple abdominal striae, secondary amenorrhea, and many other endocrine symptoms.

The vaginal smear generally shows small and large intermediate type cells, often with clustering, sometimes imitating a "progesteronic" effect.

Amenorrhea-Galactorrhea Syndromes

The concurrence of amenorrhea and a milky secretion from the nipples may occur in a number of syndromes of divergent origin, although they generally are indicative of a disturbance involving both the pituitary gonadotropins and prolactin (lactogenic hormone), and therefore point to a disturbance in the pituitary or hypothalamus.

Following childbirth, amenorrhea and galactorrhea are normally present for several months. If the mother nurses the infant the period of amenorrhea and milk secretion may be prolonged. In the early postpartum period, the smear soon becomes the atrophic type. The parabasal cells are often quite large and rich in glycogen. This is followed by a period of intermediate proliferation, which may be prolonged in the nursing mother. Gradually the normal cyclic pattern returns with the occurrence of menstruation and the return of ovulation.

When amenorrhea and galactorrhea persist for 1 year or more despite the fact that the woman is not nursing and no other cause, such as a pituitary tumor, can be found to account for the condition, it is spoken of as the Chiari-Frommel syndrome, or persistent postpartum amenorrhea and galactorrhea.

The vaginal smears from these patients show a markedly atrophic pattern that may persist for many years.

Amenorrhea and galactorrhea may occur in nonpuerperal women as the result of a pituitary tumor, usually a chromophobe adenoma, a craniopharyngioma, or another less common lesion involving this area of the brain. The term Forbes-Albright syndrome is generally applied to cases of nonpuerperal amenorrhea and galactorrhea associated with a tumor.

The vaginal smear in these cases may vary considerably. Most often the smear shows parabasal and small intermediate type cells, but occasionally there is an increase in the number of mature cells.

Women with hypogonadotropic amenorrhea and galactorrhea, for whom careful study has ruled out a lesion arising in the pituitary or brain, are classified as having del Castillo syndrome. Patients with postpill amenorrhea and a milky breast secretion are also included in this category.

The vaginal smear generally shows a preponderance of small intermediate type cells.

Pseudocyesis applies to women who develop the symptoms and many signs of pregnancy, including amenorrhea and breast secretion, on a psychogenic basis, ie, a type of conversion hysteria. From an endocrine standpoint they show evidence of a persistent corpus luteum, thus imitating the hormonal findings of early pregnancy.

The vaginal smear shows large intermediate and superficial type cells, often with folding and clumping, suggesting a "progesteronic" effect.

Syndromes of Precocious Puberty

The appearance of secondary sex characteristics during childhood, such as the development of the breasts, growth of pubic hair, and initiation of menstruation, is referred to as feminizing precocious puberty. This may result from a number of causes.

Constitutional or Idiopathic Precocious Puberty

In this condition, the hypothalamic-pituitary-ovarian mechanism begins to function at an unusually early age for no apparent reason. Ovulation, menstruation, and even pregnancy may occur in these children. Instead of the atrophic pattern of childhood, the vaginal smear shows good proliferation, and serial smears may even show a cycling pattern similar to that of the normal cycle during the reproductive years.

Lesions of the Central Nervous System

In rare instances tumors or other lesions in the region of the hypothalamus may stimulate gonadotropic function. The vaginal smear shows varying degrees of proliferation.

Feminizing Tumors of the Ovary

Estrogen-producing tumors of the ovary occurring in children, such as granulosa cell tumors, may induce pubertal changes and vaginal bleeding. In such instances, ovulation does not occur and the condition is referred to as precocious pseudopuberty. The vaginal smear shows a marked continuous proliferative or estrogenic effect, consisting of large intermediate and superficial cells with a high Karyopyknotic Index.

REVIEW EXERCISES

Indicate which of the following statements are true or false.

1. Secondary amenorrhea indicates that the patient stopped having menstrual periods after the age of 18 years.

2. In the typical Turner's syndrome the vaginal smear generally shows an atrophic pattern, and the cells are sex chromatin negative.

3. In a buccal smear showing some cells with one Barr body, some with two Barr bodies, and some with no Barr bodies, the most likely karyotype is a mosaic with an XX/XO/XY makeup.

4. In the testicular feminization syndrome the vaginal smear shows chiefly large intermediate and superficial cells. The smear is sex chromatin negative.

5. In a 1-week-old infant with ambiguous genitalia, the finding of Barr bodies in many cells on the buccal smear would be consistent with the diagnosis of congenital adrenal hyperplasia in a female.

6. In patients with secondary amenorrhea, the vaginal smear is of the atrophic pattern.

7. In women, androgens are secreted only by the adrenal cortex, while estrogens are secreted by the ovary and the adrenals.

8. A smear from the midvagina showing parabasal, intermediate, and superficial type cells in the same field can be noted in some patients with secondary amenorrhea and hirsutism.

9. Vaginal smears from patients taking combined oral contraceptives (estrogen and progesterone) generally show a high Karyopyknotic Index.

10. Proliferative patterns are found in the vaginal smears of patients with the Chiari-Frommel syndrome, anorexia nervosa, and granulosa cell tumors of the ovary.

SELECTED READINGS

deNeef J. *Clinical Endocrine Cytology.* New York, NY: Harper & Row Publishers Inc; 1965.

Frost JK. Gynecologic and obstetric cytopathology. In: Novak E, Woodruff JD, eds. *Gynecologic and Obstetric Pathology.* Philadelphia, Pa: WB Saunders Co; 1967.

Rakoff AE. Hormonal cytology in gynecology. *Clin Obstet Gynecol.* 1961;4:1045.

Rakoff AE. The vaginal cytology of gynecologic endocrinopathies. *Acta Cytol.* 1961;5:153.

Rakoff AE, Daley JG. Vaginal hormonal cytology. In: Sunderman FW, Sunderman FW Jr, eds. *Laboratory Diagnosis of Endocrine Diseases.* St. Louis, Mo: Warren H. Green Inc; 1971.

Rakoff AE, Takeda M. *Hormonal Cytology of Gynecologic Endocrinopathy.* Chicago, Ill: Tutorials of Cytology; 1974.

Wachtel E. *Exfoliative Cytology in Gynecologic Practice.* Washington, DC: Butterworth Inc; 1964.

Wied GL, Bibbo M. Evaluation of endocrinologic condition by exfoliative cytology. In: Gold JJ, ed. *Gynecologic Endocrinology.* New York, NY: Paul B. Hoeber; 1975.

CHAPTER

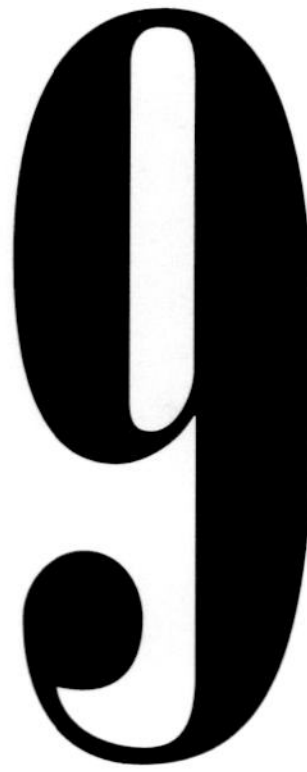

Nomenclature for Cervicovaginal Cytology

DIANE SOLOMON, MD, MIAC

CONTENTS

Terminology is an organized system or set of names. In pathology, we use diagnostic terminology as a framework for education and research, and as a vehicle for communication between the laboratory and the clinician. These different functions may or may not all be best served by one set of terms. Analysis of subtle morphologic differences and creation of multiple subgroupings of lesions may be important for investigational studies. Communication between cytologist and clinician, however, must focus on clarity and unambiguous diagnostic reporting of laboratory findings with emphasis on clinical relevance.

In addition to fulfilling different needs, terminology is not static over time; rather it evolves in parallel with increased understanding of the nature of disease and with changes in therapeutic management of patients. What follows is an overview of the evolution of terminology for cervicovaginal cytology, with special emphasis on The Bethesda System.

THE PAPANICOLAOU CLASSIFICATION

At the time large-scale cervical cytology screening was introduced in the 1950s, Papanicolaou devised a numeric system of five classes (I-V) to convey the cytologist's degree of confidence that cancer cells were present. As initially used by Papanicolaou, the numeric designations represented the following: class I, benign; class II, minor cellular abnormalities considered benign; class III, cells suspicious for but not diagnostic of cancer; class IV, cells fairly conclusive for malignancy; and class V, cells diagnostic of cancer.

As the field of cytology gained credibility and expanded as a diagnostic field, many cytopathologists advocated replacing the Papanicolaou classes with more meaningful diagnostic terms. Morphologic correlates of benign, infectious and reactive processes were described and reported. The designation "class II" proved inadequate to accommodate the diversity of benign reactive processes that were encountered in cervical specimens.

In addition, analysis of lesions identified through cervical screening programs revealed that the incidence of precancerous lesions was much greater than the projected incidence of invasive cancer. Therefore it was recognized that some lesions identified cytologically as precancerous would not necessarily progress to invasive cancer. Cytologists postulated that the key to predicting the behavior (ie, progression) of precancerous lesions lay in morphology. Cytopathologic evaluation shifted from answering the question "Is cancer present and with what degree of certainty?" to "What degree of abnormality of precursor lesion is present?"

As the concept of precursor lesions emerged, cytologists unwilling to relinquish the Papanicolaou class numbers modified the classification as originally intended, in an attempt to convert from communicating *degrees of certainty of cancer presence*, to communicating *degrees of abnormality present*. However, each laboratory created its own idiosyncratic version of the Papanicolaou classes, some including such complex subgroupings as class III A1, III A2, III B, etc. This chaotic approach to revision of the Papanicolaou classification resulted in a complete lack of consensus as to the interpretation of the specific classes I to V.

DYSPLASIA AND CARCINOMA IN SITU

Dysplasia, a term introduced first by Papanicolaou at the suggestion of Ober of the National Cancer Institute (NCI) and promulgated by Reagan, was used to designate these "less than cancer" lesions.

In this context, dysplasia was initially considered to be a lesion separate, in behavior and possibly etiology, from carcinoma in situ (CIS). As epidemiologic and other scientific evidence accumulated to support the concept of a continuum of precursor lesions, pathologists came to use mild, moderate, and severe dysplasia and CIS as terms reflecting degrees of abnormality rather than as two distinct processes. However, the artificial dichotomy between dysplasia and CIS continued to be maintained by some clinicians who placed undue confidence in the ability of the pathologist to identify specifically which lesions would progress to cervical cancer. The pathologic distinction between severe dysplasia and CIS often dictated whether hysterectomy would be performed.

Patten and colleagues meticulously studied and delineated morphologic criteria for 12 subcategories of dysplasia: three *types* of dysplasia (keratinizing, nonkeratinizing, and metaplastic), each with four *degrees* of abnormality (minimal, slight, moderate, and marked). While some claim success with reproducibility of this system, others feel that such diagnostic distinctions cannot be made with any significant level of diagnostic consistency or consensus among cytologists.

CERVICAL INTRAEPITHELIAL NEOPLASIA

Richart introduced the term *cervical intraepithelial neoplasia* (CIN) grades 1, 2, and 3 to promote the concept of a disease continuum of precursors to invasive cancer.

The morphologic criteria for the three grades of CIN are based on tissue architecture: the proportional thickness of the epithelium involved by disorderly growth and cytologic atypia. Abnormal growth restricted to the lower third of the epithelium is designated CIN 1. CIN 2 lesions involve between one third and two thirds of the epithelial lining. If more than two thirds of the epithelium demonstrate such changes, the lesion is considered CIN 3. Mild and moderate dysplasia roughly correspond to CIN 1 and CIN 2, respectively. However, CIN 3 encompasses severe dysplasia and CIS, thus eliminating this difficult and sometimes arbitrary diagnostic distinction.

Richart actually considered the grade of CIN irrelevant in determining clinical management. Rather, he emphasized that once invasion is ruled out, the size and distribution of a lesion are far more important factors in determining clinical management than is pathologic grade. Recently, Richart has proposed shifting from three grades of CIN to a two-tiered division of low-grade CIN (formerly CIN 1) and high-grade CIN (formerly CIN 2 and 3).

While the CIN classification has been widely adopted in histopathology, and to a more limited extent in cytology, some pathologists and clinicians have objected to the use of the term "neoplasia" (especially for low-grade CIN) as it is clear that not all CIN represents malignant transformation. Over time, many of these lesions either regress or fail to progress to a higher grade of abnormality.

HUMAN PAPILLOMAVIRUS AND KOILOCYTOSIS

Koilocytotic atypia, a term proposed by Koss, was recognized by Meisels to be a manifestation of genital human papillomavirus (HPV). Diagnostic features of a koilocyte include nuclear and cytoplasmic abnormalities: nuclear enlargement with hyperchromasia or nuclear pyknosis with chromatin smudging; and a well-defined perinuclear cavity associated with peripherally thickened cytoplasm.

Others, including Papanicolaou, had previously described similar morphologic changes as part of the spectrum of "atypical" or precancerous lesions, without considering these features as indicative of a distinct entity. The recognition of the association between HPV and koilocytotic atypia led to the creation of a separate diagnostic category of "HPV" or "condyloma," considered "less than" true dysplasia/CIN.

When koilocytotic changes were seen in association with "true" dysplasia or CIN, the prevailing concept was that HPV changes could be morphologically distinguished and separated. As techniques for identifying HPV have become more sensitive, HPV DNA has been found in the vast majority of cervical neoplasias studied. HPV is now considered a key link in the pathogenesis of the entire continuum of squamous precursors and cervical cancer. Scores of HPV subtypes have been identified and categorized as low-risk or high-risk types.

So-called "HPV only" or "condyloma" lesions, as a group, contain low-risk and high-risk HPV types. This same heterogeneity of viral types is also found in mild dysplasias and CIN 1 lesions. Therefore, isolation of "koilocytotic atypia" or "HPV effect" as a separate distinct entity from dysplasia/CIN may no longer be biologically valid (see "Low-Grade Squamous Intraepithelial Lesion" below).

THE BETHESDA SYSTEM

Despite the well-recognized deficiencies of the Papanicolaou classification outlined above, a survey performed in 1987 revealed that 72% of laboratories in one metropolitan area included a numerical class designation in the laboratory report. While many of these laboratories utilized descriptive diagnostic terminology in conjunction with the Papanicolaou classification, often the class number took precedence and dictated clinical management of the patient.

In addition, a proliferation of poorly defined descriptive terms such as *benign atypia, keratinizing atypia,* and *koilocytotic atypia* have been used loosely with widely varying connotations to indicate lesions demonstrating HPV and/or abnormalities "less than" dysplasia. The resulting ambiguity made it difficult to compare results from different laboratories and pathologists, and at times, jeopardized patient care.

In December 1988, the NCI sponsored a workshop to address this "diagnostic chaos" and to develop a uniform descriptive diagnostic terminology for cervicovaginal cytopathology. What emerged was not simply a listing of terms, but rather a format for reporting cervicovaginal cytologic diagnoses, which became known as The Bethesda System (TBS).

The advantages of this system can be summarized as follows: (1) TBS provides uniform diagnostic terminology to improve communication between the laboratory and the clinician, and from laboratory to laboratory; (2) the terminology is based on a current understanding of the pathogenesis and biology of cervical neoplasia; (3) the format incorporates specimen adequacy evaluation as an integral part of the report; and (4) it eliminates Papanicolaou class numbers.

Over the 2 years following the first 1988 NCI workshop, TBS became widely disseminated. However, support for TBS has not been unanimous. Individuals have provided thoughtful, critical commentary. A second meeting was convened in April 1991 to evaluate the impact, advantages, and disadvantages of TBS in actual laboratory practice. As a result of this meeting, TBS underwent emendation; the 1991 Bethesda System [**T** *9.1*] has been significantly streamlined and simplified.

TBS has three basic elements: statement of specimen adequacy, general categorization, and descriptive diagnoses.

Adequacy of the Specimen for Evaluation

A significant innovation of TBS is the inclusion of a statement of specimen adequacy as an integral part of the report. Specimens may be designated *Satisfactory, Satisfactory but limited by...*(specify), or *Unsatisfactory...*(specify). Four elements comprise the adequacy of the specimen for the detection of abnormalities of the uterine cervix:

1. Correct specimen identification is essential for evaluation. Furthermore, proper identification of the patient

Adequacy of Specimen
- Satisfactory for evaluation
- Satisfactory for evaluation but limited by...(specify reason)
- Unsatisfactory for evaluation...(specify reason)

General Categorization (optional)
- Within normal limits
- Benign cellular changes (see descriptive diagnosis)
- Epithelial cell abnormality (see descriptive diagnosis)

Descriptive Diagnoses
- Benign Cellular Changes
  - Infection
    - *Trichomonas vaginalis*
    - Fungal organisms morphologically consistent with *Candida* species
    - Predominance of coccobacilli consistent with shift in vaginal flora
    - Bacteria morphologically consistent with *Actinomyces* species
    - Cellular changes associated with herpes simplex virus
    - Other*
  - Reactive Cellular Changes Associated With
    - Inflammation (includes typical repair)
    - Atrophy with inflammation ("atrophic vaginitis")
    - Radiation
    - Intrauterine contraceptive device
    - Other
- Epithelial Cell Abnormalities
  - Squamous Cell
    - Atypical squamous cells of undetermined significance (qualify)†
    - Low-grade SIL (encompassing HPV*/mild dysplasia/CIN 1)
    - High-grade SIL (encompassing moderate and severe dysplasia, CIS/CIN 2 and CIN 3)
    - Squamous cell carcinoma
  - Glandular Cell
    - Endometrial cells, cytologically benign, in a postmenopausal woman
    - Atypical glandular cells of undetermined significance (qualify)†
    - Endocervical adenocarcinoma
    - Endometrial adenocarcinoma
    - Extrauterine adenocarcinoma
    - Adenocarcinoma, not otherwise specified
- Other Malignant Neoplasms (specify)
- Hormonal Evaluation (applies to vaginal smears only)
  - Hormonal pattern compatible with age and history
  - Hormonal pattern incompatible with age and history (specify)
  - Hormonal evaluation not possible due to...(specify)

* Cellular changes of human papillomavirus (HPV)—previously termed koilocytosis, koilocytotic atypia, or condylomatous atypia—are included in the category of low-grade squamous intraepithelial lesion (SIL).

† Atypical squamous or glandular cells of undetermined significance should be further qualified, if possible, as to whether a reactive or a premalignant/malignant process is favored.

T9.1
The 1991 Bethesda System

enhances the laboratory's ability to locate prior records and slides from the patient that may influence the current evaluation.

2. Pertinent clinical information should increase the sensitivity and reliability of the evaluation. This information may clarify otherwise uncertain cytologic findings, and it can be used to select cases for special review.
3. The cellular constituents must be interpretable for diagnostic evaluation. A variety of factors may impair or prevent such interpretation (see "Definitions and Criteria for Specimen Adequacy" below).
4. TBS defines a fully Satisfactory specimen as containing both squamous cells and endocervical or squamous metaplastic cells (see "Definitions and

Criteria for Specimen Adequacy" below). These cellular elements form the microscopic basis for the assumption that the transformation zone has been sampled. Presence of both squamous and endocervical cells does not guarantee, however, adequate sampling of the transformation zone. Conversely, an optimal specimen from a postmenopausal woman may lack endocervical cells due to limitations of patient anatomy, not poor technique. The clinician ultimately determines what is adequate sampling for an individual patient based on integrating information from clinical history, visual inspection of the cervix, and the cytopathology report.

Definitions and Criteria for Specimen Adequacy

Satisfactory for evaluation indicates that the specimen has the following: appropriate labeling and identifying information; relevant clinical information; adequate numbers of well-preserved and well-visualized squamous epithelial cells; and an adequate endocervical/transformation zone component (from patient with a cervix).

Well-preserved and well-visualized squamous epithelial cells should be spread over more than 10% of the slide surface. An adequate endocervical/transformation zone component should, as a minimum, consist of two clusters of well-preserved endocervical and/or squamous metaplastic cells, each cluster composed of a minimum of at least five appropriate cells. This definition applies to specimens from both premenopausal and postmenopausal women with a cervix, except in the situation of marked atrophy where metaplastic and endocervical cells often cannot be distinguished from parabasal cells. In cases of marked atrophic changes, the absence of an identifiable endocervical/transformation zone component does not affect the specimen adequacy categorization of a specimen otherwise determined to be *satisfactory for evaluation*.

A specimen is *satisfactory for evaluation but limited by...* if any of the following apply: lack of pertinent clinical patient information (age, date of last menstrual period as a minimum; additional information as appropriate); partially obscuring blood, inflammation, thick areas, poor fixation, air-drying artifact, contaminant, etc, which precludes interpretation of approximately 50% to 75% of the epithelial cells; or lack of an endocervical/transformation zone component as defined above.

Satisfactory for evaluation but limited by... indicates that the specimen provides useful information; however, interpretation may be compromised. A report of *Satisfactory for evaluation but limited by an absence of endocervical cells/transformation zone component* does not necessarily require a repeated smear. Patient factors, such as location of the transformation zone, age, pregnancy, and previous therapy, may limit the clinician's ability to obtain an endocervical sample. The ultimate determination of specimen adequacy rests with the clinician, who must correlate the findings described in the cytopathology report with the clinical knowledge of the individual patient.

A specimen is *unsatisfactory for evaluation...* if any of the following apply: lack of patient identification on the specimen and/or requisition; a technically unacceptable slide defined as one that is broken and cannot be repaired, or cellular material that is inadequately preserved; scant squamous epithelial component (well-preserved and well-visualized squamous epithelial cells spread over less than 10% of the slide surface); obscuring blood, inflammation, thick areas, poor fixation, air-drying artifact, contaminant, etc, which precludes interpretation of approximately 75% or more of the epithelial cells. The *unsatisfactory...* designation indicates that the specimen is unreliable for the detection of cervical epithelial abnormalities and should be repeated.

Specimen adequacy is evaluated in all cases. However, any epithelial abnormality is of paramount importance and must be reported regardless of compromised specimen adequacy. If abnormal cells are detected, the specimen is never categorized as *unsatisfactory*. Such cases may be considered *satisfactory* or *satisfactory but limited by...* based on the above outlined criteria.

General Categorization

The general categorization is provided as a clerical device to aid clinicians in prioritizing cases for review or to assist laboratories in compiling statistical information; it should not be used as a substitute for a descriptive diagnosis. Three broad diagnostic groupings are included: *Within Normal Limits*; *Benign Cellular Changes*; and *Epithelial Cell Abnormality*. If both an infectious process and an epithelial abnormality are identified, the specimen should be categorized according to the most clinically significant lesion, ie, epithelial cell abnormality.

Descriptive Diagnoses

There are four categories of descriptive diagnoses: Benign Cellular Changes, Epithelial Cell Abnormalities, Other Malignant Neoplasms, and Hormonal Evaluation.

Benign Cellular Changes

This category includes infection and reactive changes. Although the main purpose of cervicovaginal cytology screening has been the detection of cervical cancer precursors, reporting findings of infectious or reactive conditions provides valuable clinical information pertinent to patient management.

Infection includes organisms that may be identified by cytologic evaluation. To indicate that the cytopathologic diagnosis of microorganisms is neither as sensitive nor as definitive as microbiologic culture, TBS includes qualifying phrases such as organisms *morphologically consistent with* and *cellular changes associated with* [an organism]. However, with attention to diagnostic criteria, excellent specificity can be achieved for the cytopathologic diagnosis of fungal elements, *Trichomonas vaginalis*, and herpes simplex virus. *Trichomonas* and fungi are identified directly by visualization of the organism; herpes simplex virus induces characteristic nuclear changes that can be recognized. Note that HPV is not included under the category of infection but under the category of epithelial cell abnormalities.

In reactive changes, cells will manifest morphologic changes in response to a variety of traumatic insults, such as infection, inflammation, and radiation. It is important to recognize benign reactive features to avoid overinterpretation and resulting false-positive diagnoses. Cellular changes may include increase in nuclear size, increase in number and prominence of nucleoli, binucleation, cytoplasmic vacuolization, perinuclear halos (distinct from HPV-induced koilocytosis), and polychromasia. However, nuclear chromatin distribution and nuclear contours remain regular, and marked hyperchromasia is not seen.

Repair is characterized by flat, monolayer sheets of cells that may demonstrate marked nuclear changes consisting of increased nuclear size, anisonucleosis (variably sized nuclei), prominent single to multiple nucleoli, granular chromatin, and mitotic figures. Spider-like cytoplasmic projections may be seen in metaplastic cells. Reparative changes may be seen in either squamous metaplastic or columnar endocervical epithelium. Often, the changes are so extensive that it becomes very difficult to differentiate between the two types of epithelium. Three important features to note to avoid overcalling these cells are (1) preservation of nuclear polarity, which gives a streaming look to the cellular clusters; (2) cohesive monolayered sheets of cells without significant nuclear overlap; and (3) few if any single abnormal cells. Predisposing factors include severe cervicitis, cryotherapy, conization, and previous biopsy.

Epithelial Cell Abnormalities

Epithelial abnormalities are divided into those of squamous and glandular cell origin. "Atypia" has long been an overused term meaning anything from benign reactive changes to preinvasive cellular changes. Cytopathologists have equivocated on the interpretation of some cases by employing the vague term "inflammatory atypia." With such a diagnosis, clinicians have been uncertain as to appropriate follow-up. In TBS, "atypia" is *not* to be used for specimens that are interpreted as benign but demonstrate cellular changes associated with, for example, inflammation, *Trichomonas vaginalis*, or *Candida* species.

The diagnosis *atypical squamous cells of undetermined significance* is restricted to those cases in which cellular changes exceed those of benign, reactive processes, but which fall short of a definitive diagnosis of squamous intraepithelial lesion (SIL). Laboratories should strive to minimize use of this term; it is not a license for equivocation.

Atypical squamous cells of undetermined significance demonstrate nuclear enlargement approximately two to three times the size of a normal intermediate squamous cell nucleus. The nuclei may be normochromatic or slightly hyperchromatic; importantly, the chromatin remains evenly distributed and nuclear outlines are typically smooth.

Atypical squamous cells of undetermined significance encompass a variety of diagnostic dilemmas, including cases of probable marked atypical reactive/reparative changes that cytologically go beyond the range of confidence that the changes are unequivocally benign; cases in which there are features suggestive of SIL, but criteria for definitive diagnosis are lacking; and atypical cellular changes associated with atrophy. When possible, the diagnosis of atypical squamous cells of undetermined significance should be further qualified as to whether a reactive or SIL process is favored. In the context of atrophy, the cytopathologist may want to recommend a trial of estrogen followed by repeated smear to further evaluate the atypical cells. Such comments may help guide the clinician in patient management.

Hyperkeratosis, *parakeratosis*, and *dyskeratosis* are descriptors that have been used inconsistently in the past and are not included in TBS terminology. The classification of cellular changes that use these descriptors depends on the cytoplasmic and nuclear alterations present. Anucleate but otherwise unremarkable mature polygonal squamous cells ("hyperkeratosis") may indicate a benign reactive cellular change. Alternatively, inadvertent contamination of the specimen with vulvar material or skin from the fingers of the specimen collector may also yield anucleate squames. Miniature polygonal squamous cells with dense, orangeophilic or eosinophilic cytoplasm and small pyknotic nuclei ("parakeratosis") usually represents a benign reactive change and should not be considered an epithelial cell abnormality. However, cells shed singly or in three-dimensional clusters that demonstrate increased nuclear size or chromasia ("dyskeratosis" or "atypical parakeratosis") should be categorized as atypical squamous cells of undetermined significance or SIL, depending on the extent of the nuclear abnormalities.

In TBS, *low-grade SIL* and *high-grade SIL* encompass the spectrum of precursors to squamous carcinoma of the cervix. Low-grade SIL includes changes of HPV and mild dysplasia/CIN 1. High-grade SIL incorporates moderate dysplasia/CIN 2, severe dysplasia/CIN 3, and carcinoma in situ/CIN 3.

The inclusion of HPV within SIL requires the use of strict criteria for the diagnosis to avoid overdiagnosis and unnecessary treatment of women for nonspecific morphologic changes. Overdiagnosis of HPV, in part due to overinterpretation of any cytoplasmic halo as "koilocytosis" and use of "nonclassic" cytologic signs of condyloma, is a significant problem. Cells diagnostic of HPV effect demonstrate nuclear abnormalities as well as cytoplasmic perinuclear cavitation. Specimens with subtle changes that fall short of definitive SIL may be categorized as atypical squamous cells of undetermined significance suggestive of SIL.

Although occasional borderline cases of SIL occur, the majority of cases can be classified as either low- or high-grade SIL by close study of nuclear and cytoplasmic features. Low-grade SIL is characterized by nuclear enlargement at least three times the size of a normal intermediate cell nucleus. Although the nucleus is hyperchromatic, the chromatin is uniformly distributed or it may appear degenerated and smudged if associated with cellular changes of HPV. Features that favor a high-grade lesion include increased numbers of abnormal cells, higher nuclear/cytoplasmic ratios, greater irregularities in the outline of the nuclear envelope and nuclear chromatin distribution, and increased number of chromocenters.

The appearance of the cytoplasm may also assist in determining whether a borderline case is low- or high-grade SIL. Low-grade SIL changes typically involve squamous cells with "mature" intermediate/superficial type cytoplasm with polygonal borders. Cells of high-grade SIL have a more immature type of cytoplasm, either "soft"/finely vacuolated or dense/metaplastic, with rounded cell borders.

High-grade SIL also encompasses lesions previously termed "pleomorphic dysplasia," "keratinizing dysplasia," or "atypical condyloma." These lesions are composed of single cells or clusters of cells with enlarged hyperchromatic nuclei and abundant but abnormally keratinized cytoplasm. Such specimens may show variation in nuclear size (anisokaryosis) and cellular shapes (including elongate/spindle and caudate/tadpole cells). In contrast to invasive carcinoma, nucleoli and a tumor diathesis are not seen.

The rationale for the two-tier SIL terminology is based on current knowledge of the pathogenesis of cervical cancer, including inherent limitations of light-microscopic morphologic diagnosis to distinguish lesions and predict progression; the molecular virology of HPV; and the clinical behavior and management of cervical lesions.

Numerous studies have demonstrated the lack of reproducibility in subdividing SIL into four or five categories: HPV and CIN 1, 2, and 3; or HPV, slight, moderate, and severe dysplasia, and CIS. Perhaps the most difficult distinction by light microscopy is that between HPV and slight dysplasia/CIN 1.

Recent HPV molecular analyses have revealed similar heterogeneous distribution of low- and high-risk HPV types in both "HPV only" and CIN 1 lesions. By contrast, high-grade SIL shows a more homogeneous pattern of expression of high-risk HPV types, notably HPV 16.

Longitudinal studies of "HPV only" and slight dysplasia/CIN 1 lesions have shown virtually identical rates of progression to high-grade lesions. Therefore, if "HPV alone" and slight dysplasia/CIN 1 cannot be reliably distinguished morphologically, and if these lesions demonstrate similar patterns of behavior, then it is reasonable to assume that they should be managed similarly. Management of high-grade lesions is based principally on the size, location, and extent of the abnormality rather than the pathologic grade of CIN 2 or CIN 3.

However, it is emphasized that TBS is a flexible format and *does not preclude the addition of further subclassification of a lesion for those cytopathologists who wish to retain the degrees of dysplasia or grades of CIN.*

Squamous cell carcinoma, as used in TBS, indicates a probable invasive tumor with marked irregularities in chromatin distribution, prominent nucleoli, and/or a tumor diathesis. Subtypes of keratinizing, large cell nonkeratinizing, and small cell are not included in TBS lexicon; pathologists are free to append these descriptors. (Note that small cell tumors with neuroendocrine differentiation are more properly categorized under "Other Malignant Neoplasms.")

The presence of cytologically unremarkable endometrial cells in a postmenopausal patient not receiving exogenous hormones should be communicated to the clinician. Previous reference to endometrial cells "out of phase in a menstruating woman" (in the 1988 version) has been dropped for two reasons: (1) the low yield of pathologic abnormalities on work-up of these patients; and (2) increased numbers of specimens with endometrial cells "out of phase" due to inadvertent sampling of lower uterine segment epithelium by cervical brush instruments.

Atypical glandular cells of undetermined significance include glandular cells that demonstrate changes beyond those encountered in benign reactive processes; however, these changes are insufficient for a diagnosis of invasive adenocarcinoma. This diagnosis should be further qualified, if possible, to indicate whether the cells are thought to be of endocervical or endometrial origin. If the origin of the cells cannot be determined, the diagnosis of atypical glandular cells of undetermined significance is used.

Atypical endocervical cells of undetermined significance include a broad morphologic spectrum, ranging from atypical-appearing reactive processes to adenocarcinoma in situ. If possible, this diagnosis should be further qualified as to whether a reactive or a premalignant/malignant process (adenocarcinoma in situ) is favored. *Atypical endocervical cells of undetermined significance, probably reactive*, demonstrate nuclear enlargement three to five times normal and slight hyperchromasia. A honeycombed pattern with distinct cell borders is often maintained. *Atypical endocervical cells of undetermined significance, probably adenocarcinoma in situ*, are characterized by cellular strips and rosettes demonstrating elongate, overlapping nuclei with moderately coarse chromatin and hyperchromasia. In some cases it may be difficult to differentiate SIL with gland involvement from AIS. Additionally, squamous and glandular intraepithelial lesions may coexist.

Benign tubal metaplasia may also demonstrate crowded sheets of glandular cells with enlarged nuclei as well as cell fragments with nuclear palisading, mimicking some of the morphologic features of adenocarcinoma in situ. However, cellular strips and rosettes are less numerous in tubal metaplasia and the nuclear chromatin tends to be more finely granular. The most helpful criterion, however, is the presence of cilia on such cells.

Criteria for separating *atypical endometrial cells of undetermined significance* into "probably reactive" or "probably premalignant/malignant" categories are not well defined; therefore, this diagnosis is not subdivided further. Atypical endometrial cells are usually present in small clusters and show some nuclear enlargement and hyperchromasia with less cytoplasm than seen in endocervical cells.

Invasive adenocarcinoma is suggested by the presence of marked nuclear chromatin and nuclear envelope irregularities, and/or a background tumor diathesis. The type of adenocarcinoma—endocervical, endometrial, or extrauterine—should be indicated if possible.

Other Malignant Neoplasms

This category includes rare tumors such as undifferentiated small cell carcinoma, melanoma, lymphoma, and sarcoma.

Hormonal Evaluation

Hormonal evaluation communicates whether the pattern is compatible or incompatible with age and history provided.

RECOMMENDATIONS

When deemed appropriate, the cytopathologist may choose to provide a suggestion for further patient evaluation, *without stipulating a specific procedure*. In the event of a nondiagnostic specimen, the cytopathologist may recommend how a more diagnostic specimen might be obtained at the next opportunity. In general, these comments make a positive contribution to patient care and are appreciated by the majority of physicians.

SELECTED READINGS

Cecchini S, Confortini M, Bonardi L, et al. "Nonclassic" signs of cervical condyloma. *Acta Cytol.* 1990;34:781-784.

Hudson EA, Coleman DV, Brown CL. The 1988 Bethesda System for reporting cervical/vaginal cytologic diagnoses. *Acta Cytol.* 1990;34:902.

Kiviat N, Koutsky L, Critchlow C, et al. Prospective evaluation of clinical utility of reporting changes of condyloma separately from those of low-grade dysplasia. The Bethesda System Second Conference, Bethesda, Md, April 1991.

Kline TS, Solomon D. Guidelines for specimen adequacy: a plea for workable definitions. *Diagn Cytopathol.* 1991;7:1-2.

Koss LG. Dysplasia: a real concept or a misnomer? *Obstet Gynecol.* 1978;3:374-379.

Koss LG. The new Bethesda System for reporting results of smears of the uterine cervix. *JNCI.* 1990;82:988-991.

Koss LG, Durfee GR. Unusual patterns of squamous epithelium of the uterine cervix and pathologic study of koilocytotic atypia. *Ann N Y Acad Sci.* 1956;63:1245-1261.

Kurman RJ, Malkasian GD Jr, Sedlis A, Solomon D. Clinical commentary: from Papanicolaou to Bethesda. *Obstet Gynecol.* 1991;77:779-782.

Maguire NC. Current use of the Papanicolaou class system in gynecologic cytology. *Diagn Cytopathol.* 1988;4:169-176.

Malkasian GD Jr. Cytopathological interpretation and medical consultation. *JAMA.* 1989;262:942.

McGregor JA. Letter to the editors. *J Reprod Med.* 1990;35:541-542.

Meisels A, Fortin A. Condylomatous lesions of the cervix and vagina, I: cytologic patterns. *Acta Cytol.* 1976;20:505-509.

National Cancer Institute Workshop. The 1988 Bethesda System for reporting cervical/vaginal cytologic diagnoses. *JAMA.* 1989;262:931-934.

National Institutes of Health. Report of the 1991 Bethesda Workshop. *JAMA.* 1992;267:1892.

Papanicolaou GN. A survey of the actualities and potentialities of exfoliative cytology in cancer diagnosis. *Ann Intern Med.* 1949;31:661-674.

Papanicolaou GN. *Atlas of Exfoliative Cytology.* Cambridge, Mass: Harvard University Press; 1954.

Patten SF Jr. *Diagnostic Cytology of the Uterine Cervix.* 2nd ed. Basel, Switzerland: S Karger; 1978.

Reagan JW. Presidential address. *Acta Cytol.* 1965;9:265-267.

Reagan JW, Seidemann IL, Saracusa Y. The cellular morphology of carcinoma *in situ* and dysplasia or atypical hyperplasia of the uterine cervix. *Cancer.* 1953;6:224-235.

Richart RM. Cervical intraepithelial neoplasia. *Pathol Annu.* 1973;3:301-328.

Richart RM. A modified terminology for cervical intraepithelial neoplasia. *Obstet Gynecol.* 1990;75:131-133.

Richart RM. Natural history of cervical intraepithelial neoplasia. *Clin Obstet Gynecol.* 1968;5:748.

Sherman ME, Schiffman MH, Kurman RJ, Erozan YS, Wacholder S. The Bethesda System: interobserver reproducibility of cytopathologic diagnoses. The Bethesda System Second Conference, Bethesda, Md, April 1991.

Soloway HB, Belliveau RR. The Bethesda Classification System: a counterintuitive approach to data presentation. *Hum Pathol.* 1991;22:401-402.

Stoler MH. Correlations of HPV gene expression with The Bethesda Classification of low grade squamous intraepithelial lesions. The Bethesda System Second Conference, Bethesda, Md, April 1991.

Vooijs GP. Does the Bethesda System promote or endanger the quality of cervical cytology? *Acta Cytol.* 1990;34:455-456.

Willett GD, Kurman RJ, Reid R, Greenberg M, Jenson AB, Lorincz AT. Correlation of the histologic appearance of intraepithelial neoplasia of the cervix with human papillomavirus types. *Int J Gynecol Pathol.* 1989;8:18-25.

CHAPTER 10

Inflammation

Marluce Bibbo, MD, ScD, FIAC
George L. Wied, MD, FIAC

CONTENTS

MICROBIOLOGIC CLASSIFICATION

The microbiologic classification performed on cytologic samples, although not as accurate as that performed on bacteriologic cultures, can provide the clinician with valuable information [**T** *10.1*]. In assessing the vaginal flora, the adequacy of the cellular sample should also be evaluated. Only vaginal smears prepared from secretions obtained from the fornix or the lateral or posterior portion of the vagina are suitable for microbiologic classification. Another important factor in diagnostic accuracy is the microscopic magnification used for viewing. The x40 high dry objective is recommended for the discrimination of the various microorganisms.

Döderlein's bacilli, which encompass a heterogeneous group of bacilli, are normal constituents of the vaginal flora. To demonstrate the heterogeneity of these bacilli, Miravete isolated 71 strains of *Lactobacillus* from acid vaginal secretions and found that 69% were *L acidophilus*, the only species capable of hydrolyzing glycogen.

Enzymes of Döderlein's bacilli may cause cell destruction. This bacterial cytolysis begins with destruction of the cytoplasm. The smears become crowded with cellular debris, free nuclei, and Döderlein's bacilli [**I** *10.1*]. This type of cytolysis may be inhibited by intravaginal administration of bacteriostatic agents or by douching with distilled water. Bacterial cytolysis is limited to intermediate cells. Superficial cells are not cytolyzed because they are resistant to the cytolytic effects of Döderlein's bacilli. Parabasal cells usually occur in hormonal conditions in which few or no Döderlein's bacilli are present.

The category of mixed bacteria comprises mixtures of rods and/or cocci, which can only be properly identified by culture. In asymptomatic adults, mixed bacteria are a normal finding.

Coccoid bacteria are frequently observed either exclusively or in the presence of trichomonads and/or leptothrix. A change in the staining reaction of the cells (pseudoeosinophilia) and a slight relative increase in nuclear pyknosis (pseudopyknosis) frequently accompany the presence of coccoid bacteria and often preclude hormonal evaluation of smears.

Careful microscopic examination may reveal clusters of pairs or individual pairs of bean-shaped cocci in the cytoplasm of polymorphonuclear leukocytes. This finding in itself is not diagnostic of gonorrhea. It does, however, warrant follow-up studies with Gram's stain and culture and may be a useful observation for the clinician.

Micrococcus species include a large number of coccoid organisms that may cause vaginitis. One of these, *Staphylococcus aureus*, may cause the toxic shock syndrome. *Gardnerella vaginalis* may cause vaginitis and may be identified in the cell sample when "clue" cells are found. Studies have shown that when these cells are found in cytologic smears, *G vaginalis* may be confirmed by culture in over 87% of the cases. The Papanicolaou-stained smears of patients with *G vaginalis* generally show a few pus cells, a

Döderlein's bacilli
 With cytolysis
 Without cytolysis
Mixed bacteria
Cocci or coccoid bacteria
Gardnerella vaginalis
Leptothrix
Actinomyces
***Chlamydia* species**
Trichomonads
Fungi
Viruses
Other microorganisms (rare findings, eg, pinworm and ameba)
No microbiologic classification possible (scanty material

* The prevalence figures of these microorganisms are as variable as the population groups screened.

T *10.1*
*Microbiologic Classification Used at the University of Chicago**

lack of lactobacilli, a background of many small rods, an "clue" cells [**I** *10.2*].

"Clue" cells are epithelial cells covered with adhere small bacilli that are uniformly spaced and grain appearing. Some of the cells are only partially covered b adherent bacilli. Characteristic clumps of small rods in th background are of additional diagnostic value. Som nonspecific inflammatory changes have been note Although occasionally bacterial organisms, such as dipl theroids, and cocci will adhere to epithelial cells an mimic the clue cells of *G vaginalis*, their distinction generally not difficult.

Leptothrix (actinomycetes) vary in number and siz They are thin, gray, segmented, hairlike structures th may branch but do not form spores [**I** *10.3*]. In Pap smear actinomycetes occur as filamentous branching structures i irregular, spidery bodies of various sizes. Filaments radia from a central, dark, dense core and branch at acute angl in typical sulfur granules that usually are surrounded b inflammatory cells and histiocytes [**I** *10.4*].

Actinomycetic organisms have been described wit increased frequency in patients in whom intrauterin devices (IUDs) have been implanted. Actinomycetes occu in association with many different kinds of IUDs o pessaries; the organisms are more frequently commens than pathogenic. However, they do have the ability t become invasive, and pelvic actinomycotic infections hav been reported.

The chlamydial organisms cause trachoma, psittacosi and lymphogranuloma venereum, as well as venereall transmitted genital tract infections and inclusion conjun tivitis. These organisms have been called by a number c different names, including *Bedsonia*, *Miyagawanella*, an trachoma inclusion conjunctivitis (TRIC) agents. For man years they were classified as viruses. Now it is clear that they are, indeed, bacteria. However, because of their peculiar life cycle, they have been placed in their own order, which consists of one genus, *Chlamydia*, with two species, *C psittaci* and *C trachomatis*.

The life cycle of chlamydial organisms begins when small elementary bodies infect a host cell by inducing active phagocytosis. During the next 8 hours, these small bodies reorganize into larger, reticulated initial bodies, which then divert the cell's synthesizing functions to their own metabolic needs and begin to multiply by binary fission. About 24 hours after infection, these larger organisms begin reorganizing into infective elementary bodies. At about 30 hours, multiplication ceases, and by 35 to 40 hours, the disrupted host cell dies, releasing new elementary bodies that can infect other host cells and thus continue the cycle.

Within the female genital tract, the anatomic site most commonly infected is the cervix. Chlamydial organisms can cause cervicitis but need not cause disease. They appear to be a specific parasite of squamocolumnar cells, and thus they grow only within the transitional zone and the endocervix.

Chlamydia-infected cells show intracytoplasmic changes. Initially, *Chlamydia* particles occur as fine, acidophilic coccoid bodies. This stage is followed by localization, condensation, and transformation of these particles into fine vacuoles and larger inclusions. These inclusions tend to be cyanophilic or basophilic. *Chlamydia* inclusions generally reveal uniform size, molding, distinct outlines, central condensation (target formation), and perinuclear distribution and should be distinguished from other degenerative vacuoles, secretions, and fluid accumulation in the cells [▮*10.5*].

Chlamydia-infected cells are often classified as atypical. They occur singly or in small groups of cells, with distinct outlines. Columnar and metaplastic cells usually are involved. The nuclei of the *Chlamydia*-infected cells are enlarged and hyperchromatic with uniformly distributed chromatin, which suggests increased growth activity or repair process. Nucleoli are rare and inconspicuous. The cellular changes suggestive of *Chlamydia* infection are subject to confirmatory studies.

Trichomonas vaginalis may be diagnosed in Papanicolaou-stained smears by its small pear-shaped form, faint gray- or pink-staining reaction, small oval eccentric hypochromatic nucleus, and eosinophilia of the cytoplasm of parabasal cells in the cytologic sample [▮*10.6*]. Trichomoniasis is usually associated with coccoid bacteria and leptothrix, and rarely with fungi. Trichomonads usually induce inflammatory changes, but occasionally may be found without any host reaction. Trichomonads are frequently misdiagnosed in cytologic specimens. The flagellae are lost during fixation and staining, leading to false-negative readings for trichomonads. Conversely, degenerated leukocytes, cellular fragments, parabasal cells with karyolysis, and granulated mucus on atrophic smears may be the cause of erroneous diagnoses of trichomonads.

The great majority of mycotic vulvovaginitis is due to *Candida albicans*, although *Candida glabrata*, *Geotrichum candidum*, and other species of fungi can also cause inflammation of the female reproductive tract [▮*10.7*].

Specific identification of fungi is not possible from the cytologic smear. The presence of yeast cells, budding yeast cells, pseudomycelium, or mycelial elements can be reported, and sometimes this may be enough for a presumptive diagnosis of fungal infection.

In true mycelial formation, the protoplasm is continuous between the main stem and the branches. *Candida* organisms are yeast and reproduce by budding. The buds elongate and form pseudomycelia. *Geotrichum* reproduces by forming true mycelia and spores (arthrospores). The presence of encapsulated yeast in a smear may indicate the presence of *C glabrata*.

Herpes simplex, herpes zoster, aberrant vaccinia, cytomegalovirus, adenovirus, condyloma acumination, verruca vulgaris, and molluscum contagiosum may induce cell changes. These changes are primarily due to the intracellular location of viruses.

Well-established cytologic changes are present in herpesvirus infection. Initially, coarse clumping and granulation of the nuclear chromatin material are noted with the later appearance of small intranuclear vacuoles [▮*10.8*]. These changes are initially confined to single epithelial cells. As infection progresses, the entire nucleus assumes a homogeneous, ground-glass appearance with margination of the chromatin. The formation of large syncytia and multinucleated cell groups by the coalition of individually affected cells is also apparent at this stage [▮*10.9*]. Molding of the nuclei is often present. The final stage of the infection process is characterized by partial or complete fragmentation (karyorrhexis) of the nuclei followed by complete karyolysis, resulting in the appearance of aggregates of amphophilic cytoplasmic remnants.

The clinical significance of herpesvirus infection is venereal transmission and particular association with gonorrhea, risk of neonatal infection, risk of spontaneous abortion, and possible association with carcinoma of the cervix.

Herpes zoster may affect the vulva. The cytologic diagnosis is made by examining scrapings from margins of the vesicles, and cytologic features are similar to those of herpes simplex.

Genital infection with vaccinia virus may occur following vaccination, autovaccination, or contact contamination. The cytologic diagnosis is based on the presence of eosinophilic elementary bodies in the cytoplasm of the affected cells.

Cytomegaloviruses are important causes of fetal damage and unrecognized intrauterine infection. Detection of these viral infections in smears is feasible and is based on the presence of prominent, single, cyanophilic intranuclear inclusions, which often give the cells an "owl's eye–like" appearance.

Cellular changes compatible with adenovirus infection have been observed in smears. The epithelial cells exhibit multiple or single cyanophilic inclusions.

Condyloma acuminata are a relatively common finding in the female genital tract. Lesions are found on the vulva, perineum, vagina, and cervix. Cellular changes occur in squamous or metaplastic cells; some cells may show degenerative features. The cytoplasm stains irregularly. Nuclei may be single but are often double and sometimes multiple. They are enlarged, and the chromatin is smudged or pyknotic. Karyorrhexis is frequently seen. No nucleoli are present [▮*10.10*, ▮*10.11*].

Special types of cells most frequently found in cervical condylomata are the koilocyte, dyskeratocyte, and parabasal cell. The koilocyte is a mature squamous cell containing one or two slightly enlarged hyperchromatic nuclei. The chromatin structure usually is not discernible because it is either smudged or pyknotic. Surrounding the nuclei is an almost empty cavity that has irregular, sharply cut borders. The cytoplasm peripheral to this cavity is very dense and stains irregularly. The dyskeratocyte is a small squamous cell with an enlarged, dense, sometimes pyknotic nucleus and dense cytoplasm of a brilliant orange color when stained with orange G 6 by the Papanicolaou technique. When dyskeratocytes occur singly, they have been called miniature squamous cells. However, they are most frequently seen in large, tridimensional clusters in cases of condyloma of the cervix. In these clusters, the nuclei are often double and larger than nuclei of superficial cells. The parabasal cell has a normal nuclear/cytoplasmic ratio, one or two dark nuclei with indistinct chromatin structure, and amphophilic cytoplasm. These cells must be differentiated from dysplastic and neoplastic cells in which the chromatin structure is well preserved and the nuclear membrane can be easily observed. Any of these cell types may predominate. Although the koilocyte is the most typical cell, it is not found in all cases of condyloma. Often only dyskeratocytes are present; sometimes dyskeratocytes and parabasal cells are seen; and sometimes all these cell types can be observed on the same smear.

Other microorganisms observed in Pap smears are considered to be unusual findings. During childhood, vaginitis may be due to intestinal parasites or their ova. The most common parasite is *Enterobius vermicularis*, but the occurrence of ascaris should also be considered.

Bilharzia ova and miracidia occasionally may be seen in vaginal smears of patients who live or have lived in countries where the disease is endemic.

Uncommon protozoa found in cytologic samples from the female genital tract include *Vorticella*, *Entamoeba histolytica*, and *Balantidium coli*. There are also reports of various species of filariae in vaginal smears.

Occasionally, vinegar eels (*Turabatrix aceti*) may be found in smears from patients who have douched with vinegar. Arthropods, such as water fleas or mites, also may be observed in vaginal smears.

Several contaminants, such as *Alternaria*, *Hormodendrum*, *Gaffkya*, and *Aspergillus* species, pollen, or other vegetable cells and hair of the carpet beetle [▮*10.12*], may be found in vaginal cell samples.

INFLAMMATORY REACTIONS

The site and type of inflammatory reaction may be identified from the cell sample. An acute inflammatory reaction is characterized by the presence of abundant well-preserved neutrophils and epithelial cells of various degrees of maturity showing inflammatory changes. When the lesion is localized, these features are found in only one or two of the sites of the routine vaginal, cervical, and endocervical smears; when generalized, they are found in all three.

In chronic follicular cervicitis, a diffuse or localized lymphocytic infiltration of the cervical stroma occurs. In the cytologic sample, an admixture of mature and immature lymphocytes, plasma cells, histiocytes, and occasionally reticular cells are found [▮*10.13*].

Inflammatory exudates containing abundant histiocytes or plasma cells are associated with chronic inflammation. Multinucleated histiocytes are commonly observed in samples from menopausal and postmenopausal women and patients undergoing radiation therapy.

Inflammation induces distinct changes in epithelial cells. The cytoplasmic changes are vacuolization, decreased staining intensity, polychromasia, perinuclear halos, and irregularity of shape. The nuclear changes include binucleation or multinucleation, vacuolization, chromatin clumping, karyopyknosis, and karyorrhexis.

Factors that predispose to inflammation are traumatic injury, decrease of the vaginal acidity, epithelial atrophy, irradiation, and neoplasia. Atrophic vaginitis may occur as a result of natural menopause, castration, or other ovarian dysfunction.

Patients with neoplasia are susceptible to secondary infection. Variable numbers of inflammatory cells and abnormal flora are often found in smears from patients with invasive neoplasms.

IUDs, acting as foreign bodies, may induce inflammatory reactions in the endometrial cavity. The string attached to the IUD can also induce atypical changes of the endocervical epithelium. The glandular cells of endocervical origin usually appear in clusters and show vacuolization, engulfing of polyps, moderate variation in nuclear size and shape, and hyperchromatic cells. The squamous metaplastic cells exhibit large vacuoles in the cytoplasm that push the nuclei toward the periphery, a slight increase in nuclear size, and bland chromatin pattern. Reparative cell changes and inflammatory background also may be seen.

Endometrial cells occur singly or in clusters and are shed throughout the menstrual cycle. When in clusters, they sometimes exhibit large cytoplasmic shape. More often, endometrial cell clusters have cells exhibiting scant cytoplasm, uniformity in nuclear size and shape, and some hyperchromasia. In the presence of endometritis, the endometrial cells exhibit degenerative cell changes and have an accompanying inflammatory background. In the differential diagnosis of adenocarcinoma, the following are salient features: tumor diathesis, variation in nuclear size and shape, and clearing of the chromatin and nucleoli.

Some bizarre cells are also exfoliated; the origin of this is not clear. These cells show increased nuclear/cytoplasmic ratio, hyperchromasia, and nucleoli, looking like carcinoma in situ cells. Differential features from carcinoma in situ include few cells, bland and hyperchromatic chromatin, nucleoli, and multinucleation.

TISSUE REPAIR

Cells derived from reparative processes have varying degrees of differentiation. They may originate from columnar, metaplastic, or squamous epithelium [▮*10.14*-▮*10.16*], and they may be isolated or predominantly arranged in sheets. The total number of cells varies considerably. In cells of epithelial origin, the cytoplasm is usually cyanophilic, sometimes eosinophilic, and less often indeterminate. A moderate degree of anisocytosis is present. The nuclear chromatin pattern is predominantly uniformly finely granular with chromocenters or coarsely granular. Generally, the cells contain eosinophilic macronucleoli, which may be single or multiple. Most of the nucleoli are regular in configuration, but irregular nucleoli are occasionally found. Mitotic figures may be present.

The presence of cell aggregates in the cytologic sample may at times cause difficulties in the evaluation of a specimen, especially in those cases exhibiting macronucleoli. A large nucleolus reflects the active engagement of the cells in protein synthesis; thus, it may be present either in benign regenerative processes or in neoplasias. Close scrutiny of the arrangement of the cells in sheets, of the predominant delicate chromatin pattern, and of the thread-like structures visible between the nuclei, in some cases, will help differentiate these cells from malignant tumor cells.

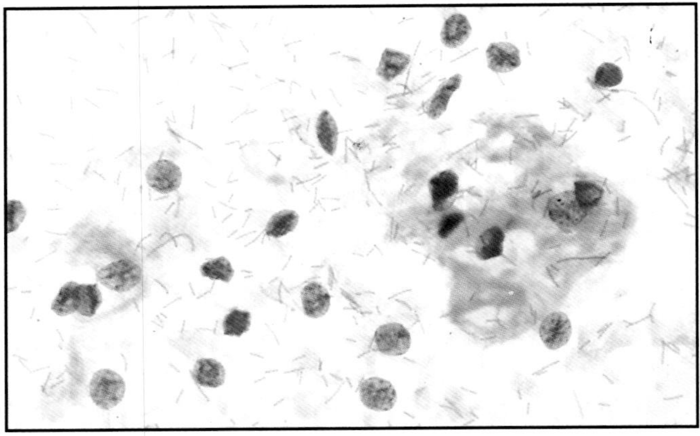

10.1
Döderlein's bacilli (x400).

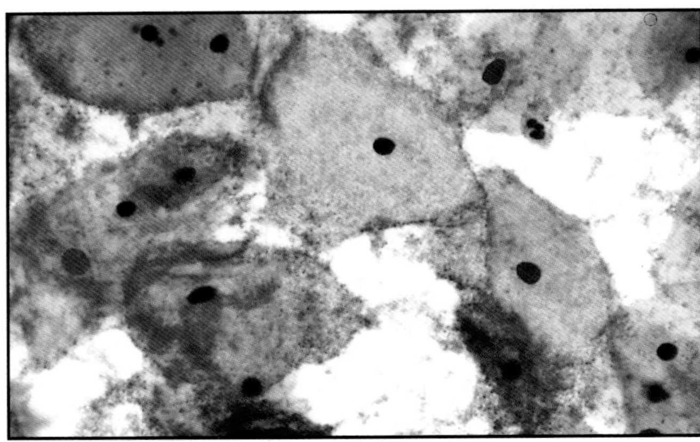

10.2
"Clue" cell in a patient with Gardnerella vaginalis *(x400).*

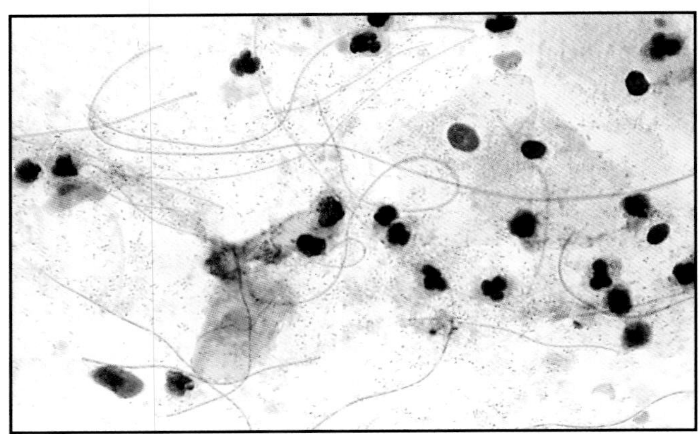

10.3
Leptothrix (x400).

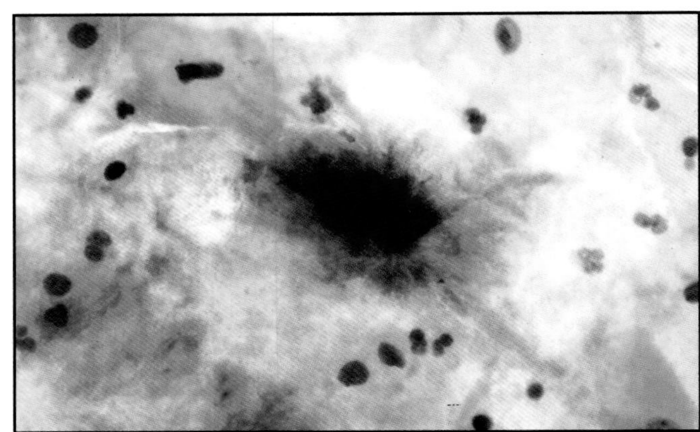

10.4
Actinomycetes (x400).

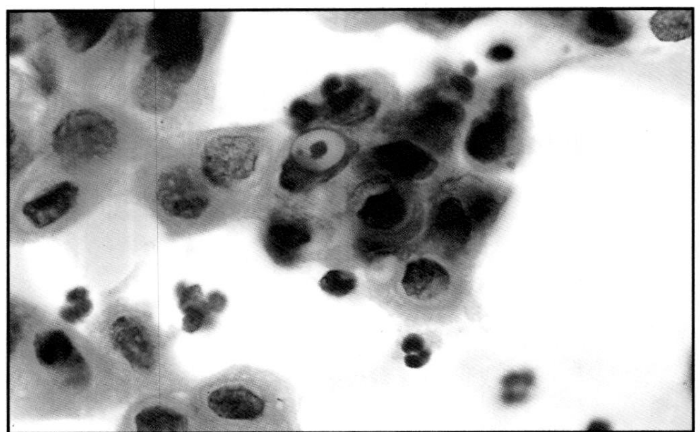

10.5
Chlamydia, *inclusion bodies (x650).*

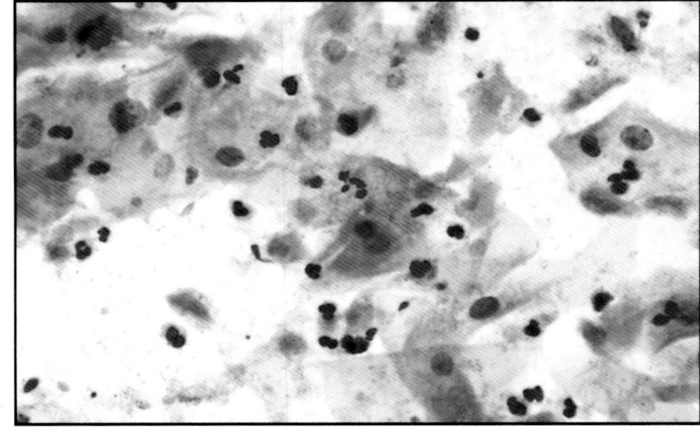

10.6
Trichomonas vaginalis *(x400).*

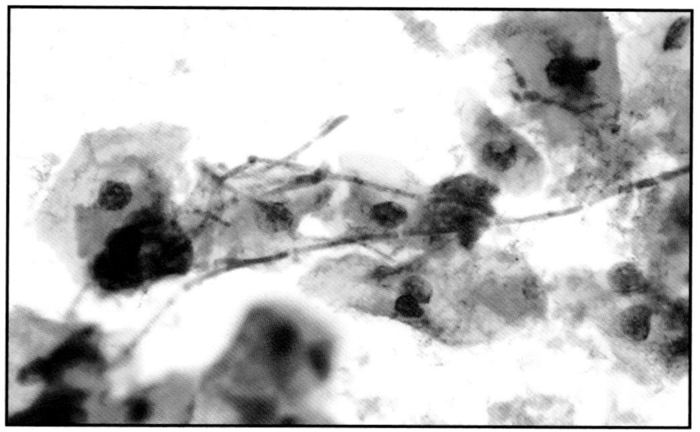

10.7
Candida species (x400).

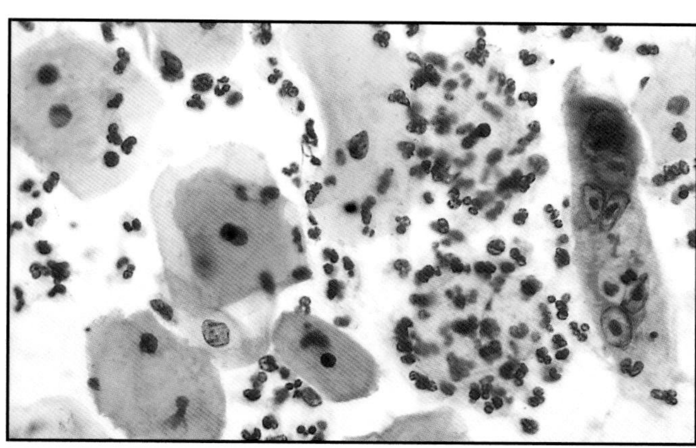

10.8
Herpesvirus, inclusion bodies (x400).

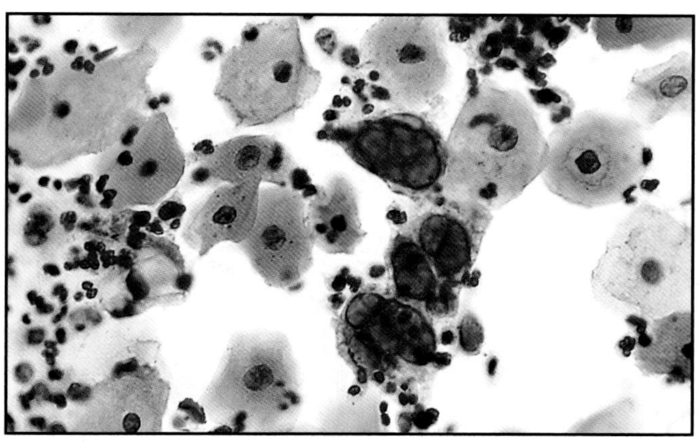

10.9
Herpesvirus, ground-glass appearance (x400).

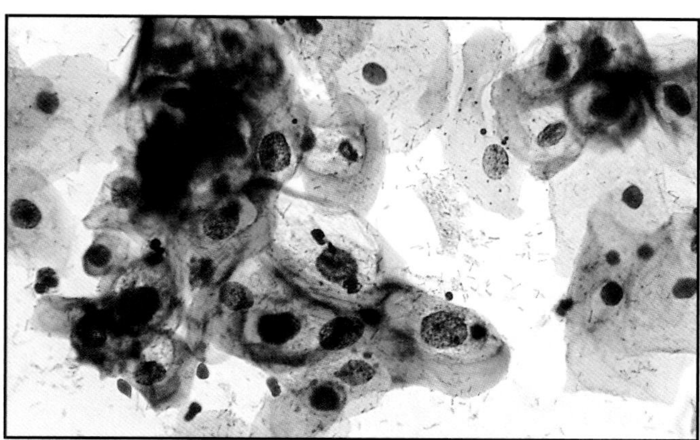

10.10
Condyloma acuminatum (x400).

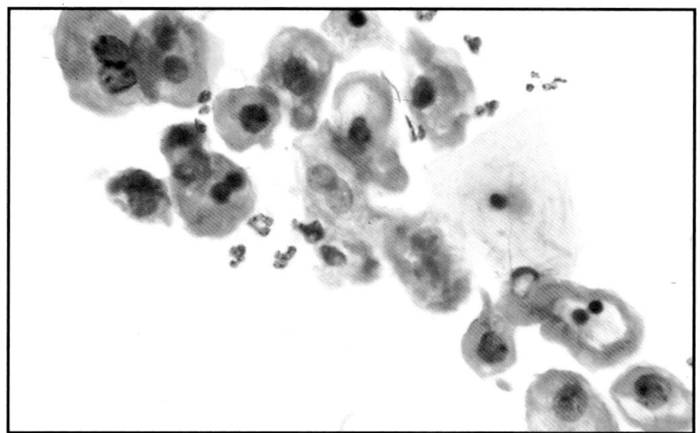

10.11
Condyloma acuminatum (x400).

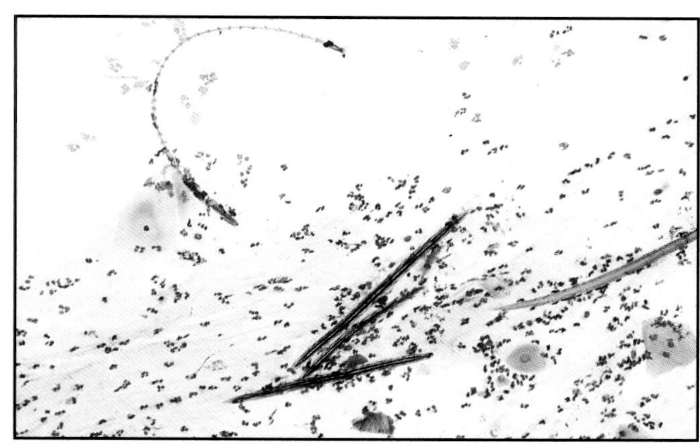

10.12
Hair of the carpet beetle (x400).

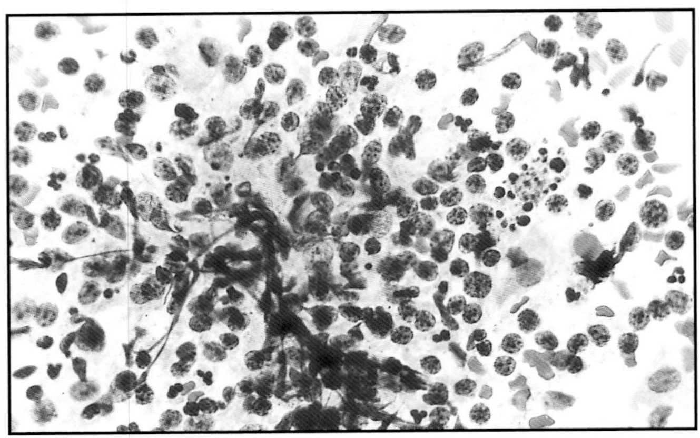

10.13
Follicular cervicitis (x400).

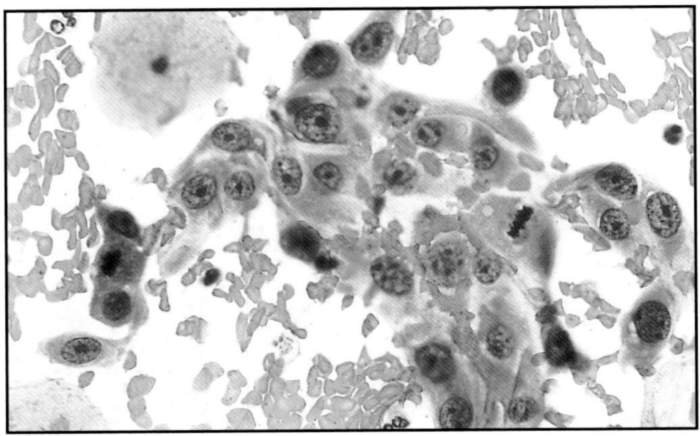

10.14
Tissue repair (x400).

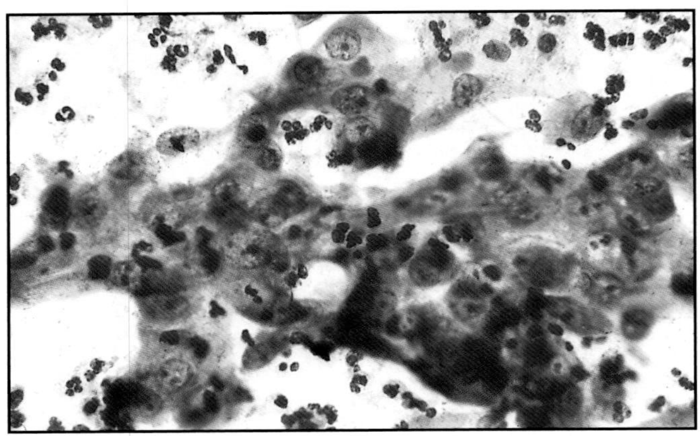

10.15
Tissue repair (x400).

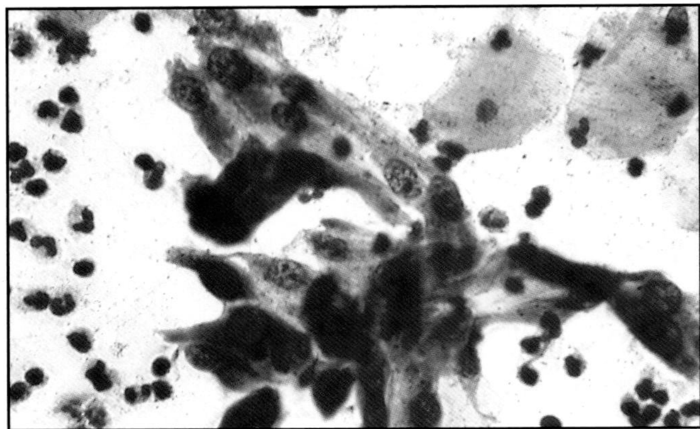

10.16
Tissue repair (x400).

REVIEW EXERCISES

1. What kinds of microorganism can be identified in the cytologic sample from the female genital tract?
2. Which cells are affected by cytolysis, and what causes this type of cellular destruction?
3. What are "clue" cells, and what does their presence usually indicate?
4. Describe the life cycle of chlamydial organisms.
5. Describe the cytologic features of *Actinomyces* species.
6. Which main types of viral infection may involve the female genital tract?
7. What are the cytologic features of herpes simplex infection?
8. Describe the main cytologic features of inflammation of the female reproductive tract.
9. Describe the cytologic features of tissue repair.

SELECTED READINGS

Bibbo M, Keebler CM, Wied GL. The cytologic diagnosis of tissue repair in the female genital tract. *Acta Cytol.* 1971;15:133-137.

Bibbo M, Keebler CM, Wied GL. *Diagnostic Cytology.* Baltimore, Md: Williams & Wilkins Co; 1978:454-463.

Gardner HL, Kaufman RH. *Benign Diseases of the Vulva and Vagina.* 2nd ed. St. Louis, Mo: CV Mosby Co; 1980.

Geirrson G, Woodworth FE, Patten SF, et al. Epithelial repair and regeneration in the uterine cervix, I: an analysis of the cells. *Acta Cytol.* 1977;21:371-378.

Gupta PK. Microbiology, inflammation and viral infections. In: Bibbo M, ed. *Comprehensive Cytopathology.* Philadelphia, Pa: WB Saunders Co; 1991.

Gupta PK, Hollander DH, Frost JK. Actinomycetes in cervico-vaginal smears: an association with IUD usage. *Acta Cytol.* 1976;20:295-297.

Gupta PK, Lee EF, Erozan YS, et al. Cytologic investigations in *Chlamydia* infection. *Acta Cytol.* 1979;23:315-320.

Josey YW, Nahmias A, Naib ZM. Viral and virus-like infections of the female genital tract. *Clin Obstet Gynecol.* 1969;12:161.

Koss L. *Diagnostic Cytology and Its Histopathologic Basis.* 3rd ed. Philadelphia, Pa: JB Lippincott Co; 1979.

Lewis JF, O'Brien S. Diagnosis of *Haemophilus vaginalis* by Papanicolaou smears. *Tech Bull Regist Med Tech.* 1969;39:34-37.

Meisels A, Fortin R. Condylomatous lesions of the cervix and vagina, I: cytologic patterns. *Acta Cytol.* 1976;20:195-201.

Miravete AP. Estudios sobre flora vaginal, IX: classification de lactobacilli de origen vaginal. *Rev Latin Am Microbiol.* 1967;9:11-14.

Patten SF Jr. *Diagnostic Cytopathology of the Uterine Cervix.* 2nd ed. Basel, Switzerland: S Karger; 1978. Monographs in Clinical Cytology.

Rosebury T. *Microorganisms Indigenous to Man.* New York, NY: McGraw-Hill Book Co Inc; 1962.

Widholm O. Gynecologic infections during childhood and adolescence. *Int J Gynaecol Obstet.* 1970;8:457-466.

Wied GL, Bibbo M. Microbiologic classification on the cellular sample in management of patients with vaginal infections. *J Reprod Med.* 1972;9:1-16.

HAPTER

11

Diseases of the Uterine Cervix

TANLEY F. PATTEN, JR, MD, PHD, FIAC

CONTENTS

The nonkeratinizing stratified squamous and simple columnar epithelia covering the uterine cervix not only respond to various internal hormonal stimuli and/or metabolic states, but also to a continually changing external environment, resulting in a variety of morphologic responses that depart from normal. Basically, these morphologic responses of the cervical epithelia may be characterized as protective, destructive, reparative or regenerative, and neoplastic. With the exception of neoplasia, the term "benign proliferative reaction" may be applied to most other responses of the cervical epithelia to external stimuli. These benign reactions may result in some degree of epithelial and/or cellular "atypia" in that specific morphologic alterations are present that represent a departure from normal [▮*11.1*-▮*11.6*]. Those tissue and cellular alterations associated with atypia must be recognized by the cytotechnologist and the pathologist as specific entities, and in some instances distinguished from the morphologic features of neoplasia.

BENIGN PROLIFERATIVE REACTIONS

Protective Reactions

The stratified squamous and columnar epithelia of the uterine cervix are limited in the manner in which they may respond to external stimuli as a protective mechanism. A mature, nonkeratinizing, stratified squamous epithelium covering the vagina and cervix retains the potential for further differentiation as a protective mechanism. This potential may be realized in those situations in which the vagina and/or ectocervix are subjected to chronic irritation of considerable magnitude. An excellent example is uterine prolapse or descensus. Under these circumstances, the epithelium increases its protective role by producing a greater number of cells (hyperplasia), resulting in a greater overall thickness. In addition, granular cell and keratin layers may develop, resulting in a morphologic pattern of epithelium virtually indistinguishable from skin or epidermis. This process of added differentiation has been cited as an example of true "epidermization." Clinical examination of the vagina or uterine cervix under these circumstances may reveal white, plaque-like areas known as leukoplakia. Its presence is detected in cellular samples by the identification of numerous anucleate squames, the morphologic features of which have been described previously. The identification in routine cytologic samples of anucleate squames alone, particularly in irregular sheets, warrants an interpretation of "cellular changes present consistent with hyperkeratosis" [▮*11.1*].

Another protective reaction involving the stratified squamous epithelium is also characterized by a type of hyperdifferentiation. It may exist alone or in combination with hyperkeratosis. It is manifested by the formation of multiple layers of compact, miniature squamous cells wi pyknotic nuclei. This surface reaction can be sharp demarcated from the underlying normal epithelium, ar because it resembles a similar process observed in the sk or epidermis, it is referred to as parakeratosis. It may ori nate in the so-called intraepithelial zone and represent abortive attempt at keratinization. In the cellular samp parakeratosis may be recognized by the presence of min ture superficial squamous cells presenting as isolated ce or in sheets [▮*11.2*]. Their cytoplasmic staining reaction usually orangeophilic or eosinophilic.

While the cytologic identification of cells deriv from hyperkeratosis and/or parakeratosis may not be clinical significance in many instances, similar surfa changes are associated with squamous intraepithel lesions and may mask an underlying condyloma, dysplasia, or even an invasive cancer. A form of parak atosis more commonly associated with neoplas processes is that manifested by the presence of pleom phic (elongate and caudate forms) parakeratotic cel Therefore, persistence of either of these benign protecti reactions would warrant further clinical investigation exclude an underlying abnormal process.

Several processes mimic parakeratosis. The mo common occurs in postmenopausal patients who have atrophic cellular hormonal pattern. Degeneration of in vidual atrophic squamous cells results in the presence miniature eosinophilic or orangeophilic cells with pykno as well as fragmented nuclei [▮*11.3*, left]. However, the cy plasm of these cells is granular or finely vacuolated ratl than structureless as in true parakeratosis. Karyorrhexis seldom observed in the parakeratotic cell. The second situ tion occurs in women who, during their reproductive yea are taking birth control pills, particularly those with a re tively high progesterone component. In such patients, sp imens acquired during the second half of the menstru cycle from the endocervical canal may contain peculi parakeratotic-like cells lying in strings of mucus [▮*11* right]. It has been demonstrated that such cells probab represent degenerating endocervical columnar epithel cells. Their cytoplasm usually appears granular a evidence of karyorrhexis may be present.

The most common protective reaction of the uteri cervix is squamous metaplasia. Because squamous me plasia is a normal physiologic process, its cytologic ma festations do not depart from normal. Its histologic a cytologic features have been described elsewhere. T entire concept of squamous metaplasia is extremely imp tant to an understanding of the processes of squamo carcinogenesis in the uterine cervix and, therefo extremely important in diagnostic cytopathology. Brief from the standpoint of the cytoplasmic morphology, ea stage of the physiologic squamous metaplastic process mimicked by a comparable abnormal or neoplas process. For example, the cytoplasmic morphology of ce originating from reserve cell hyperplasia is identical to th of abnormal cells arising from a high-grade intraepithel lesion such as carcinoma in situ. From the standpoint of diagnostic cytopathology, the biologic and morphologic clues to the distinctions between normal and neoplasia reside primarily in the nucleus, not the cytoplasm.

Since most cytologic samples from the uterine cervix contain cells derived from immature and/or mature squamous metaplasia, the uniformity of their nuclei provides an excellent standard reference for comparing nuclear sizes (approximately 50 μm^2). In the absence of squamous metaplasia, the size of the nucleus of the intermediate squamous cell may be equally useful as a standard (approximately 35 μm^2). Again, the cytoplasm only provides information relative to the parentage or maturity of a cell. The nucleus reflects the biologic activity and potential of a cell. As stated previously, most abnormal squamous cells observed in the presence of "atypia" or neoplasia of the cervical mucosa possess cytoplasmic areas or characteristics observed in the spectrum of normal squamous epithelium, reserve cell hyperplasia, or squamous metaplasia. Consequently, attention to nuclear size (area) and morphology permits a more accurate assessment of the cell in relation to the reaction or process of origin.

Degenerative and Destructive Reactions

The cellular aspects of degeneration are related in most instances to inflammation, although physical and chemical trauma to the cervical epithelia may result in similar morphologic alterations. Alteration of normal cell morphology by inflammatory agents may be of a specific or nonspecific type. The details relating to specific agents are described elsewhere (Chapter 10). However, in addition to cell destruction, which includes cytolysis, karyorrhexis, and karyolysis, significant alterations important in diagnostic cytopathology occur chiefly in the nucleus. Such alterations include binucleation, nuclear enlargement, and chromocenter formation. In most instances, these nuclear alterations can be recognized as manifestations of inflammation and can be distinguished from other forms of atypia or early cervical neoplasia. Epithelial reactions secondary to destruction, electrocautery, or cryocautery may result in self-limited significant degrees of nuclear enlargement and hyperchromasia, which, in the absence of adequate clinical history, may be indistinguishable from certain changes of early cervical neoplasia.

Reparative and Regenerative Reactions

The cellular manifestations of epithelial repair and regeneration [▮*11.4*] are discussed in detail elsewhere (Chapter 10). However, in conjunction with the spectrum of benign proliferative reactions, the salient features of the reparative/regenerative reactions must be reviewed because the morphologic manifestations may be confused with those of invasive cancer. Reparative/regenerative reactions involve both squamous and columnar epithelia. The principal morphologic manifestation is significant nuclear enlargement in association with prominent nucleolar formation. Nucleoli may be single or multiple, variable in size, and often irregular in shape. The affected cells are identified almost exclusively in some form of cell aggregate, usually a sheet or syncytial-like arrangement. Three features usually associated with the cellular manifestations of an invasive process are not observed in the presence of a so-called reparative reaction. These are nuclear hyperchromasia in association with an irregular chromatin distribution, numerous isolated abnormal cells, and evidence of cell and/or tissue destruction (host response or tumor diathesis).

CYTOLOGIC ATYPIA

Falling between the cellular manifestations of normal and neoplastic epithelia are a range of cellular alterations related in terms of The Bethesda System of classification as changes secondary to infection and reactive and reparative processes. These changes, which have been alluded to previously, manifest themselves principally as alterations in nuclear size and/or morphology. Reactive cellular changes manifested by nuclear enlargement are observed, in addition to various types of inflammation, secondary to folic acid deficiency, ionizing radiation, chemotherapy, intrauterine contraceptive devices, and other physical or chemical traumas to the cervical mucosa. So-called reparative reactions may be observed in the presence of nonspecific inflammation, following radiotherapy, electrocautery, cryocautery, or laser cautery. Under circumstances in which nuclear enlargement can be directly related to an inflammatory, reactive, or reparative process, the biologic relationship to carcinogenesis is at best nebulous. The foregoing morphologic alterations must be distinguished from those of neoplasia, particularly the relatively early cellular alterations associated with squamous neoplasia, so-called squamous atypia, which will be defined later. In the United States, the term "atypia" has been applied principally to the lower end of the spectrum of cellular abnormality and chiefly to inflammatory, reactive, or reparative reactions. Conversely, particularly in Europe, "atypia" commonly encompasses the entire spectrum of intraepithelial neoplasia.

THE BIOLOGY OF NEOPLASIA

An Analogy

A tumor is defined as any localized swelling or mass that occurs in tissue. Like other lesions, a tumor is composed of living cells. Since it often constitutes a new growth of cells, it is therefore also called a neoplasm. Some tumors, or neoplasms, are relatively innocuous growths and are said to be benign tumors. Others are more harmful and are designated as malignant tumors.

Many similarities exist between objectionable plants or weeds and tumors. Although some weeds are more objectionable than others, they are all undesirable. Similarly, some tumors are slow growing and have few serious complications. For this reason, they are called benign tumors. However, they are neither desirable nor without consequences. There are no desirable tumors, just as there are no desirable weeds. A garden plant growing in a carefully tended lawn is a weed, even though it looks like the plants that are carefully tended in the garden. A benign tumor may closely resemble its parent tissue, but the parent tissue, normal in some sites, is out of place in a tumorous growth. Unlike a weed, a benign tumor is often surrounded by a thick shell of tissue, which is called a capsule. This capsule tends to limit the tumor's ability to grow and spread. The essential features of a benign tumor are slow growth, a structure often resembling that of the normal parent tissue, and encapsulation.

Crabgrass is one of the common destructive weeds. This type of weed is more like a malignant tumor. Early in its growth, crabgrass is relatively innocuous in its appearance. It only has two leaves, which closely resemble the blades of the surrounding grass. Similarly, a malignant tumor may have an innocent appearance early in its growth, and to the naked eye, may look like the normal surrounding tissue. At an early stage in its growth, crabgrass can be pulled out easily and, similarly, a malignant tumor can be eradicated more easily early in its development.

Crabgrass can grow unnoticed at a rapid rate, spreading out from the innocent-appearing initial shoot. A rapid rate of growth is also characteristic of a malignant tumor, and the growth may occur without giving signs or symptoms of its presence until it has spread some distance into the normal tissue. Unless eradicated, the crabgrass sends out claw-like tentacles, or extensions, that crowd out and destroy the desirable grass. Likewise, this invasion also characterizes the growth of a malignant tumor that extends into and destroys surrounding healthy tissue. The infiltrating cell cords extending out from the main mass of the malignant tumor are reminiscent of the legs extending out from a crab. Because of this, a malignant tumor is sometimes called cancer (meaning "crab") or carcinoma (crab-like tumor).

Unless checked by midsummer, crabgrass may devastate a lawn and create an appearance quite different from that of its innocuous nature during the early stages of development. Similarly, a carcinoma when examined under the microscope has an ominous appearance. The cancer cells in many instances do not resemble the normal cells, but have the features of primitive or extremely immature cells. Ultimately crabgrass is damaged by the first frost, but not before it has developed seeds that are shed only to germinate again the next year. Similarly, a cancer may reproduce by seeding. Like seeds, the cancer cells may be carried in the bloodstream or the lymphatic channels to set up other malignant growths. These are called metastases, and the process of seeding is referred to as metastasis. Cells may also fall from the tumor to implant and grow in a site that fulfills the requirement of a fertile soil. This is also referred to as seeding or implantation. In contrast to a benign neoplasm, a malignant tumor, or a cancer, is characterized by the following: a rapid rate of growth; a structure that is not representative of normal tissue but of primitive tissue; an infiltrating type of growth that is not restricted by encapsulation; and the process of seeding, or metastasis.

Terminology

In the foregoing analogy of crabgrass to neoplasia of the squamous epithelia of the uterine cervix, the morphologic stages of the squamous neoplastic process in this site have been arbitrarily characterized or subclassified. In the recently proposed Bethesda System, these stages include squamous atypia of undetermined significance, low- and high-grade squamous intraepithelial lesions, and squamous cell carcinoma. The fundamental rationale for this classification included the following: elimination of the often confusing Papanicolaou classification; a requirement for a statement of cytologic specimen adequacy; subclassification of intraepithelial lesions that might provide more widespread improved interpretive correlation between the cellular and tissue samples; and improved communication for proper management of intraepithelial lesions.

While further subclassification is not justifiable from the standpoint of the proper clinical management of a majority of patients with squamous intraepithelial lesions, the spectrum of morphologic changes encompassed by the category of high-grade squamous intraepithelial lesion (HGSIL) warrants further subclassification for a more specific understanding of squamous carcinogenesis in the uterine cervix and its cellular manifestations. Low-grade squamous intraepithelial lesions (LGSIL) may be classified as slight (mild) dysplasia or cervical intraepithelial neoplasia type 1 (CIN 1), with or without the manifestations of human papillomavirus (HPV). On the other hand, HGSILs encompass the categories of moderate dysplasia (CIN 2), marked (severe) dysplasia (CIN 3), and carcinoma in situ (CIN 3) with or without the manifestations of HPV. For the purposes of this discussion, the terms "dysplasia" and "carcinoma in situ" will continue to be emphasized, as the descriptive and morphometric parameters required for proper cellular interpretation have been clearly defined and tested over the years.

Dysplasia and carcinoma in situ represent a continuum and spectrum of morphologic lesions of the uterine cervical squamous epithelium in which the individual cells deviate from normal. Some of these epithelial reactions retain to a varying degree the characteristics of a maturing stratified squamous epithelium. These reactions are termed "dysplasia." The more dedifferentiated stratified reactions are usually called "carcinoma in situ." It is impossible to predict the outcome of any given intraepithelial abnormality in the uterine cervix. Those reactions referred to as dysplasia tend, as a group, to possess a relatively low potential for progression to carcinoma in situ or invasive cancer (approximately 30%-40%). Those lesions classified as carcinoma in situ possess a greater risk of developing into invasive cancer. However, like dysplasia, carcinoma in situ does not invariably progress to cancer (approximately 50%). Early or microinvasive cancer may originate from either dysplasia or carcinoma in situ. However, the latter is more likely to constitute the source of invasion (approximately 65%-70%).

From the standpoint of cytopathology, early in the process of carcinogenesis, only a limited degree of cellular abnormality may be apparent. Similar morphologic changes may be induced by noncarcinogenic stimuli such as inflammation or folic acid deficiency. At this stage in the evolutionary process, it is impossible to predict the biologic outcome, such as in the case of atypical squamous cells of undetermined significance. Morphologic variations from the normal are more readily recognized as the process of carcinogenesis proceeds. While the probability of the development of invasive cancer increases as carcinogenesis proceeds, the morphologic features of any particular stage cannot as yet be used to predict the progression of any given lesion. At present, no accurate morphologic criteria are available for distinguishing those intraepithelial lesions that will end in cancer from those that will have a more favorable prognosis.

The intraepithelial, neoplastic lesions of the uterine cervix constitute a broad spectrum of abnormal histologic patterns that may contribute to the diversity of abnormal cells in the cellular sample. A morphologic subclassification for these squamous intraepithelial lesions provides a logical basis for optimal correlation between the cytologic and histologic sample. Recent studies have demonstrated that a classification scheme with only two intraepithelial subclasses, such as The Bethesda System, provides higher levels of correlation in the average laboratory. However, provided the prerequisites of an adequate cellular sample and well-preserved cellular detail, the cytotechnologist and cytopathologist trained in the use of analytical and morphometric criteria can usually recognize certain morphologic features that permit a relatively accurate morphologic subclassification (approximately 95%+ correlation of subclasses of intraepithelial lesions). This obviously provides a more realistic framework for communication between the laboratory and the clinician.

In general, abnormal cells originating from squamous intraepithelial lesions of the uterine cervix can be subclassified on a morphologic basis into two groups: (1) a squamous group of varying maturity and bearing a resemblance to cells that might arise from superficial, intermediate, and superficial deep spinous layers of the normal squamous mucosa; and (2) those that more closely resemble the so-called reserve cells or very immature squamous metaplastic cells. When related to the tissue reaction of origin, the latter arise from intraepithelial lesions in which no differentiation takes place and cytoplasmic borders are inconspicuous (syncytial-like arrangement). On the basis of nuclear and cytoplasmic volumes, such lesions may be further subclassified as being composed of relatively large, intermediate, and small primitive cell types. Most pathologists would agree that these lesions fall within the classic definition of carcinoma in situ of the uterine cervix. Those intraepithelial lesions that contain evidence of squamous cell (cytoplasmic) differentiation similarly would be expected to give rise to abnormal cells with evidence of squamous differentiation. Thus, on the basis of an evaluation of an abnormal cell population, one can obtain rather specific information on the differentiation characteristics of the parent lesion(s).

This method of morphologic subclassification is based on the premise that a majority of both normal and abnormal cells observed in the cellular sample originate from the upper levels of the epithelium of origin. The evaluation of cytoplasmic differentiation in optimal cytologic samples, in combination with careful analysis of nuclear structure, permits relatively accurate subclassification and correlation between cells and tissue.

SQUAMOUS INTRAEPITHELIAL LESIONS

Atypical Squamous Cells

Excluded from the category of atypical squamous cells of undetermined significance are abnormal squamous cells originating from inflammatory, reactive, or reparative processes. Rather, the term "noninflammatory squamous atypia" seems appropriate for these abnormal squamous cells, since there is no apparent basis for the nuclear changes observed. While for many years we have considered these changes to be those of "early neoplasia," only recently has evidence emerged to suggest that noninflammatory squamous atypia may be an early manifestation of the human papillomavirus (HPV).

As introduced earlier, it is important in diagnostic cytopathology to establish certain normal cell nuclei as reference nuclei for estimating nuclear areas. In samples from the uterine cervix, the normal intermediate squamous cell nucleus possesses an area of 36 ± 13 μm^2 and relative nuclear area of 4%. Perhaps more applicable to most squamous intraepithelial lesions is the mean nuclear area of normal immature squamous metaplastic or atrophic squamous cells (50 μm^2). Those cells designated as characteristic of noninflammatory squamous atypia are generally the size of an intermediate squamous cell with a mean nuclear area of 98 ± 22 μm² with a relative nuclear area of approximately 8% [▮*11.5*]. In general, the squamous nuclei should be considered atypical when the area is approximately twice that observed in a normal immature squamous metaplastic cell nucleus or three times the nuclear area of a normal intermediate squamous cell. The nuclei derived from dysplasia in which cell maturation resembles that of an intermediate squamous cell possess a nuclear area three to four times that observed in immature squamous metaplastic cells (178 ± 32 μm² and relative nuclear area of 14%). In most instances, the chromatinic material of the nucleus in squamous atypia is finely granular, uniformly distributed, and only rarely hyperchromatic.

A 20-year follow-up of a group of 20,000 cyclic patients with noninflammatory squamous atypia showed a progression to or association with a more advanced process in approximately 10% of patients followed up from 1 to 20 years. This might have been anticipated, since indeed atypical squamous cells appear to represent the earliest morphologic manifestation of cervical neoplasia. Therefore, these women appear to be at greater risk for developing more significant lesions of squamous neoplasia and should be monitored closely for relatively long periods.

Other forms of atypia involving immature metaplastic cells [▮*11.6*] with nuclear changes less than those of dysplasia have also been reported to "progress" to more advanced lesions of squamous neoplasia, also in approximately 10% of cases.

Squamous Intraepithelial Lesion (SIL)—Dysplasia

In the uterine cervix, the term dysplasia is applied to a spectrum of heteroplastic lesions involving stratified squamous or squamous-like (metaplastic) epithelium. As the term implies, this group of reactions is characterized by malformation or disordered development, manifested morphologically by variations in cytoplasmic maturation and association with certain nuclear abnormalities. Fundamentally, the dysplastic lesions are characterized by the following: an increase in the content of primitive cells; premature keratinization of component cells; abnormal differentiation of the uppermost cell layers; evidence of cytoplasmic maturation or cell borders in the upper levels; mitotic activity above the basal cell layer; and abnormally large nuclei. Thus, the altered stratified squamous epithelium of dysplasia has an increased content of primitive cells (hyperplasia) in association with abnormally large nuclei in the upper layers of the epithelium. There may or may not be evidence of active cellular proliferation. While the normal layering or polarity of the cells may be maintained, this may be altered in some cases. In the upper layers of the epithelium, varying degrees of differentiation or maturation are noted and cell borders are distinct. Abnormal differentiation may be manifested as so-called isolated cell keratinization (dyskeratosis) or as small keratohyaline pearls. Overlying these lesions or reactions may be parakeratosis and/or hyperkeratosis.

Lesions of the uterine cervix characterized as dysplasia are usually localized to that portion of the cervical mucosa anatomically related to the external cervical os or so-called "native squamous epithelium" or mature squamous metaplastic epithelium of the initial transformation zone. Less commonly, dysplasia may involve portions of the transformation zone lying in the endocervical canal, including, in some cases, extension into so-called underlying gland spaces. Because of this, cells from dysplasia are more abundant in cell samples collected directly from the ectocervix and region of the external cervical os. The content of abnormal cells is affected by the severity of the dysplastic reaction, the interval between samplings, variations in technique, and the sampling method utilized. Samples obtained by aspirating the contents of the posterior vaginal fornix or by irrigation of the vaginal canal may or may not contain cells from a dysplastic lesion. The paucity of abnormal cells from dysplasia in samples obtained by these methods may be, in part, because the cells are relatively differentiated and lack the decreased mutual adhesiveness characteristic of cancer cells. Therefore, in the presence of dysplasia, comprehensive sampling of the existing epithelial abnormalities is best achieved by a combined scraping of the ectocervix and an aspiration or brushing of the endocervical canal. The latter sample is most useful in documenting the presence of dysplasia involving the endocervical canal and excluding the presence of in situ or invasive cancer.

Abnormal cells originating from dysplasia most often occur singly but may be observed in aggregates or sheets. In a sheet, the cells are more or less regularly arranged in relation to one another and usually possess distinct cell borders. Within the spectrum of dysplasia, the cells are usually polygonal, round, or oval in configuration. Less often, isolated irregular cell forms may be identified with elongate or caudate configurations with discrete cell borders. The mean cytoplasmic area of cells originating from dysplasia is 1089 ± 311 μm². Many of the cells are comparable in size to normal intermediate and superficial squamous cells (1604 ± 312 μm²), whereas others possess cytoplasmic areas more reminiscent of the squamous metaplastic cell (502 ± 98 μm²). Samples containing dysplastic cells predominantly in the range of normal squamous cells tend to originate from a more mature dysplastic reaction. Similarly, samples with dysplastic cells possessing cell areas more reminiscent of squamous metaplastic cells are more likely to have arisen from a reaction composed of relatively immature cells. The cytoplasmic staining reaction is most often cyanophilic and less often eosinophilic or indeterminate.

The nucleus reflects the abnormal nature of the cell originating in a squamous intraepithelial lesion or dysplastic reaction. Nuclear enlargement may be pronounced. Some of the largest nuclei observed in any abnormality involving the uterine cervix occur in the presence of dysplasia. The reported mean nuclear area is 167 ± 38 μm^2, resulting in a calculated relative nuclear area of 16 ± 4%. The nucleus of the dysplastic cell is usually hyperchromatic and possesses a finely granular chromatin pattern that is evenly distributed throughout the nucleus. However, one or more coarse aggregates of chromatinic material (chromocenters) may be present, becoming increasingly prominent in dysplastic cells resembling immature squamous metaplastic cells of round or oval configuration. Discrete, eosinophilic nucleoli are inconspicuous except when abnormal cells are obtained from the deeper layers of a dysplastic reaction or when a dysplastic reaction lies adjacent to a focus of microinvasion. In approximately 75% of intraepithelial lesions possessing the features of dysplasia, cellular evidence of overlying parakeratosis is noted. In approximately 50%, cellular evidence indicates an associated hyperkeratosis. These surface reactions are more frequently observed in those squamous intraepithelial lesions having the coexisting cytopathic features of human papillomavirus. A significant percentage of cases of dysplasia will possess some abnormal cell changes reflective of HPV. These changes have been described elsewhere.

Rationale for Subclassification of Dysplasia

Squamous intraepithelial lesions of the uterine cervix, including dysplasia, as previously stated, represent a broad spectrum of intraepithelial histologic and comparable cytologic patterns possessing differing morphologic characteristics and, on the basis of various studies, in a general sense, differing biologic potentials. Many years ago, Papanicolaou introduced the term "dyskaryosis" to describe the abnormal nuclear morphology in cells originating from squamous intraepithelial lesions. Although the term is not in general use today, its basic concept is still applicable in the context of learning and understanding cellular morphology in cervical carcinogenesis. In essence, Papanicolaou related observed dyskaryotic changes to the cytoplasmic characteristics of cells that might arise from various levels of normal nonkeratinizing stratified squamous epithelium. Thus, he referred to superficial and intermediate cell dyskaryosis, parabasal cell dyskaryosis, and basal cell dyskaryosis. Subsequently, at the recommendation of a colleague, he offered the suggestion that the newly introduced term "dysplasia" might similarly benefit from the addition of a descriptive prefix such as "intermediate cell dysplasia."

In practice, abnormal cells of a superficial or intermediate dyskaryotic type are usually referred to as originating from a slight or mild dysplasia (LGSIL or CIN 1); those of parabasal dyskaryotic type as marked or severe dysplasia (HGSIL or CIN 3); and intermediate gradations between the two as moderate dysplasia (HGSIL or CIN 2). Over the years, this method of classifying abnormal cells in the cervical cell sample has permitted some degree of correlation with the tissue reaction of origin. However, this classification makes no provisions for quantitating differences in nuclear structure or admixtures of abnormal cells originating from different morphologic lesions in different anatomic sites. Therefore, an approach that recognizes quantitative differences within the spectrum of squamous intraepithelial lesions would provide a more realistic basis for learning and understanding the cellular spectrum, and also permit improved correlation between the tissue and cellular samples in many instances for improved patient treatment.

A classification scheme that combines an evaluation of cellular (cytoplasmic) differentiation and probable biologic activity as reflected in nuclear morphology might be more easily quantitated. From the standpoint of cellular differentiation, the spectrum of squamous intraepithelial lesions of the uterine cervix, and more particularly lesions encompassed by the term dysplasia, tend to mimic the types of normal squamous epithelium (ie, mature nonkeratinizing and the various stages of metaplastic stratified squamous epithelium). Obviously, the nucleus of a cell may serve as a morphologic indicator of biologic activity. In the context of the process of carcinogenesis, abnormal cells with nuclear chromatin patterns resembling those of normal intermediate squamous cells could be anticipated to be the least biologically active. In contrast, those with clumping of the chromatinic material, more reminiscent of the cancer cell, might be considered to be more biologically active. Thus, for abnormal cells originating in an intraepithelial lesion designated as dysplasia, the chromatin pattern will usually vary according to the biologic nature of the parent lesion.

In addition, it has been well documented that during the process of carcinogenesis, as the biologic severity of the lesion increases, the individual cells progressively become less cohesive. Therefore, based on comprehensive cell sampling techniques, the number of abnormal cells originating from dysplasia in most instances reflects the extent and severity of the lesion in the cervical mucosa. Given a relatively uniform sampling technique, when abnormal cells are few in number, a dysplasia might be interpreted as "slight or mild" (LGSIL or CIN 1), whereas a cellular sample containing large numbers of abnormal cells might be interpreted as "marked or severe" (HGSIL or CIN 3). In evaluating the content of abnormal cells originating from a lesion designated as dysplasia, the following should be considered: total content of abnormal cells; the maturity of the cytoplasm; and nuclear morphology including size and chromatin pattern. On these bases, utilizing comprehensive cellular samples from the uterine cervix in association with optimal preservation of cytologic features, it is possible to arrive at a reasonably specific conclusion in any specific case with respect to possible anatomic site of origin, degree of differentiation, and potential biologic severity. The manner and form in which this information is transmitted to the clinician will vary depending on the experience and/or philosophy of each individual pathologist, laboratory, or community.

To provide a more rational approach to cytodiagnosis beyond the "it's such-and-such because I say so" or "it's such-and-such because it looks like it" approaches, the following subclassification of lesions in the category of dysplasia by morphometric information may be useful to the student as well as practitioner of cytopathology.

Nonkeratinizing Dysplasia

Nonkeratinizing dysplasia includes well-differentiated dysplasia, slight or mild dysplasia, superficial and intermediate cell dyskaryosis, and LGSIL (CIN 1) [▮*11.7*, ▮*11.8*]. This morphologic variant is the most common form of dysplasia, observed seven times more frequently than the so-called metaplastic form and 25 times more frequently than the so-called keratinizing or pleomorphic type. Biologically, nonkeratinizing dysplasia is least apt to progress to in situ or invasive cancer. In one study, of those dysplasias antedating the development of carcinoma in situ, only 13 were classified initially as nonkeratinizing. The anatomic site of origin of most mature or nonkeratinizing dysplasias is in the region of the initial transformation zone or squamocolumnar junction. Cells originating from nonkeratinizing dysplasia are predominantly polygonal in configuration with a cell area of 1264 ± 201 μm^2. The nuclei are large (178 ± 32 μm^2) and occupy relatively small portions of the total cell area (14%). The cytoplasmic staining reaction is cyanophilic in 75% of the abnormal cells and eosinophilic in approximately 25%. The chromatin pattern has been described as uniformly finely granular and hyperchromatic in 87% of the cells analyzed. The chromatin pattern is uniformly finely granular with prominent chromatin clumping in 13% of the abnormal cells. Approximately 10% of the abnormal cells are observed in sheets. In some instances, cell samples may contain hundreds of abnormal squamous cells with the foregoing features. Under such circumstances, it is probably prudent to consider the presence of a dysplastic lesion of moderate to marked severity or HGSIL.

Metaplastic Dysplasia

Metaplastic dysplasia includes moderately differentiated dysplasia, moderate to marked dysplasia, parabasal cell dyskaryosis, and high-grade squamous intraepithelial lesions (CIN 2-3) [▮*11.9*, ▮*11.10*]. This form of dysplasia comprises approximately one eighth of all such lesions. On the other hand, approximately 85% of those dysplasias antedating the appearance of carcinoma in situ are of the relatively immature metaplastic type or admixtures of the nonkeratinizing and metaplastic forms at the time of initial detection. The progression rate of this form of dysplasia to carcinoma in situ has been reported to be in the range of 30% to 40%. The anatomic site of origin of the so-called metaplastic form of dysplasia is the proximal or upper portions of the transformation zone. Coexistence of nonkeratinizing and immature metaplastic types of dysplasia finds the more mature former type lying toward the external cervical os and the more immature latter forms lying toward the endocervical canal. The abnormal cells originating from this intraepithelial lesion resemble the squamous metaplastic cells with a mean cell area of 492 ± 109 μm^2. The nuclei are small compared with those of nonkeratinizing dysplasia (156 ± 35 μm^2). The relative nuclear area is approximately 32%. The nuclei in this form of dysplasia are approximately two to three times the size of the nuclei in normal squamous metaplastic cells (50 μm^2). The cell configurations are predominantly round or oval with occasional small polygonal forms. The cytoplasmic staining reaction is principally cyanophilic and not infrequently dense due to the three-dimensionality of the cells. From the standpoint of subclassification, the nuclear chromatin pattern, while predominantly uniformly finely granular and hyperchromatic, frequently contains evidence of chromatin clumping or chromocenter formation. The latter is more often observed in cells originating from a more severe dysplasia of metaplastic type or CIN 3. A uniformly distributed, coarsely granular chromatin pattern is not observed with any frequency in so-called metaplastic dysplasias. In most instances, the abnormal cells lie in an isolated fashion on the slide, but occasional aggregates are observed, principally in a sheet-like arrangement. Rarely, the aggregate may appear syncytial-like and originate from a lesion classified as marked or severe dysplasia.

Keratinizing Dysplasia

Keratinizing dysplasia is also known as pleomorphic dysplasia [▮*11.11*, ▮*11.12*]. This form of dysplasia is relatively uncommon, comprising approximately one thirtieth of all cases. As is true of so-called keratinizing squamous cell carcinoma, this intraepithelial lesion was more common 25 to 30 years ago. From the standpoints of recognition and proper clinical management, it is the most difficult of the intraepithelial lesions. This form of dysplasia usually has its anatomic origin on the ectocervix, probably in zones of so-called native squamous epithelium rather than in the transformation zone. With sampling by an Ayre-type spatula, keratinizing or pleomorphic dysplasia resides against a background of abnormal cells from a coexisting nonkeratinizing dysplasia. Also noted are cellular evidence of hyperkeratosis and/or parakeratosis, the presence of abnormal cells with irregular configurations, and, not infrequently, cellular evidence of an HPV cytopathic effect. The classic presentation of keratinizing dysplasia is not an orangeophilic cytoplasmic staining reaction alone but rather a presentation of abnormal squamous cells in which approximately 22% possess elongate (spindle-shaped) and/or caudate (tadpole-shaped) configurations. The cell and nuclear areas are so variable that they are relatively meaningless in relation to the other variants of dysplasia. Approximately 44% of the cells possess an eosinophilic or orangeophilic staining reaction. Reflecting the degeneration occurring in the intraepithelial lesion of origin, perhaps secondary to HPV, approximately 15% of the nuclei are opaque or pyknotic. Often, it is difficult, if not impossible, to distinguish between a severe surface reaction of keratinizing dysplasia and an underlying keratinizing squamous cell carcinoma. A significant number of keratinizing squamous cell cancers of the uterine cervix may possess an overlying surface lesion that might ordinarily be classified as a slight or mild dysplasia. Similarly, little is known of the progression rates of this form of dysplasia to invasive cancer. Consequently, even the mildest form of keratinizing or pleomorphic dysplasia is biologically highly unpredictable and must be managed aggressively to exclude the development or presence of invasive cancer. In general, the more advanced keratinizing or pleomorphic dysplasias are considered to represent a more differentiated form of carcinoma in situ than that classically described for the uterine cervix. They are often termed well-differentiated or keratinizing carcinoma in situ.

Carcinoma In Situ

Carcinoma in situ implies that the lesions are intimately related to cancer and, therefore, with regard to the stages of carcinogenesis in the uterine cervix, are more apt to antedate the appearance of invasive cancer than was the abnormal surface reaction termed dysplasia. Despite the foregoing well-documented evidence, some expert gynecologic pathologists and cytopathologists state emphatically that there is no documented evidence that abnormal cells arising from lesions classified as in situ cancer and those classified as marked or severe dysplasia can be differentiated on a cellular or biologic basis. It is certainly valid that there is relatively little basis, with respect to clinical management, that the two be distinguished. However, from the standpoint of cytotechnologist and pathologist education and training, it is important to recognize distinct morphologic patterns within the continuum of cervical neoplasia and the biologic potential of lesions classified as carcinoma in situ vs those of marked or severe dysplasia. Again, a majority of microinvasive carcinomas of the uterine cervix arise from intraepithelial lesions possessing the histologic and cytologic features of classic carcinoma in situ, not dysplasia.

Those intraepithelial lesions designated as carcinoma in situ of the uterine cervix are described in the medical literature as preinvasive cancer, noninvasive cancer, incipient cancer, surface cancer, intraepithelial cancer, and intramucosal cancer. In retrospect, it is too bad that these lesions and their representative cytologic counterparts were labeled as carcinoma or cancer because they lack two essential morphologic and biologic prerequisites, namely, the nuclear morphology of true cancer cells and the biologic capability for invasion or infiltration. Therefore, those who refer to abnormal cells arising from these intraepithelial lesions as cancer cells are in error. Perhaps Ayre was correct from a philosophical standpoint in referring to the spectrum of squamous intraepithelial lesions as "the precancer cell complex" or "nearocarcinoma."

Those intraepithelial lesions known as carcinoma in situ involve the surface epithelium of the uterine cervix and, in many instances, the underlying gland-like spaces. Replacement of the columnar epithelium of these underlying structures by these intraepithelial processes, although at times extensive, is not regarded as invasion in the usual sense of the word. Carcinoma in situ has a predilection for the lining mucosa of the endocervical canal in the proximal transformation zone since invariably a coexisting dysplastic reaction is present in the distal portions in a majority of cases. In many patients with evidence of an invasive squamous cell carcinoma, there is a surface lesion resembling that of carcinoma in situ. Therefore, patients with carcinoma in situ must be examined carefully to exclude the presence of an invasive process elsewhere in the uterine cervix. Intraepithelial lesions characterized as carcinoma in situ possess a multilayered epithelium composed entirely of primitive, anaplastic squamous cells. Active cellular proliferation is reflected in the frequency of mitotic division. The layering or polarity of the cells is different from that observed in normal stratified squamous epithelium. The long cell axis is often vertical to the mucosa and may be inconstant. With the exception of several layers of flattened cells at the surface, cell boundaries or evidence of cytoplasmic differentiation are absent, even in the higher layers of the epithelium. In most instances, a basal or germinal cell layer cannot be identified. A similar epithelial lesion may involve the so-called glands of the uterine cervix beneath the sites of surface involvement.

Although there is still some controversy regarding whether cells originating in carcinoma in situ are distinctive, there is no solid evidence to refute the concept that the cellular changes are specific and characteristic of this entity. With experience and careful adherence to the definitions of dysplasia and carcinoma in situ as outlined, it is possible in a significantly high percentage of cases to recognize the squamous intraepithelial lesion known as carcinoma in situ on the basis of the cellular changes.

Cells from carcinoma in situ are usually abundant in material collected by scraping the portio vaginalis of the uterine cervix and sampling the contents of the endocervical canal by aspiration or brushing. In such material, the abnormal cells are usually in excess of 500 per slide. In many instances, the abnormal cell count exceeds 1000 per slide. With other collection techniques, fewer cells may be represented. Depending on the collection technique utilized, abnormal cells originating in carcinoma in situ may be either isolated or arranged in aggregates. Aggregates of abnormal cells are more commonly observed in samples obtained by scraping the ectocervix or brushing the endocervical canal, whereas isolated cells are more frequently present in specimens obtained by aspirating the contents of the endocervical canal or posterior vaginal fornix. Aggregates in the presence of carcinoma in situ have a syncytial-like arrangement in that the component cells are irregularly arranged in relation to one another and they possess indistinct cell borders when examined by light microscopy. A syncytial-like arrangement is identified at some site in the cytologic sample in most cases. Its absence should give pause to an outright interpretation of carcinoma in situ on a cellular basis.

The cells of carcinoma in situ are relatively small compared with mature squamous cells and abnormal cells originating from dysplasia. The mean cell diameter has been reported as 20.8 µm and the mean area as 310 to 352 μm^2. Wied has reported a mean cell area of 381 ± 112 μm^2. The cell area is relatively comparable with that of immature squamous metaplastic cells. The cells are usually round or oval, and there is little cell pleomorphism. The cytoplasmic boundary, whether in syncytial-like arrangements or isolated, is usually indistinct. The staining reaction of the cytoplasm is invariably cyanophilic. Consideration of cellular area and configuration underscores the primitive nature of cells from carcinoma in situ. However, cytoplasmic features alone contribute little toward distinction between normal primitive cells, such as those that might arise from immature squamous metaplasia or reserve cell hyperplasia, and those from carcinoma in situ. For this distinction, nuclear morphology is the prime factor.

The nuclei of cells derived from carcinoma in situ are relatively large (109 μm^2) when compared with nuclei of immature squamous metaplasia and reserve cell hyperplasia (50 μm^2). Dependent on the morphologic variant of carcinoma in situ, the nuclear area ranges from 60 to 200 μm^2. Obviously, the relative nuclear area is variable, depending on the type of in situ cancer from which the cells originate, and ranges from 32% to 75%. While the basic chromatin pattern of the dysplastic cell is finely granular, that of the abnormal cell originating in carcinoma in situ is finely granular with irregular chromatin clumping to frankly coarsely granular chromatin. These chromatin patterns reflect the immaturity and increased biologic activity of these cells. Chromocenters or basophilic "false nucleoli" are observed with considerable frequency in abnormal cells originating in carcinoma in situ. However, circumscribed intranuclear masses that have a distinct eosinophilic staining reaction are rare. They are regarded as micronucleoli because of their size. Large, circumscribed eosinophilic intranuclear masses, or macronucleoli, are not observed in cells originating from carcinoma in situ, and their absence constitutes a significant differential diagnostic feature in distinguishing in situ from frank invasive cancer.

Morphologic Variants of Carcinoma In Situ

Like dysplasia, the intraepithelial lesions defined as carcinoma in situ are represented by a spectrum of morphologic patterns. While basically a lesion composed of primitive or anaplastic cells, variations in cytoplasmic mass and nuclear size result in a varied morphology. Each variant sheds cells that are relatively distinct morphologically. By the criteria of nuclear size, carcinoma in situ may be subdivided into the following types: large, intermediate, and small cell. These three variants of carcinoma in situ represent the intraepithelial lesions from which a majority of invasive cancers originate. Again, the most common form of dysplasia giving rise to invasive cancer is the keratinizing or pleomorphic variant.

Carcinoma In Situ, Large Cell Type

This variant of carcinoma in situ is reminiscent of the histologic features of a severe dysplastic reaction with respect to the thickness of the epithelium (number of cell layers) and relative maturity of the cells composing the abnormal epithelium [▮*11.13*, ▮*11.14*]. However, well-defined cell margins are absent, and the nuclei are relatively large in relation to the cytoplasmic mass. In the cellular sample, abnormal cells originating from large cell carcinoma in situ are relatively few in number with only scattered isolated cells and syncytial-like aggregates reflecting the tissue of origin. The cells are slightly larger than immature squamous metaplastic cells, possessing a mean cell area of 435 μm^2. The nuclei resemble those observed in cells arising from so-called nonkeratinizing dysplasia ranging in size from approximately 150 to 200 μm^2 with a mean nuclear area of 164 μm^2. The calculated relative nuclear area is 38%, although in some cells it approaches 65% to 70%. The nuclear chromatin pattern is hyperchromatic, with a majority of the nuclei having a finely granular, evenly distributed pattern. Approximately 15% of the nuclei may possess a regularly arranged, coarsely granular pattern. Coexisting with the abnormal cells originating from large cell carcinoma in situ is a predominance of abnormal cells from dysplasia. This variant of carcinoma in situ appears to have increased in frequency over the years, now comprising approximately 20% of all in situ cancers of the uterine cervix.

Carcinoma In Situ, Intermediate Type

This variant appears to be the dominant form of in situ cancer of the uterine cervix, comprising approximately 70% of cases [▮*11.15*, ▮*11.16*]. While isolated abnormal cells are invariably present, the usual cellular presentation is syncytial-like aggregates or "microbiopsies." The cells are round or oval in configuration. They are reminiscent of cells originating from very immature squamous metaplasia, but they possess ill-defined cell margins in contrast with the sharply defined cell margins associated with differentiated squamous cells. The mean cell area of this variant is 190 μm². The mean nuclear area is 95 μm² with a relative nuclear area of 50%. The nuclei are hyperchromatic, with a majority having either a finely granular pattern with clumping or a uniformly coarsely granular pattern. The latter appears in approximately 30% of the nuclei. Frequently, a coexisting dysplasia with squamous metaplastic cytoplasmic features is present.

Carcinoma In Situ, Small Cell Type

The cells from this variant of carcinoma in situ usually occur as small, loosely arranged, syncytial-like aggregates of relatively small cells reminiscent of so-called reserve cells with a mean cell area of 95 μm² [▮*11.17*]. Whereas the nuclei are predominantly round and relatively uniform in the large and intermediate types of in situ cancer, the nuclei of the small cell variant are often oval or elongate, presumably due to compression by a high mitotic rate within the tissue of origin. Similarly, the chromatin pattern is predominantly uniformly coarsely granular in well-preserved specimens. This pattern is suggestive of the nuclei of cells approaching impending prophase. In that context, dissolution of the nuclear envelope may be observed and is indicative of impending prophase. The nuclei are relatively small, as would be expected from the cytoplasmic area, the mean nuclear area being 68 μm² with a range of 60 to 80 μm² and a calculated mean relative nuclear area of 72%. This variant of carcinoma in situ appears to have decreased in frequency over the past 30 years, now comprising about 10% of cases.

The chromatin patterns in abnormal cells originating from those intraepithelial lesions classified as dysplasia and carcinoma in situ possess a uniform or even distribution whether finely granular, finely granular with chromocenter formation, or coarsely granular. Similarly, true micronucleoli are, for all practical purposes, not observed in the classic presentation of these intraepithelial lesions.

Again, abnormal cells derived from a carcinoma in situ rarely comprise the entire abnormal cell population. In most instances, abnormal cells from a coexisting dysplasia are represented in the screening pattern. Such cells would be expected to exhibit a varied morphology, dependent on the spectrum or degree of maturation of intraepithelial lesions present in the uterine cervix. Cells originating from squamous metaplasia, reserve cell hyperplasia, hyperkeratosis, or parakeratosis may be associated with the presence of a coexisting dysplasia. Cellular evidence of HPV may or may not be present. All three morphologic variants of carcinoma in situ may coexist and be represented in the cellular sample. As is true of most normal or physiologic surface reactions in the uterine cervix, such as squamous metaplasia, the most primitive or immature abnormal intraepithelial lesion is found highest in the endocervical canal and the most mature closest to the ectocervix.

In addition to the three foregoing variants of carcinoma in situ, which represent the most common intraepithelial precursor lesions for microinvasive carcinoma, the so-called keratinizing dysplasias represent a fourth type of intraepithelial precursor lesion for the development of microinvasive squamous cell carcinoma. It is often referred to as squamous, well-differentiated, or keratinizing carcinoma in situ.

MICROINVASIVE SQUAMOUS CELL CARCINOMA

Microinvasive carcinoma [▮*11.18*] refers to a microscopic epithelial penetration of the cervical stroma from an overlying squamous intraepithelial lesion (carcinoma in situ or, less often, dysplasia). Microinvasion usually originates from an abnormal surface epithelium and less frequently from an abnormal epithelial lesion that has extended into underlying gland-like spaces. When microinvasive carcinoma is limited in extent, the invading foci are single or multiple and tend to be in continuity with the overlying epithelial lesion. With greater depths of penetration, a multifocal origin is more commonly observed, and the infiltrating cords of cells are less readily traced to the surface epithelium. At the site of stromal penetration, the epithelial cords are surrounded by a distinctive stromal infiltrate of leukocytes. In biopsy specimens, potential sites of microinvasion may be represented by foci of cellular "differentiation" in the deep layers of an otherwise primitive or anaplastic surface lesion. In addition to cytoplasmic eosinophilia and apparent increase in cytoplasmic mass, the nuclei may assume the features more often associated with frank cancer in the foregoing zones of potential stromal penetration.

On the basis of cellular morphology, it is frequently possible to suggest the presence of an early or microinvasive process. When the cellular pattern is suggestive of early invasion, this should be reported to the clinician. In most instances, foci of microinvasive carcinoma are not readily recognized by even the most skilled colposcopist. The cellular changes are often distinctly different from those commonly associated with classic carcinoma in situ or invasive squamous cell carcinoma. When considered in relation to the extent of stromal infiltration by an abnormal intraepithelial lesion, the cellular changes are more reminiscent of those of carcinoma in situ when the degree of infiltration or penetration is limited. This is in contrast with the cellular features of those lesions with a greater extent of stromal penetration, and the abnormal cell population possesses features more reminiscent of frank cancer.

The earliest cellular changes associated with a microinvasive cancer are superimposed on a cellular pattern most often suggestive of carcinoma in situ. These include a relative increase in the number of abnormal cells identified in syncytial-like aggregates, the presence of distinct eosinophilic micronucleoli in most abnormal cell nuclei possessing the cytoplasmic features of classic in situ cancer, and an alteration of the chromatin pattern characterized by change from a uniform to an irregular distribution, sometimes referred to as "nuclear clearing." The magnitude of the changes in nuclear morphology is directly proportional to the extent of infiltration. In most instances, abnormal cells originating from foci of microinvasive carcinoma, in which there is stromal penetration to a depth of 3 mm from the epithelial-stromal junction, possess nuclear features that are indistinguishable from those associated with frank cancer.

Finally, the abnormal cells with these features do not originate directly from the zones of stromal penetration. Rather, the distinctive nuclear changes develop in a preexisting surface squamous intraepithelial lesion most likely just prior to the active process of stromal penetration. If cells were to be obtained from the foci of early penetrating epithelium, their nuclear structure most likely would resemble that of frank cancer.

INVASIVE SQUAMOUS CELL CARCINOMA

Like its precursors, squamous cell carcinoma of the uterine cervix is characterized by varying morphologic patterns. Some have their origins on the portio vaginalis and tend to arise from intraepithelial lesions possessing the features of keratinization and cellular pleomorphism. Often, this form of invasive cancer forms a bulky outgrowth from the uterine cervix, sometimes referred to as an exophytic growth pattern. Because of its tendency to produce keratin, this type of invasive cancer is referred to as keratinizing squamous cell carcinoma [▮*11.19*, ▮*11.20*]. In the past, keratinizing carcinoma of the uterine cervix represented approximately 40% of the cases, but it presently comprises less than 20% of invasive cancers. The most common morphologic variant of squamous cell carcinoma of the uterine cervix, in many respects, resembles the normal stratified squamous epithelium of the cervix and, for this reason, has been termed large cell nonkeratinizing squamous cell carcinoma [▮*11.21*, ▮*11.22*]. This form of invasive cancer has its origin in the distal portions of the endocervical canal near the external cervical os. It tends to arise from an intraepithelial lesion, resembling carcinoma in situ of the large cell or intermediate type. Its growth pattern is generally not exophytic, as with the keratinizing cancers, but is rather endophytic. While previously approximately equal in occurrence with keratinizing carcinoma, this form now comprises over 70% of the cases of invasive cancer of the uterine cervix. A third morphologic variant of invasive carcinoma of the uterine cervix has its origin, in most instances, high in the endocervical canal, apparently arising from an abnormal intraepithelial lesion most often resembling small cell carcinoma in situ. Because of the relatively small size of the component cells and growth pattern in the cervical stroma, this form of cervical cancer has been termed small cell or anaplastic carcinoma, which implies a squamous origin [▮*11.23*, ▮*11.24*]. Recent studies have shown that many of these small cell neoplasms of the uterine cervix are malignant neuroendocrine tumors resembling the small cell cancers of the lung. However, on a cytologic basis, it is impossible to recognize the neuroendocrine features of this group of invasive cancers without the application of immunocytochemical techniques or electron microscopy. Although now distinguished from squamous cell carcinomas and considered as a separate group with other neuroendocrine tumors such as the carcinoids, it remains convenient to consider them in the context of the invasive squamous cell cancers because logically there should be an invasive counterpart to the anaplastic small cell variant of in situ cancer. Whereas so-called small cell cancers of the cervix comprised approximately 20% of all cases 30 years ago, its occurrence today is in the range of 5% to 10%.

The basis for any morphologic subclassification of a particular variety of cancer is an attempt to provide some uniformity in reporting for statistical purposes as well as to yield information relative to its potential behavior after appropriate therapy. In that context, the aforementioned classification of squamous cell carcinoma of the uterine cervix appears to satisfactorily meet both criteria. In general, large cell nonkeratinizing carcinoma has an extremely favorable 5-year survival rate after therapy, approaching approximately 80% for all cases. Conversely, small cell carcinomas of the uterine cervix have an extremely poor 5-year survival rate, approaching less than 5% in recent years. Keratinizing squamous cell carcinoma of the uterine cervix possesses an overall 5-year survival rate intermediate between the foregoing variants, approaching 50% overall. Therefore, with a predominance of large cell nonkeratinizing carcinomas, survival for patients developing invasive cancer of the uterine cervix today is more optimistic than it was 25 years ago.

General Cytologic Features of the Malignant Tumor Cell

Although functionally and chemically, certain differences are apparent between normal cells and those making up a malignant tumor, as yet there is no known substance or characteristic that is present in all malignant tumor cells and absent in all benign or normal cells. Recent advances in immunocytochemistry, however, give promise for the future. In the practice of cytology the identification of a malignant tumor cell becomes more certain when distinguishing morphologic characteristics are more numerous. Similarly, the identification is more accurate when based on a study of many cells rather than a single cell. Although under certain circumstances a few seriously altered cells may be of great significance, the interpretation is generally more accurate when based on many cells having the characteristics of a malignant tumor cell. No single feature of the malignant tumor cell is in itself diagnostic.

Nuclear enlargement and an alteration in the nuclear/cytoplasmic ratio (relative nuclear area) are important characteristics of the malignant tumor cell. This can be appreciated by comparing the nuclear size of a malignant tumor cell with that of a normal counterpart, if present. Nuclear enlargement has been attributed to many factors, including increased DNA content, an increase in the number of chromosomes, and the process of endomitosis. Nuclear enlargement may also be associated with certain degenerative changes, in cells originating in benign proliferative reactions, and in abnormal intraepithelial lesions antedating the development of frank cancer.

Variation in nuclear size may be observed in the cells of some malignant tumors. This is of greater significance when observed in the cells of a so-called microbiopsy or cell aggregate in the cytologic sample. This may also be apparent when comparing the nuclear sizes of isolated cells. The observation is more significant in the presence of marked variations in nuclear size. It is not completely clear why some malignant neoplasms possess a heterogeneous cellular composition and others a homogeneous cellular content, although the latter may represent a monoclonal origin.

Alterations in nuclear chromatin structure and hyperchromasia are important diagnostic morphologic features of the malignant tumor cell. Hyperchromasia may be related to an increase in the amount of chromatinic material or a change in its character. It is desirable to compare the nuclear staining of the abnormal cells with that of coexisting normal cells. The chromatin pattern of the malignant tumor cell may be aggregated in coarse masses of various sizes and shape and may differ in its distribution from one site to another within the nucleus. The aberrations are many and varied. Large discrete DNA masses or chromocenters may be conspicuous in some neoplastic cells. In some tumor cells, there may be depositions of chromatinic material beneath the nuclear envelope (chromatinic membrane). Some studies have suggested that these changes may be related to polyploidy; in other instances, they may be evidence of initial cell degeneration.

Variations in nuclear shape are observed in many malignant tumor cells. This may, in part, be related to cellular shape but not necessarily. Lobulated, bizarre, or other abnormal nuclear configurations may occur. In some instances, these abnormal configurations may be secondary to incomplete mitoses. In general, these variations are more commonly associated with rapidly growing malignant tumors.

Macronucleoli are large, circumscribed eosinophilic intranuclear bodies that are observed in some tumor cells. The nucleolar area of cancer cells may be four to five times as great as that of normal cells. One or more enlarged nucleoli may be observed. When the macronucleoli are both enlarged and abnormal in shape, they are of greater diagnostic significance. However, nucleolar enlargement is also characteristic of regenerating cells, and this feature in itself is not diagnostic of the malignant tumor cell. The true nucleolus should be distinguished from large basophilic intranuclear masses or chromocenters that commonly occur in the cells of many benign proliferative reactions.

Multinucleation is of only limited value in the identification of the malignant tumor cell unless the component nuclei are markedly varied in size, shape, or structure. Multinucleation may occur in epithelial cells, histiocytes, and cells derived from benign proliferative reactions.

Mitosis, or evidence of cell division, is uncommon in isolated tumor cells. While nuclear chromatin patterns suggestive of an impending prophase are observed with some frequency, it is unusual to observe isolated tumor cells in anaphase or metaphase. On the other hand, an abnormal cell division may be of some diagnostic significance.

Indistinct cell boundaries are observed in many malignant tumor cells, as well as in some normal cells. This may be related to the presence of microvilli over the surface of the cell, as demonstrated by electron microscopy. This feature is more commonly associated with undifferentiated malignant tumors, whereas cells derived from more differentiated malignant tumors are more likely to have distinct cell boundaries.

Variations in cell size can be appreciated by examining the cells of small tissue fragments or cell aggregates. Some malignant tumor cells are varied in size while others are more uniform. Most are smaller than their normal counterparts, although there are exceptions to this.

Variation in cell shape may be outstanding in some malignant tumors. The bizarre, elongate, caudate, and otherwise irregular forms are easily identified. Their configuration is significant only when associated with altered nuclear structure. Of the malignant neoplasms arising in the uterine cervix, those associated with abnormalities of keratinization are most likely to be associated with bizarre forms. Bizarre cellular forms may also originate from various nonepithelial malignant neoplasms of the female genital tract, such as sarcomas of the uterine corpus.

The cytoplasmic staining reaction is seldom an important diagnostic feature. However, an orange, yellow, or eosinophilic cytoplasmic stain is common in cells originating from malignant tumors possessing morphologic evidence of keratinization. Most malignant tumor cells, like primitive cells, possess a cyanophilic cytoplasm.

Abnormal cell groupings of various types may be observed in cellular samples. These represent changes in the inter-relationships of cells. In squamous cell carcinoma of the uterine cervix, the groupings or "microbiopsies" reflect the arrangement of the cells in the malignant tumor. These minute tissue fragments or cell aggregates provide considerable information about the neoplasm. The most common arrangement observed in the cellular sample in the presence of a malignant neoplasm is that of a syncytial-like aggregate.

The host response to the presence of a malignant neoplasm may be of considerable diagnostic importance when reflected in the cellular sample. This so-called tumor diathesis is characterized by the presence of eosinophilic or cyanophilic granular debris, cellular detritus, and hemosiderin. While certain benign conditions involving the uterus may produce similar material in the cytologic sample, this is rare. However, a host response in the absence of cellular abnormality is not in itself diagnostic.

General Cytologic Features of Squamous Cell Carcinoma

Compared with superficial squamous cells, cells originating in squamous cell cancer of the uterine cervix are relatively small, having a mean cytoplasmic area of 229 ± 83 μm^2. Depending on the type of specimen and the nature of the cancer present, the number of cancer cells present on a slide varies considerably. Some cancer cells occur isolated (51%), while many are arranged in some form of cell aggregate (49%). Approximately 41% of the abnormal cells are observed in syncytial-like arrangements. The configuration of the malignant tumor cells depends to some extent on the type of cancer that exists. Approximately 75% of the abnormal cells are round or oval, the remaining being caudate, elongate, or otherwise irregular in form. About 25% of the cancer cells have a cytoplasm that stains orange, red, yellow, or eosinophilic. An additional 25% of the cells have an indeterminate cytoplasmic staining, which is neither clearly eosinophilic nor cyanophilic. In 50% of the cells, there is a cyanophilic staining reaction, which is more commonly associated with less-differentiated tumors. The nucleus of the cell originating in squamous cell cancer of the uterine cervix averages more than twice the size of that of the normal intermediate squamous cell or 77 ± 27 μm^2. In relation to the apparent size of the cell, the nucleus is relatively large in the squamous cancer cell (35%). The nuclear shape, in part, reflects the shape of the cell. As a result, in cells of squamous cell cancer, there are significant numbers of ovoid or somewhat elongate nuclei (64%). Nuclear hyperchromatism is a prominent feature in the cells of squamous cell carcinoma. In about 25% of the cells the nuclear chromatin pattern is finely granular, while in 50% there is a coarse granularity to the chromatinic material. Whether finely or coarsely granular, there is invariably an uneven distribution of the chromatinic material or nuclear clearing. In about 25% of the cells, the nuclear mass is either translucent or opaque without definite structure. Such cells are malignant tumor cells that are undergoing degeneration. Discrete macronucleoli are observed in more than 10% of the cells originating from squamous cell cancers of the uterine cervix. The basis for the identification of relatively few cancer cells with nucleoli is that cell samples are generally obtained from the biologically less active surface of the neoplasm rather than from zones of active growth deep in the cervical stroma. At least some of the cells observed in cell samples from patients with invasive cancer originate in coexisting surface changes that may resemble dysplasia and or carcinoma in situ. Evidence of degeneration and inflammation are common, depending on the nature of the cancer and its stage of development.

The Cytologic Subclassification of Squamous Cell Carcinoma

In addition to permitting a more critical evaluation of the cellular sample, the chief objective for the subclassification of invasive cancer on a cellular basis is its potential prognostic value. An adequate cellular preparation represents a comprehensive sample of any lesion involving the uterine cervix. Because of this, it may be more representative of an abnormal process in certain cases than a tissue sample of limited size. Under such circumstances, the histologic classification may be of limited value for predicting survival, whereas on the basis of a specific interpretation of the cellular sample, more accurate information on the potential biologic behavior of the neoplasm is possible.

In keratinizing squamous cell carcinoma, the abnormal cell population in the presence of this variant of cervical cancer includes many large cells that are highly variable in size and configuration [▮*11.19*, ▮*11.20*]. In the presence of a keratinizing cancer, a host response or tumor diathesis is usually not conspicuous in contrast to that observed in cellular preparations derived from other types of invasive cancer of the uterine cervix. The mean cell area is 275 ± 107 μm^2, which demonstrates that this form of invasive cancer is characterized by relatively large cells. The relatively large standard deviation underscores the prominent variation in cell population. Cellular pleomorphism is the distinguishing feature of keratinizing carcinoma, with approximately 15% of the tumor cell population being represented by elongate and caudate forms. A majority of the abnormal cells derived from keratinizing cancer are isolated, with approximately 13% occurring in syncytial-like aggregates. In most instances, the latter are not pleomorphic but are more reminiscent of a nonkeratinizing cancer. Cytoplasmic orangeophilia or eosinophilia is a prominent feature of cells originating from keratinizing cancer. The nuclei are intermediate in size, with a mean nuclear area of 77 ± 28 μm^2. However, a mean relative nuclear area of 29% implies that the cytoplasm of the altered cells is relatively more abundant than that of other forms of invasive cancer. The nuclear chromatin is finely granular in 22% of the abnormal cells and coarsely granular in 59%. An opaque or translucent nucleus is identified in 19% of the cells, most probably reflecting a degenerative process. This nuclear alteration is observed only rarely in the other variants of squamous cell cancer of the uterine cervix.

Cellular evidence of hyperkeratosis and/or parakeratosis may be observed in a significant number of preparations from keratinizing carcinoma. Frequently, abnormal cells presumed to be originating from an invasive keratinizing carcinoma may in fact be arising predominantly from a severe surface intraepithelial lesion possessing the characteristics of a keratinizing dysplasia. Therefore, in the absence of relatively large numbers of abnormal pleomorphic forms, abnormal cells with coarsely granular chromatin patterns, and macronucleoli or abnormal cells in syncytial-like aggregates, a definitive cytologic interpretation of an invasive process may not be possible. In cases where differentiation between a keratinizing intraepithelial or invasive process may not be possible on the basis of the cellular evidence, a diagnosis of "marked keratinizing dysplasia (keratinizing carcinoma in situ), keratinizing squamous cell carcinoma cannot be excluded" may be justified.

Abnormal cells originating from large cell nonkeratinizing squamous cell carcinoma are observed in association with a tumor background or diathesis in most cases, which reflects the host's response to the invasive neoplastic process [▮*11.21*, ▮*11.22*]. The cells are relatively large and somewhat variable in size, with a mean cell area of 256 ± 69 μm^2. While many of the abnormal cells are isolated, a significant number occur in syncytial-like aggregates (23%). Although the cytoplasmic staining reaction may be variable, the predominant reaction is cyanophilic. Cytoplasmic lysis is prominent in the presence of nonkeratinizing cancers, resulting in the identification of numerous "free" or "striped" abnormal nuclei in most cases. Their presence in the screening pattern may be helpful in suggesting that an abnormal process is present, but they in themselves are not diagnostic. A definitive interpretation of cancer should always be founded on features present in intact cells. The nuclei are relatively large, with a mean area of 88 ± 30 μm^2, and are usually characterized by a hyperchromatic, irregularly coarsely granular chromatinic pattern. Macronucleoli may be conspicuous, with their identification in approximately 24% of the abnormal cells (Reagan's original analytic study reported 24 macronucleoli per slide or case).

The abnormal cell population in small cell carcinoma includes many small, relatively uniform cells, with a mean area of 169 ± 37 μm^2 [▮*11.23*, ▮*11.24*]. They are usually associated with evidence of an abnormal host response or tumor diathesis. The cells are usually observed in a loose syncytial-like arrangement, although differences in sampling techniques might result in a greater population of isolated cells. The cytoplasmic staining reaction is usually cyanophilic. The nuclei of cells derived from small cell cancers are relatively small, with a mean nuclear area of 65 ± 13 μm^2. While not a particularly prominent feature of the other variants of cervical cancer, the nuclei of the small cell or anaplastic type are frequently oval, which probably reflects extracellular pressure due to a relatively high rate of proliferation within the neoplasm. The nuclear chromatin is predominantly hyperchromatic and irregularly coarsely granular, as reflected by approximately 80% of the cells. While these neoplasms are now classified within the neuroendocrine group of small cell tumors and therefore are presumably related to the small or oat cell carcinomas of the lung, the nuclear structure observed in classic oat cell carcinomas are not observed in the small cell cancers of the uterine cervix, nor is the nuclear pattern of the so-called intermediate type of small cell cancer of the lung. Nucleoli occur with about the same frequency as they do in cells derived from a nonkeratinizing carcinoma. Because of the nuclear size and dense chromatin pattern, it is often difficult to appreciate the presence of the nucleoli.

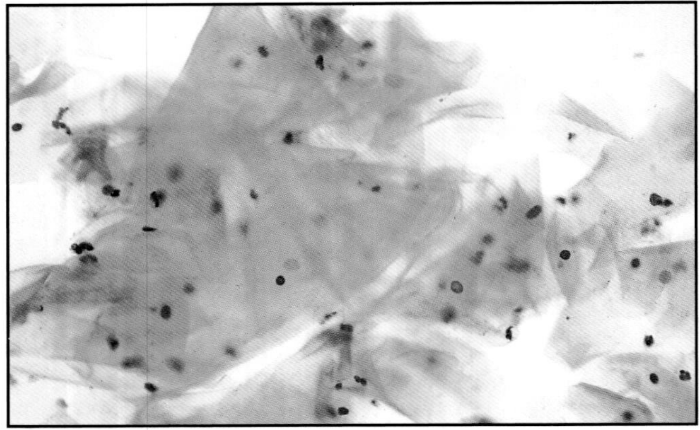

11.1
Anucleate squames derived from hyperkeratosis (x400).

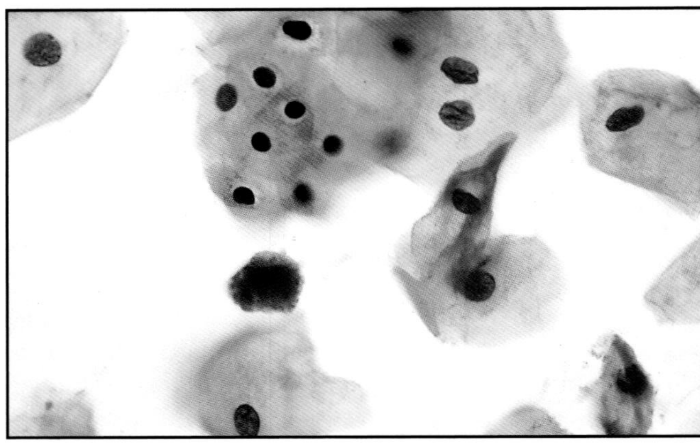

11.2
Miniature squamous cells with pyknotic nuclei derived from parakeratosis (x400).

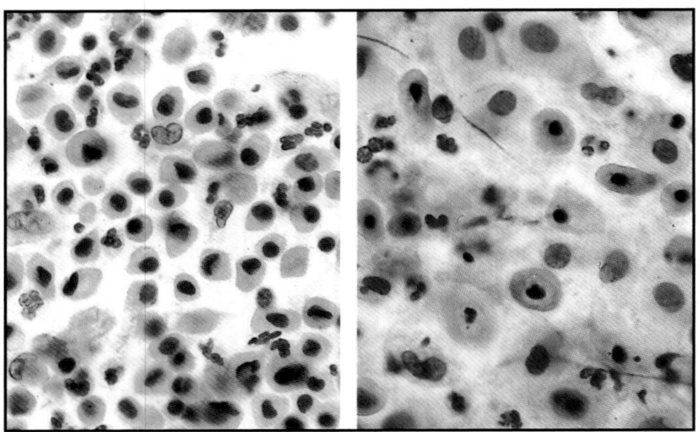

11.3
Left, Parakeratotic-like epithelial changes in degenerating atrophic squamous cells observed in postmenopausal patients (x400). Right, Parakeratotic-like epithelial reaction ("pseudoparakeratosis") secondary to oral contraceptives (x400).

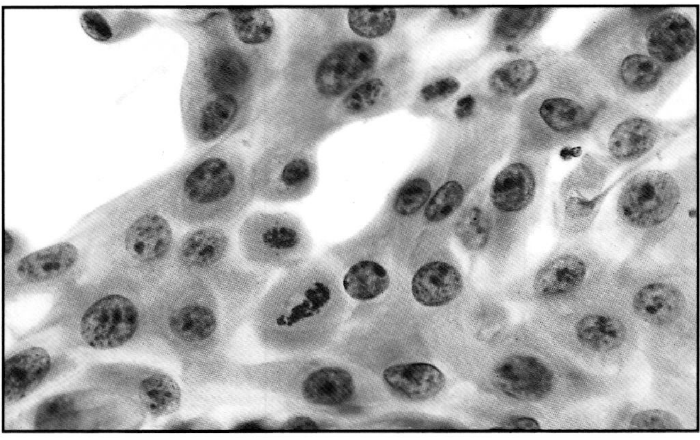

11.4
Atypical squamous cells derived from so-called benign epithelial reparative reaction. Note prominent nucleoli (x400).

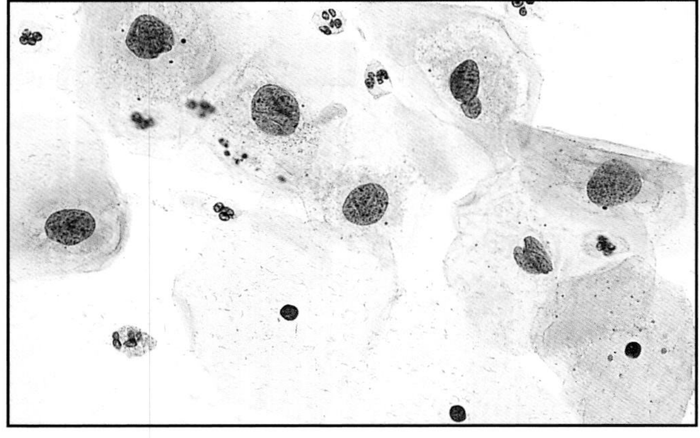

11.5
Atypical cells of squamous type "of undetermined significance" (x400).

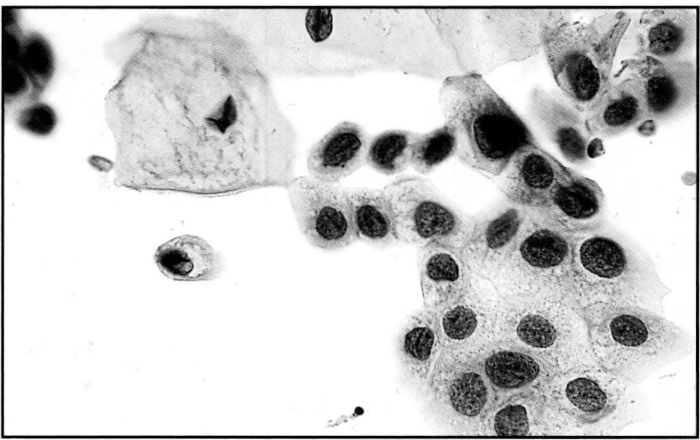

11.6
Atypical cells of immature squamous metaplastic type "of undetermined significance" (x400).

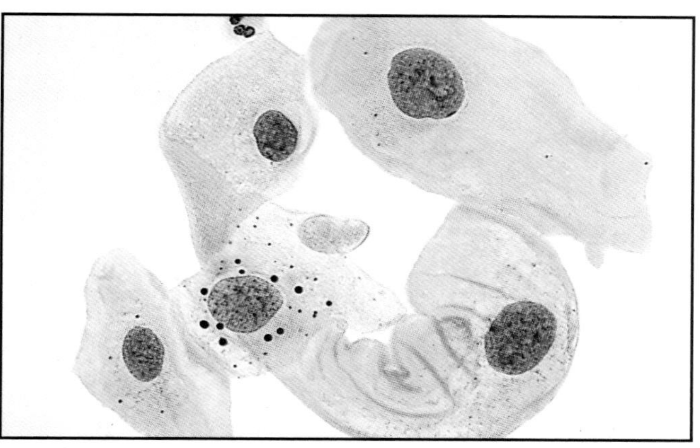

11.7
Abnormal squamous cells derived from slight (mild) dysplasia (LGSIL, CIN 1) (x400).

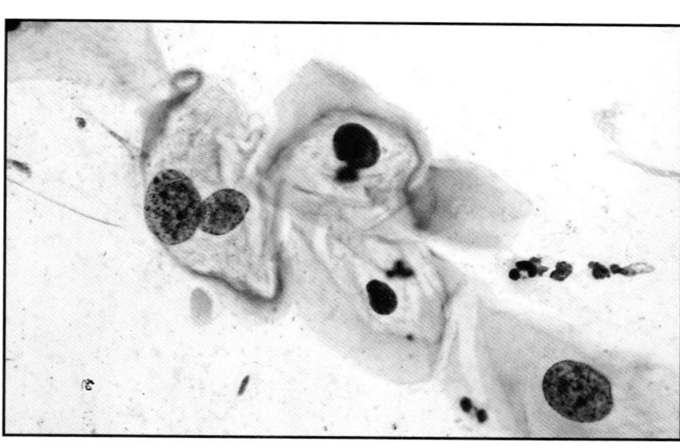

11.8
Abnormal squamous cells derived from slight (mild) dysplasia with coexisting HPV cytopathic effect (LGSIL, CIN 1) (x400).

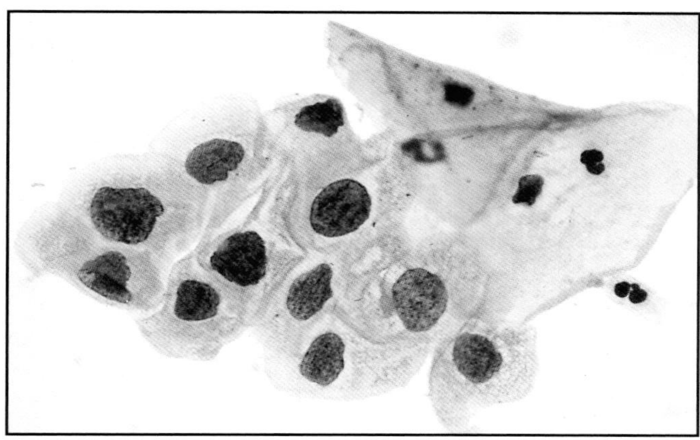

11.9
Abnormal squamous cells derived from moderate dysplasia (HGSIL, CIN 2) (x400).

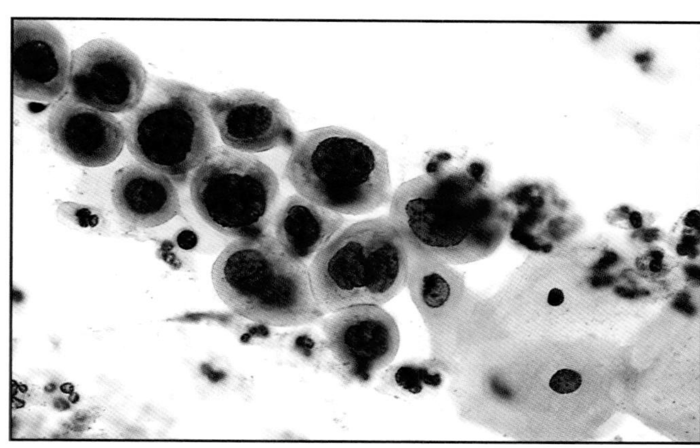

11.10
Abnormal squamous cells derived from marked (severe) dysplasia (HGSIL, CIN 3) (x400).

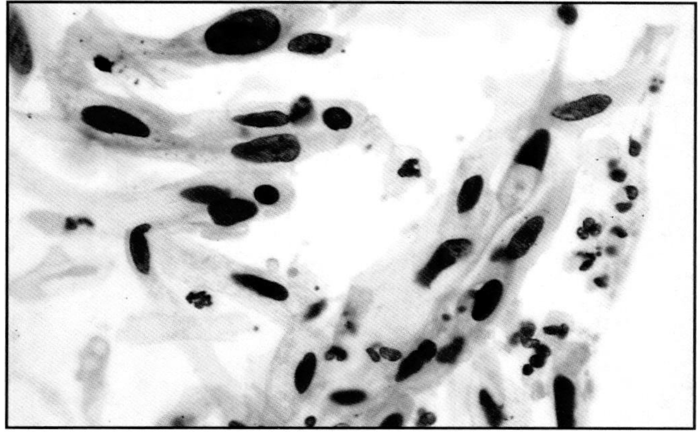

11.11
Abnormal squamous cells derived from moderate to marked dysplasia, keratinizing or pleomorphic type (HGSIL, CIN 2-3) (x400).

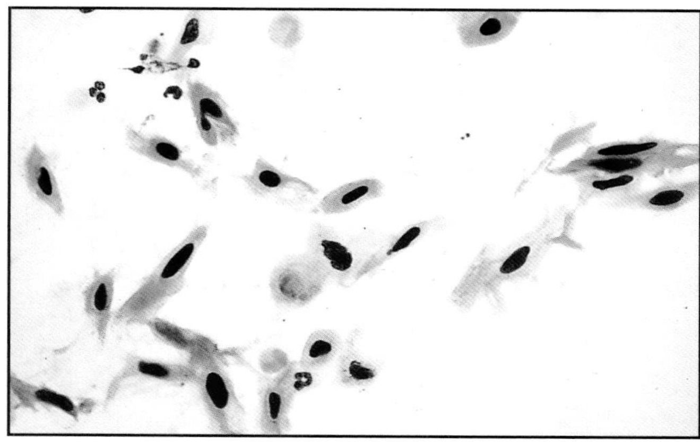

11.12
Abnormal or pleomorphic parakeratosis observed in association with keratinizing or pleomorphic dysplasia. Note miniature caudate and elongate forms (x400).

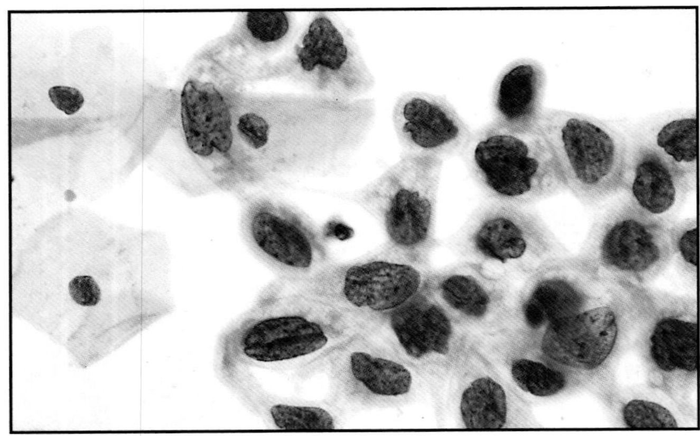

▌11.13
Abnormal anaplastic squamous cells derived from carcinoma in situ, large cell type (HGSIL, CIN 3) (x400).

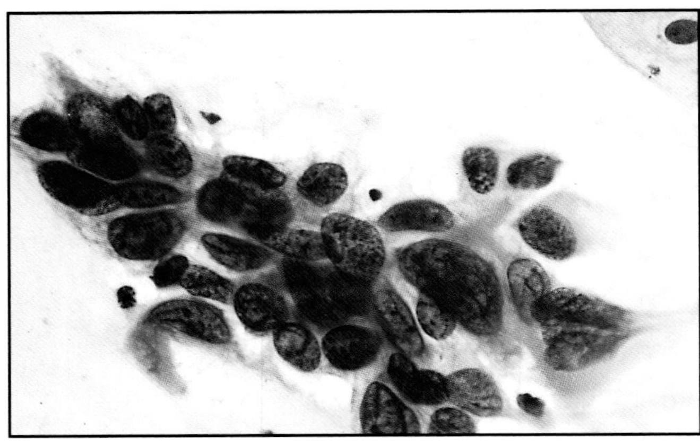

▌11.14
Abnormal anaplastic squamous cells derived from carcinoma in situ, large cell type (HGSIL, CIN 3) (x400).

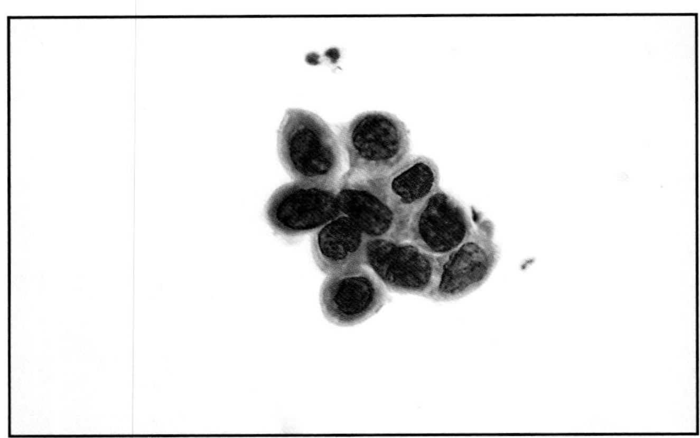

▌11.15
Abnormal anaplastic squamous cells derived from carcinoma in situ, intermediate type (HGSIL, CIN 3) (x400).

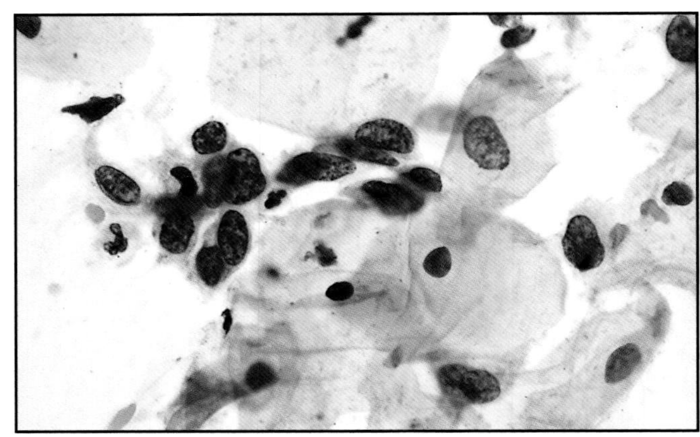

▌11.16
Abnormal anaplastic squamous cells derived from carcinoma in situ, intermediate type. Note uniformly coarse chromatin pattern (HGSIL, CIN 3) (x400).

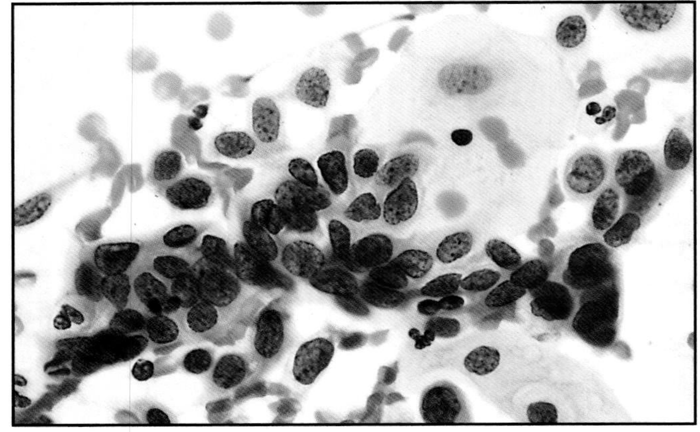

▌11.17
Abnormal anaplastic squamous cells derived from carcinoma in situ, small cell type (HGSIL, CIN 3) (x400).

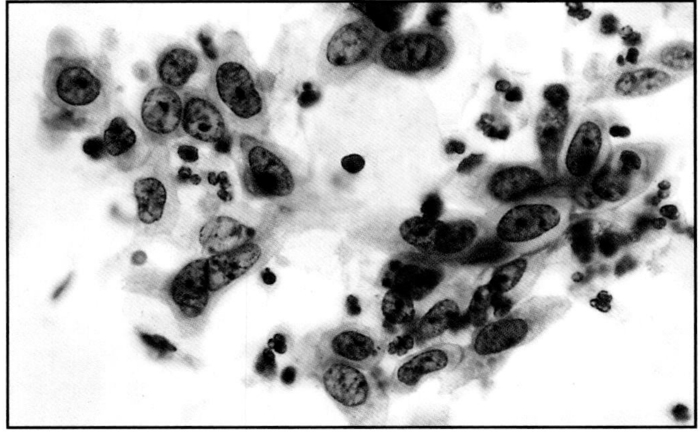

▌11.18
Abnormal anaplastic squamous cells derived from microinvasive squamous cell carcinoma. Note micronucleoli and irregular chromatin distribution (x400).

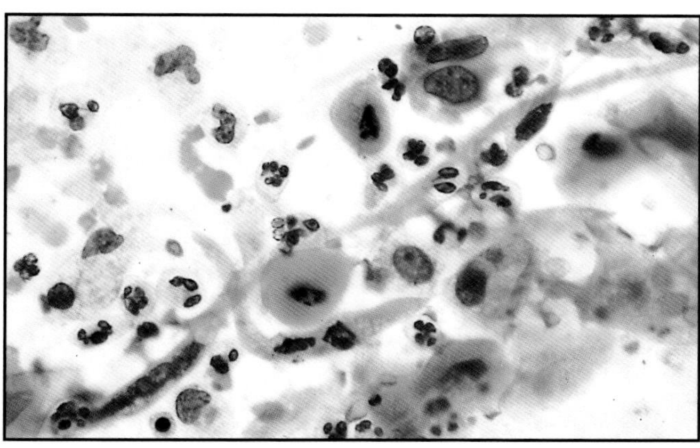

▮*11.19*

Malignant tumor cells derived from squamous cell carcinoma, keratinizing type (x400).

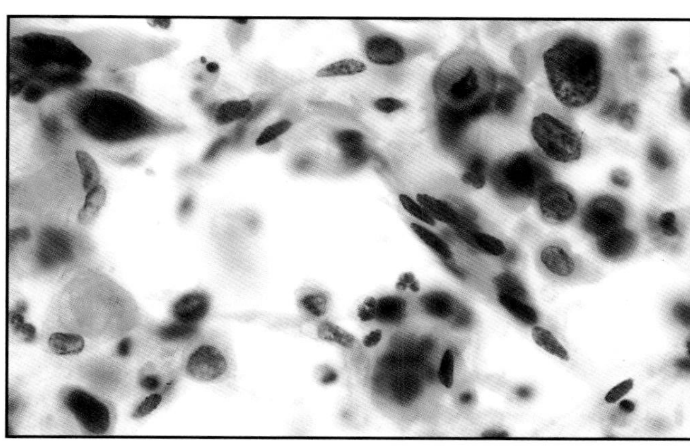

▮*11.20*

Malignant tumor cells derived from squamous cell carcinoma, keratinizing type (x400).

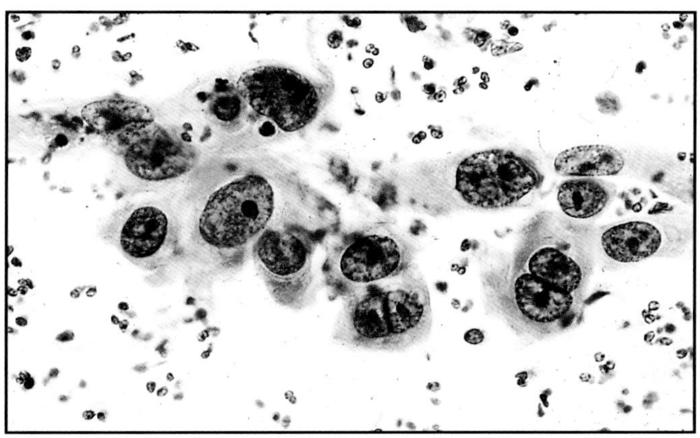

▮*11.21*

Malignant tumor cells derived from squamous cell carcinoma, large cell nonkeratinizing type (x400).

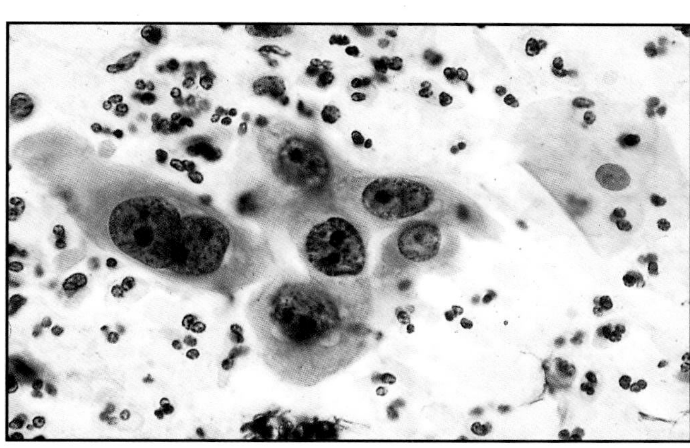

▮*11.22*

Malignant tumor cells derived from squamous cell carcinoma, large cell nonkeratinizing type (x400).

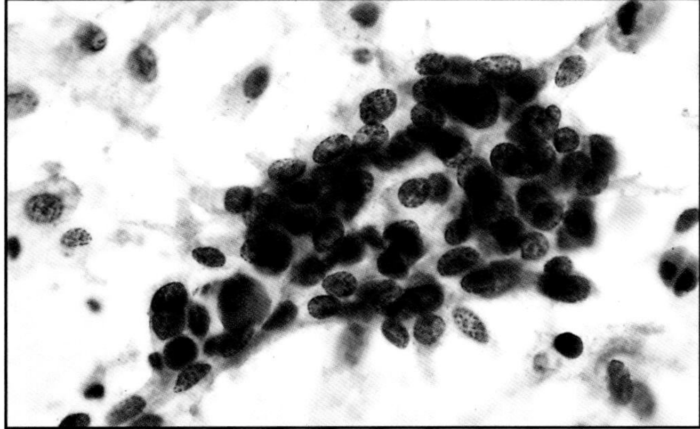

▮*11.23*

Malignant tumor cells derived from small cell carcinoma of the uterine cervix (x400).

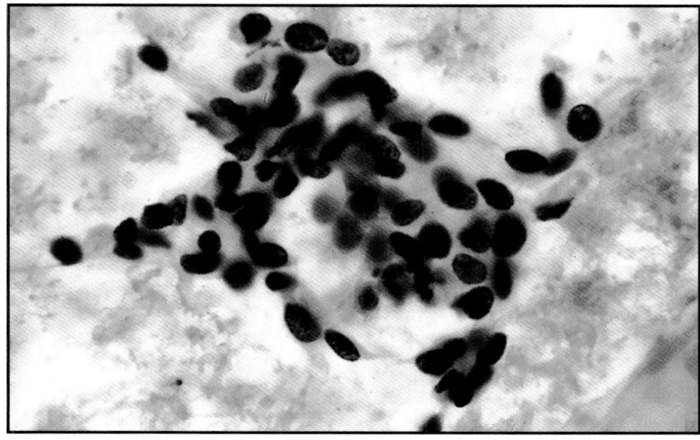

▮*11.24*

Malignant tumor cells derived from small cell carcinoma of the uterine cervix (x400).

REVIEW EXERCISES

1. From a differential diagnostic standpoint, compare the cellular features of the following.
   a) Small cell carcinoma
   b) Normal deep endometrial stromal cells
   c) Carcinoma in situ, small cell type

2. In terms of the following features, compare in chart form the three morphologic variants of squamous cell carcinoma of the uterine cervix.
   a) Probable surface intraepithelial lesion of origin
   b) Probable anatomic location in the uterine cervix
   c) Cell size
   d) Nuclear size
   e) Relative nuclear area
   f) Cellular pleomorphism
   g) Syncytial-like aggregates
   h) Macronucleoli
   i) Chromatin pattern
   j) Tumor diathesis

3. What are the main distinguishing cellular features of those squamous intraepithelial lesions classified as dysplasia and carcinoma in situ?

4. What are the cellular features that sometimes help distinguish abnormal cells originating from an early or microinvasive carcinoma of the uterine cervix from those originating from classic carcinoma in situ and advanced invasive carcinoma?

SELECTED READINGS

Ayre JE. *Cancer Cytology of the Uterus*. New York, NY: Grune & Stratton; 1951:130-218.

Bonfiglio TA. Cytopathology of dysplasia, carcinoma in situ and invasive carcinoma of the uterine cervix. In: Astarita RW, ed. *Practical Cytopathology*. New York, NY: Churchill Livingstone Inc; 1990:60-82.

Ng ABP, Reagan JW. Microinvasive carcinoma of the uterine cervix. *Am J Clin Pathol*. 1969;52:511-529.

Ng ABP, Reagan JW, Lindner EA. The cellular manifestation of microinvasive squamous cell carcinoma of the uterine cervix. *Acta Cytol*. 1972;16:5-13.

Patten SF Jr. Benign proliferative reactions of the uterine cervix. In: Wied GL, Keebler CM, Koss LG, Reagan JW, eds. *Compendium on Diagnostic Cytology*. 6th ed. Chicago, Ill: Tutorials of Cytology; 1990:83-87.

Patten SF Jr. *Diagnostic Cytopathology of the Uterine Cervix*. 2nd ed. Basel, Switzerland: S Karger; 1978:3. In: Wied GL, ed. Monographs in Clinical Cytology.

Patten SF Jr. Dysplasia of the uterine cervix. In: Lewis GG, Wentz WB, Jaffe RM, eds. *New Concepts in Gynecological Oncology*. Philadelphia, Pa: FA Davis Co; 1966:33-44.

Patten SF Jr. Morphologic subclassification of preinvasive cervical neoplasia. In: Wied GL, Keebler CM, Koss LG, Reagan JW, eds. *Compendium on Diagnostic Cytology*. 6th ed. Chicago, Ill: Tutorials of Cytology; 1990:105-113.

Reagan JW. The nature of the cells originating in so-called "precancerous" lesions of the uterine cervix. *Obstet Gynecol Surv*. 1958;13:157-179.

Reagan JW, Bell BA, Neuman JL, Scott RB, Patten SF Jr. Dysplasia in the uterine cervix during pregnancy: an analytical study of the cells. *Acta Cytol*. 1961;5:17-29.

Reagan JW, Hamonic MJ. The cellular pathology in carcinoma in situ: a cytohistopathological correlation. *Cancer*. 1956;9:385-402.

Reagan JW, Hamonic MJ. Dysplasia of the uterine cervix. *Ann N Y Acad Sci*. 1956;63:1236-1244.

Reagan JW, Hamonic MJ, Wentz WB. Analytical study of the cells in cervical squamous cell cancer. *Lab Invest*. 1957;6:241-250.

Reagan JW, Patten SF Jr. Analytical study of cellular changes in carcinoma in situ, squamous cell cancer, and adenocarcinoma of the uterine cervix. *Clin Obstet Gynecol*. 1961;4:1097-1125.

Reagan JW, Patten SF Jr. Dysplasia: a basic reaction to injury in the uterine cervix. *Ann N Y Acad Sci*. 1962;97:662-682.

Reagan JW, Seidemann IL, Patten SF Jr. Developmental stages of in situ carcinoma in uterine cervix: an analytical study of the cells. *Acta Cytol*. 1962;6:538-546.

Reagan JW, Seidemann IL, Saracuse Y. The cellular morphology of carcinoma in situ and dysplasia or atypical hyperplasia of the uterine cervix. *Cancer*. 1953;6:224-235.

van Niekerk WA. Cervical cytological abnormalities caused by folic acid deficiency. *Acta Cytol*. 1966;10:67-73.

Vooijs GP. Benign proliferative reactions, intraepithelial neoplasia and invasive cancer of the uterine cervix. In: Bibbo M, ed. *Comprehensive Cytopathology*. Philadelphia, Pa: WB Saunders Company; 1991:153-230.

Wentz WB, Lewis GG. Correlation of histologic morphology and survival in clinical cancer following radiation therapy. *Obstet Gynecol*. 1965;26:228-232.

CHAPTER 12

Human Papillomavirus Infections

Alexander Meisels, MD, FRCPC, FIAC

CONTENTS

The human papillomaviruses (HPVs) are small (55 nm) DNA viruses of the Papova family. They comprise a group of nearly 70 types, which differ from one another by at least 50% of DNA homology as determined by reassociation of heterologous DNA in liquid phase followed by S/nuclease digestion. The circular DNA contains approximately 7900 base pairs. HPVs cannot be cultured in vitro. For this reason, much of what is known today has been obtained by methods of molecular DNA or RNA hybridization, for which the standard has been the Southern blot technique. Newly developed and extremely sensitive techniques using gene amplification by polymerase chain reaction (PCR) are opening further research possibilities, particularly in the field of epidemiology.

Papillomaviruses are common viruses that infect many mammals but are not transmitted from one species to another. They are also site-specific: skin HPVs only rarely produce mucosal lesions, and vice versa. About 25 HPV types are found in the female genital tract. Types 6 and 11 produce warty lesions on the external genitalia, known as condylomata acuminata, but these HPV types can also be found in some of the flat intraepithelial lesions of the cervix. They are considered to have very little oncogenic association. Types 16 and 18 and associated types are found in intraepithelial lesions and in invasive carcinomas of the cervix, vagina, vulva, and perineal and perianal areas, as well as of the penis, and are therefore considered to have a high oncogenic association.

The mode of transmission of HPVs is usually sexual intercourse, although the possibility of transmission through fomites must be considered, since these viruses are resistant and capable of surviving outside of the organism.

Because of their close association with premalignant and malignant lesions of the cervix, most authors concur that HPVs play a significant role in the genesis of carcinoma of the lower genital tract. Therefore, the presence of HPVs must be detected as early as possible, since the lesions they produce are thought to be the first step in a continuum that leads to cancer. These findings justify screening with cellular samples all sexually active women.

CYTOLOGIC ASPECTS OF HUMAN PAPILLOMAVIRUS INFECTIONS

HPV infection is diagnosed on the cell spread by the presence of two pathognomonic changes in squamous cells: koilocytosis and dyskeratosis.

The koilocyte [▮*12.1*, ▮*12.2*] is a mature squamous cell characterized by a large perinuclear clear space or cavity. The cytoplasm in the periphery is dense and sometimes displays an amphophilic staining. The nucleus is always abnormal: it is often enlarged and hyperchromatic, with indistinct, or smudged, chromatin structure. No nucleoli or nuclear or cytoplasmic inclusion bodies are present in these cells. Binucleation is common, and multinucleation is also often seen.

The dyskeratocyte [▮*12.3*, ▮*12.4*] is a mature squamous cell that contains one or two, sometimes several, nuclei morphologically similar to the nuclei of koilocytes. There is no perinuclear cavity—the cytoplasm is uniformly dense and orangeophilic. Dyskeratocytes (ie, abnormal keratinization) are usually shed in dense clusters, with much overlapping and crowding.

A smear diagnostic for HPV infection may contain koilocytes, dyskeratocytes, or both. These are the "classic" signs for HPV infection. Sometimes amphophilic parabasal cells with degenerated nuclei can be observed, but these usually occur on smears that also contain koilocytes or dyskeratocytes. Recently, "nonclassic" signs of HPV infection have been described in retrospective studies of patients with proven HPV infection, ie, binucleation, "mild" koilocytosis, "mild" dyskeratosis, etc. However, a cytologic diagnosis of HPV infection should only be made when the cellular pattern is undisputable. A false-positive diagnosis of this sexually transmitted disease that may cause cancer can have devastating psychologic, social, and medical consequences for the patient and her sexual partner. Care should therefore be exercised so that an accurate diagnosis is reported. A written report that a cell study is "suggestive" of HPV infection is meaningless and should be avoided. If the cellular pattern is not conclusive, then it is preferable to indicate that the cell study contains "squamous cellular changes of undetermined significance" and ask for a repeat smear in 6 months. No serious damage will be done by this conservative attitude.

SQUAMOUS INTRAEPITHELIAL LESIONS AND HUMAN PAPILLOMAVIRUS

When the cellular changes are limited to those of koilocytosis and/or dyskeratosis, then the proper diagnosis would be "low-grade squamous intraepithelial lesion (SIL) (HPV infection)." HPV effect can also be seen associated with high-grade SIL. The classic example of this association is what I called the "atypical condyloma" [▮*12.5*], in which the cells are mature, dyskeratotic, and contain enlarged hyperchromatic nuclei. This cellular pattern is reminiscent of the keratinizing invasive squamous carcinomas. The differential diagnosis can be difficult. In general, in the high-grade SIL with HPV effect, the cells are shed in dense clusters with much overlapping, whereas in keratinizing carcinomas, the cells tend to be isolated or in small groups. The chromatin is smudged but can be almost pyknotic in high-grade SIL, whereas in carcinomas, when the nuclei are not pyknotic, the chromatin is clearly visible. The nuclear membrane is not perceptible in high-grade SIL with the HPV effect but is usually visible in carcinomas.

In other cases the smears contain cells of the type described in high-grade SIL with HPV effect, associated with cells typical of pure high-grade SIL [❚ *12.6*]. The latter will be of the parabasal type, with cyanophilic cytoplasm, an increased nuclear/cytoplasmic ratio, and an irregular, hyperchromatic nucleus with clearly defined chromatin structure.

The caution recommended for the diagnosis of HPV infections applies not only to studies performed on smears but also to those done on tissues. Overdiagnosis of koilocytosis is often due to the misinterpretation of glycogen-laden cells. The rule that for a positive diagnosis the nuclei must be abnormal and hyperchromatic, with indistinct chromatin structure, unapparent nuclear membrane, and no nucleoli, applies even more rigorously to cells in tissue sections. Additionally, binucleation is often found in true HPV-related changes. Koilocytosis is a descriptive term and should not be used as a diagnosis. The proper diagnostic term is "low-grade SIL (HPV)."

Other techniques to reveal HPV infections, both on smears and in tissue sections, include demonstration of virus particles by electron microscopy or by immuno(cyto)histochemistry against an HPV group antigen. Although these techniques prove the presence of the virus when the results are positive, a negative finding is meaningless, because only about 50% of true HPV infections give positive results with these techniques. Molecular hybridization, preferably preceded by gene amplification (PCR), is the most sensitive technique available for detecting the presence and determining the precise type of HPV.

Whether there is any clinical value in establishing the type of HPV present in a patient remains debatable. Although types 6 and 11 are purported to be less oncogenic than types 16 and 18, they still represent a sexually transmitted disease and should probably be treated. Gynecologists usually treat cervical lesions according to their extension rather than their severity. Local destruction by laser vaporization, loop electrosurgery, or cryosurgery is the treatment of choice for all SILs, irrespective of grade, if there is no indication of early invasion and the lesion can be visualized completely by colposcopic examination.

In some cases, several types of HPV may coexist in the same patient (eg, types 11 and 16). Low-grade SIL may contain types 16 or 18, so neither the morphology nor the HPV type should influence the treatment of the patient or allow for prognostic deductions.

WILL MOLECULAR TECHNIQUES REPLACE THE CELL SPREAD AS A SCREENING PROCEDURE?

It has been postulated that screening all women for the presence of HPV using PCR would identify those at high risk for cancer of the cervix. Only women who tested positive would then be followed up by conventional methods. This reasoning supposes that HPV is the *only* cause of cancer of the cervix, which has never been established. Furthermore, it is not known what percentage of women will test positive in any given population. The number could be high, probably in the range of 10% to 30%. Most of these women will never develop any lesion, and results of their cell sample and colposcopic examination will remain negative. However, patients alerted to the fact that they harbor a sexually transmitted, potentially oncogenic virus will in all likelihood demand treatment. Yet no treatment is available for the HPV infection per se. The patient will have to be told that nothing more can be done for her, and that she should present herself for periodic checkups. Such a situation will prove frustrating for both the patient and her physician.

The cell sample only detects between 15% and 40% of patients proven by hybridization to harbor HPV. These are patients who actually have a lesion that can be determined by colposcopy and histologic study. These are the only women who can be adequately treated. The cytodiagnostic technique, therefore, remains the most efficient method of routine screening for HPV. It is not likely that another technique will replace it in the foreseeable future.

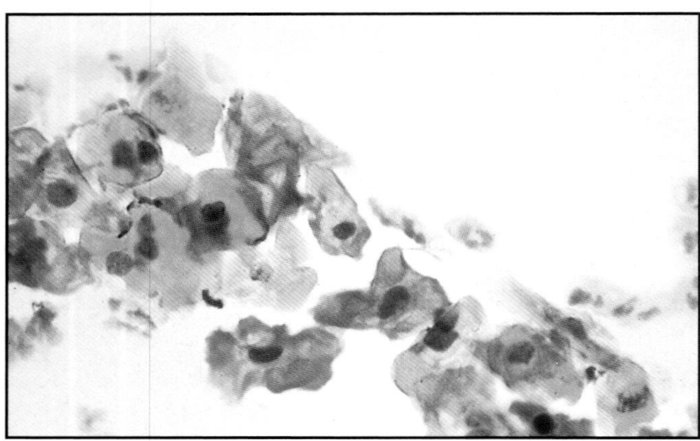

12.1

Low-power view of a group of koilocytes. Note the perinuclear clearing and the dense amphophilic cytoplasm. The nuclei are hyperchromatic, without any chromatin detail. Several cells contain two nuclei.

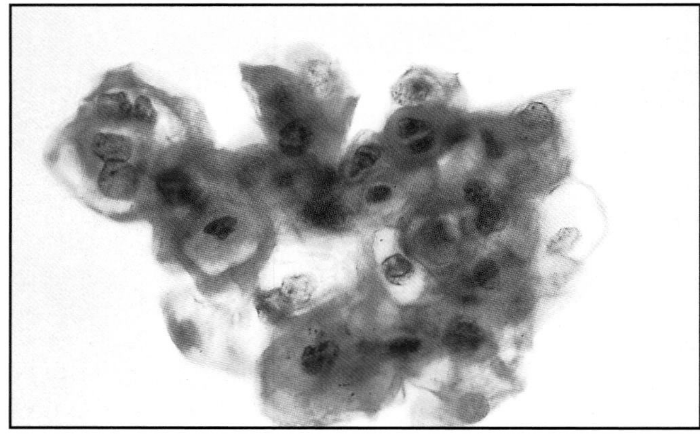

12.2

High-power view of a cluster of koilocytes. Binucleation is clearly seen here. The nuclei are enlarged and show signs of degeneration. The perinuclear clearing or cavity has sharply defined borders.

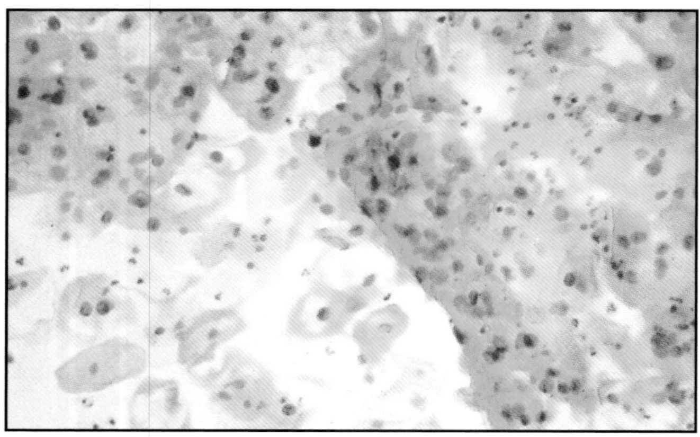

12.3

Low-power view of an aggregate of dyskeratotic cells. The nuclei are similar to those found in koilocytes, some of which can also be seen. The central aggregate is made up of squamous cells with densely stained orangeophilic cytoplasm, without perinuclear clearing.

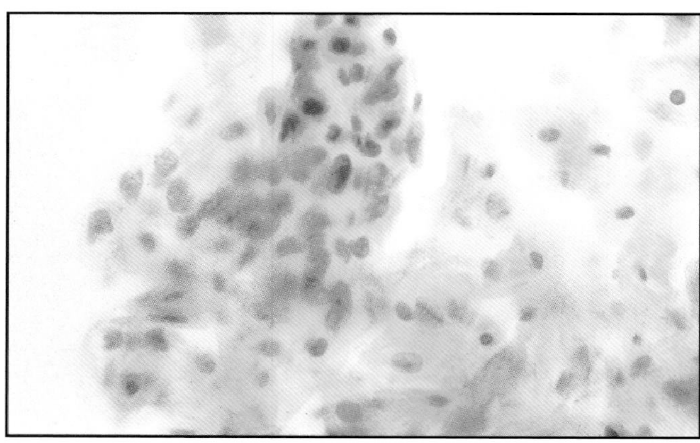

12.4

High-power view of a group of dyskeratotic cells. Hyperchromasia and binucleation are clearly visible. Dyskeratotic cells tend to clump together in three-dimensional aggregates.

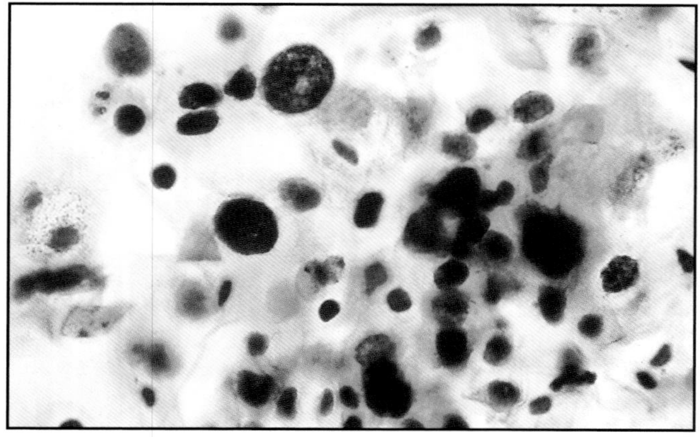

12.5

High-grade squamous intraepithelial lesion (SIL) with HPV effect. It may be difficult to differentiate this lesion from invasive keratinizing carcinoma.

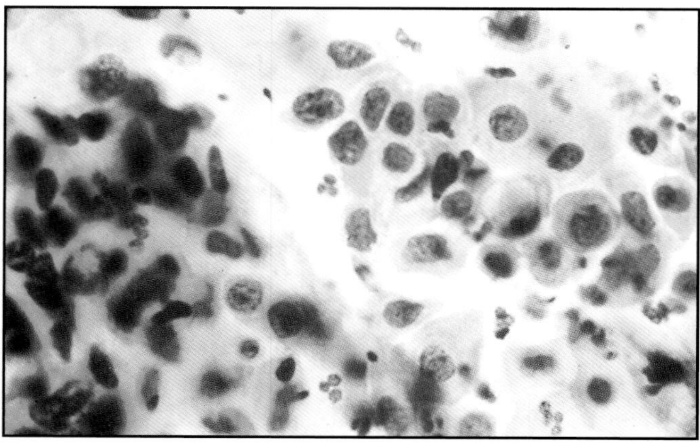

12.6

High-grade SIL without HPV (parabasal cells) associated with the mixed type (high-grade SIL with HPV effect). This pattern may be confused with early stromal invasion.

SELECTED READINGS

De Villiers EM. Heterogeneity of human papillomavirus group. *J Virol.* 1989;63:4898-4903.

Ley C, Bauer HM, Reingold A, et al. Determinants of genital human papillomavirus infection in young women. *J Natl Cancer Inst.* 1991;83:997-1003.

Meisels A, Fortin R. Condylomatous lesions of the cervix and vagina, I: cytologic patterns. *Acta Cytol.* 1976;20:505-509.

Meisels A, Morin C. *Cytopathology of the Uterine Cervix.* Chicago, Ill: ASCP Press; 1991.

National Cancer Institute Workshop. The 1988 Bethesda System for reporting cervical/vaginal cytological diagnoses. *JAMA.* 1989;262:931-934.

Nuovo GJ, Nuovo J. Should family physicians test for human papillomavirus infection? An opposing view. *J Family Pract.* 1991;32:188-191.

Reid R, Lorincz AT. Should family physicians test for human papillomavirus infection? An affirmative view. *J Family Pract.* 1991;32:183-188.

Schiffman MH, Bauer HM, Lorincz AT, et al. Comparison of Southern blot hybridization and polymerase chain reaction methods for the detection of human papillomavirus DNA. *J Clin Microbiol.* 1991;29:573-577.

Schneider A, Meinhardt G, De Villiers EM, Gissmann L. Sensitivity of the cytologic diagnosis of cervical condyloma in comparison with HPV-DNA hybridization studies. *Diagn Cytopathol.* 1987;3:250-255.

CHAPTER 13

Glandular Diseases of the Uterus

ALAN B. P. NG, MD, FIAC

CONTENTS

In the United States and some other parts of the world, there has been a decrease in the frequency of squamous cell cancer of the uterine cervix and an absolute and relative increase in the frequency of endometrial and endocervical adenocarcinoma. Today, adenocarcinoma of the uterus is more frequently encountered than cervical squamous cell cancer in regions with successful screening programs, constituting about 60% of the uterine cancers. Of the adenocarcinomas, 77% are of endometrial origin and 23% originate in the endocervix. Over 20% of cervical cancers are of glandular type. This changing trend has focused attention on the detection of glandular tumors of the uterus and indicates a growing need for the improved detection of endometrial and endocervical carcinoma and their precursors. If this is to be achieved by means of the cellular approach, unlike the detection of cervical squamous cell cancer and its precursors, the cellular detection of glandular neoplasms, especially of endometrial origin, requires more care in sampling, more clinical information, and greater experience on the part of the microscopist.

SAMPLING TECHNIQUES

Cytologic sampling techniques that are optimal for the detection of cervical squamous cell cancer and its precursors are not equally effective in detecting glandular lesions, particularly endometrial diseases.

Cellular sampling techniques used for routine screening must obtain the sample easily, cause minimal discomfort to the patient, and result in an adequate number of representative cells in an optimal state of preservation to allow for consistent and definitive evaluation. Optimal collection depends in part on whether the collecting instrument obtains a sample from a site at or close to the potential lesion.

Cellular samples obtained by aspirating the posterior vaginal fornix, cervical canal (and cervical scrape), and endometrial cavity are used for the detection of adenocarcinoma and its precursors of the endometrium and endocervix. Although samples from the posterovaginal fornix are readily obtained, endometrial cells are infrequently identified, usually limited in number, and in a deteriorated state, making accurate evaluation difficult. In contrast, samples obtained directly from the endometrial cavity consistently contain a large concentration of cells in an optimal state of preservation. Compared with endometrial curettings, aspiration can be performed in the doctor's office or outpatient clinics and does not require a general anesthetic. Major complications, such as uterine perforation, are rare. However, the collection necessitates sterile conditions, is relatively expensive and time-consuming, requires more complex instrumentation, and creates more discomfort when compared with routine Pap smears. The endometrial sample is also more difficult to interpret; additionally, it is difficult to differentiate normal from pathologic hyperplasia, and pathologic hyperplasia from well-differentiated adenocarcinoma on a cellular basis in an endometrial sample. Aspiration is not cost-effective for mass screening, and should be used solely for women at high risk for the development of endometrial cancer, and for women in whom endometrial disease is suspected, eg, when endometrial cells are present in a cervical sample from perimenopausal or postmenopausal women.

Short of direct endometrial sampling, the endocervical sample is the next most valuable cytologic technique for detecting endometrial cancer and, to a lesser extent, endometrial hyperplasia. As the endocervical canal is in close proximity to the endometrial cavity, endometrial cells collected from this location tend to be better preserved and are relatively more abundant when compared with those collected by vaginal and ectocervical samples. Thus the endocervical sample together with the routine ectocervical sample are not only ideal in the evaluation of cervical squamous and endocervical lesions, but are also suitable for the detection of endometrial cancer and its precursors, short of applying the more complex endometrial sampling procedure.

Numerous types of endocervical and endometrial samplers are now commercially available; however, some of them are relatively expensive. Often, a modified Ayre-type spatula with an extended elongated tip is adequate for sampling the endocervix and secretions in the canal as well as the ectocervix. This is much more economical than most endocervical samplers. The use of a nonabsorbable cotton swab to collect material from the endocervical canal is generally inferior, as the sample usually contains a limited number of representative cells and the cells tend to be distorted.

CLINICAL INFORMATION

When the cellular sample is obtained for the purpose of evaluating the endometrium, pertinent clinical information must be provided. The age of the patient and the type of sample should be recorded. The cells of the endometrium respond to the endogenous and exogenous hormonal stimuli, and it is necessary to evaluate the cell changes in relation to the stimuli. To evaluate endogenous hormonal stimulation it is necessary to know the date of onset of the last menstrual period and the date the cellular sample was obtained. The menopausal status should be provided, and the use of any exogenous hormones should be cited, as this may alter the appearance of the sample.

The following additional information may also be important in evaluating the sample. An intrauterine device may affect the appearance of the cellular sample. Any recent intrauterine instrumentation alters the appearance of the sample. Where relevant, the clinical diagnosis and the existing complaint should be noted on the requisition form. Often this reveals the nature of the clinical problem. When this is known it may be possible to resolve the problem on the basis of the cellular evidence. While some of this information will not be applicable in every case, the significance of the cellular evaluation is directly related to the amount of pertinent information provided.

SIGNIFICANCE OF SPONTANEOUSLY DESQUAMATED NORMAL ENDOMETRIAL CELLS

Considerable experience is required to recognize the normal features of endometrial cells, partly because endometrial cells are small and minor structural changes may be significant. Their cellular appearance changes in response to hormonal stimulation, and there are several types of epithelial cells as well as superficial and deep stromal cells. Based on the evaluation of 270,000 consecutive cases where each case consisted of a cervical scrape and endocervical aspiration, 5427 (2.0%) of cases contained normal or abnormal endometrial cells; normal-appearing endometrial cells were seen in 4712 (1.8%) of the cases; 1688 (0.6%) contained endometrial cells when the specimens were collected during the first half of the menstrual cycle and 3024 (1.2%) during the second half of the cycle or postmenopausal period; hyperplastic endometrial cells were reported in 594 (0.2%) of cases; and malignant endometrial cells were recorded in 121 (0.04%) of cases. Of the cases that contained normal or abnormal endometrial cells, the endometrial cells were seen in 99.8% from the endocervical aspirate sample and only 24% from the cervical scrape sample.

Under normal conditions, endometrial cells are more frequently encountered in samples collected in the first half of the menstrual cycle. As might be anticipated, in samples collected from the cervical canal or the posterovaginal fornix, endometrial cells are more frequently observed on days 1 to 5 of the menstrual cycle and less frequently on days 6 to 12. During the first few days of the cycle, not only are endometrial cells frequently seen, they are seen in large numbers consisting of small and large aggregates as well as single cells with a bloody background and inflammatory cells. The number of endometrial cells is in the thousands. During the latter part of the first half of the cycle, the number of endometrial cells present progressively decreases. When normal endometrial cells are shed in the second half of the cycle or postmenopausal period, they are usually relatively few in number.

The presence of endometrial cells in samples obtained during the first half of the cycle is due to physiologic shedding, and when seen in the second half of the cycle and in the postmenopausal period is related to abnormal shedding of the endometrium and must be explained. The frequency and nature of abnormal change are dependent on the age of the woman at the time of detection. The abnormal desquamation of apparently normal endometrial cells may also be encountered under the following conditions: during the immediate postpartum period, in impending or early abortion, in abnormal bleeding related to the endometrium, in the presence of endometritis, in women wearing intrauterine devices, following recent intrauterine instrumentation, in women receiving hormonal therapy, in submucous myoma, in cervical or vaginal endometriosis, and in endometrial adenomatous polyps. A large percentage of cases of abnormal shedding of normal-appearing endometrial cells apparently have no associated clinical findings; however, on subsequent investigation with endometrial curettings, some showed endometrial polyps or benign endometrial changes such as anovulation and endometritis. In endometrial hyperplasia and less frequently in adenocarcinoma, normal-appearing endometrial cells are shed alone or with abnormal endometrial cells. To evaluate the significance of normal endometrial cells it is essential to have pertinent clinical information.

In a study of 696 women in which normal-appearing endometrial cells were observed either in the second half of the menstrual cycle or during the postmenopausal period, endometrial tissue was obtained for evaluation within 6 months of cellular examination. Of the 192 subjects in the 20- to 29-year-old group, the endometrium appeared within normal limits in 89%. Adenomatous polyps of the endometrium were observed in 9.2% and abnormal endometrial hyperplasia in 2% of the women. Invasive adenocarcinoma was not observed in this age group. Of the 237 women in the 40- to 49-year-old group, the endometrium was within normal limits in 63%, adenomatous polyps were encountered in 28%, endometrial hyperplasia in 7%, and adenocarcinoma in 2%. Among those 49 years and younger, in whom the endometrium appeared within normal limits, a history of either contraceptive therapy, estrogen therapy, use of intrauterine device, submucous myoma, or dysfunctional uterine bleeding was recorded in a large number of the subjects. Among the 188 women in the 50- to 59-year-old group, 44% had a normal endometrium. Adenomatous polyps of the endometrium were observed in 41%, endometrial hyperplasia in 11%, and adenocarcinoma in 4%. Of the 76 women who were over 59 years of age, only 40% had an endometrium typical for their age and 29% had adenomatous polyps. In contrast, 18% had endometrial hyperplasia, and adenocarcinoma was observed in 13%. Thus, endometrial cancer and its precursors were encountered in about one third of the women who were over 59 years of age and in approximately 18% who were in the 50- to 59-year-old group in which the cellular samples contained apparently normal endometrial cells.

In subjects with normal-appearing endometrial cells in whom subsequent investigation showed adenocarcinoma, epithelial cells of endometrial origin were observed in 96% and stromal cells were identified in only 4%. In the presence of endometrial hyperplasia and adenomatous polyps of the endometrium, 91% of the specimens contained normal-appearing epithelial cells of endometrial origin and 9% contained stromal cells without recognizable epithelial cells. In those cases in which the endometrium appeared within normal limits, the cellular samples contained endometrial epithelial cells in 85%, while stromal cells without epithelial cells were recognized in 15%.

CYTOLOGY OF BENIGN GLANDULAR LESIONS

Benign endometrial changes commonly seen include the various causes of dysfunctional bleeding secondary to hormonal imbalance, exogenous hormonal effects and pregnancy changes, intrauterine device effects, endometritis, polyps, and benign tumors such as a submucous leiomyoma. Cytologic specimens from either direct endometrial samples or cervical or vaginal aspirates are not usually used and are not optimal in the diagnosis of benign endometrial conditions. With few exceptions, the characteristic cytologic features of benign endometrial lesions have not been documented. However, benign endometrial lesions may sometimes shed endometrial cells that appear within normal limits and are slightly atypical or reactive; these characteristics may be confused with and must be differentiated from malignant or premalignant changes. Sometimes, benign endometrial lesions shed normal-appearing endometrial cells at a time they are not normally expected in vaginal or cervical aspirates.

Decidua or deciduoid cells in cellular samples are seen in association with pregnancy, exogenous progesterone effect, and contraceptive hormones, and occasionally in late secretory phase. Multinucleated syncytial trophoblastic cells are sometimes present in samples in association with pregnancy. Cytotrophoblastic cells are less characteristic and have some of the features of decidua cells. Occasionally, Arias-Stella cells are seen in cell samples and are often difficult to differentiate from atypical benign columnar cells and may be mistaken for malignancy. Oncocytic cells are sometimes seen in conjunction with a reactive endometrium.

When tissue fragments are present in endometrial samples they are best processed and interpreted as histologic tissue specimens, and in these cases a definitive diagnosis of a benign endometrial lesion can be accurately made on its histologic basis.

The most common endocervical lesions are degenerative and regenerative changes of endocervical cells, which produce various cytologic features and cytologic atypias. Those relating to changes that may mimic adenocarcinoma are dealt with later in this chapter.

Microglandular hyperplasia of the endocervix seldom sheds cells, and the endocervical cells that are desquamated are few and often appear within normal limit or show slight atypia but lack malignant characteristics.

PRECURSORS OF ENDOMETRIAL ADENOCARCINOMA

Pathology

Hyperplasia of the endometrium may be physiologic or abnormal. Abnormal endometrial hyperplasia, manifested in the surface epithelium or glands, may have a unicentric or multicentric focus of origin in the endometrium. Diffuse involvement of the endometrium may occur and is usually associated with an endometrium showing unopposed estrogenic effect. Microscopically, endometrial lesions implicated in the genesis of the endometrial carcinoma include cystic hyperplasia [▮*13.1*], adenomatous hyperplasia, atypical hyperplasia, and adenocarcinoma in situ. An associated squamous metaplasia may be observed with the hyperplasia. All of these lesions are said to have the potential for progressing to invasive adenocarcinoma. The malignant propensity is high for adenocarcinoma in situ and atypical hyperplasia (hyperplasia with atypia), very low for cystic hyperplasia, and intermediate for adenomatous hyperplasia (hyperplasia without atypia). There is evidence to indicate that an increase in the incidence of endometrial hyperplasia is associated with the rising frequency of adenocarcinoma.

Each of the hyperplastic changes has a distinctive microscopic appearance, but transitions between them are frequent. In cystic hyperplasia, there is an overgrowth of endometrial tissue consisting of normal sized and dilated glands separated by hyperplastic stroma [▮*13.1*]. The glands are usually lined by tall columnar and sometimes ciliated cells with evidence of mitoses. The nuclei are usually basal and infrequently intermediate in location. Micronucleoli are rarely evident. There is abundant stroma separating the dilated glands. In adenomatous hyperplasia there are outpouchings of the proliferating endometrial glands forming bud-like projections that may become pinched off to form small nests of closely packed glands. These glands, however, have the same staining qualities as the surrounding proliferating endometrium. The slightly enlarged nuclei are usually basally located and less frequently intermediate in location. Micronucleoli are infrequent.

Atypical hyperplasia is usually characterized by large and normal-sized glands that are closely related but separated by definite stroma. The glandular epithelial cells are frequently enlarged and stratification of the cells is evident. Papillary infoldings of the epithelium may be present but are usually not pronounced. The nuclei are enlarged and appear round or oval; they are usually basal or intermediate in location, often stratified, and may have an altered polarity. Mitosis may be observed. Micronucleoli may be encountered in the epithelium. These changes do not involve the glandular epithelium uniformly. Atypical hyperplasia may be a progression of adenomatous hyperplasia and often occurs in the presence of adenocarcinoma in situ or invasive adenocarcinoma.

Endometrial adenocarcinoma in situ is characterized by an increased number of glands. There is no invasion of the endometrial stroma or the myometrium. The affected glands are separated by limited amounts of endometrial stroma. Back-to-back glands and bridging of the epithelium do not usually occur. Papillary infoldings and reduplications of the glandular epithelium are frequently observed. Stratification of the cells is common. The epithelium lining the glands is of the tall columnar type. There is some altered cellular polarity. The cells have an eosinophilic or amphophilic cytoplasm. The enlarged oval nuclei are basal, intermediate, or superficial in location and have increased granular chromatin. Micronucleoli are frequent; however, macronucleoli are unusual. Mitoses are not common.

Recently, a new classification and terminology for pathologic hyperplasia has been proposed: hyperplasia without atypia, simple and complex; and hyperplasia with atypia, simple and complex. Anovulatory changes, cystic hyperplasia, and some early adenomatous hyperplasias are called hyperplasia without atypia, simple type.

Most adenomatous hyperplasia with crowding of glands is classified as hyperplasia without atypia, complex. Most atypical hyperplasia and adenocarcinoma in situ are classified as hyperplasia with atypia, complex; few are classified as simple.

The Cells of Endometrial Hyperplasia

The presence of endometrial hyperplasia may be related to minor changes in the structure of the endometrial cells. Unless the microscopist is experienced, the cellular alterations may be overlooked when the sample contains only a few characteristic cells. Samples collected directly from the endometrial cavity contain a large concentration of cells.

In general the abnormal cells spontaneously desquamated from endometrial hyperplasia are few in number and their shedding is inconstant. In the premenopausal woman abnormal endometrial cells are more readily identified at times when physiologic shedding is not observed. The period from day 15 to 24 in the menstrual cycle is the most opportune time to appreciate the abnormalities. The spontaneous desquamation of endometrial cells in postmenopausal women is frequently associated with a variety of lesions related to endometrial hyperplasia. The cellular abnormalities observed in endocervical aspirates from women with endometrial hyperplasia and adenocarcinoma in situ include cellular and nuclear enlargement, nuclear hyperchromasia, alterations in nuclear chromatin, and the presence of nucleoli. The degree of cellular abnormality is related to the severity of the endometrial abnormality. The altered cells are often accompanied by erythrocytes and evidence of an estrogenic effect, while the milieu associated with endometrial cancer is not observed in endometrial hyperplasia and adenocarcinoma in situ.

Cellular samples from women with cystic hyperplasia contain few cells. The specimens have an average of 107 abnormal cells per slide and a mean of five cell groups. There is a slight increase in the cellular and nuclear size. The mean cell area is 89 μm^2 and the mean nuclear area is 42 μm^2. Nuclear changes are minimal. There is a slight hyperchromasia and the chromatin granules often appear more conspicuous in the nuclei; however, the basic chromatin pattern resembles that of normal proliferative endometrial cells, observed in 95% of the cells. An irregular distribution of the finely granular chromatin is observed in only 5% of the cells. Micronucleoli are rare, being evident in 2% of the abnormal cells. In addition to the abnormal endometrial epithelial cells, stromal cells are evident in 89% of the cases. Many of the endometrial cells appear within normal limits. An adverse host response usually associated with an invasive adenocarcinoma is not evident.

In adenomatous hyperplasia of the endometrium, the cellular changes are often comparable with those of cystic hyperplasia [▮*13.2*]. The cellular samples have an average of 142 abnormal cells and eight cell groupings per slide. The mean cell area is 98 μm^2 and the mean nuclear area is 49 μm^2. Hyperchromasia and increased nuclear granularity are more readily observed in the nuclei. A uniformly finely granular chromatin is observed within the nucleus in 89% of the cells, while 11% are considered to have an irregular distribution. A single micronucleolus is identified in 6% of the cells. In addition to the abnormal epithelial cells, 83% of the specimens also contain endometrial stromal cells. Some endometrial cells appear within normal limits. The diathesis usually associated with invasive adenocarcinoma is not evident.

The cellular features of atypical hyperplasia of the endometrium [▮*13.3*] are more conspicuous and characteristic than those observed in cystic and adenomatous hyperplasia. The degree of cellular abnormality approaches that observed in adenocarcinoma in situ and grade I endometrial adenocarcinoma. There is an average of 245 abnormal cells per slide and a mean of 12 cell groupings. The mean cell area is 114 μm^2 and the mean nuclear area is 52 μm^2. Nuclear hyperchromasia and increased nuclear granularity are evident. The nuclear chromatin is finely granular and evenly distributed in 77% of the cells, irregularly finely granular in 22% of the cells, and the nuclei appear pyknotic in 1%. A total of 17% of the cells contain a single nucleolus. These are usually considered to be micronucleoli; macronucleoli are rarely observed. Stromal cells are identified in 29% of the cases evaluated. Few of the endometrial cells appear within normal limits. The milieu usually associated with frank cancer is not evident.

The cells derived from endometrial adenocarcinoma in situ have many features observed in cells of grade I endometrial adenocarcinoma. In specimens with endometrial adenocarcinoma in situ, there is an average of 305 abnormal cells per slide and an average of 13 cell groups per slide. The mean cell area is 125 μm^2 and the mean nuclear area is 57 μm^2. In contrast to cells derived from invasive adenocarcinoma, the nuclei of the cells derived from adenocarcinoma in situ appear more hyperchromatic and chromatin granules appear more conspicuous. The chromatin is evenly finely granular in 53% of the cells, and irregularly finely granular in 43%. A pyknotic nucleus is observed in 4% of the cells. Nucleoli are identified in 32% of the cells. They are usually micronucleoli and single, while macronucleoli are rarely observed. Stromal cells are observed in less than 20% of the cases. Very few endometrial cells appear within normal limits. An adverse host response consisting of cellular detritus, exudate, and fresh altered erythrocytes is not evident.

In endocervical cell samples, cells derived from cystic and adenomatous hyperplasia of the endometrium more closely resemble those of normal endometrial cells. Conversely, to some degree, the cellular abnormalities of atypical hyperplasia and adenocarcinoma in situ more nearly resemble those associated with grade I endometrial adenocarcinoma. The observations are in keeping with the overall trends in endometrial carcinogenesis.

As biologic potential and differences between cystic and adenomatous hyperplasia and those between atypical hyperplasia and adenocarcinoma in situ are not markedly significant, from the practical point of view it is possible to group the comparative cytologic changes of grade I endometrial carcinoma from its precursors [**T***13.1*].

The precursors of endometrial adenocarcinoma can be detected in cell blocks or direct cell films prepared from endometrial aspirates or washings. When tissue fragments are obtained the diagnosis of endometrial hyperplasia or adenocarcinoma in situ may be made on the basis of histopathologic criteria [**I***13.1*]. Optimal cell films prepared from endometrial aspiration contain an abundance of normal or hyperplastic cells. Although only limited information is presently available about the cellular characteristics of the precursors of endometrial carcinoma in endometrial aspirates, the features are essentially similar to those described in endocervical aspirates. However, far more skill is needed to detect hyperplastic cells from endometrial samples.

ENDOMETRIAL CARCINOMA

Histopathology

Adenocarcinoma may originate from any site occupied by the endometrium showing varying stages of precursor changes or, less frequently, from a preexisting benign polyp. On macroscopic examination, with a unicentric focus of origin, the endometrium may appear normal or may be characterized by a circumscribed overgrowth tissue. As carcinogenesis proceeds, the endometrium becomes thickened, polypoid, and may be papillary. Ultimately, necrosis and hemorrhage may occur. While diffuse involvement of the endometrium may be the end result of adenocarcinoma having a unicentric focus of origin, it is more likely to be related to carcinogenesis with multicentric foci of origin. This may account for two thirds of the endometrial adenocarcinomas.

Essential for the microscopic diagnosis of endometrial adenocarcinoma is a loss of the normal endometrial pattern. The glands are usually increased in number, more closely spaced, and have little or no discernible intervening stroma. While variable in size and shape, the glands are often smaller than their normal prototypes. The glandular pattern is less conspicuous in the more anaplastic neoplasms. While the cellular changes are related to the differentiation of the neoplasm, the basic epithelium is of the columnar type. It may be simple or stratified and the cellular polarity is usually altered. The cells and their nuclei are usually larger than their normal counterparts. The nucleus is usually round or oval with an

Cellular Features	Cystic Hyperplasia and Adenomatous Hyperplasia	Atypical Hyperplasia and Adenocarcinoma In Situ	Adenocarcinoma Grade I
No. of cells	+	++	+++
Cell area	+	++	+++
Nuclear area	+	++	+++
Hyperchromasia	++	++	+
Uniform chromatin	+++	++	–
Irregular chromatin	–	+	+++
Micronucleoli	–	+	+++
Tumor diathesis	–	–	++

– to +++ indicates increasing change of each variable.

T*13.1*
Comparative Cellular Features of Endometrial Carcinoma and Its Precursors

abnormal chromatin. Nucleoli of varying size and number may be present. Necrosis and hemorrhage may be evident and, as a result of necrosis, psammoma bodies may occur, although these are present in only 1% of the cases.

Certain pathologic factors are significant in the management and prognosis of endometrial carcinoma, including Broders' histologic grade, histologic types, and extent of growth at the time of detection.

Tumors having cells that resemble those of the normal parent tissue are said to be differentiated, while those composed predominantly of primitive cells are said to be poorly differentiated or dedifferentiated. In general, neoplasms having a differentiated structure are usually less malignant than those characterized by a poorly differentiated cellular content. The most widely used method for evaluating the differentiation of a malignant tumor is that described by Broders. With this method of histologic grading, several different factors are taken into consideration. Of these the most important is the differentiation of the cells, although the frequency of mitosis and the character of the infiltrative growth are also considered. Based on a study of 520 cases of endometrial carcinoma from 1949 to 1973, 37% of the cases were grade I neoplasms, 42% were grade II neoplasms, 15% were grade III neoplasms, and 6% were grade IV neoplasms. The 5-year survival was 92.6% for grade I neoplasms, 87.6% for grade II neoplasms, 30.2% for grade III neoplasms, and 23.1% for grade IV neoplasms.

Of the histologic types of carcinoma, the typical (endometrioid) adenocarcinoma constitutes about 60% of cases; adenocarcinoma with a benign-appearing squamous component (adenoacanthoma), 20%; adenocarcinoma with a malignant squamous component (adenosquamous carcinoma), 10%; papillary serous adenocarcinoma, 7%; clear cell carcinoma, 1%; and the other 2% of cases represent secretory carcinoma, pure mucinous carcinoma, neuroendocrine tumor, and ciliated cell carcinoma. Sometimes, various components are seen in the same tumor. In adenoacanthoma, the glandular component is usually well differentiated. In adenosquamous carcinoma, the glandular component is usually moderately differentiated. The 5-year survival was 77.1% for endometrioid adenocarcinoma, 100% for secretory carcinoma, 50% for clear cell carcinoma, 42.1% for serous papillary carcinoma, 78.2% for adenoacanthoma, and 27.7% for adenosquamous carcinoma.

Knowing the extent of the endometrial cancer is important to determine management and prognosis. Through direct extension, the adenocarcinoma may involve the full thickness of the myometrium, the peritoneum, uterine tubes, ovaries, and the cervix and/or vagina, as well as other pelvic organs. Of 489 cases, in 269 (55%) the adenocarcinoma was limited to the endometrium (extent A), in 117 (24%) there was extension into the inner one half of the myometrium (extent B), in 49 (10%) there was penetration of more than one half the thickness of the myometrium (extent C), and in 54 (11%) there was extrauterine involvement (extent D). In other studies, the uterine tubes were involved in 5% and the ovaries in 12% of the cases. Direct extension to the uterine cervix occurred in 10% of the cases and the vagina was involved in 4% of the cases. The lymphatic system of the uterus may facilitate the spread of uterine adenocarcinoma to pelvic and para-aortic lymph nodes, to other pelvic organs, and to the lower female genital tract. Hematogenous spread with distant metastasis may be evident.

Women with neoplasms limited to the endometrium (extent A) had an 88% 5-year survival. When the neoplasm had involved less than one half the thickness of the myometrium (extent B) the 5-year survival was 72%. With involvement of more than one half the thickness of the myometrium (extent C) the 5-year survival was only 27%. The 5-year survival was 14% for cases with extrauterine involvement (extent D).

Malignant mixed müllerian tumors (mixed mesodermal tumors) of uterus consist of tumors of epithelial and mesenchymal components. The most common epithelial component is an adenocarcinoma and/or squamous cell cancer. The sarcoma component may be of stromal type (homologous) or elements not seen in the uterus (heterologous). The most common heterologous components include rhabdomyosarcoma, bone, cartilage, glial tissue, and undifferentiated sarcoma.

THE CELLS OF ENDOMETRIAL ADENOCARCINOMA BASED ON SPONTANEOUS DESQUAMATION

Considerable information may be obtained about a uterine neoplasm by analyzing the cellular changes in a suitable cellular sample. This may include the detection of the neoplasm, the characteristics of the cancer, its site of origin, and its distribution. Of all the features that have been attributed to the cells of endometrial carcinoma, the most important are the size of the cell and nucleus, the appearance of the nuclear structure, the appearance of the nucleolus, the inter-relationship of the cells, and the milieu in which they exist [▮*13.4*-▮*13.6*]. In malignant cells the cellular relationship is lost and there is a loss of nuclear polarity. The growth pattern and the differentiation of the neoplasm are related to the appearance of the cellular sample. Papillary adenocarcinoma sheds more than twice the number of neoplastic cell compared with carcinoma lacking this growth pattern. The cell groups range from compact cell balls to aggregates having a papillary arrangement. The samples contain an average of 54 abnormal cells per square centimeter. These occur singly or in groups. An average of 2.9 groupings are observed per square centimeter.

The abnormal cells and their nuclei are larger than their normal counterparts. Abnormal cells have a mean area of 149 μm^2. The cells are usually round or oval and only 3% have a columnar configuration. In endometrial carcinoma involving the uterine cervix the cervical aspiration may contain neoplastic cells with a columnar configuration. Except for this location, desquamated cells from endometrial carcinoma are seldom columnar in shape. Most of the cells have an indistinct cell outline and the cytoplasm is usually scanty. The cytoplasm is cyanophilic in 53% of the cells, eosinophilic in 31%, and indeterminate in 16%. The cytoplasm is diffusely and finely vacuolated in 65% of the cells, homogeneous in 31%, and granular in only 4%. Discrete cytoplasmic vacuoles are observed in only 17% of the cells. It is difficult to determine how frequent this is related to cell secretion and how often it reflects degeneration.

The mean nuclear area is 68 μm². On average the nuclear area represents 46% of the cell area. The nucleus is often observed in an eccentric position. It is oval in 69% of the cells, round in 19%, and irregular or indented in 12%. Unlike the chromatin in the nucleus of the normal endometrial cell, the nuclear chromatin of the neoplastic cell is clumped and the interchromatinic areas are more conspicuous. In 97% of the neoplastic cells the chromatin is irregularly finely granular, in 2% the chromatin is coarsely granular, and in 1% the nuclei are pyknotic. Although some degree of hyperchromasia characterized almost all the cells, this is not as pronounced as observed with squamous cell carcinoma. Discrete nucleoli are identified in 88% of the cells. Of the total population with nucleoli, 60% have a single nucleolus and 28% have multiple nucleoli. Although larger than normally observed, the nucleolus is considered to be a micronucleolus in 74% of the cells and a macronucleolus in 14%. The nucleoli are usually round and only infrequently irregular in configuration.

The milieu in which the neoplastic cells exist is often characteristic. It includes exudate, transudate, fresh and altered erythrocytes, fibrin, cellular detritus, and histiocytes. These features are observed in over 90% of the specimens, being more conspicuous in the presence of dedifferentiated and more advanced carcinoma. The cytohormonal pattern in postmenopausal women with endometrial adenocarcinoma is not significantly different from that observed in a comparable group of presumably normal postmenopausal women. Other authors maintain that there is cellular evidence to suggest an increased estrogenic effect in postmenopausal women with endometrial adenocarcinoma.

CELLULAR MORPHOLOGY IN RELATION TO GRADE

The appearance of the desquamated cells is directly related to the differentiation of the parent neoplasm. For the most part these changes can be related to the malignant character of the cells and involve the relationship of the nucleus and cytoplasm. Cytoplasmic changes relating to differentiation per se are in the minority. There are significant differences in the desquamation of the malignant tumor cells, the measured cellular and nuclear areas, the frequency of cytoplasmic vacuoles, and the intimate structure of the nucleus. Some of the most notable differences are summarized as follows: Cellular preparations from women with grade I endometrial adenocarcinoma [▮*13.4*] contain an average of 346 malignant tumor cells and an average of 18 cell groups per cell film. As determined by planimetry, the mean area of the malignant tumor cells is 132 μm². Large, discrete cytoplasmic vacuoles are identified in 22% of the cells. The nuclei have an average area of 60 μm² and occupy on the average 45% of the cellular area. Distinct nucleoli are observed in 73% of the cells. Seventy percent of the cells have micronucleoli, while 3% have macronucleoli. All of the nucleoli are round in configuration and none are irregular. Within the cell films, there is an associated tumor diathesis in 90% of the grade I adenocarcinomas.

Cellular preparations from women with grade II endometrial adenocarcinoma [▮*13.5*] contain an average of 620 malignant tumor cells and an average of 37 malignant tumor cell groupings in each cell film. The malignant tumor cells have a mean area of 151 μm². Only 16% have discrete cytoplasmic vacuoles. The nucleoli have a mean area of 67 μm² and occupy on the average 45% of the cellular area. Nucleoli are identified in 97% of the cells. In 86% of the cells there are micronucleoli, and in 11% the forms are classified as macronucleoli. The nucleoli are round in all but 0.3% of the cells, in which they are irregular in configuration. An associated tumor diathesis is observed in 94% of the grade II adenocarcinomas.

Cell films from patients with grade III endometrial adenocarcinomas [▮*13.6*] have an average of 606 malignant tumor cells and 34 cell groups. The malignant tumor cells have a mean area of 176 μm². Discrete cytoplasmic vacuoles are observed in 11% of the cells. The nuclei have a mean area of 85 μm² and on the average the nucleus occupies 48% of the area of the malignant tumor cell. All of the cells considered to be malignant tumor cells have nucleoli. In 64% of the cells there are micronucleoli, and in 36% macronucleoli are observed. In 99% of the cells the nucleolus is round, and in 1% it is irregular. A tumor diathesis is usually evident in cell films with grade III adenocarcinomas.

Cell films from women with grade IV endometrial adenocarcinoma contain an average of 607 malignant tumor cells and an average of 31 malignant tumor cell groupings. The malignant tumor cells have a mean area of 198 μm². Only 6% of the cells have discrete cytoplasmic vacuoles. The nuclei of the malignant tumor cells have a mean area of 92 μm² and occupy on the average 46% of the cell area. All the nuclei evaluated contained nucleoli. In 55% of the cells there are micronucleoli, and in 45% there are macronucleoli. In 85% of the cells the nucleoli are round, and in 15% they are irregular in configuration. An associated tumor diathesis is usually observed in cell films with grade IV adenocarcinomas.

CELLULAR MORPHOLOGY IN RELATION TO CELL TYPE

With few exceptions it is difficult to cytologically diagnose specific cell types of adenocarcinoma of the endometrium. Usually the cellular features reflect the endometrial origin and the degree of differentiation of the tumor, but not the specific histologic subtypes of the carcinoma.

Secretory Adenocarcinoma

The cellular features of secretory adenocarcinoma are basically those of a typical grade I endometrial adenocarcinoma and are not distinctive of a secretory cancer. Some cells may show more distinct cytoplasmic vacuoles that may represent secretion and may be due to degenerative changes. A tumor diathesis is often absent or inconspicuous.

Mucinous Adenocarcinoma

Most mucinous (intestinal) carcinomas of the endometrium are relatively well differentiated, representing grade II tumors. In some cell samples, the malignant cells contain more conspicuous cytoplasm with large distinct vacuoles that contain a homogeneous pale slightly eosinophilic fluid representing mucin secretion. Although these vacuoles may be difficult or impossible to differentiate from degenerative changes, the vacuoles from degeneration have clear vacuoles and often contain neutrophils. Often the vacuoles of mucinous carcinoma are so large that they distend the cell borders, and occasionally signet-ring cells are seen. When mucin is extensive, the smear during preparation is sticky and the cell sample has a pale homogeneous streaky background representing extracellular mucin. The latter is indistinguishable from mucin produced by endocervical cells.

Clear Cell Adenocarcinoma

This is usually a poorly differentiated adenocarcinoma representing grade III and, less frequently, grade IV neoplasms, and is often not distinctive for clear cell type. Some of the cells have a moderate amount of cytoplasm, which appears diffusely vacuolated or granular and is fragile. A clear cytoplasm seen in tissue specimen is seldom seen in cellular samples. The enlarged nuclei often contain multiple nucleoli, and macronucleoli are common. The cellular changes resemble clear cell carcinomas derived from the cervix, vagina, and ovary.

Serous Papillary Adenocarcinoma

Most tumors of this type are grade III adenocarcinomas; less frequently they are grade II or IV neoplasms. The basic cellular changes are those described for these grades. However, the characteristic feature of this tumor is that the cell aggregates appear predominantly papillary in form and in different sizes and shapes [▮*13.7*]. The papillary groupings may appear as small compact round cell balls, elongated sausage-like tight groups with peripheral molding of the cellular border, and irregular tight clusters of cells with radiating papillary fronds. Occasionally, when viewed at its proper perspective, a central core of connective tissue with or without capillaries representing the stalk of the papilla may be identified in some cell aggregates. Psammoma bodies are also more likely to be encountered. Papillary forms may be seen in other histologic types of adenocarcinoma but is usually not conspicuous. For comparable grades, tumors that are predominantly papillary in type shed more cells than nonpapillary tumors.

Undifferentiated Carcinoma

The cytologic features of these tumors are those described for a grade IV adenocarcinoma.

Adenoacanthoma

The abnormal cells analyzed in the presence of adenoacanthoma are not significantly different from the cells identified in other endometrial adenocarcinomas. The appearance of the cells reflects the differentiation of the glandular component. While metaplastic squamous cells are identified in most samples, it is difficult to relate the cells to the neoplasm rather than to an origin in the uterine cervix. Only when metaplastic squamous cells occur in continuity with the desquamated cells from adenocarcinoma is there reason to suspect adenoacanthoma.

Mixed Adenosquamous Carcinoma

In adenosquamous carcinoma, both malignant glandular and squamous components are evident. In one study malignant tumor cells were identified in 54 (93%) of the 58 cellular samples. Cells derived from endometrial adenocarcinoma were observed in all the cell samples [▮*13.8*, ▮*13.9*]. Forty (74%) of the samples contained both malignant glandular and malignant squamous cells, whereas 14 (26%) of the cell samples had only malignant cells derived from endometrial adenocarcinoma. Of the 40 samples containing malignant cells from both glandular and squamous components, cells of glandular origin were preponderant in 28 samples, whereas in 8 samples malignant squamous cells were more conspicuous. In the remaining 4 samples, cells of both epithelial components were equally conspicuous.

Malignant Mixed Müllerian Tumor

This tumor consists of an admixture of malignant epithelial and malignant mesenchymal components where the sarcoma cells often predominate. The most common epithelial component is of glandular type and is often associated with a malignant squamous component. The most common sarcoma components are stromal sarcoma or fibrosarcoma (homologous type or carcinosarcoma) and rhabdomyosarcoma, whereas bone, cartilage, and glial tissue are less frequently present (heterologous type). Cell samples may contain malignant glandular component of endometrial type with or without squamous component, and/or sarcoma cells of stromal, striated muscle or other sarcoma cell types. The number of abnormal cells is usually not abundant in cell samples. A tumor diathesis is evident.

In malignant mesenchymal or müllerian tumors, spontaneous desquamation of malignant cells tends to occur singly and rarely in aggregates, whereas malignant epithelial tumors tend to shed cells singly and in aggregates. However, in direct endometrial samples, sarcoma may appear as single cells, aggregates, and microfragments. When fragments are present and processed, as for surgical specimens, a definitive diagnosis can be rendered more readily.

In spontaneous desquamation, stromal sarcoma cells are seen singly and are two to three times the size of normal deep stromal cells. They appear round to oval with scanty cytoplasm that stains weakly cyanophilic or indeterminate. The enlarged nuclei are round with fine granular chromatin showing irregular distribution, and often a nucleolus is evident. Heterologous sarcoma cells are most frequently of skeletal muscle origin [▮*13.10*]. These cells are seen singly, often showing a moderate degree of pleomorphism in cell size and shape. The cells may be as big or bigger than normal squamous cells and as small as stromal sarcoma cells. Bizarre, elongate, or caudate forms may be observed, with a moderate amount of dense cytoplasm that stains cyanophilic and sometimes a greenish tinge. The nuclei are enlarged to two to four times the nucleus of normal squamous cells and are usually round or oval; irregular forms are infrequently seen. Binucleation or multinucleation is common. The chromatin pattern can be variable: it may be finely or coarsely granular with or without an irregular distribution. Nucleoli tend to be prominent and big.

CELLULAR MORPHOLOGY IN RELATION TO EXTENT OF CARCINOMA

Cellular changes in relation to the extent of endometrial carcinoma depend on the extent of endometrial mucosa involvement by cancer; the extent of invasiveness of the cancer into the myometrium, pelvis, and elsewhere; and the degree of extension into the cervix. Focal involvement of the endometrial mucosa by cancer, usually representing early disease, is much less likely to shed cells, and if cells are shed they are usually limited in number. Most focal cancers are well differentiated and are often associated with precursor changes or normal endometrium. Cell samples obtained from focal cancers that contain endometrial cells have few cells and may show a combination of normal, hyperplastic, and malignant well-differentiated adenocarcinoma cells. A tumor diathesis is more likely to be absent and if present is inconspicuous. In some cases, there is evidence of precipitated protein with a watery background. Focal poorly differentiated adenocarcinoma is less frequently encountered and also tends to shed less cells showing features of a poorly differentiated adenocarcinoma.

In contrast, tumors with extensive involvement of the endometrial mucosa and invasion into the myometrium are more prone to shed cells in greater numbers, and a tumor diathesis is more frequently encountered and more pronounced. There is a relationship between the invasiveness of an endometrial cancer and the differentiation of the neoplasm. Poorly differentiated cancers are usually more invasive. When there is involvement of the endocervix by endometrial carcinoma, it may sometimes be difficult to differentiate it from a primary endocervical endometrioid adenocarcinoma in cellular samples. Usually the cellular characteristics of the parent tissue of origin assist in their differentiation.

SAMPLES FROM THE ENDOMETRIAL CAVITY

The appearance of endometrial carcinoma cells in specimens obtained from the endometrial cavity depends on the method used in processing. When macroscopically recognizable fragments are obtained, they are processed by the cell block technique and are evaluated with the same criteria used in the histologic study of surgical specimens, which are well documented [▮*13.8*]. The rest of the specimen is smeared or concentrated in a glass slide and stained with the Papanicolaou stain and evaluated as a cytologic specimen. The specimens obtained may contain malignant cells occurring singly, in aggregates, or in microfragments; hyperplastic endometrial cells occurring in aggregates or microfragments and, less frequently, singly; and even benign endometrial cells occurring singly, in aggregates, or in microfragments. A tumor diathesis is usually present if cancer is extensive and aggressive, with hemorrhage and necrosis.

When single cells or cell groups are present, the criteria are similar to those described for malignant cells that spontaneously desquamate into the endocervical canal or vaginal fornix [▮*13.9*]. However, the malignant cells from direct endometrial samples are abundant, and cell aggregates are larger and the cellular details are better preserved, facilitating interpretation. Microfragments vary in size and shape from single abnormal whole or partial glands to large sheets or fragments of tumor cells. The gland openings are crowded or compressed and vary in size and shape. Papillary folds or diffuse sheets of tumor cells with no glandular stomas may be evident, especially in undifferentiated tumors. The malignant cells in the glands, papillae, or sheets are crowded with overlapping cells or cell stratification; and the cellular and nuclear polarity are altered and irregularly arranged in relationship to one another. The shape of the cells, especially when viewed within glands, are low columnar or cuboidal; however, most cells appear round or oval. Strips of abnormal cells are also encountered. The cells and nuclei are enlarged and the cellular and nuclear size increase with increasing lack of differentiation. There is some variation in size of cells and nuclei. Due to the crowding of the cells, the cytoplasm is often inconspicuous, and overlapping and crowding of the enlarged nuclei with the long axis irregularly arranged are evident. The chromatinic material is slightly more granular and irregularly distributed. Nucleoli are seen and their frequency, size, and number increase with increasing dedifferentiation of the tumor. Mitotic activity may be seen in some of the cells. Many of the larger cell aggregates tend to have a sheet-like appearance and are less likely to be large three-dimensional cell balls. Clusters of foam cell histiocytes are often observed, and psammoma bodies are rarely identified.

Sometimes, morules and, less frequently, sheets of benign-appearing squamous metaplastic cells are seen within abnormal glands or contiguous to them, representing an adenoacanthoma. Sheets of malignant squamous cells may be seen contiguous to or separate from malignant glandular cells representing an adenosquamous carcinoma. In serous papillary carcinoma there are papillary cell groupings and fragments of papillary tissue in the specimen. The cytoplasm of clear cell carcinoma may be moderately abundant with clear or foamy cytoplasm. Hobnail cells may be seen within glands. Mucinous carcinomas may be recognized cytologically when large cytoplasmic vacuoles stain a pale eosinophilic color.

CERVICAL ADENOCARCINOMA

There has been an increase in the frequency of endocervical adenocarcinoma. Today 15% to 25% of all cervical cancers are endocervical adenocarcinomas. The steps in carcinogenesis are similar to those of squamous cell cancer. Even some agents, such as human papillomavirus, herpes, and smoking, have been implicated in genesis of endocervical adenocarcinoma. Other factors such as hormones may also play a part. The major pathway involves a spectrum of changes in the endocervical columnar epithelium designated as endocervical columnar dysplasia, adenocarcinoma in situ, microinvasive adenocarcinoma, and outspoken endocervical adenocarcinoma. Adenocarcinoma may also arise without precursor or has a very short precursor phase. The basic cell is the subcolumnar reserve or multipotential cell, which undergoes mutagenic changes into different phases of carcinogenesis, giving rise to the typical endocervical adenocarcinoma or its subtypes. Up to 50% of precursors of adenocarcinoma and invasive adenocarcinoma are associated with an abnormal squamous epithelial lesion showing cervical intraneoplastic or invasive changes.

In a review of 162 consecutive cases, endocervical adenocarcinoma constituted 131 (81%); microinvasive adenocarcinoma, 9 (5.5%); adenocarcinoma in situ, 19 (11.7%); and endocervical dysplasia, 2 (1.2%).

Precursor lesions of endocervical adenocarcinoma are being recognized with increasing frequency; however, its frequency is still less than for outspoken cancer. This may indicate that there should be an increased awareness in the detection of precursor lesions of endocervical adenocarcinoma in cytology and tissue specimens. It is important to ensure that endocervical material is sampled in cytologic specimens. It is also important to have a high cervical cone for comprehensive tissue evaluation in suspected precursor or early endocervical adenocarcinomas. Colposcopic directed or punch biopsies may not be adequate to evaluate the whole endocervix. Colposcopic examination does not contribute to detection in most cases.

Histopathology

The histologic features of invasive adenocarcinoma and adenocarcinoma in situ of cervix are well defined; however, that of endocervical dysplasia and microinvasive adenocarcinoma are less clearly delineated.

Invasive Adenocarcinoma

Primary adenocarcinoma of the uterine cervix may originate from the epithelium of the surface of the uterine cervix, from the glands or clefts, and less frequently from mesonephric rests, or rarely from endometriosis. On macroscopic examination, adenocarcinoma may resemble other cancers of the uterine cervix.

The spread of cervical adenocarcinoma is similar to that of squamous cell cancer. By direct extension the neoplasm may replace the uterine cervix, or spread to the endometrium, the myometrium, the vagina, the peritoneum, and pelvic organs. Lymphatic and blood vascular involvement may occur earlier in cervical adenocarcinoma than in squamous cell cancer. Spread to pelvic and aortic lymph nodes occurs with considerable frequency, and distant metastasis may occur.

Microscopically, adenocarcinoma of the uterine cervix is associated with a loss of the glandular pattern and epithelial alteration. There may be associated precursor changes. In well-differentiated neoplasms there is only limited alteration in the glandular pattern, while in dedifferentiated adenocarcinoma glandular patterns become inconspicuous. The glands are increased in number, variable in size, and often small and closely approximated. There may be prominent infolding of the glandular epithelium and a papillary appearance may be observed. The cells are larger than their normal prototype, usually having a columnar or cuboidal form. Polygonal or bizarre configurations, although infrequent, are observed more often in dedifferentiated neoplasms. The nucleus is usually enlarged, round or oval, and rarely irregular. The nuclear chromatin is granular and more conspicuous than in the cells of endometrial adenocarcinoma. Micronucleoli or macronucleoli are frequently observed. Macronucleoli are more conspicuous in the cells of dedifferentiated neoplasms. In one series of cervical adenocarcinoma, 27% were classified as grade I, 36% as grade II, 25% as grade III, and 12% as grade IV.

Approximately 45% of primary endocervical adenocarcinomas are considered to be of the typical endocervical type (including adenoma malignum and mucinous types); 45% are mixed carcinomas, where the majority are adenosquamous carcinomas and less frequently are mucoepidermoid, signet-ring cell, or glassy cell carcinomas; 5% are clear cell carcinomas; and the remaining 5% are composed of uncommon types, including endometrioid type (2%), adenoacanthoma, serous papillary, adenoid cystic, and mesonephric carcinomas. Metastatic adenocarcinomas infrequently involve the cervix; and they include primary from the endometrium, ovary, lower genital tract, gastrointestinal tract, urinary bladder, pancreas, breast, and, less frequently, other sites (eg, lung or skin melanomas).

In adenoma malignum or minimal deviation adenocarcinoma, the abnormal glands are lined by well-differentiated cancer cells or cells with minimum cytologic abnormality. The glands are large or normal sized and are separated by fibrous bands. They are located within and outside the normal confines of normal endocervical glands. Clear cell adenocarcinoma morphology is similar to that seen in the vagina, endometrium, and ovary, and is of müllerian origin. The tumors are solid, cystic, or papillary; the latter two patterns may be lined in part by "hobnail" cells. The clear appearance of the cytoplasm is the result of glycogen removed in the processing of the tissue. Most are poorly differentiated. All forms of mixed carcinomas are aggressive cancers and have a poorer prognosis when compared with the typical endocervical types.

In one study, the 5-year survival for adenocarcinoma of cervix was 45.5% for adenoacanthoma, 38.9% for endocervical type adenocarcinoma, 31.6% for clear cell carcinoma, 25.0% for adenoid cystic carcinoma, and 20.4% for mixed adenosquamous cancer. The extent and degree of differentiation of the tumor are other important prognostic factors. Thus, for endocervical type adenocarcinoma the 5-year survival rate was 47.2% for well-differentiated tumors (grades I and II) and 15.8% for poorly differentiated cancers (grades III and IV). The 5-year survival rate was 90% for clinical stage Ia (microinvasive) disease, 65.4% for stage Ib, 38.5% for stage II, 7.1% for stage III, and 0.0% for stage IV disease.

Adenocarcinoma In Situ

In adenocarcinoma in situ, there are abnormal cells lining the epithelium of surface and/or glands; however, the normal interrelationships of the glands are maintained and there is no infiltration into the stroma. The surface epithelium may appear papillary. The abnormal glands are normal in size or enlarged, and papillary infolding may be observed; however, outpouchings or back-to-back crowding of small glands are absent or inconspicuous. Part of the whole gland may be involved.

The abnormal cells may be single layered or stratified. They are slightly larger than their normal counterpart, and variation in cell size and shape is not conspicuous. Columnar form is maintained, while cuboidal form is less frequently present. A sharp demarcation usually distinguishes normal from abnormal epithelium. The nuclei appear crowded, enlarged, and elongated, and are variable in their location from cell to cell, forming a pseudostratified pattern. The nuclei are more hyperchromatic and possess a more granular chromatin than normal. Nucleoli, usually micronucleoli and less frequently macronucleoli, are observed. Mitoses are frequently encountered. There is usually no tumor necrosis or inflammatory response contiguous to the abnormal glands or surface epithelium. Subtypes frequently seen are adenosquamous carcinoma in situ, and less frequently are mucinous, clear cell, and endometrioid types.

Endocervical Columnar Dysplasia

Endocervical dysplasia shows changes less severe and less extensive than those observed in adenocarcinoma in situ. The involved glands are normal or enlarged. Surface papillary and papillary infoldings of glands are usually not seen. The atypical cells may wholly or partly involve surface and glandular epithelium. Stratification is seldom present. The cells are columnar and are slightly larger than normal. The nuclei are slightly enlarged and elongated and appear less crowded than those of adenocarcinoma in situ, and show some variable location from cell to cell. The nuclei are hyperchromatic with a finely granular chromatin. Micronucleoli are inconspicuous.

Microinvasive Adenocarcinoma

The histologic diagnosis of early infiltration of columnar cells into cervical stroma can be made when one of the following changes is identified: (1) A small cluster of abnormal columnar cells from an adenocarcinoma in situ penetrates through the basement membrane into cervical stroma and evokes a host inflammatory reaction. (2) Infiltration occurs by single or small clusters of small crowded back-to-back adenocarcinoma in situ glands by budding or outpouchings into contiguous stroma with an associated inflammatory reaction and/or desmoplasia. (3) The bridging of papillary infoldings within adenocarcinoma in situ glands forming back-to-back small glands causes an expansive growth of the parent gland with an associated inflammation and/or desmoplasia. (4) Small focal infiltration is present when abnormal glands are identified beyond the anatomic confines of normal endocervical glands.

The upper limit of microinvasive cancer, before a lesion is designated an outspoken adenocarcinoma, has not been clearly defined. A tumor should be designated an outspoken adenocarcinoma when some or all of the following findings are evident in early invasive cancer: (1) Invasive cancer is located deeper than the normal anatomic location of normal endocervical glands. (2) There is a confluence of one or more groups of early invasive glands. (3) There is a depth of infiltration of more than 5 mm, as measured from the base of the surface mucosa irrespective of the site of origin. (4) There is extensive superficial disease with confluence and/or unequivocal evidence of tumor involving lymphatics and/or blood vessels.

THE CELLS OF ENDOCERVICAL ADENOCARCINOMA AND ITS PRECURSORS

Endocervical Adenocarcinoma

As for squamous cancer, the criteria of malignancy in cellular samples include altered cellular relationship, nuclear changes, and adverse host response to cancer (tumor diathesis). The shape and cytoplasmic characteristics reflect the origin of the cell type. Changes in abnormal cells include altered cellular relationship, increase in cellular and nuclear size, and some variation in cellular and nuclear size. The chromatin is granular and is irregularly distributed within the nucleus; the chromatin pattern tends to be different from cell to cell. Nucleoli, which may be small or large and single or multiple, and tumor diathesis are present. The cytoplasm appears granular and tends to stain slightly eosinophilic or cyanophilic with the EA-65 stain.

The malignant cells are usually numerous and may occur singly or in aggregates. The aggregates may appear as irregular syncytia of different sizes, strips, or rosettes. Tight cell ball groupings are less frequently encountered. Depending on the perspective in which the cells are viewed, the abnormal cells may appear columnar, cuboidal, round, or oval. Bizarre forms are rare. When in strips or rosettes, the enlarged nuclei are irregularly arranged. In well-differentiated adenocarcinoma, strips and rosettes are more frequently identified and the malignant cells tend to be columnar. With increasing lack of differentiation, malignant cells in aggregates tend to form syncytia masses; the cells and nuclei become bigger; the cells become less columnar and tend to be cuboidal, round, and oval; and nucleoli become bigger and multiple.

Based on an analysis of the cells observed in samples from 43 women with proven disease [▮*13.11*, ▮*13.12*], an average of 13,700 abnormal cells are identified in each cell film. The concentration of abnormal cells observed is large compared with that in endometrial carcinoma. In part this is related to the use of samples obtained by cervical aspiration—the method of choice in the detection of cervical adenocarcinoma. Abnormal cells occur in an isolated state and also in groups. An average of 218 malignant tumor cell groups are observed. The arrangement of the cells is often characteristic. There are often loose groupings in which the cells retain a side-by-side arrangement, although rosette-like arrangements also are observed.

The abnormal cells have a mean area of 186 μm^2. Using the EA-65 stain, cytoplasmic staining is eosinophilic in 80% of the cells, cyanophilic in 10%, and indeterminate in 10%. Although the configuration of the altered cells is varied, 58% of the cells have a columnar configuration. This configuration is more characteristic of endocervical than endometrial adenocarcinoma in samples obtained by cervical aspiration. In 26% of the altered cells there is a delicate cytoplasmic vacuolization and in 74% there is a characteristic granular cytoplasm, which is less commonly observed in cells of endometrial carcinoma. Only 9% of the cells had discrete cytoplasmic vacuoles. A minority of the vacuoles contained leukocytes.

The abnormal cells have a mean nuclear area of 91 μm^2. The configuration of the nucleus is round in 20% of the cells, oval in 76%, and indented in 4%. The nuclear chromatin that is irregularly distributed is finely granular in 91% of the cells, coarsely granular in 8%, and opaque in 1%. Although nuclear hyperchromasia is observed, it is less pronounced than in the cells of squamous cell cancer. Nuclei without pyknosis usually have demonstrable nucleoli. There are micronucleoli in 62% and macronucleoli in 38% of the cells. In 24% of the cells they are single and in 76% they are multiple, with multiple nucleoli more characteristic of the cells of cervical rather than endometrial adenocarcinoma. A tumor diathesis is observed in 85% of the cases.

Except for certain cell types, the cytologic characteristics of the various histologic subtypes of adenocarcinoma of the cervix are not readily delineated and they reflect the degree of differentiation of the cancer in cell samples. The cytologic features of adenoma malignum are those of a well-differentiated endocervical adenocarcinoma. Distinct cytoplasmic mucinous vacuoles are seen in mucinous adenocarcinoma, which is usually well differentiated. In endocervical endometrioid adenocarcinoma, the malignant cells have many of the features of endometrial adenocarcinoma, except that the number of malignant cells are more numerous, the aggregates are loose and less likely to be molded and compact, and the cells tend to have a more columnar or cuboidal form when compared with their counterpart in the endometrium. On objective evaluation it may be difficult to distinguish this type of primary cervical cancer from secondary involvement of the cervix by primary endometrial and endometrioid ovarian cancer.

In clear cell carcinoma, the malignant cells appear poorly differentiated and are relatively large, oval, or polygonal in form, with ill-defined cell borders. They tend to occur in loose aggregates, and sometimes some appear papillary and singly. There may be a moderate amount of cytoplasm in some cells, which stains weakly cyanophilic or indeterminate and appears finely and diffusely vacuolated. The malignant nuclei are large, round, and centrally placed. A central macronucleolus is evident in many cells. True mesonephric adenocarcinoma shows some of the features of clear cell carcinoma; however, the cells appear smaller and nucleoli are not as large.

In adenosquamous carcinoma, the glandular component usually resembles that associated with adenocarcinoma of endocervical type of varying differentiation and the squamous component is of large cell type in 52% of cases, keratinizing type in 33% of cases, and small cell type in 15% of cases. In the signet-ring cell type, some cells of the glandular component have a signet-ring appearance and stain positive for mucin. In glassy cell carcinoma, the malignant cells appear poorly differentiated and are polygonal in shape with a granular slight eosinophilic cytoplasm. The enlarged nuclei have more conspicuous granular chromatin but no significant clumping. A macronucleolus is usually seen in each cell. In some cases, eosinophils may be numerous in the cell samples. This neoplasm may be confused with squamous cell cancer, large cell type, in both histopathologic and cellular samples. Adenoacanthoma of the endocervix may be diagnosed when benign-appearing squamous cells are seen with malignant glandular cells in the same aggregate.

The cellular features of cervical adenoid cystic carcinoma are that of an endocervical small cell type, and when these cells occur in syncytial form they may be mistaken for small cell cancer.

Adenocarcinoma In Situ

Cell samples from women with endocervical type adenocarcinoma in situ contain a moderate number of abnormal endocervical columnar cells [▮*13.13*-▮*13.16*]. The number of abnormal cells is dependent on the extent of disease. Associated normal or reactive endocervical cells are often present. The abnormal cells occur predominantly in cell aggregates, and abnormal single cells are few. The groupings consist of an admixture of strips, rosettes, and syncytia with indistinct cell borders. When they occur in syncytia, the borders of the aggregates show scanty cytoplasm and the nuclei at the margins of aggregates form an irregular edge due to the varying levels in which the nuclei are positioned within the stratified epithelium, giving them a frayed or feathery appearance to the edges of the aggregates.

The abnormal endocervical cells are larger than their normal counterpart, measuring approximately 200 μm², and are comparable in size to well-differentiated adenocarcinoma cells. They tend to appear uniform in size; however, sometimes cell size may vary from aggregate to aggregate due to the perspective in which the abnormal columnar cells are viewed. Cell borders are indistinct. The cells may appear columnar, cuboidal, or round to oval in form. The cytoplasm is moderate or scanty depending on from which perspective the cells are viewed. It stains weakly cyanophilic or weakly eosinophilic and is usually finely granular.

The slightly enlarged nuclei in abnormal cell groups appear crowded and have an inconsistent nuclear polarity. When cells appear in strips, there is nuclear stratification where the nuclei are observed at different levels of the cells with an irregular nuclear polarity. In circular groups or rosettes, the nuclei tend to be basally located; however, the polarity is altered. The mean nuclear area is 75 μm² and the nuclei tend to be uniform in size and round or oval, and show slight to moderate hyperchromasia due to increased fine granularity of the chromatin and multiple chromocenters. The fine granularity of the chromatin is usually uniformly distributed within the nucleus, and irregular distribution is seen in a small number of cells. Micronucleoli are seen in about 15% of abnormal cells, and macronucleoli are less frequently encountered. A tumor diathesis is absent; however, an associated inflammatory exudate is frequently seen.

Up to 50% of cases of adenocarcinoma in situ are associated with squamous dysplastic and carcinoma in situ cells, justifying the diagnosis of adenosquamous carcinoma in situ. Adenocarcinomas in situ of mucinous, endometrioid, and clear cell type have also been encountered.

Differential features between adenocarcinoma in situ and invasive endocervical adenocarcinoma include the number of abnormal cells, cellular distribution, the type of cellular aggregates, some nuclear differences, and diathesis. Generally, in adenocarcinoma in situ the abnormal cells are fewer and tend to occur in aggregates with few single cells, whereas in invasive adenocarcinoma there are more abnormal cells and many single cells, as well as aggregates in the cell sample. The aggregates in adenocarcinoma in situ tend to appear as strips and rosettes, and in a feathery pattern, whereas in invasive adenocarcinoma, these types of groupings are less conspicuous. The nuclei of invasive cancer show more irregular distribution of the chromatin, and nucleoli are more frequently encountered and tend to be larger than in adenocarcinoma in situ. A tumor diathesis is usually present in invasive cancer and absent in adenocarcinoma in situ.

Endocervical Columnar Dysplasia

The abnormal cells have some of the features of adenocarcinoma in situ but the degree of abnormality is less conspicuous. Samples from endocervical dysplasia contain much fewer abnormal cells with smaller strips or part rosettes with no significant stratification. Feathery aggregates are not usually seen. The cells and nuclei tend to be slightly enlarged, nuclei are more granular and hyperchromatic with none or very few showing nuclear clearing, and small nucleoli are infrequently seen. A tumor diathesis is also absent.

Microinvasive Adenocarcinoma

Usually the cytologic features are that of an adenocarcinoma in situ and less frequently of an outspoken well-differentiated adenocarcinoma. In addition to adenocarcinoma in situ cytologic features, sometimes additional features are present that may suggest microinvasion. Small aggregates of abnormal endocervical cells that appear squamoid with an oval-polygonal shape, granular slightly eosinophilic cytoplasm with the EA-65 stain, and enlarged nuclei with a prominent nucleolus suggest microinvasion. In a cell sample containing predominantly adenocarcinoma in situ cells with no tumor diathesis and an occasional group of cells showing outspoken adenocarcinoma, microinvasion may be considered.

CELLS ORIGINATING IN EXTRAUTERINE NEOPLASMS

Malignant tumor cells observed in cellular samples from the posterovaginal fornix, the cervical canal, or endometrial cavity are usually derived from primary uterine neoplasms and less frequently originate in extrauterine cancers. Extrauterine malignant neoplasms shedding cells into the vagina or uterus are usually of the glandular type and only rarely are squamous cell cancers, sarcomas, lymphomas, or leukemias. The ability to recognize malignant glandular cells of extrauterine origin is important, as it will determine the nature of the investigation. Furthermore, in patients with known extrauterine cancer, the presence of malignant cells in uterine samples provides information about the extent of the neoplasm. Occasionally, evidence of extrauterine neoplasm is first appreciated in a routine cellular sample.

Of 66 cell samples containing malignant cells from women with proven extrauterine cancer, the primary tumor was in the ovary in 28 (42%) of the patients, in the gastrointestinal tract in 13 (20%), in uterine tube in 5 (8%), in the pancreas in 4 (6%), in the urethra in 3 (5%), in the breast in 3 (5%), and in the peritoneal mesothelium in 2 (3%). Other primary neoplasms included one each from the urinary bladder, gallbladder, and lung. In one case of leukemia, there was a uterine involvement by leukemic cells. In four cases, there was diffuse carcinomatosis involving the peritoneal cavity and the primary site of the origin could not be determined. Of the 13 primary tumors in the gastrointestinal tract, 9 were located in the rectosigmoid colon, while the descending colon, appendix, small bowel, and stomach were each represented by 1 case. In 62 of the 66 cases, the primary tumor was related to the organs of the pelvis and/or abdominal cavity. In only 4 cases was the primary tumor located elsewhere.

In addition to the site of origin of the primary tumor, there are other factors considered important in influencing the desquamation of malignant cells of extrauterine origin into the vagina or uterus. These include extent and location of the neoplastic spread, ascites, and patency of the uterine tube. At the time of cellular detection, 38 (58%) of the 66 cases had ascites, 49 (74%) had evidence of tumor involvement in the pelvis and peritoneum, and 18 (27%) had proven metastasis to the mucosa of the uterus and/or vagina. Of the 18 cases with verified secondary cancers of the uterus or vagina, there was involvement of the vagina in 12 cases, the cervix in 5 cases, and the endometrium in 6 cases. Neoplasms originating in the colon or urethra involved the vagina by direct extension, while metastasis by vascular or transtubal routes occurred with other neoplasms. All the uterine tubes available for study were patent so there was a potential route for the passage of the malignant tumor cells into the uterus.

The tumor cells in endocervical, vaginal, or uterine samples may originate either directly from the primary tumor or its metastasis in the pelvis and/or the abdominal cavity passing through the lumens of the uterine tubes. Under these circumstances, evidence of an adverse host response is usually absent in the cellular sample [▌*13.17*, ▌*13.18*]. In cell samples containing malignant cells of extrauterine origin, a tumor diathesis was observed in 13 (20%) while a tumor diathesis was not evident in 53 (80%) of the 66 cases. In all 13 cases having a tumor diathesis there was vaginal and/or uterine metastasis with mucosal involvement and ulceration. In contrast, only 8% of the cell samples from women with primary endometrial adenocarcinoma did not have a tumor diathesis. Similarly, only 15% of the cell samples from women with proven primary endocervical adenocarcinoma lacked a tumor diathesis. When elements originating in a poorly differentiated adenocarcinoma are observed without an associated tumor diathesis, extrauterine origin should be considered.

As few as 10 malignant tumor cells are evident in one cell film while counts in excess of 1500 are observed in other samples. The mean cell count is 150 cells and 12 cell groupings per sample. The cellular characteristics of malignancy evident in each cell sample are usually those associated with poorly differentiated carcinoma. On the basis of variables evaluated, there is usually no significant correlation between the cellular changes and the specific type of the malignant tumor. Infrequently, the arrangement and morphology of the cell aggregates sometimes reflect the tissue of origin and the differentiation of the parent tumor. An ovarian origin should be considered when malignant cells of extrauterine origin are arranged in a papillary pattern. A papillary pattern is less frequently encountered in primary neoplasm of the pancreas and mesothelium. A primary ovarian tumor should be considered in the presence of psammoma bodies; however, psammoma bodies have been associated with primary endometrial carcinoma, mesothelioma, and neoplasms of the pancreas, lung, thyroid, kidney, and skin appendage.

Except for a lack of tumor diathesis, the cellular characteristics of neoplasms originating in the uterine tube have many of the features of endometrial adenocarcinoma. Evidence of a watery transudate in the cell film may be observed. A primary mammary carcinoma should be suspected when malignant cells of extrauterine origin occur in a linear arrangement. Tall columnar cells with elongated nuclei arranged in a palisading pattern reflect a relatively well-differentiated adenocarcinoma of the colon. In a case of leukemia with infiltration of the myometrium, mucosa of the cervix, and endometrium, the cell sample contains numerous abnormal immature and mature lymphocytes. The immature cells of the lymphocytic series have scant cytoplasm, and the enlarged hyperchromatic nuclei have an altered chromatin. Nucleoli are evident in some cells. There is no evidence of phagocytosis, and reticular cells are not observed.

DIFFERENTIAL DIAGNOSIS OF UTERINE ADENOCARCINOMA

Endocervical Compared With Endometrial Adenocarcinoma

In samples collected from the endocervical canal, there are significant differences between the cell population of endometrial and endocervical adenocarcinoma. In the presence of endocervical adenocarcinoma, cell films prepared from the cervical aspirate contain an average of 13,700 malignant tumor cells and 218 malignant tumor cell groupings per cell sample. Comparable samples collected from women with endometrial adenocarcinoma have an average of 538 malignant tumor cells and 28 malignant tumor cell groupings per cell sample. As compared with the cells originating in endometrial adenocarcinoma those derived from endocervical adenocarcinoma are in general somewhat larger. For comparable differentiation, the malignant tumor cells of endometrial adenocarcinoma have an average mean area of 149 μm^2 while those originating from the uterine cervix have a mean area of 186 μm^2. In large part this can be attributed to differences in the size of the normal prototypes.

Among the cells derived from endocervical adenocarcinoma 58% have a columnar configuration, while only 4% of the cells from endometrial adenocarcinoma have such a configuration. Differences in cytoplasmic staining as observed with the EA-65 stain are important. In endocervical adenocarcinomas, the cytoplasm is eosinophilic in 80% of the cells, cyanophilic in 10% of the cells, and indeterminate in staining in 10% of the cells. Of the cells originating from endometrial adenocarcinoma, 31% are eosinophilic, 53% are cyanophilic, and 16% are indeterminate in staining. In the presence of endocervical adenocarcinoma, 74% of the cells are characterized as having granular cytoplasm while in 26% the cytoplasm is considered to be diffusely and finely vacuolated. Among the cells shed from endometrial adenocarcinoma, 65% have a finely vacuolated cytoplasm, 31% have an amorphous cytoplasm, and only 4% have a granular cytoplasm. The cytoplasm of the cells derived from endocervical adenocarcinoma is more commonly eosinophilic and granular; in contrast, that derived from endometrial adenocarcinoma is more commonly cyanophilic and finely vacuolated.

The mean nuclear area is 91 μm^2 in cells of endocervical adenocarcinoma and 68 μm^2 in cells derived from endometrial adenocarcinoma. Differences in nuclear structure are also evident. While most of the cells have a finely granular chromatinic material, those originating in the uterine cervix are characterized by a chromatinic material having a relatively larger particle size than is usually observed in endometrial adenocarcinoma. This is reflected in a relatively more conspicuous hyperchromasia in the nuclei of endocervical adenocarcinoma when compared with those of endometrial adenocarcinoma. Differences in the size and number of the nucleoli are also of importance. Multiple nucleoli are recognized in 76% of the cells derived from endocervical adenocarcinoma as compared with 29% from endometrial neoplasms. Macronucleoli are identified in 38% of the cells from endocervical adenocarcinoma and in 15% from endometrial adenocarcinoma. The differences described between endometrial and endocervical adenocarcinomas are statistically significant.

Uterine Adenocarcinoma Compared With Extrauterine Adenocarcinoma

Most extrauterine adenocarcinomas are poorly differentiated and are usually not associated with a tumor diathesis in vaginal and uterine samples (endocervical and endometrial), whereas a tumor diathesis is usually associated with a poorly differentiated endometrial or endocervical adenocarcinoma. Together with pertinent clinical information this is the most important reliable variable. Other differences reflecting the parentage of the neoplastic cells and cellular pattern may also assist in their differentiation.

Uterine Adenocarcinoma Compared With Cervical Squamous Carcinoma

Reflecting the parentage of cellular origin, endocervical adenocarcinoma has aggregates showing palisading, acinar, papillary, and loose groupings of columnar or cuboidal shaped cells, whereas malignant squamous cells occur in syncytia with round, oval, or irregular shaped cells. The cytoplasm of endocervical carcinoma cells tends to have a finely granular and less frequently a finely vacuolated cytoplasm with often an eosinophilic tinge using the EA-65 stain. In contrast, malignant squamous cells tend to have a homogeneous cyanophilic cytoplasm, except for the keratinizing type where some of the cells stain eosinophilic and orangeophilic. The nuclei of malignant glandular cells of cervix appear generally less hyperchromatic and granular with more nucleoli when compared with malignant squamous cells.

Small cell cancer and its precursors of the cervix may be confused with well-differentiated adenocarcinoma of the endometrium. In well-differentiated adenocarcinoma of endometrium the samples contain relatively few cell aggregates and appear as loose altered acinar or tight clusters with molded peripheral borders, and the cells may be cuboidal with eccentric nucleus, and the chromatin is irregularly finely granular with micronucleoli. The cytoplasm is finely vacuolated. In small cell carcinoma, the cell sample contains many cells occurring singly and in aggregates, the aggregates are in syncytial form, the nuclei are more hyperchromatic with more granular chromatin, and nucleoli are less conspicuous. The cytoplasm is scanty and granular. Nucleoli and tumor diathesis are absent in small cell carcinoma in situ.

Large cell type of squamous carcinoma may be confused with poorly differentiated adenocarcinoma of endometrium. Although cell samples from poorly differentiated adenocarcinomas may contain sheet-like or syncytial cell aggregates, papillary groups and tight cell ball clusters may be present as well. The cytoplasm remains finely vacuolated, the chromatinic material remains relatively finely granular, and macronucleoli are conspicuous. In contrast, cell samples from large cell nonkeratinizing squamous cell carcinoma contain many more abnormal cells occurring singly or in syncytia with no papillary or tight cell ball pattern. The cytoplasm stains denser and homogeneous, the nuclei are more hyperchromatic and the chromatin is more granular with more conspicuous nuclear clearing, and macronucleoli are less conspicuous.

Irradiated malignant cells in cell samples may sometimes be difficult to evaluate as to cell type and origin of tumor. Malignant glandular cells may lose their characteristic features and mimic cells of squamous type, and malignant squamous cells may take on characteristics of a glandular component.

Benign Lesions Simulating Adenocarcinoma

The most common entity that is often confused for adenocarcinoma is regenerative endocervical, parabasal, or immature squamous metaplastic cell aggregates of the cervix. When compared with adenocarcinoma, regenerative cervical cells are relatively larger than malignant endometrial cells and comparable in size with malignant endocervical cells; there are few single cells and most reactive endocervical cells tend to occur in aggregates, which are sheet-like and often show irregular cytoplasmic processes. Mitotic figures and inflammatory cell infiltrate are often seen in the sheets of cells. When there is a monolayer of cells, the cytoplasm is moderately abundant, may appear vacuolated, and the nuclear/cytoplasmic ratio is variable but usually low. Often some cells in the sheets appear relatively normal while others appear atypical. The nuclei are enlarged and often macronucleoli are evident. However, irregular distribution of chromatinic material is inconspicuous or absent. Although there may be a hemorrhagic inflammatory background in the cell sample, a tumor diathesis is usually absent. These reactive cells usually disappear when inflammation subsides on repeated cell studies following treatment.

Degenerative changes, especially in immature metaplastic cells of the cervix, may be confused for adenocarcinoma. The most common degenerative change is the presence of cytoplasmic vacuoles. These vacuoles in small metaplastic cells may push the nucleus to one side and when seen in aggregates may be mistaken for adenocarcinoma. The cytoplasm of metaplastic cells has a densely staining homogeneous cyanophilic cytoplasm, and even with the presence of degenerative cytoplasmic vacuoles a thin rim of dense-staining cytoplasm usually is still recognizable. The nuclei of metaplastic cells are uniformly granular with no nuclear clearing or nucleoli.

Arias-Stella cells have been rarely described and are difficult to differentiate from other atypical cell types in cervical and endometrial samples. They are relatively easy to appreciate in endometrial samples containing tissue fragments, and in cellular samples they lack the cytologic features of malignancy. Syncytial trophoblasts are multinucleated cells in cervical and endometrial samples. Cytotrophoblasts are more difficult to identify except when tissue fragments are present. They have many of the features of decidua cells.

The presence of bare nuclei of endocervical origin occurring singly and in aggregates has been mistaken for adenocarcinoma. The nuclei are relatively uniform in size and shape and appear bland with no nucleoli. An interpretation of adenocarcinoma or other cellular abnormality should not be made primarily on bare or free nuclei. Artificial changes in endocervical columnar cells and in cells derived from benign processes induced by improper collection, fixation, or staining may produce changes simulating adenocarcinoma that include cellular and nuclear enlargement, cytoplasmic vacuolization, chromatin alterations such as irregular clumping of chromatin material and nuclear clearing, and nuclear inclusions. Great caution should be taken in interpreting cells in poorly prepared specimens. When detailed study is difficult or impossible, it is advisable to report such a specimen as "unsatisfactory for proper evaluation" and a repeated cell study should be requested.

ACCURACY OF DETECTING UTERINE ADENOCARCINOMA AND ITS PRECURSORS

A variety of factors have bearing on the ultimate accuracy achieved in the cellular detection of uterine adenocarcinoma and its precursors. Processes and their anatomic sites of origin, which exist in the host, are important. Cervical stenosis may reduce or prevent the desquamation of cells from the endometrium and may make it difficult to obtain an endocervical lavage. In general, precancerous lesions are less likely to shed a significant number of cells than their malignant counterparts. Papillary tumors shed more cells than their nonpapillary counterparts. Poorly differentiated adenocarcinomas shed a greater number of cells than well-differentiated neoplasms. Inflammation and necrosis tend to increase the desquamation of cells in uterine adenocarcinoma. Tumors with greater involvement of the surface of the endometrium or cervix shed more cells than those of only limited size. Neoplasms that involve the cervical canal primarily or secondarily are accurately identified when studied by sampling methods that forcibly removed cells from their parent tissues.

Pertinent clinical information and the sampling method used are important factors in determining accuracy. The sampling methods that are optimal in detecting squamous cell cancer and its precursors are not equally effective in the detection of uterine adenocarcinoma and its precursors. The care used in obtaining the sample and in preparing the cell films have a direct bearing on accuracy. Additionally, the experience of the cytotechnologist and pathologist is important in determining accuracy, and experience in detecting cervical squamous cell cancer is not necessarily an indication of competence in detecting adenocarcinoma. Due to the plethora of influencing factors, it is practically impossible to achieve 100% accuracy in diagnostic cytopathology, especially endometrial and endocervical cytology.

Endometrial Carcinoma and Its Precursors

Using direct endometrial sampling, accuracy for the detection of endometrial hyperplasia when tissue fragments are obtained is over 90% and for detection of adenocarcinoma is over 95%. If no tissue fragments are present and diagnosis is based on cellular changes, the accuracy is about 50% for endometrial hyperplasia and 90% for endometrial carcinoma.

The sensitivity for the detection of endometrial hyperplasia based on spontaneous desquamation of endometrial cells (endocervical or vaginal sample) is very low and is not optimal for a screening program for the detection of endometrial hyperplasia, but it is a simple method for detecting some endometrial conditions when endometrial cells are identified in routine samples. In our experience, endometrial cells are seen in about 25% of cases in patients with adenomatous hyperplasia with atypia (atypical hyperplasia and adenocarcinoma in situ) and about 10% of cases in patients with adenomatous hyperplasia without atypia (adenomatous and cystic hyperplasia) in endocervical aspirate samples. Endometrial cells are seen in about 5% of vaginal samples for all hyperplasias. However, when endometrial cells are present, the diagnosis of endometrial hyperplasia in these cases is relatively high—up to 75% in endocervical aspirates.

The overall accuracy for the diagnosis of endometrial adenocarcinoma by vaginal samples is less than 45%. In contrast, the overall accuracy rate for the detection of endometrial carcinoma by the endocervical sample is over 70%. In up to 15% of cases only normal-appearing endometrial and hyperplastic endometrial cells are seen in the endocervical sample from patients with endometrial cancer. Furthermore, the detection rate for well-differentiated adenocarcinoma is 60% and over 80% for poorly differentiated adenocarcinoma and adenosquamous cancer.

Endocervical Adenocarcinoma and Its Precursors

The optimal sampling method for the detection of endocervical adenocarcinoma is the cervical aspiration or endocervical sample. Any sampling method that dislodges cells from the cervical canal might provide characteristic cells. Samples obtained from the posterior vaginal fornix are less satisfactory, as are self-obtained specimens from the vagina. The cervical scraping similarly is not the ideal sampling method and is of value only in advanced disease.

In one series of 70 cases of endocervical adenocarcinoma in situ, abnormal endocervical cells were observed in 66 (94%) of cases and in the remaining 4 (6%), no abnormal glandular cells were reported; however, squamous carcinoma in situ cells were identified. Of the 66 cases with abnormal endocervical cells, 56 (85%) of cases were correctly diagnosed as adenocarcinoma in situ/endocervical dysplasia and 10 (15%) were interpreted as invasive adenocarcinoma. Of 40 cases of microinvasive or early invasive adenocarcinoma, 36 (90%) showed abnormal endocervical cells and 4 (10%) showed only abnormal squamous cells and no abnormal endocervical cells. Of the 36 cases with abnormal endocervical cells, 17 (47%) were correctly interpreted as microinvasive or early invasive cancer, 12 (33%) as adenocarcinoma in situ, and outspoken adenocarcinoma in 7 (19%) of cases.

Of the 116 cases of primary adenocarcinoma of the uterine cervix evaluated by means of cervical aspiration, 113 (97%) had cellular evidence of cervical adenocarcinoma. A comparable accuracy was achieved for all the major histopathologic variants. Of 46 adenocarcinomas, malignant cells were identified in 44 (96%) of cases as were all 5 cases of adenoacanthoma. Of 54 adenosquamous cancers, malignant cells were identified in 53 (98%) of cases, and all 11 examples of clear cell cancer were recognized in the cellular sample.

Extrauterine Cancer

The objective diagnosis of extrauterine cancer is possible when there is cellular evidence of a poorly differentiated adenocarcinoma and the absence of the anticipated diathesis. A total of 33 cell samples from women with proven extrauterine cancer were evaluated. All were identified as adenocarcinoma and 27 (81%) were objectively classified as being of extrauterine origin. Six (19%) of the samples were incorrectly classified as being of uterine adenocarcinoma. Of these, five were erroneously thought to be of endometrial origin and one was incorrectly classified as primary endocervical adenocarcinoma. This study illustrates that with characteristic changes, extrauterine cancers can be identified and distinguished from primary adenocarcinoma. Many of the errors were in cases of patients with intrauterine adenocarcinoma that was secondary to or coexisted with an extrauterine cancer. This produced a diathesis that suggested a primary neoplasm.

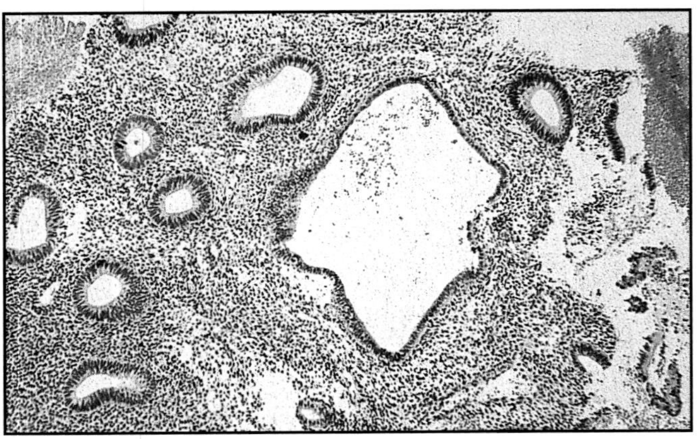

13.1
Cell block prepared from endometrial washing. Cystic hyperplasia of endometrium (x250).

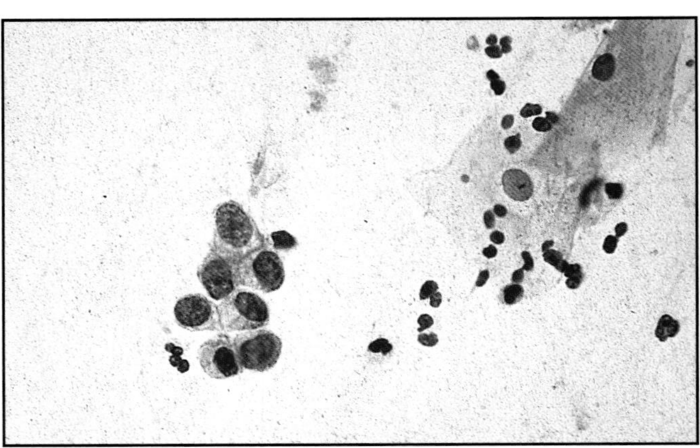

13.2
Hyperplasia of endometrium. Cervical aspirate (x500).

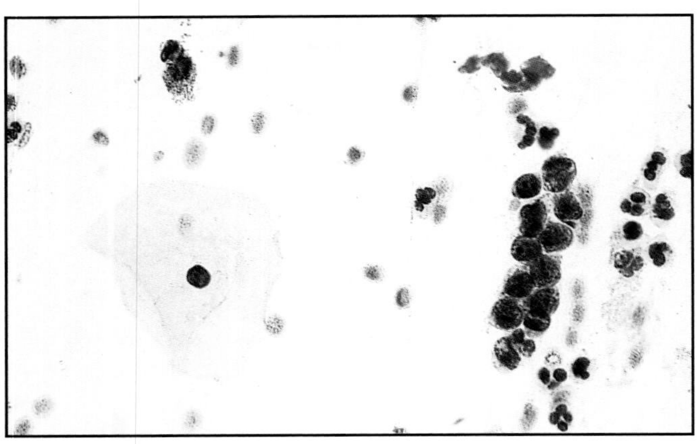

13.3
Atypical hyperplasia of endometrium. Cervical aspirate (x500).

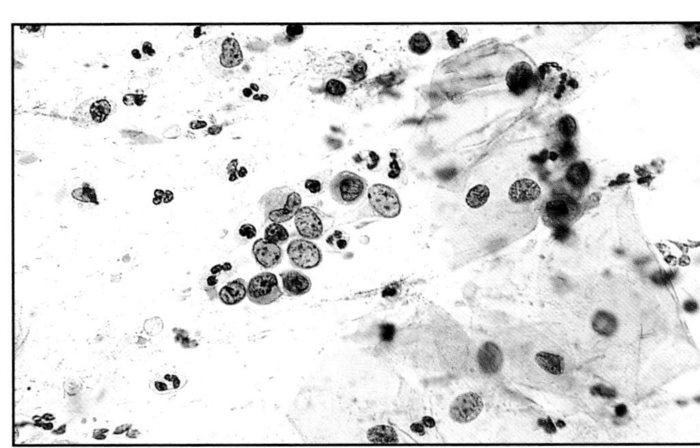

13.4
Grade I endometrial adenocarcinoma (x500).

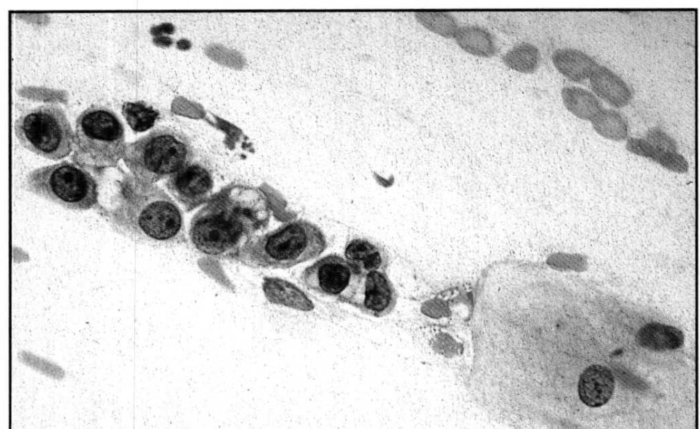

13.5
Grade II endometrial adenocarcinoma (x500).

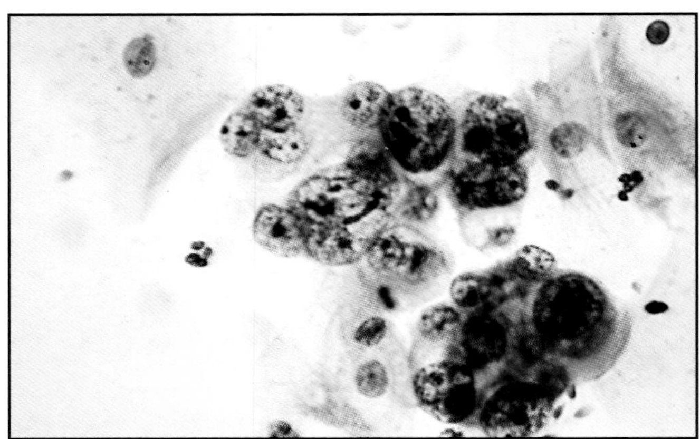

13.6
Grade III endometrial adenocarcinoma (x500).

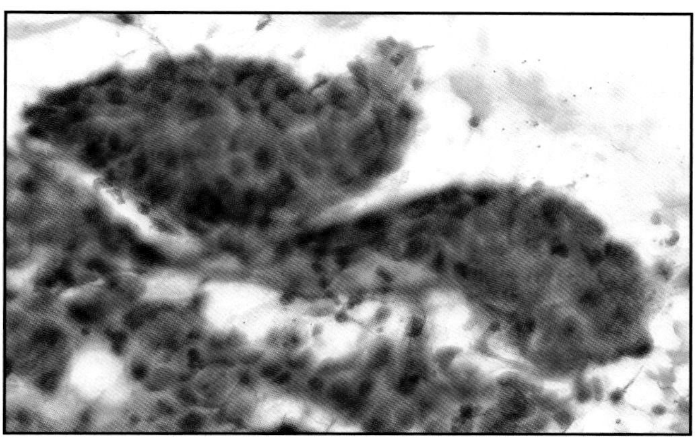

13.7

Serous papillary adenocarcinoma of the endometrium. Endocervical aspirate (x400).

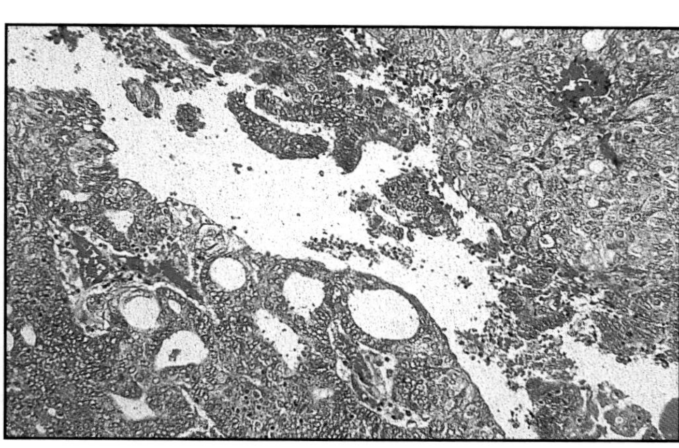

13.8

Histology of adenosquamous carcinoma of endometrium (x250).

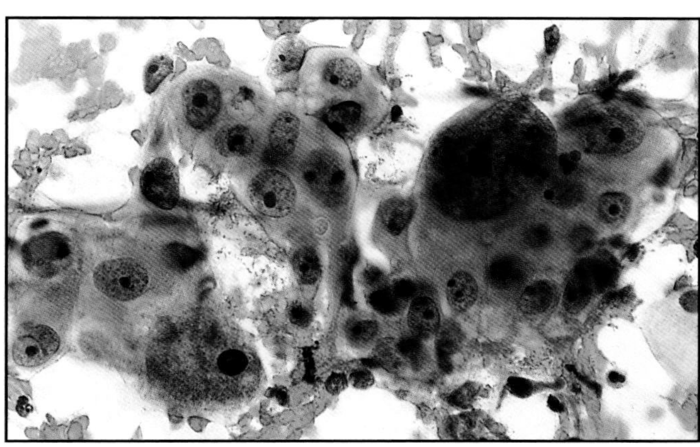

13.9

Adenosquamous carcinoma of endometrium (x500).

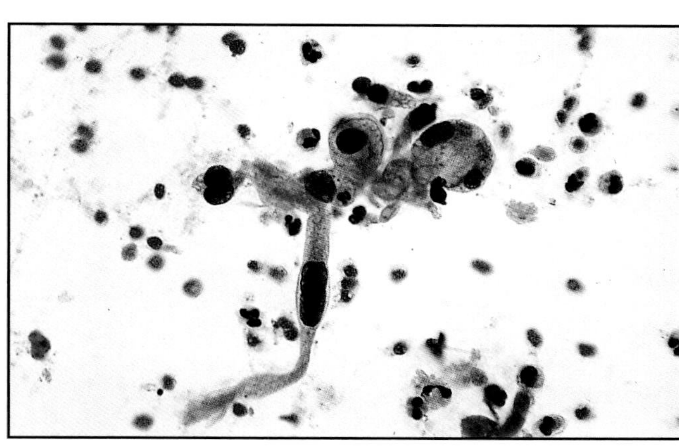

13.10

Sarcoma cells of malignant müllerian tumor of uterus. Endocervical aspirate (x500).

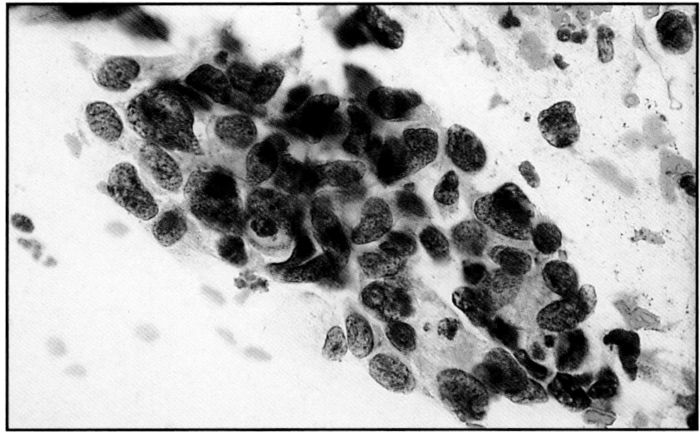

13.11

Endocervical adenocarcinoma (x500).

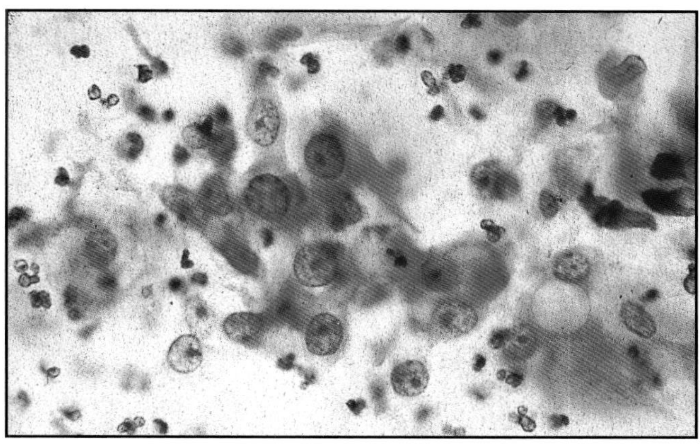

13.12

Endocervical adenocarcinoma (x500).

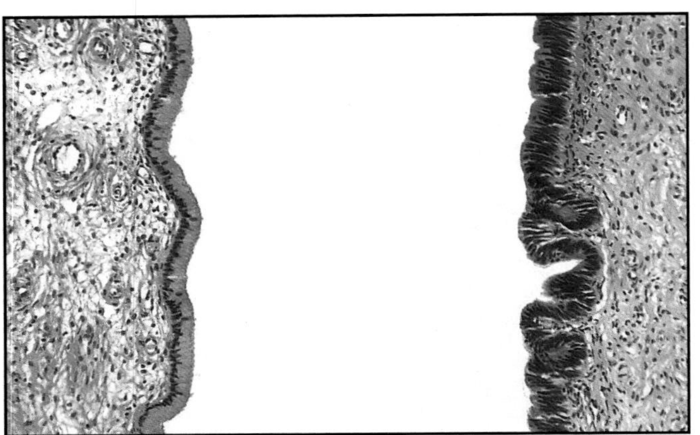

13.13
Tissue of endocervical adenocarcinoma in situ on surface epithelium on left and normal endocervical epithelium on right (x125).

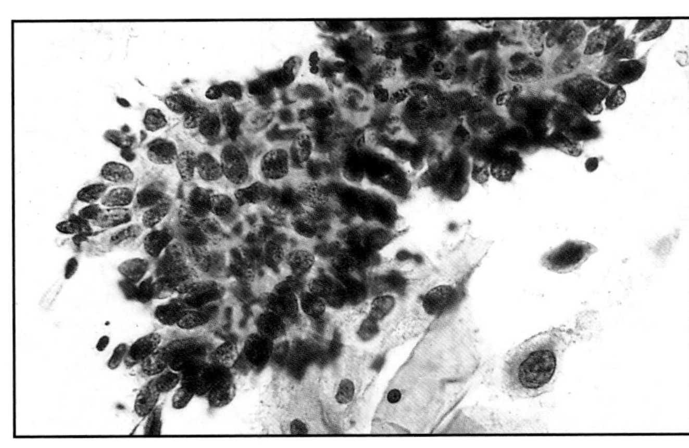

13.14
Endocervical adenocarcinoma in situ. Feathery pattern. Endocervical aspirate (x300).

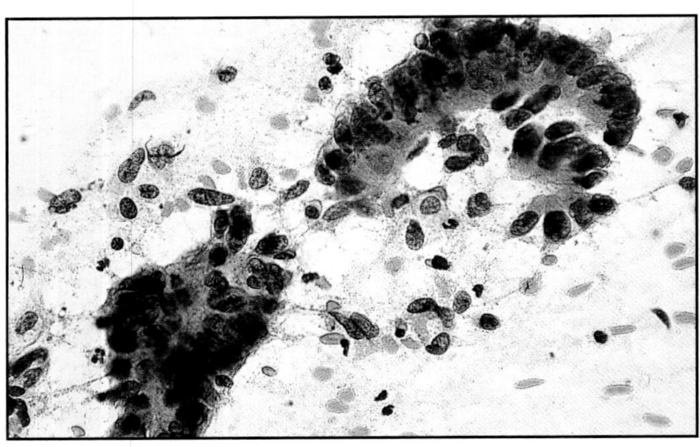

13.15
Endocervical adenocarcinoma in situ occurring in a strip. Endocervical aspirate (x200).

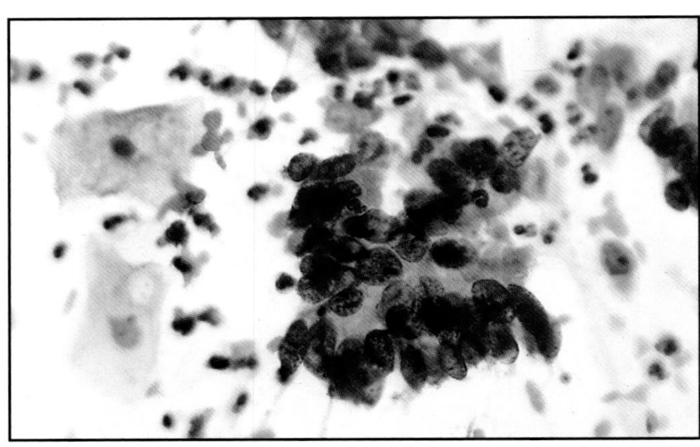

13.16
Endocervical adenocarcinoma in situ showing part of an abnormal acinar structure. Endocervical aspirate (x300).

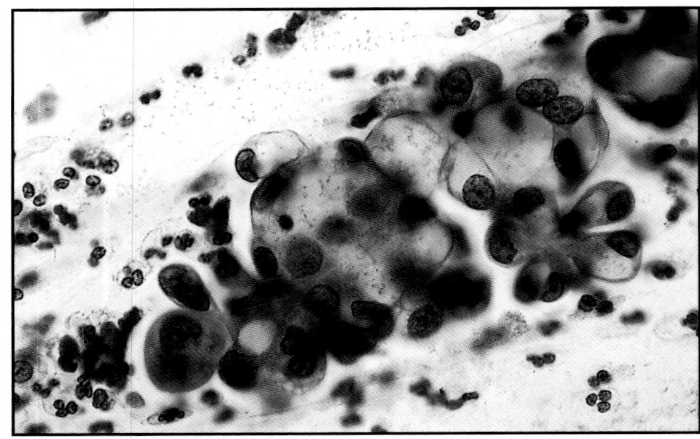

13.17
Extrauterine adenocarcinoma, primary from ovary (x500).

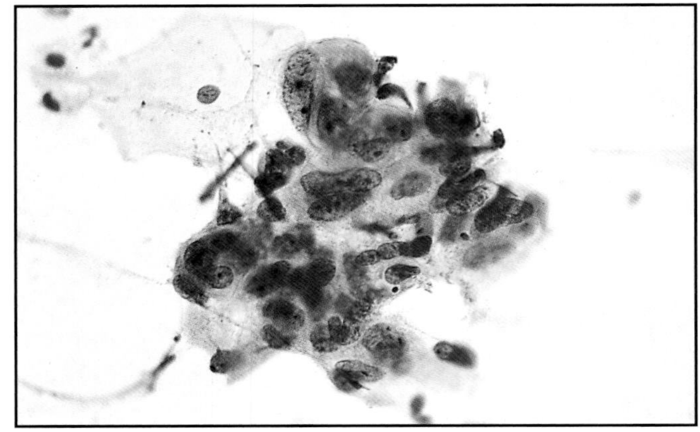

13.18
Extrauterine adenocarcinoma, primary from colon (x500).

REVIEW EXERCISES

1. Discuss the significance of identifying endometrial cells in the following cell sample from
   a) a 42-year-old woman on day 8 of the menstrual cycle.
   b) a 48-year-old woman on day 19 of the menstrual cycle.
   c) a 60-year-old postmenopausal woman.

2. Compare the findings in cellular samples from women with endometrial adenocarcinoma and atypical hyperplasia of the endometrium.

3. Discuss the differentiating cellular features of endocervical and endometrial adenocarcinoma in cell samples obtained by aspirating the cervical canal.

4. Compare the findings in cellular samples from women with primary uterine adenocarcinoma and extrauterine carcinoma.

5. Discuss the factors that have bearing on the ultimate accuracy achieved in the cellular detection of uterine adenocarcinoma and its precursors.

SELECTED READINGS

Ayer B, Pacey F, Greenberg M, Bousfleld L. The cytologic diagnosis of adenocarcinoma in situ of the cervix uteri and related lesions, I: adenocarcinoma in situ. *Acta Cytol.* 1987;31:397-411.

Cherkis RC, Patten Jr SF, Andrews TJ, Dickenson JC, Patten FW. Significance of normal endometrial cells detected by cervical cytology. *Obstet Gynecol.* 1988;71:242-244.

Ng ABP, Reagan JW, Cechner RL. The precursors of endometrial cancer: a study of their cellular manifestations. *Acta Cytol.* 1973;17:439-448.

Ng ABP, Reagan JW, Hawliczek S, Wentz BW. Significance of endometrial cells in the detection of endometrial carcinoma and its precursors. *Acta Cytol.* 1974;18:356-361.

Reagan JW, Ng ABP. *Cells of Uterine Adenocarcinoma.* 2nd ed. Basel, Switzerland: S Karger; 1973.

Wied GL, Keebler CM, Koss LG, Reagan JW, eds. *Compendium on Diagnostic Cytology.* 6th ed. Chicago, Ill: Tutorials of Cytology; 1990:18-20,139-153,162-166,176-188,194-212.

CHAPTER 14

Diseases of the Vulva and Vagina

Fadi W. Abdul-Karim, MD, MIAC

CONTENTS

Exfoliative cytology of the vulva and vagina can provide rapid diagnostic information about the nature of a lesion with little discomfort to the patient; it is not a substitute for biopsy, especially since vulvar lesions are visible and readily accessible for biopsy. The cytologic approach, however, can detect a wide variety of infectious, inflammatory, and dermatologic diseases, and can serve as an adjunct diagnostic technique for benign and malignant tumors. Vaginal cytology is used more widely in the diagnosis and follow-up of vaginal diseases and hormonal evaluation with excellent results.

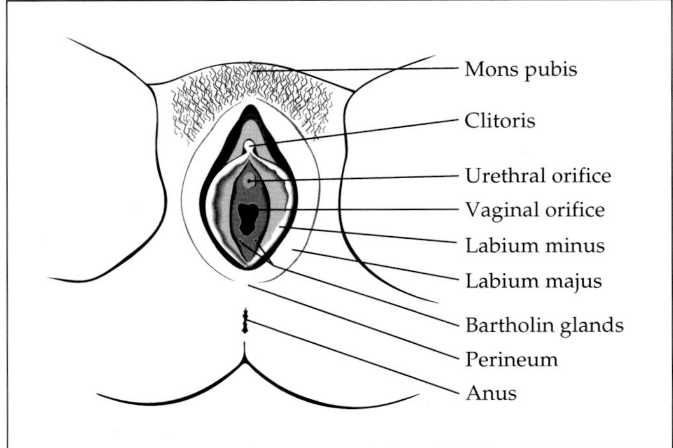

F *14.1*
External genitalia.

VULVA

Anatomy

The vulva consists of the labia majora, labia minora, mons pubis, perineum, clitoris, vestibule (urethral meatus and vaginal introitus), and Bartholin's glands. Collectively, they represent the female external genitalia [**F** *14.1*]. Prior to puberty, the labia majora, in contrast to labia minora, are inconspicuous and at puberty develop as secondary sexual characteristics.

Histology

The labia majora are folds of skin, with their appendages including hair follicles and sebaceous, sweat, and apocrine glands. The skin of the labia majora is composed of an outer lining of keratinized stratified squamous epithelium, which includes a basal layer of cells (stratum malpighii), a thin granular layer (occasionally absent), and a horny layer. The basal layer of the epidermis is continuous with that of the pilosebaceous unit and hair sheath. The surface of the labia minora is covered by nonkeratinizing squamous epithelium. This epithelium is rich in sebaceous glands; however, apocrine glands are rare, and hair follicles are absent. The vestibule is covered by stratified squamous epithelium. The vagina, urethra, and ducts of Bartholin's glands open into the vestibule. Bartholin's glands are paired tubular glands with simple mucin-producing columnar epithelia that lie in the posterior aspect of the labia majora. The main excretory ducts of the Bartholin's glands are lined by stratified squamous epithelium. Remnants of normal breast tissue are sometimes found in the vulva.

Sampling Techniques

The surface of the vulva, especially the labia majora, is physiologically dry and covered with a superficial layer of keratin. A cytologic sample of the vulva requires vigorous scraping to obtain adequate cellular material. To reduce the tendency for drying, most of the superficial lesions should be moistened by applying a wet compress prior to scraping. The wet compress removes most of the loose, degenerated cell debris and serum crust that may otherwise contaminate the smear. The initial scrape may be discarded for a more cellular second scrape that samples the deeper layers of the epithelium. Scraping can be performed with a variety of instruments, including the edge of a glass slide, scalpel blade, or a wooden or metal spatula. A moist or ulcerated lesion may be evaluated by pressing a glass slide to the lesion or by swabbing the edge of the ulcer, spreading the material on a slide, and immediately fixing the cell sample with a fixative or 95% ethanol. Cystic and subepidermal lesions of the vulva are best evaluated by fine needle aspiration biopsy technique.

Infectious Diseases

Various manifestations of bacterial, mycotic, viral, parasitic, venereal and nonvenereal diseases can be found on vulvar and vaginal scrapes.

Gonorrheal vulvitis is more common in children than adults, because the vulvar and vaginal mucosae in the pediatric age group are lined only by a few layers of squamous parabasal cells and are especially susceptible to infection. Cell studies show *Neisseria gonorrhoeae* diplococci in the cytoplasm of neutrophils or attached to the surface of squamous cells. A definitive diagnosis requires culture, which should always be done to confirm the preliminary cytologic impression.

Chancroid (soft chancre) caused by *Haemophilus ducreyi* presents as a vesiculopustule that progresses to a deep ulcer on the skin of the vulva. The diagnosis is based on examination of fresh exudate from the ulcer for the presence of numerous small, gram-negative bacilli arranged in pairs or short chains within leukocytes or lying free in the background. The cytologic findings, however, are nonspecific, and the diagnosis of chancroid requires isolation of *H ducreyi*. A skin test for chancroid is available, and the results of this will remain positive for several years after an acute infection.

The definitive diagnosis of syphilis can be aided by cytologic examination of fresh smears from syphilitic lesions by dark-field examination or by silver stain for the presence of spirochetes.

Granuloma inguinale is caused by the gram-negative bacillus *Calymmatobacterium granulomatis* and manifests as a large ulcerating lesion, which may extensively involve the vulva. Scrapings of the periphery of the ulcerative granulomatous lesions from the vulva or from rectal, inguinal, and urethral areas may reveal the bean-shaped organisms with "safety-pin" appearance in numerous multiple cystic spaces in the cytoplasm of macrophages (Donovan's bodies). Cellular debris and acute inflammatory cells are present in the background. Donovan's bodies are best evaluated by Romanowsky or silver stains. Smears from patients who have granuloma inguinale should be screened carefully because an association with squamous cell carcinoma has been reported.

Bartholin's gland infections may be the result of a variety of anaerobic or aerobic organisms. Both ductal and glandular elements may be infected, resulting in the formation of an abscess. The diagnosis may be established by fine needle aspiration cytology with appropriate cultures.

Mycotic vulvar infections are usually secondary to infection by *Candida albicans* or *Candida tropicalis*. The presence of hyphae with pseudoseptation, acute angle branching, and pear-shaped blastoconidia is diagnostic. *Torulopsis glabrata* is often present in smears from healthy women but may be a cause of mild vulvovaginitis. It can be differentiated from *Candida* by the absence of hyphae (only spores are present), variation in size, and tendency to cluster. Other superficial and deep mycotic infections are rare. Contaminating pollen and other plant bodies can mimic fungi.

Herpes simplex virus can infect skin and mucosa at various sites and is a common cause of vulvar ulcers and vesicles. Herpes simplex virus type 2, which mainly affects the genitalia, is transmitted primarily by sexual contact. Following exposure, 80% of previously unexposed females become infected. Scrapings of the margins of an ulcer or denuded base of a vesicle show typical multinucleated and isolated epithelial cells with homogeneous ground-glass nuclear appearance and discrete eosinophilic intranuclear inclusions often surrounded by a clear halo [❚*14.1*]. Cytologic methods cannot differentiate herpes simplex virus type 1 from type 2 or from varicella-zoster virus infections.

The vestibule and labial folds are the most common sites of condyloma acuminatum (venereal warts). The cytologic features of condyloma acuminatum at various sites of the female genital tract are identical. Cytologic evaluation reveals squamous cells that display paranuclear cavitation and hyperchromatic nuclei [❚*14.2*]. Hyperkeratosis and parakeratosis can be prominent.

Molluscum contagiosum is caused by a virus of the pox group and can involve the vulva and vagina. The infection, believed to be sexually transmitted, presents as localized, waxy, umbilicated lesions, which may be pruritic. Cellular samples demonstrate superficial squamous cells with large, round to oval, homogeneous, eosinophilic, intracytoplasmic inclusions (molluscum bodies) [❚*14.3*]. The nuclei are irregular, often eccentric, and degenerated or pyknotic. Without knowledge of the clinical setting, the molluscum bodies may be mistaken for artifacts or contaminants (pollen).

In geographic areas where parasitic infections are endemic, infection of the vulva and the vagina by parasites such as *Schistosoma*, *Filaria*, and *Entamoeba histolytica* (amebiasis) can be readily identified by recognizing the organism or ova on a cytologic preparation. The simplicity of the method is especially important in these countries, since more sophisticated means of diagnosis may not be available.

Inflammatory Conditions

Inflammatory diseases of the vulva and vagina are most frequently diagnosed by clinical examination or by biopsy rather than by a cytologic sample. Pemphigus vulgaris is a severe bullous dermatitis characterized by itching, acantholysis on biopsy specimens, and severe morbidity prior to adrenocorticoid therapy. Scraping the base of a freshly ruptured lesion yields intermediate basal squamous cells, either isolated or in sheets (Tzanck cells). These cells are characterized by round to oval central large nuclei, regularly distributed coarsely granular chromatin, and prominent nucleoli [❚*14.4*]. Degenerate paranuclear halos are present, as well as binucleation and multinucleation. Without correlation with the clinical setting, the cellular features of Tzanck cells might be mistaken for poorly differentiated adenocarcinoma cells, except for the overall repair-like features and the regularity of the chromatin pattern and nuclear membrane.

Bullous pemphigoid can be distinguished from pemphigus vulgaris on the basis of cytologic, histopathologic, and immunofluorescence features. Scraping of the base of a ruptured bulla or vesicle shows sheets of degenerated or semikeratinized, intermediate-type, squamous cells with central, large, single nuclei. The chromatin pattern is finely granular and regularly distributed, and nucleoli are small and inconspicuous. The background is relatively clean. Acantholytic cells (Tzanck test) are not present in bullous pemhigoid as the blisters are subepidermal. No inclusions are seen in either pemphigus vulgaris or bullous pemphigoid lesions.

Benign Tumors

Approximately 7% of all granular cell tumors involve the vulva. The majority involve the labia majora and present as a discrete, firm, raised, superficial mass. The overlying skin tends to be pigmented and sometimes ulcerated. The diagnostic exfoliated cells are usually large with sharp, well-defined cytoplasmic borders. The cytoplasm is thick and abundant, and contains numerous fine, dark, eosinophilic granules. The nucleus is regular, round, eccentrically placed, and relatively small. The chromatin is granular and uniformly distributed. Nucleoli are not prominent.

Of all papillary hidradenomas (hidradenoma papilliferum), 80% occur on the vulva and the remaining 20% involve the perianal skin. These tumors are usually asymptomatic but occasionally may ulcerate, bleed, or cause pain. This lesion is usually diagnosed by clinical examination or by biopsy rather than by cytologic examination. Histopathologically, the tumor is characterized by a papillary pattern consisting of fibrovascular stroma lined by two cell layers: superficial tall columnar cells and basal small cuboidal cells. Acinar or tubular structures may be present in variable proportions. A cytologic scrape of an ulcerated exophytic papillary lesion reveals clusters and sheets of low cuboidal to columnar cells showing little pleomorphism or atypia and resembling normal or hyperplastic breast ductal cells.

Non-neoplastic Epithelial Disorders

These lesions have been previously categorized as dystrophies and subdivided into atrophic, hyperplastic, and mixed types. Current classification of non-neoplastic epithelial disorders categorizes these legions into lichen sclerosus (lichen et atrophicus), squamous cell hyperplasia (formerly hyperplastic dystrophy), and other dermatoses.

Lichen sclerosus most frequently affects postmenopausal women. In advanced stages, the skin shows hyperkeratosis, atrophy, and a subepidermal zone of hyalinized collagen, below which is a band-like infiltrate of plasma lymphocytes and cells.

Squamous cell hyperplasia is characterized by hyperkeratosis, acanthosis, and absence of cytologic atypia. Some of these lesions show various combinations of histopathologic features and are classified as mixed. Cytologically, an increased number of anucleate squames and parakeratotic cells is observed in all these lesions. Distinction of the type of non-neoplastic epithelial disorder (dystrophy) based on cytologic appearance is not possible. Caution should be exercised in interpreting the significance of anucleate squames and parakeratotic cells, since they are present in normal skin or may overlie vulvar intraepithelial neoplastic lesions. Squamous cells in non-neoplastic epithelial disorders may demonstrate reactive changes; however, significant nuclear atypia and pleomorphism are not noted unless an underlying vulvar intraepithelial neoplastic lesion is present.

Vulvar Intraepithelial Neoplasia

Vulvar intraepithelial neoplasia (VIN) is defined as neoplastic change confined to squamous epithelium. A number of studies suggest that this lesion is becoming more prevalent in younger age groups than previously observed (ie, women 20–35 years of age). The epidemiologic profile of VIN suggests an important role for human papillomavirus (HPV) infection, and approximately 30% to 40% of patients with VIN have coexisting preinvasive or invasive lesions of the cervix or vagina. Immunodepressive disorders are present in approximately 5% of patients with VIN. Vulvar intraepithelial neoplasias are subclassified as to their severity and their potential to progress into an invasive process as follows: VIN I (mild dysplasia); VIN II (moderate dysplasia); and VIN III (severe dysplasia and carcinoma in situ). Cytologically, abnormal cells in low-grade lesions are usually polygonal, whereas those of high-grade lesions tend to be round or oval [▮*14.5*, ▮*14.6*]. The nuclear/cytoplasmic ratio increases with the severity of the lesion. Koilocytotic change is noted frequently within and adjacent to the lesions. Hyperkeratosis, parakeratosis, and pearl-like formations may also be present. In most cases, the number of abnormal cells and extent of cytologic abnormality make it possible to separate low- from high-grade intraepithelial lesions. Low-grade lesions, however, may be clinically indistinct and the cellular changes subtle. Cells of VIN III are more commonly observed in syncytial aggregates than those observed in equivalent cervical lesions. In some of these lesions, considerable variation in size and shape of the cells may be observed, and the nuclei demonstrate a prominent granular chromatin and hyperchromasia. Nucleoli are seldom seen. Confirmational biopsy is indicated, since these cellular changes may mimic those of large cell squamous cell carcinoma. The background of VIN lesions, however, is usually free of necrotic debris, which is commonly present in invasive carcinoma.

Bowenoid Papulosis

Bowenoid papulosis cannot be distinguished histopathologically from squamous cell carcinoma in situ. Clinical presentation, however, can distinguish these two lesions since bowenoid papulosis most commonly occurs in young adults and typically presents as multiple papules, small nodules, or plaques that clinically mimic verrucae or nevi. HPV has been identified in most of these lesions. The histopathologic similarities between bowenoid papulosis and squamous cell carcinoma in situ do not allow for separation of these lesions on cytologic grounds.

Malignant Tumors

Malignant tumors of the vulva account for approximately 5% of gynecologic cancers. The majority affect elderly women (mean age, 65 years) and are invasive squamous cell carcinomas, usually of keratinizing type. Histopathologically, these tumors are characterized by prominent intercellular bridges, cytoplasmic keratinization, and formation of keratin pearls. Less commonly, the tumors are large cell, nonkeratinizing, or small cell types. The cytologic characteristics of vulvar squamous carcinoma resemble those of their counterpart in the uterine cervix. Abnormal cells may occur singly or in aggregates, the latter more frequently found in keratinizing carcinomas. The cancer cells are usually polygonal, with well-defined cell borders and dense eosinophilic cytoplasm. Variation in size and shape may be prominent, as well as multinucleation and occasional elongated or tadpole bizarre forms. The nuclei may be relatively uniform or vary greatly in size and shape depending on the degree of differentiation. The nuclear/cytoplasmic ratio is high. The chromatin is irregularly, coarsely clumped [▮*14.7*]. Anucleated squames or parakeratotic cells, often with marked degeneration, are commonly found. The background of the smear characteristically shows necrotic debris and inflammatory cells.

Verrucous carcinomas present as large cauliflower-like tumors that have an indolent biologic behavior. Histopathologically, the tumor is composed of exophytic papillary fronds with surface hyperkeratosis and parakeratosis. The tumor forms bulbous rete pegs having blunt pushing borders, and it is generally well demarcated from the underlying stroma. Nuclear pleomorphism is mild or absent. Mitoses are rare. Cytologic smears from verrucous carcinomas typically show sheets of hyperkeratotic and parakeratotic cells and aggregates of squamous cells with little cellular or nuclear pleomorphism. The diagnosis of verrucous carcinoma is not possible on a cytologic basis because the findings are nonspecific and overlap with those of pseudoepitheliomatous hyperplasia and condyloma acuminatum. A biopsy specimen that includes the base of the lesion is necessary for diagnosis.

Basal cell carcinoma of vulva constitutes 2% to 3% of vulvar malignant tumors and occurs predominantly in elderly patients. The histopathologic features are similar to those of basal cell carcinomas found at other sites. The tumor is composed of infiltrating nests of small uniform cells with distinct peripheral palisading of the outermost layer. Only few cases have been described cytologically. Scraping of the lesion yields numerous sheets of small uniform cells with a scant amount of poorly defined cytoplasm and occasional peripheral palisading [▮*14.8*]. The nuclear/cytoplasmic ratio is high, and the nuclei are relatively uniform in size and shape. The chromatin pattern is coarsely granular and irregularly distributed, which imparts significant hyperchromasia. Nucleoli may be seen. These cellular characteristics must be confirmed by biopsy for a definitive diagnosis. The background of the smear is usually clean except when the tumor is ulcerated.

Extramammary Paget's disease occurs predominantly in white elderly women in the sixth and seventh decades of life and involves the vulvar, perineal, or perianal regions. It presents as well-demarcated erythematous or eczematous lesions that may be multifocal and frequently ulcerate. Histopathologically, Paget's disease is characterized by the presence of large, pale, vacuolated cells with mucicarmine-positive cytoplasm that are interspersed in the epidermis. Signet ring forms and intracytoplasmic melanin granules may occasionally be present. Only 30% of patients with vulvar Paget's disease have demonstrable invasive carcinoma. Cytologically, Paget's cells present as isolated or loose aggregates of abnormal glandular cells with a moderate amount of amphophilic cytoplasm [▮*14.9*]. The nuclei are enlarged and contain one or more prominent nucleoli. Signet ring forms and engulfing of one tumor cell by another are commonly observed. Cytologic examination does not allow for distinction between pure epithelial involvement and the presence of underlying invasive adenocarcinoma. Pigmented Paget's cells may be differentiated from melanoma cells by the demonstration of positive mucin staining and negative immunohistochemical staining for melanin.

Malignant melanoma of vulva accounts for 8% to 11% of all vulvar malignancies and is the second most common malignant tumor of the vulva following squamous cell carcinoma. Vulvar melanomas have a peak age incidence in the sixth to eighth decade and occur most often in whites. The clinical presentation is usually that of a mass accompanied by bleeding or pruritus. Most of the lesions are pigmented, with the superficial spreading form being the most frequent histopathologic variant and nodular melanoma being the least common. As with melanomas of the skin at other sites, the prognosis correlates strongly with the level of invasion. Cytologically, melanomas are characterized by the presence of isolated or loosely aggregated large pleomorphic cells, with abundant cytoplasm and large, round to oval nuclei [▮*14.10*]. Binucleation and multinucleation are frequently noted. The nuclear membranes are thick, the chromatin is abnormally clumped, and prominent nucleoli are frequently present. Intracytoplasmic melanin granules and clusters of free melanin pigment deposits may be observed in pigmented lesions. When pigment is abundant, it may obscure the nucleus.

Metastatic tumors of the vulva constitute approximately 8% of all vulvar malignancies. Metastases to the vulva are much less common than those to the vagina. They most frequently arise from carcinomas of the cervix followed by those of the endometrium, urethra, and kidney. Other frequent secondary tumors include malignant lymphoma, malignant melanoma, neuroblastoma, and cancers of the ovary, lung, rectum, and breast. Characteristically, metastatic tumors are localized to the dermis and subcutis and are rarely sampled by vulvar scraping except when ulcerated. The cellular characteristics of these lesions resemble those of the primary neoplasm.

Bartholin's gland carcinoma accounts for 2% to 7% of all vulvar malignancies and occurs predominantly in the fifth or sixth decade. Approximately one third of patients, however, are younger than 40 years of age. The most common symptom is a palpable mass or pain. Various histopathologic patterns have been described, including, most commonly, squamous cell carcinoma and adenocarcinoma, followed by undifferentiated, transitional cell, adenoid cystic, and adenosquamous carcinoma. When vulvar or vaginal ulceration exists, a large number of well-preserved abnormal cells may be recovered by scraping the lesion. None of the histopathologic subtypes are unique for the Bartholin's gland, and the cytologic patterns are not distinctive and vary according to subtype present. In general, the diagnosis of Bartholin's gland adenocarcinoma should be considered in the presence of numerous, large, malignant, mucin-producing columnar cells in the absence of a demonstrable endocervical or endometrial primary tumor [▮*14.11*].

VAGINA

Anatomy

The vagina is a tubular organ, about 10 cm long, that extends from the uterine cervix to the vestibule. The portio vaginalis protrudes into the internal end of the vagina. The fornices are recesses in the upper portion of the vagina between the cervix and vagina.

Histology

The internal surface of the vagina and the surface of the portio vaginalis are covered with a stratified squamous epithelium. This epithelium is hormonally sensitive and its thickness differs with age. In childhood, it is composed of few cell layers; however, after menarche and during the childbearing years, the epithelium thickens and becomes stratified. After menopause, as a result of loss of estrogenic stimulation, the epithelium becomes thin and atrophic. Squamous cells and debris exfoliating from this stratified squamous epithelium may accumulate mainly in the posterior vaginal fornix when the patient is prone. These cells show cyclic changes according to the ovarian cycle.

Sampling Techniques

To reduce the likelihood of contamination and increase the effectiveness of the scraping, most vaginal cytologic samples should be obtained prior to manipulation of the cervix. Excess mucous secretion covering the vaginal mucosa should be removed by cotton balls. The vagina may be cytologically examined by aspiration of the posterior fornix or by direct smears of a lesion. In detecting vaginal adenosis, circumvaginal scraping of the upper vagina may be performed. A more effective method, however, is a four-quadrant downward scraping of the vaginal mucosa in the anterior, posterior, and lateral vaginal walls.

Infectious Diseases

Infections of the vagina are caused by the same spectrum of organisms and viruses that affect the cervix (Chapter 11). These include *Neisseria gonorrhoeae*, *Gardnerella*, *Leptothrix*, *Candida albicans*, and herpesvirus. In addition, a number of parasitic organisms may be associated with vaginitis, including trichomonads, and, less commonly , *Entamoeba histolytica*, *Balantidium coli*, *Enterobius vermicularis*, and *Schistosoma*. These organisms cause the same cytologic changes in the vagina that they do elsewhere in the female genital tract. The vaginal epithelium is most susceptible to infection when there is absence of full maturation or presence of atrophic vaginitis. Trauma may predispose the epithelium to infections, with associated inflammatory reactions and repair. While cytologic studies may show certain characteristic findings, cultures remain the most definitive method of diagnosis for the majority of infectious organisms.

Vaginitis emphysematosa is characterized by the presence of gas-filled spaces of varying sizes in the lamina propria and epithelia of the vagina and cervix. Pregnancy and infections by *Trichomonas* appear to be predisposing factors. Histopathologically, these spaces have no cell lining except for the presence of multinucleated giant cells or inflammatory cells. Cell samples may depict these giant cells, inflammatory cells, and reparative epithelial changes.

Inflammatory and Miscellaneous Conditions

Cell scrapings from patients with atrophic vaginitis usually reveal numerous intermediate or atrophic squamous cells. Allergic reactions yield numerous eosinophils in addition to the nonspecific acute and chronic inflammatory cell background. Few cases of malacoplakia involving the vagina, cervix, and Bartholin's gland have been reported. The disease manifests as multiple yellow nodules involving the vaginal mucosa. Histopathologically, malacoplakia is characterized by the presence of numerous large histiocytes containing the characteristic

Michaelis-Gutmann bodies, which are round, basophilic, concentrically lamellated, and often calcified structures measuring up to 20 µm in diameter. Samples scraped from such lesions typically show numerous histiocytes with the diagnostic intracytoplasmic inclusions.

Following hysterectomy, an acute inflammatory reaction and granulation tissue proliferation may appear in the wound at the vaginal vault. Cytologically, reparative epithelial changes may be prominent in a background of acute and chronic inflammatory cells. This reparative change can mimic persistent or recurrent neoplasm.

Cervical, vulvar, and urethral lesions may often be misinterpreted by the patient as sources of vaginal discharge. A thorough clinical history and pelvic examination usually can identify the source of discharge.

Benign Neoplasms and Tumor-like Conditions

The majority of vaginal cysts are trauma-related inclusion cysts lined with squamous mucosa. They also contain keratinous debris. Other vaginal cysts are frequently müllerian remnants, usually occur in the anterior lateral wall, and are lined with cuboidal or low columnar epithelium, which may include mucus-secreting and ciliated cells. Scrapes of such lesions yield normal-appearing squamous epithelial cells or uniform cuboidal cells. Needle aspiration cytology may be more valuable in evaluating the origin and nature of these cysts. Endometriosis of the vagina is uncommon and seldom evaluated cytologically.

Fibroepithelial (stromal) polyps present as pedunculated polypoid masses occurring in the lower lateral vagina or near the introitus. Microscopically, they are covered with "normal," intact, stratified squamous epithelium and have loose or edematous fibrovascular connective tissue cores that contain large, atypical, often multinucleated, fibroblastic cells. Cytologic scrapes reveal normal, squamous mucosa without atypia. Other benign tumors of the vagina include fibromas, leiomyomas, and hemangiomas, which are rarely evaluated by cytologic means.

Vaginal Intraepithelial Neoplasia

Vaginal intraepithelial neoplasia (VAIN) is characterized by neoplastic change confined to the squamous epithelium and is graded similarly to cervical intraepithelial neoplasia (CIN). The risk factors for VAIN are believed to be similar to those for CIN. It is estimated that up to 85% of VAIN cases are associated with previous or concurrent history of cervical or vulvar preinvasive or invasive lesions. There is also an association with HPV infection, similar to that reported for the cervix and vulva. VAIN has also been reported in immunodepressed patients and in patients who have undergone radiotherapy, usually in conjunction with synchronous lesions in the cervix and vulva. VAIN changes usually involve the upper vagina or apex, less frequently the middle or lower third, and multicentric foci of origin are not uncommon. The histopathologic and cellular changes in VAIN are indistinguishable from their counterparts in the uterine cervix. The majority of patients with VAIN are asymptomatic, and routine screening is the most effective way of detecting these changes. Cytologically, the abnormal cells show varying degrees of cellular differentiation, mitotic activity, and nuclear atypia encompassing the spectrum of changes observed in CIN. Once a cytologic abnormality is detected, the diagnostic strategy for VAIN is similar to that for CIN; colposcopic examination is used to identify affected areas, followed by multiple biopsies.

Radiotherapy to the lower genital tract is strongly associated with the development of VAIN. The cytologic changes are similar to those described for postirradiation cervical changes; cellular and nuclear enlargement, cytoplasmic polychromasia, vacuolation, and multinucleation are commonly observed. After a latency period of several months to years, varying degrees of intraepithelial abnormalities, termed postradiation dysplasia, may be observed. The abnormal cells are round to oval or polygonal and have irregular shapes, cytoplasmic polychromasia, and enlarged nuclei [▮*14.12*]. The nuclear chromatin is finely granular but may be irregularly clumped, and chromocenters may be evident. Nucleoli are uncommon. These changes are frequently associated with a persistence or recurrence of the primary cancer for which radiation therapy had been administered. Patients developing these changes within 3 years after initiation of radiation therapy are more likely to develop recurrence compared with those developing the change after a longer period.

Malignant Neoplasms

Primary malignant neoplasms of the vagina are rare, comprising 1% to 2% of all malignant tumors of the female genital tract. Squamous cell carcinoma is the most frequent and usually presents as an ulcerated nodule or exophytic growth in the upper third of the vagina of elderly women. Secondary involvement by squamous cell carcinoma of the cervix or vulva is much more frequent than primary vaginal carcinoma, which by definition must occur without involvement of the cervix or vulva. In patients who have had previous carcinomas of the cervix or vulva, a disease-free interval of at least 5 years should be documented prior to considering the vaginal neoplasm as primary. Histopathologically, most vaginal squamous cell carcinomas are of the large cell, nonkeratinizing type. Cytologic preparations exhibit features similar to those described for cervical squamous carcinoma, with varying degrees of differentiation. The cellular changes associated with primary vaginal squamous cell carcinoma are indistinguishable from those of secondary involvement.

Verrucous squamous cell carcinomas rarely occur in the vagina. Scrapes usually reveal abundant hyperkeratotic or parakeratotic cells and aggregates of squamous cells with little pleomorphism. A biopsy is necessary to establish the correct diagnosis.

Primary adenocarcinomas of the vagina, excluding clear cell carcinoma, are extremely rare. Numerous histopathologic variants, including those having adenoid cystic, mucinous components and mixed adenosquamous carcinoma, have been cytologically identified. On the basis of cellular evidence alone it may be impossible to distinguish primary vaginal adenocarcinoma from much more frequent secondary neoplasms. Adenoid cystic carcinoma may on occasion be distinguished from adenocarcinoma of endometrial or endocervical origin by the formation of rosettes of small cells containing central mucoid globules, which stain a distinct red by the Wright-Giemsa method.

Malignant Melanoma

Malignant melanoma of the vagina is extremely rare. The histopathologic and cytologic features of vaginal melanoma are similar to those described for the vulva.

Embryonal Rhabdomyosarcoma

Embryonal rhabdomyosarcoma (sarcoma botryoides) is the most frequent malignant vaginal neoplasm in infants and children. Most occur before the age of 2 years and 95% occur in patients younger than 5 years of age. The neoplasm has a grape-like appearance, may distend the vagina, and may protrude from the vaginal orifice. Histopathologically, it is distinguished by the presence of numerous spindle-shaped or round primitive rhabdomyoblastic cells present in a band-like zone in the subepithelial area ("cambium zone"). The malignant cells in the deeper layers are usually present in a myxoid background and show varying degrees of differentiation. The cytologic features for rhabdomyosarcoma have been mainly described in fine needle aspirate smears that characteristically show numerous small cells in cohesive clusters or scattered singly. These tumor cells are round to oval or elongated with varying amount of cytoplasm, which presents as a tail-like projection or as a broad band [▮*14.13*]. Nuclei are eccentric, and macronucleoli may occasionally be noted. Immunohistochemical and electron microscopic studies are helpful in establishing the diagnosis. Although rhabdomyosarcoma may be suspected on the basis of cellular evidence, a specific diagnosis requires confirmation by biopsy. Recurrent or persistent neoplasms may be more readily identified by cellular studies.

Metastatic Tumors

The most common malignant tumor of the vagina is metastatic carcinoma, which may occur either through direct extension or hematogenous/lymphatic spread. The most common sites of origin include the uterine cervix, endometrium [▮*14.14*], ovary [▮*14.15*], large intestine, and urinary bladder. Histopathologically and cytologically, most metastatic diseases show the same degree of differentiation as the primary tumor. Metastatic implants may be associated with ulceration and tumor diathesis, making it impossible to differentiate them cytologically from primary vaginal tumors. Correlation with the clinical history cannot be overemphasized.

Vaginal Adenosis

Vaginal adenosis is defined as the presence of glandular epithelium, resembling either endocervical or tuboendometrial epithelium in the vagina. Adenosis is the most common change found in women exposed in utero to diethylstilbestrol (DES) and has been reported to occur in 35% to over 90% of the female offspring in exposed women. From the late 1940s to the late 1950s, DES was commonly administered as a synthetic estrogen to women in the early stages of pregnancy to prevent spontaneous abortion. The drug was subsequently found to be ineffective and was condemned for use in pregnancy in 1977 by the Food and Drug Administration.

The incidence of adenosis in women not exposed to DES varies markedly, ranging from 0% to 41%. Other changes attributed to DES exposure have included cervical erosions, genital ridges, cervical hoods, and clear cell carcinoma of vagina. Adenosis most frequently involves the upper third of the anterior vaginal wall and manifests initially as a surface change with subsequent involvement of the lamina propria. The diagnosis of adenosis is accomplished by colposcopic examination, by cytologic studies, and most specifically by biopsy.

The majority of adenosis cases are of the endocervical type. In cellular samples of adenosis obtained by vaginal scraping before cervical manipulation, columnar epithelial cells that resemble endocervical cells and occur individually or in a honeycomb and picket-fence arrangement are identified [▮*14.16*]. In the majority of cases, adenosis undergoes spontaneous involution. With time, squamous metaplasia occurs on the surface and subsequently involves deeper glandular epithelium. Cellular samples obtained at this stage reveal immature or mature squamous metaplastic cells with or without associated columnar epithelial cells [▮*14.17*]. Residual droplets of mucin may be identified in some of these metaplastic cells. Occasional anucleated squames relating to associated hyperkeratosis may be present. Adenosis has been noted to coexist with clear cell adenocarcinoma in 95% of cases, but it is not considered to be a precursor lesion. Although squamous intraepithelial lesions have been described in DES-exposed women, there is no documented evidence that significant epithelial abnormalities are more common in these women than in non–DES-exposed women. Rare atypical variants of adenosis having variable nucleocytoplasmic abnormalities have been described. In all such cases, a biopsy is mandatory to establish the diagnosis.

Clear Cell Adenocarcinoma

Clear cell adenocarcinoma of the vagina accounts for 1% of all invasive carcinomas of the female genital tract. The mean age of patients with clear cell adenocarcinoma of the vagina is 19.5 years of age, with a range of 7 to 29 years. Two thirds of the patients have a history of maternal exposure to DES, especially before the 18th week in utero. The risk of developing clear cell adenocarcinoma in DES-exposed women from birth to age 34 years has been estimated to be 0.1%. The neoplasm usually occurs in the upper third of the anterior vaginal wall. Several histopathologic patterns may be observed, including tubulocystic, solid, and papillary types. Clear cell adenocarcinoma often is observed in association with adenosis; however, progression of adenosis to cancer has not been clearly documented. Cytologically, the cells derived from clear cell adenocarcinoma may be isolated or occur in aggregates. The cytoplasm is often fragile, poorly stained, and vacuolated, and contains abundant glycogen [▮*14.18*]. The nucleus is enlarged, round or oval, and hyperchromatic. Bulging of the nuclei toward the glandular lumen occurs, which prompts the designation of hobnail cells. The nuclear chromatin is irregularly clumped and finely or coarsely granular. One or more macronucleoli may be observed. The smear background may vary from being clean to exhibiting neutrophils, blood, and debris.

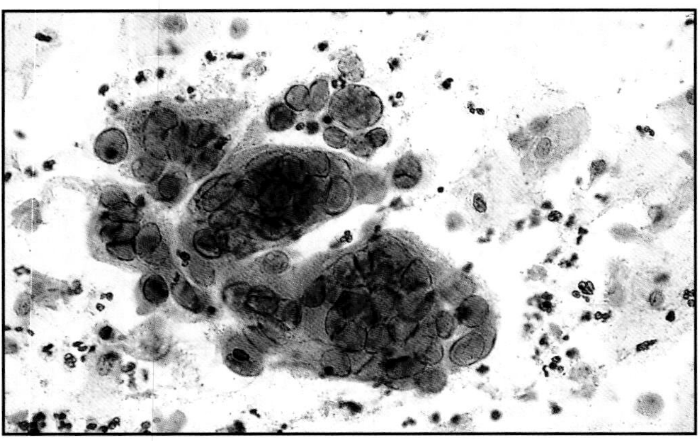

14.1

Herpes genitalis infection. Multinucleated cells with ground-glass nuclear chromatin and intranuclear inclusions (Papanicolaou, x500).

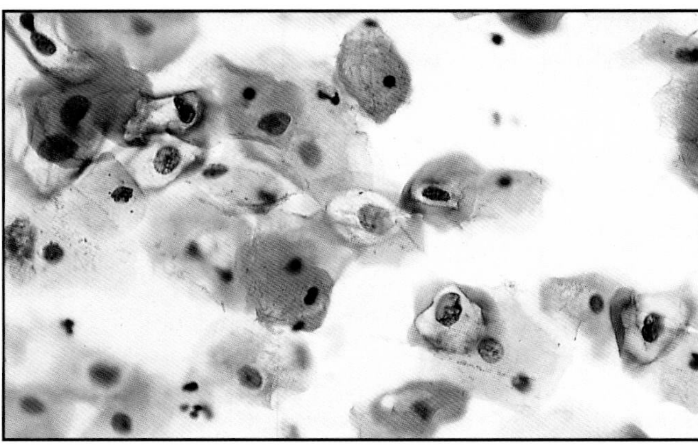

14.2

Condyloma acuminatum. Intermediate squamous cells with koilocytotic change (Papanicolaou, x500).

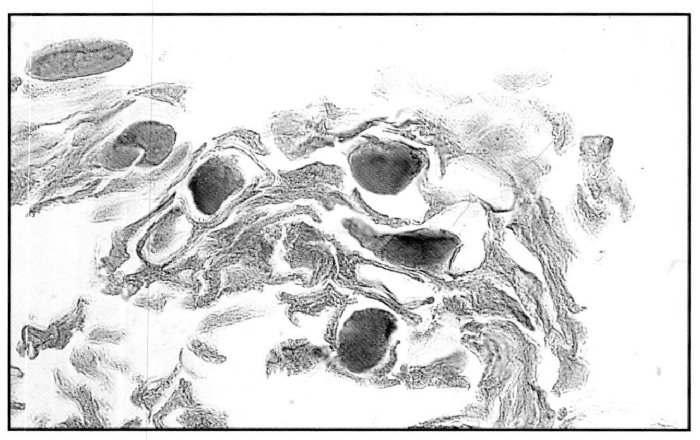

14.3

Molluscum contagiosum. Molluscum bodies with eosinophilic intracytoplasmic inclusions and eccentric pyknotic nuclei (hematoxylin-eosin, x500).

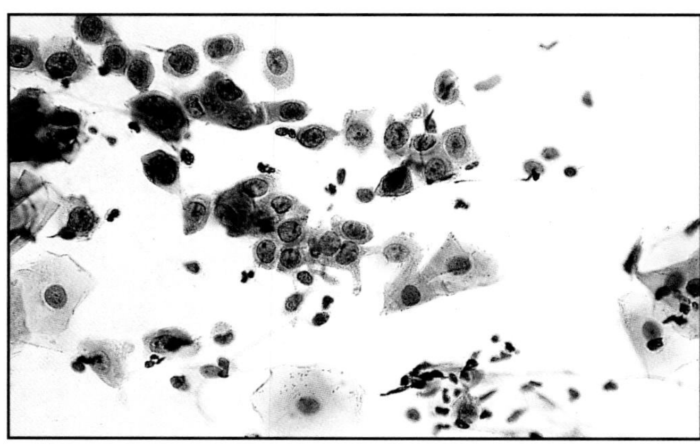

14.4

Pemphigus vulgaris. Isolated loose aggregates of acantholytic cells (Tzanck cells) (Papanicolaou, x500).

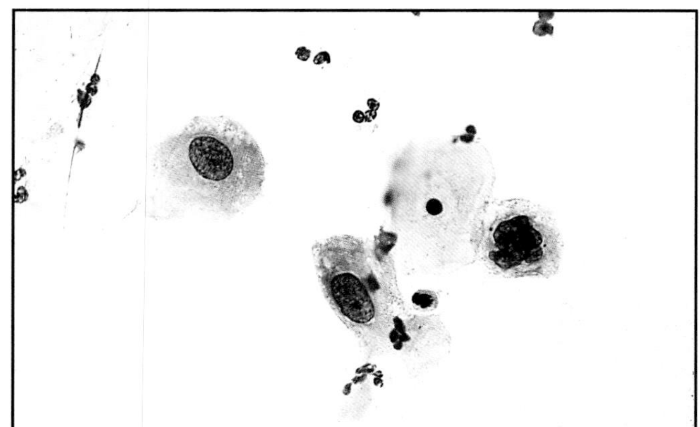

14.5

Vulvar intraepithelial neoplasia (VIN I). Abnormal polygonal cells with high nuclear/cytoplasmic ratio; the chromatin pattern is fine and evenly distributed.

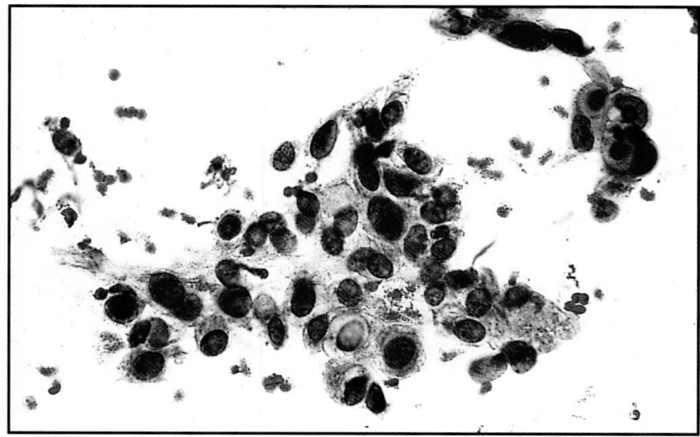

14.6

Vulvar intraepithelial neoplasia (VIN III). Syncytial aggregates of round to oval hyperchromatic cells with high nuclear/cytoplasmic ratio; background is clear (Papanicolaou, x500).

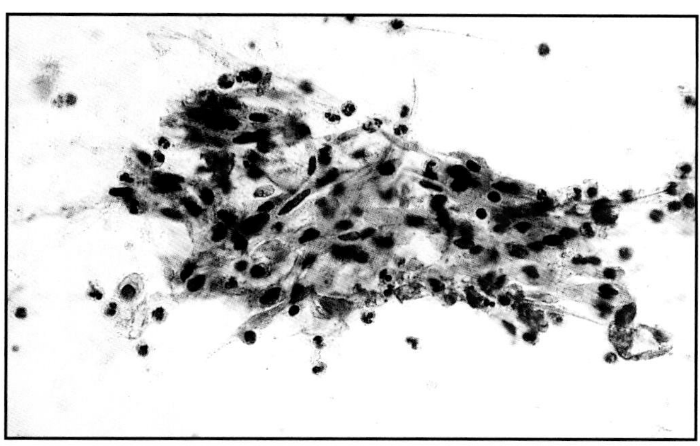

14.7

Keratinizing squamous carcinoma. Aggregates of spindle-shaped malignant squamous cells showing hyperchromatic nuclei with irregular chromatin pattern. The background shows cell debris and inflammatory cells (Papanicolaou, x500).

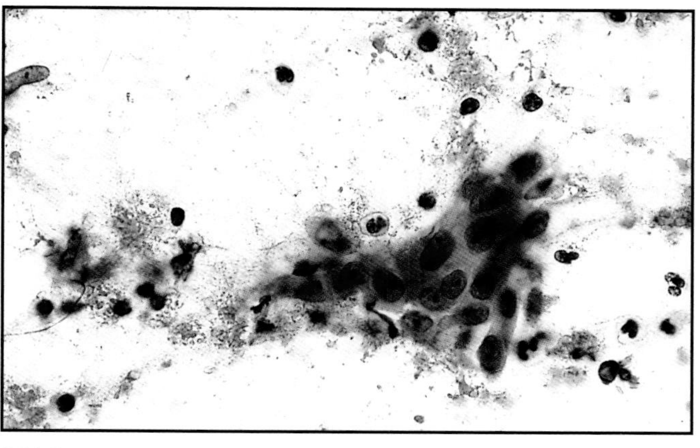

14.8

Basal cell carcinoma of vulva. An aggregate of small, relatively uniform cells with scanty cytoplasm, and conspicuous nucleoli (Papanicolaou, x500).

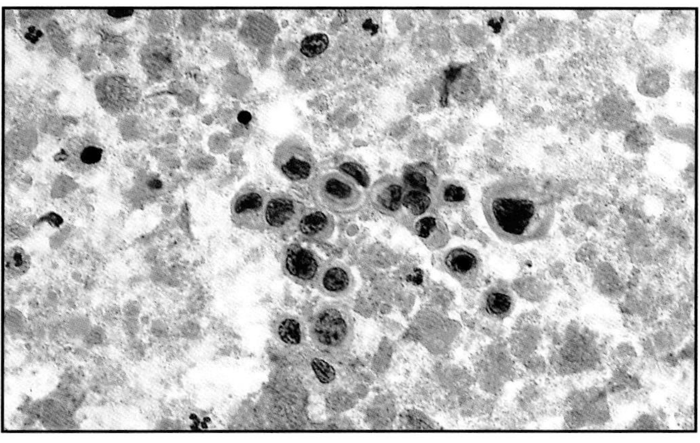

14.9

Paget's disease of vulva. Isolated malignant glandular cells with eccentric nuclei. The lesion was ulcerated (Papanicolaou, x500).

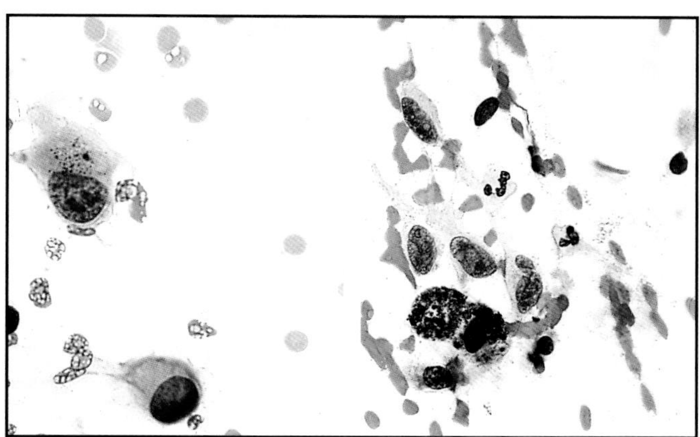

14.10

Malignant melanoma of vulva. Isolated (left) and loosely aggregated (right) pleomorphic cells with abundant cytoplasm and eccentric nuclei with prominent nucleoli. Melanin pigment is present (Papanicolaou, x500).

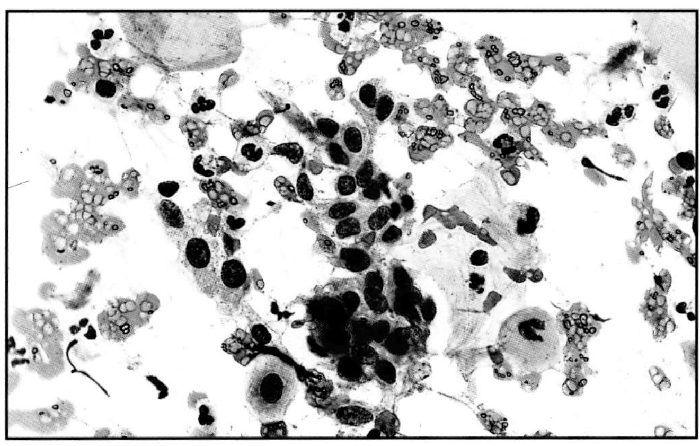

14.11

Bartholin's gland adenocarcinoma. Malignant cuboidal columnar glandular cells in loose aggregates and a three-dimensional cluster (Papanicolaou, x500).

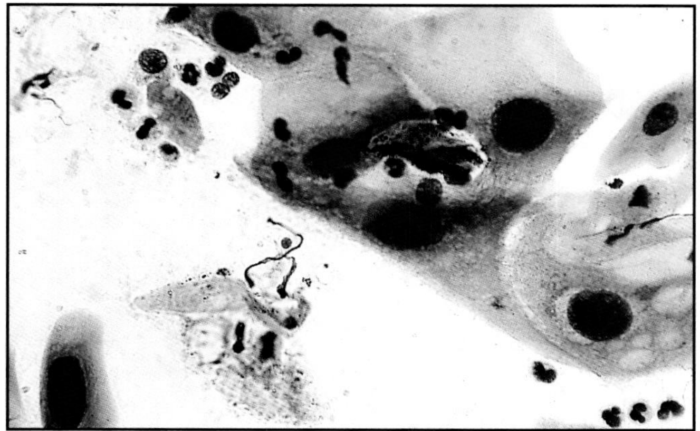

14.12

Postradiation dysplasia of vagina. Sheets of dysplastic cells with cytoplasmic polychromasia and vacuolization (Papanicolaou, x500).

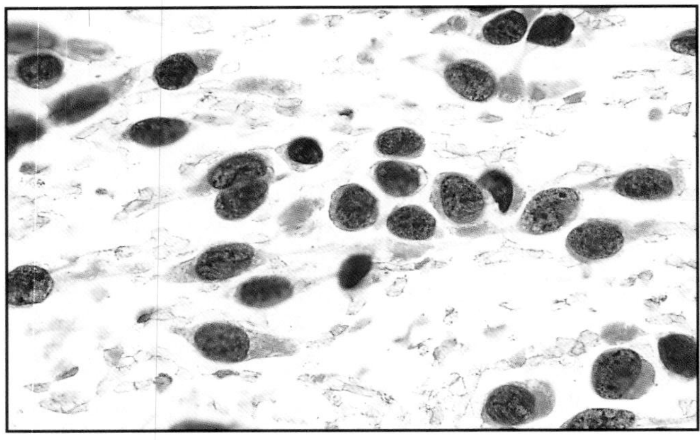

▮*14.13*

Sarcoma botryoides. Elongated sarcoma cells with eccentric nuclei and tail-like projection of the cytoplasm (Papanicolaou, x500).

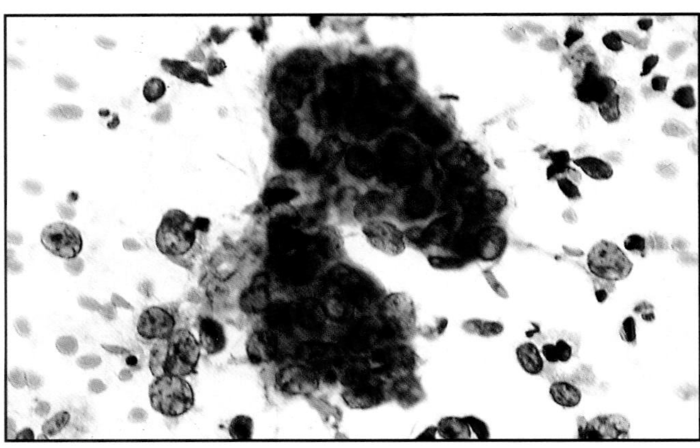

▮*14.14*

Metastatic adenocarcinoma involving vagina from endometrial adenocarcinoma (Papanicolaou, x500).

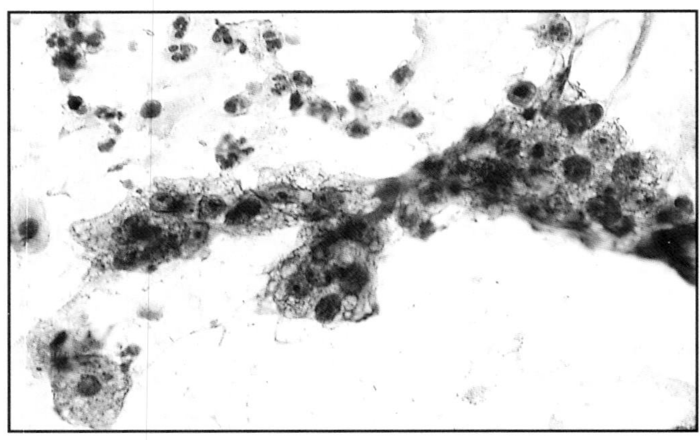

▮*14.15*

Metastatic adenocarcinoma involving vagina from primary ovarian adenocarcinoma (Papanicolaou, x500).

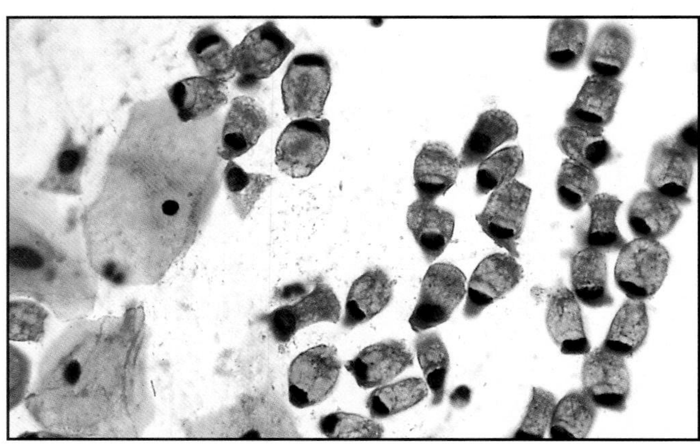

▮*14.16*

Adenosis of the vagina. Numerous, tall, columnar, mucin-producing cells (Papanicolaou, x500).

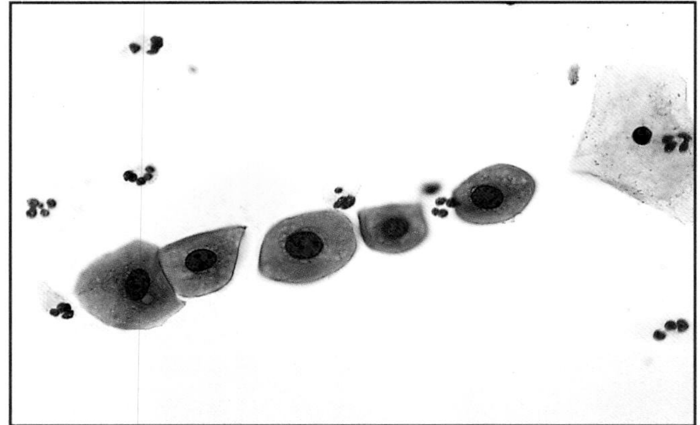

▮*14.17*

Adenosis of the vagina. Metaplastic cells derived from squamous metaplasia of endocervical-type mucosa (Papanicolaou, x500).

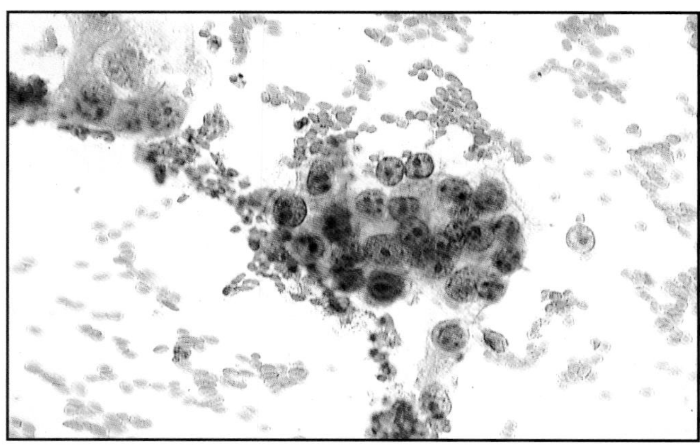

▮*14.18*

Clear cell adenocarcinoma of the vagina. Clusters of malignant glandular cells with vacuolated cytoplasm, large nuclei, and prominent nucleoli (Papanicolaou, x500).

SELECTED READINGS

Copeland LJ, Sneige N, Gershenson DM, et al. Bartholin gland carcinoma. *Obstet Gynecol.* 1986;67:794.

Fu YS, Reagan JW. *Pathology of the Uterine Cervix, Vagina, and Vulva.* Philadelphia, Pa: WB Saunders Co; 1989. Major Problems in Pathology.

Fu YS, Reagan JW, Richert RM, et al. Cytologic diagnosis of diethylstilbestrol-related genital tract changes and evaluation of squamous cell neoplasia. In: Herbst AC, Bern HA, eds . *Developmental Effects of Diethylstilbestrol (DES) in Pregnancy.* New York, NY: Thieme-Stratton; 1981.

Heustis DG. Vaginal and vulvar cytology. In: Astarita RW, ed. *Practical Cytopathology.* New York, NY: Churchill Livingstone; 1990:47-60.

Masukawa T, Friedrich EG. Cytopathology of Paget's disease of the vulva: diagnostic abrasive cytology. *Acta Cytol.* 1978;22:476-478.

Mazur MT, Hsueh W, Gersell DJ. Metastases to the female genital tract: analysis of 325 cases. *Cancer.* 1984;53:1978-1984.

Mitchell MF. Diagnosis and treatment of preinvasive disease of the female lower genital tract. *Cancer Bull.* 1990;42:71-76.

Naib ZL. *Exfoliative Cytopathology.* 3rd ed. Boston, Mass; Little, Brown and Co; 1985:233-256.

Reagan JW, Ng ABP. Vaginal and vulvar disease. In: Wied GL, Keebler CM, Koss LG, et al, eds. *Compendium on Diagnostic Cytology.* 6th ed. Chicago, Ill: Tutorials of Cytology; 1988:71-82.

Sandburg EC. Benign cervical and vaginal changes associated with exposure to stilbestrol in utero. *Am J Obstet Gynecol.* 1976;125:777-789.

Sorenson K, Somrak TM. Vulva, vagina. In: Bibbo M, ed. *Comprehensive Cytopathology.* Philadelphia, Pa: WB Saunders Co; 1991:285-296.

CHAPTER

15

Respiratory Tract

WILLIAM W. JOHNSTON, MD, FIAC

CONTENTS

The study of diseases of the respiratory tract by cytologic methods is not a recent development but rather had its origins in scientific practices of the 19th and early 20th centuries. The studies of Walshe, Beale, Hampeln, and Dudgeon are particularly noteworthy. The work of Papanicolaou in establishing the credibility of cytologic methods made possible the widespread use of cellular specimens for evaluation of diseases of the respiratory tract. Currently, the number of specimens from the respiratory tract being examined in a general cytopathology laboratory is exceeded only by the number of those from the female genital tract.

This chapter covers the cytologic and cytopathologic principles that relate to the gross and microscopic anatomy and pathology of the respiratory tract, especially the lungs. Included are discussions of the role of sputum, bronchial washings and brushings, bronchoalveolar lavages, and fine needle aspirates (FNAs) in contributing to the diagnosis of various disease entities.

ANATOMY

The major function of the respiratory system—gaseous exchange—is admirably reflected in its anatomy. A pair of lungs enclosed in an expansile cage of bone and muscle promotes the oxygenation of the blood and the removal from it of carbon dioxide. A series of converging tubes, the bronchioles and bronchi, which unite to form the trachea, connects the alveolar sacs (where gaseous exchange occurs) to the upper respiratory tract. The upper respiratory tract is composed of the nose, olfactory apparatus, paranasal sinuses, pharynx, and larynx. The major purposes of the upper respiratory tract are cleansing and regulating the temperature of the inspired air prior to its entrance into the lungs. Two other vital functions include olfaction and voice production.

The oral cavity and portions of the pharynx and nose are lined by a nonkeratinizing stratified squamous epithelium. A less thick squamous epithelium covers the vocal cords. Although the morphologic examination of specimens from these areas does not constitute a component of the discipline of respiratory cytology, superficial and intermediate squamous cells are constantly exfoliating and, therefore, will be commonly present in sputum and bronchial specimens. The trachea, bronchi, and parts of the upper respiratory tract are lined by a pseudostratified, columnar epithelium composed of three major types of cells. The most common ones are columnar cells that extend from the basement membrane to the lumen. Their free borders contain cilia. Less frequently seen are goblet cells that produce mucus. Just above the basement membrane may be seen reserve cells that are small and polygonal [**F** *15.1*]. Bronchioles, defined as bronchi less than 3 mm in diameter, are lined by a single layer of columnar or cuboidal epithelium composed of at least three cell types: ciliated columnar cells, goblet cells, and nonciliated Clara cells [**F** *15.2*]. The thin-walled alveolar air sacs are lined by alveolar cells or pneumocytes designated as type I and type II. The type II cells are believed to manufacture surfactant, a surface-active material that prevents collapse of the air sacs on expiration.

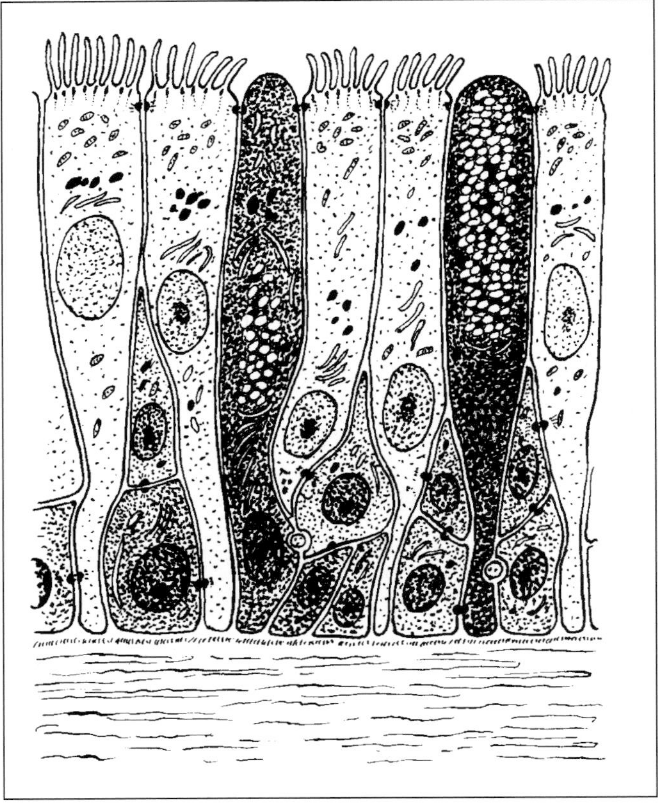

F *15.1*
Epithelium lining the trachea and bronchi shows ciliated columnar cells, nonciliated mucus-producing cells, and primitive reserve cells at the basement membrane.

TYPES OF CELLULAR SPECIMENS

The following types of cellular specimens and techniques for cellular preparation are those most commonly used in the contemporary cytopathology laboratory. The relationships between the cellular preparation and the patterns of cellular presentation within that preparation must be appreciated.

Sputum

Sputum is the product of interaction between the mucociliary apparatus and immune system of the host

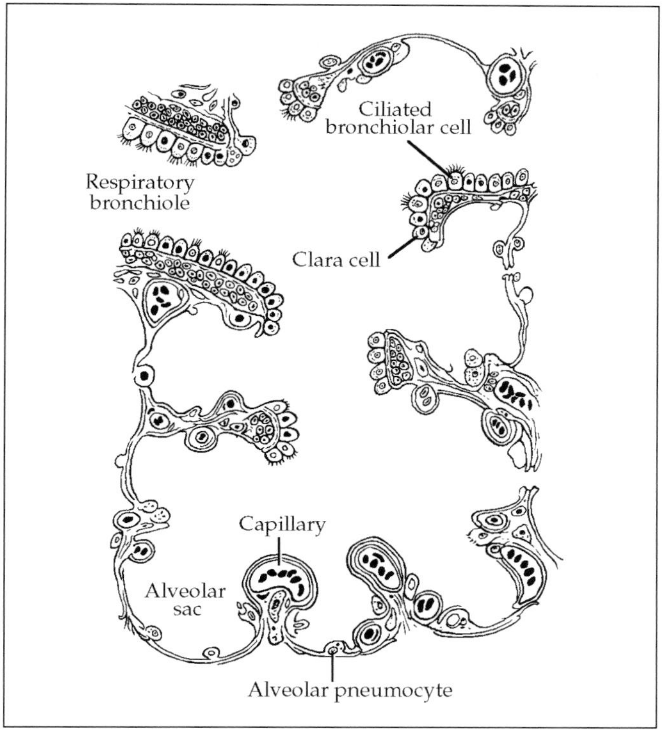

F15.2

Terminal respiratory bronchioles and alveolar network with the major cell types encountered.

and the animate and inanimate invaders from the environment. Sputum, which is composed predominantly of mucus, also contains a large variety of cellular and noncellular materials produced by the host and substances that have been inhaled. It is the most frequently examined specimen obtained from the respiratory tract.

A number of cytopreparatory techniques are used in preparing sputum for examination. The simplest method is one in which a fresh, early morning specimen of sputum produced by a deep cough is collected and brought immediately to the laboratory without any fixation. It is examined grossly for tissue fragments and other suspicious material. Smears from this material and other areas of the sputum randomly sampled are prepared and fixed in 95% ethanol. These smears, as well as all other specimens discussed in this section, are stained by the traditional Papanicolaou method. This method of sputum preparation has the advantage of revealing cells and other components that exhibit excellent preservation and staining. If the transmission of unfixed material to the laboratory is impossible, prefixed sputum may be obtained by instructing the patient to expectorate into a small widemouth jar half-filled with 70% ethanol.

Saccomanno described a method of cytopreparation of sputum that has gained wide popularity in recent years. It involves the collection of sputum in a mixture of 50% ethanol and 2% polyethylene glycol (Carbowax). Collections may involve a single specimen, or the same container may be used for collections of multiple specimens from the same patient over a period of hours or even days. In the laboratory, the specimen is broken up in a Waring-type blender, and smears are prepared from the centrifuged cell button. This technique has several major advantages, including concentration of cells and the possibility of preparing teaching slides from interesting cases. A disadvantage is the difficulty in achieving preservation of cellular and tissue organelle structures.

In those patients who cannot produce sputum spontaneously by deep coughing, a specimen of sputum can be induced. The basic principle involves the inhalation of a solution that has been aerosolized. The inspired vapor stimulates mucus production. One popular method employs a heated (37°C) solution of 15% sodium chloride and 20% propylene glycol. After inhaling these vapors for approximately 20 minutes, the patient will usually produce copious satisfactory sputum.

Bronchoscopy

The development of the rigid bronchoscope in the late 19th century formed the foundation of a technology by which the mucosal surfaces of the bronchi could be directly visualized and sampled for both tissue and cellular evaluation. In more recent years this technology has been improved by the introduction of flexible catheters advanced into the bronchi under fluoroscopic control and, perhaps even more importantly, by the development of the flexible fiberoptic bronchoscope.

After introducing the bronchoscope into the lower respiratory tract, the examiner has several options for taking direct samplings from the visualized areas. Specimens may be obtained by means of a suction apparatus that aspirates secretion. Washings from the visualized areas may also be obtained and collected by instilling 3 to 5 mL of a balanced salt solution through the bronchoscope and reaspirating the resulting material. Biopsies may also be performed for histologic examination. Once the bronchoscope is removed, direct smears may be made with immediate fixation in 95% ethanol. The aspirates and washings may be treated in several different ways. They may be centrifuged and smears prepared from the cell buttons; they may be subjected to membrane filter-preparation; or they may be centrifuged and the resulting buttons embedded in paraffin for histologic sectioning. More recently, many laboratories have added preparations made by the cytocentrifuge. In my experience, a judicious combination of direct smears, membrane filter preparations, and cytocentrifuge preparations of the aspirates and washings yields the best diagnostic results.

The development of the flexible fiberoptic bronchoscope has made it possible for the operator to view much smaller bronchi of the lung than was formerly possible with the rigid tube bronchoscope alone. With this flexible apparatus, the examiner may both visualize and brush a suspected lesion and submit the resulting cytologic material for laboratory examination. The preparation of cellular specimens from the bronchial brush is similar to those techniques used for bronchial aspirates and washings.

Bronchoalveolar Lavage

Bronchoalveolar lavage (BAL) involves the infusion and reaspiration of a sterile saline solution in distal segments of the lung via a fiberoptic bronchoscope. This technique has been utilized in the therapy of such diseases as pulmonary alveolar proteinosis, cystic fibrosis, pulmonary alveolar microlithiasis, and asthma. More recently, it has proved to be of value in the diagnosis of pulmonary disease. Although BAL has been employed in the detection of lung cancer and the evaluation of interstitial lung disease, perhaps its most important diagnostic application is the detection of opportunistic infections in immunocompromised hosts. The cytopreparatory techniques for BAL are similar to those employed for bronchial material.

Fine Needle Aspirates

In recent years, the evolution of highly sophisticated radiologic imaging techniques, which have made possible the precise visualization and localization of masses in the lung, in combination with the reintroduction of a sampling technique of such visualized lesions by the insertion of a fine-bore needle, have revolutionized diagnostic cytopathology of the lung. In this procedure, a fine needle attached to a syringe is passed through the chest wall or bronchial wall into the pulmonary mass visualized either by fluoroscopy, computed tomography, or bronchoscopy. The aspirated cellular specimen is examined by conventional cellular techniques. The importance and usefulness of fine needle aspiration (FNA) are rapidly gaining wide recognition throughout the world, and it has the potential to become the premiere tool for the evaluation of pulmonary lesions.

Although some variation exists among institutions in their policies on indications for the performance of FNA, the following are those most generally practiced: (1) suspected lung cancer that is inoperable; (2) a solitary pulmonary mass suspected of being the source of probable metastatic disease; (3) a solitary pulmonary nodule and known primary malignancy outside of the lung; (4) a patient who refuses exploratory thoracotomy for suspected lung cancer; (5) multiple pulmonary masses; (6) an undiagnosed pulmonary mass; (7) a suspected superior sulcus tumor; (8) a patient who fails to respond to appropriate antituberculosis therapy; (9) a suspected infectious process, particularly in the immunocompromised patient; and (10) any patient with suspected lung cancer on whom five consecutive early morning deep-cough specimens of sputum and one bronchial brushing or washing have been negative for malignant tumor cells.

The contraindications for FNA are as follows: (1) patients who are debilitated, uncooperative, or have uncontrollable cough; (2) hemorrhagic diathesis, anticoagulation therapy, suspected vascular lesion, or pulmonary hypertension; and (3) *Echinococcus* cyst. Complications have included pneumothorax, hemoptysis, and hemothorax.

The general technique of FNA came into use at Duke University Medical Center (Durham, NC) in the early 1970s. Of the total number of aspirates examined from all body sites, 30% have been from the lung. The current policy at the medical center is to consider any patient found with a demonstrable radiographic abnormality in the lung fields as a potential candidate for FNA. The decision to proceed with the aspiration is based on the level of suspicion that the visualized nodule or density represents cancer or an infectious process, and on the morphologic evidence provided by prior cytologic and histologic specimens obtained from the respiratory tract. All aspirations are performed by a radiologist using fluoroscopy or computed tomography.

Transbronchial FNA is a special modification of needle aspiration for those cases in which the lung neoplasm has not invaded through the mucosa into the bronchial lumen and thus is not accessible through sputum or bronchial brushing. This procedure involves the insertion of a flexible needle through the fiberoptic bronchoscope, penetration of the bronchial wall, and aspiration of cytologic material lying beyond.

In the preparation of the cellular specimen from a fine needle aspirate, the most important principle is that the diagnostic cellular material should be within the barrel of the needle and not the syringe. To ensure that this relationship remains undisturbed, the needle should be disconnected from the syringe, the syringe refilled with air, and the syringe and needle reconnected. The contents of the needle can now be expelled onto a slide or into a small amount of any solution desired. Excellent smears are easily prepared by the following steps: (1) gently lay one slide over the slide holding the drops of expelled material; (2) use the weight of the upper slide to spread the material; (3) pull the slides apart horizontally; and (4) quickly drop the slides into 95% ethanol or agitate them rapidly for air-dried smears.

At Duke University Medical Center, the following procedure is used. A 22-gauge Chiba needle with a 20-mL syringe is inserted percutaneously into the lung mass. From the aspirate, four direct smears are prepared: two for immediate wet fixation in 95% ethanol and staining with the Papanicolaou method and two for air-drying and staining with a Romanowsky method. The remaining aspirate is then mixed with 10 mL of balanced salt solution and brought to the laboratory for further procedures. The cellular suspension is centrifuged, and aliquots are processed for membrane filters, direct smears, cytocentrifuge specimens, and cell blocks. For immediate consultation, the smears being air-dried are evaluated for cellularity. By this procedure, the radiologist can be given an immediate assessment of the cellular content of the aspirate and, therefore, an implied assessment of whether the aspirate is satisfactory for diagnosis. If it is determined to be hypocellular, the aspiration can be repeated immediately. When extensive necrosis is observed, the radiologist is advised to obtain additional material from the periphery of the nodule, where well-preserved tumor cells are more likely to be found. The presence of bacteria, fungi, or inflammation are reported immediately to the radiologist so that appropriate cultures can be obtained. Based on the findings in the air-dried preparation, the specimen can be evaluated for additional cytochemical or immunocytochemical stains or for electron microscopic evaluation.

Although the cytologic presentation of the major types of lung cancer in FNAs will be discussed in the appropriate subsections, one important point is worth emphasizing. The morphology of lung tumors in these specimens is essentially the same as that in sputum and bronchial material, but with one additional characteristic: the FNA, because of direct sampling within the tumor by the needle, should contain large numbers of cancer cells and tissue fragments. The cell block becomes a useful vehicle for the study of the latter. Not infrequently, microbiopsies of tissue will be available for evaluation in these preparations. Indeed, the presence of only small numbers of putative tumor cells in an FNA should be a significant warning to the pathologist to exert extreme caution in rendering a conclusive cancer diagnosis. This is the setting in which a false-positive diagnosis of cancer is most likely to occur.

CYTOLOGY OF THE NORMAL RESPIRATORY TRACT AND CYTOPATHOLOGY OF NON-NEOPLASTIC DISEASES

Cells of Epithelial Origin

The normal epithelial components of sputum are squamous epithelial cells, which exfoliate from the oral cavity and pharynx, and respiratory columnar epithelial cells, which exfoliate most frequently from the upper respiratory passages, bronchiolar epithelium, and alveolar epithelium. The recognizable cells shed from the tracheobronchial tree may be of two types. The most common type is the ciliated columnar cell. These cells are characteristically seen in bronchial washings, aspirates, brushings, BALs, and FNAs. They should not be present in large numbers in sputum except in postbronchoscopy specimens or in situations involving extensive damage to the respiratory epithelium. The individual cell is characterized in profile by a columnar or prismatic shape ending in a tail. The nucleus is oriented toward the tail end and shows a finely granular chromatin pattern with one or more small nucleoli. Cilia with a terminal plate are present [❚*15.1*].

A second, less commonly encountered type of epithelial cell shed from the tracheobronchial tree is the mucus-producing bronchial cell, also called a goblet cell. Such cells are readily recognized by the presence of either single or multiple vacuoles that distend the cytoplasm and distort the nuclear shape. These vacuoles are filled with mucus produced by the cell [❚*15.2*, left]. These goblet cells are more common in patients with chronic tracheobronchial disease, such as asthmatic bronchitis, chronic bronchitis, and bronchiectasis.

So-called irritation forms of bronchial epithelium may occur in response to a wide variety of insults, varying from microorganisms to environmental toxins. Such irritation forms are characterized by marked nuclear enlargement, coarsening of the chromatin pattern, and one or more enlarged nucleoli [❚*15.2*, right]. An extremely common response to irritation is the presence of multinucleation; however, the nuclei are small and are mirror images of one another [❚*15.3*]. Although such cells may appear after a wide variety of insults, they are most commonly seen after instrumentation.

Hyperplasia of the respiratory epithelial cells may occur in association with a number of chronic diseases of the lung, including bronchiectasis, chronic bronchitis, and asthma. The papillary tissue fragments exfoliating from hyperplastic bronchial epithelium were first noted in a patient with chronic asthmatic bronchitis. The condition was diagnosed incorrectly as adenocarcinoma. These fragments have been reported as occurring in the sputum from 42% of cases of asthmatic bronchitis. The cytologic presentation is that of papillary clusters of cells partially covered on the surface by well-differentiated, ciliated respiratory epithelium. Some nuclear molding between individual cells is noted, although chromatin and nucleolar structures remain relatively unremarkable. At times, nuclear detail may be obscured because of the thickness of the tissue fragment. A varying number of vacuolated mucus cells may also be present in these fragments. The key to their benignancy is found in the finely granular chromatin pattern, regular uniform nucleoli, and presence of cilia [❚*15.4*].

The least frequently encountered epithelial components in material from the respiratory tract are cells exfoliating from the terminal bronchioles and from the alveoli. Although a number of modern laboratory techniques enable the differentiation of a variety of subtypes of terminal bronchiolar and alveolar cells, conventional light microscopic examination of cytologic specimens does not permit the appreciation of these various cell types. Indeed, the terminal bronchiolar and alveolar cells in their normal forms are probably not recognized in cytologic material. These cells are relatively small and, when present in cytologic material, appear as rounded single cells with finely vacuolated cytoplasm and centrally placed nucleoli with one to two small nucleoli [❚*15.5*]. With such morphology these cells are usually interpreted as alveolar macrophages. In the presence of insult, however, they may enlarge and produce differential diagnostic problems. In such circumstances, they may be present as small cellular clusters composed of enlarged cells with prominent nucleoli. Hyperdistended vacuoles may be present in the cytoplasm [▮*15.6*, ▮*15.7*].

Differential diagnosis of bronchiolar and alveolar cells, then, becomes a rather formidable problem of determining whether these cells are the result of benign disease processes (such as pulmonary fibrosis, thermal injury, thromboembolism with or without pulmonary infarction, anthracosis, or organizing pneumonia) or whether they are actually derived from a bronchoalveolar carcinoma. Pulmonary infarcts are cited in the literature as being particularly prone to give rise to such cells; however, in my experience, they are most frequently encountered in association with pneumonias of various forms and etiologies.

Squamous metaplasia probably represents an attempt of the host to repair an epithelial surface damaged by various environmental living and nonliving toxic agents. The most frequently encountered environmental toxin associated with the development of squamous metaplasia is cigarette smoke. Cigarette smoking, the development of squamous metaplasia, and their possible relationship to the pathogenesis of bronchogenic carcinoma have become of paramount interest to medicine.

The evolution of the metaplastic process begins with a proliferation of reserve cells such that a multilayered epithelium between the columnar epithelial cells and the basement membrane is produced. As these reserve cells gradually mature, an epithelium is produced that more and more resembles squamous epithelium, with cell flattening, karyopyknosis, and keratin production. In cytologic materials, reserve cell hyperplasia is recognized by the presence of tissue fragments composed of small, uniform, tightly coherent cells possessing darkly stained nuclei and a thin rim of faintly cyanophilic cytoplasm. Nuclear molding occurs, but uniformity exists throughout the fragment. There is no tendency toward fragmentation of the cluster [▮*15.8*]. At times, reserve cell hyperplasia may be alarming in appearance and must be distinguished from small cell undifferentiated carcinoma. Other small cell neoplasms, notably leukemias and lymphomas, should not be confused with reserve cell hyperplasia, because they characteristically shed into the bronchopulmonary material as single cells.

Cells from squamous metaplasia may occur as single cells or as small tissue fragments. As fragments, they are grouped in a uniform, monolayered, cobblestone-like arrangement with striking uniformity between the cells. Although they resemble maturing squamous cells, they are smaller and possess a higher nuclear/cytoplasmic ratio. Because squamous metaplasia mimics maturing squamous epithelium, metaplastic cells of varying degrees of maturity may be present. The cytoplasmic staining characteristic may vary from a deep cyanophilia to an orangeophilia, which indicates maturation and keratinization of the cytoplasm [▮*15.9*]. The nuclei may be intensely karyopyknotic.

Squamous metaplasias are capable of undergoing changes characterized by increasing degrees of nuclear abnormality. These metaplasias exhibit an increase in the nuclear/cytoplasmic ratio, a thickening of the nuclear membrane, an increasing granularity and hyperchromasia of the chromatin, and the appearance of nucleoli. These abnormalities have been called by various names, including atypical squamous metaplasia and squamous metaplasia with dysplasia. They have been observed in the presence of chronic irritation of the tracheobronchial tree particularly by cigarette smoking, and they are believed by many investigators to antedate the appearance of bronchogenic carcinoma. In about 60% of patients, however, these atypical metaplastic cells are associated with non-neoplastic conditions of the lungs, most notably pneumonia.

Severe alterations in cells may occur in response to irradiation therapy and anticancer chemotherapy. These cells may be so markedly atypical and so easily mistaken for neoplastic cells that knowledge of treatment history is necessary to differentiate between the conditions. Cellular changes in response to ionizing irradiation may involve both squamous cells and columnar cells and are characterized by cytomegaly with both cytoplasmic and nuclear enlargement, multinucleation, macronuclei, and cytoplasmic vacuolization [▮*15.10*, left]. Cells resulting from chemotherapy are prone to occur singly and to be characterized by cytomegaly, hyperchromasia, and macronuclei. Cells of the tracheobronchial epithelium, the terminal bronchiolar epithelium, and the alveolar epithelium may be involved [▮*15.10*, right]. These cells can be recognized by their tendency to be roughly rectangular in shape.

Cells of Nonepithelial Origin

Although long debated, it is now established that the pulmonary alveolar macrophage originates in the bone marrow. The presence of this characteristic cell, most frequently laden with particles of carbon, is mandatory in determining if a specimen of sputum is satisfactory for diagnostic interpretation. Pulmonary alveolar macrophages are recognized by the eccentric position of the nucleus, the abundant foamy cytoplasm, and the phagocytized material, usually carbon. On occasion, the nuclei may assume a bean shape and show one or more nucleoli [▮*15.11*, left]. Binucleated and multinucleated giant cell macrophages are occasionally encountered [▮*15.11*, right]. These latter cells may be seen in association with chronic lung disease of many varieties, including sarcoidosis, tuberculosis, and other granulomatous diseases, but they are not diagnostic and may be seen in respiratory material in the absence of clinical disease. Large vacuoles containing fat have been reported in these macrophages in the presence of lipoid pneumonia.

Other cells that originate from circulating blood and may be seen in bronchopulmonary material include lymphocytes, eosinophils, neutrophils, and plasma cells. Lymphocytes may be associated with a chronic inflammatory process or with the rupture of a lymphoid follicle in the wall of a bronchus. The lymphocytes often stream out in strands of mucus, mimicking the exfoliation pattern of small cell undifferentiated carcinoma. Eosinophils are seen most frequently in association with asthmatic bronchitis as well as in any disease that has a component of allergy. Plasma cells are commonly encountered in chronic inflammatory exudates.

Cellular specimens obtained by FNA may contain a variety of cells unique to them because of the anatomic route followed by the needle as it is inserted percutaneously into the lung. Thus, such a specimen may contain squamous epithelial cells, cells from various skin appendages, fibro-fatty connective tissue, striated muscle, capillaries, and mesothelium. The latter occurs in monolayered sheets and may be a pitfall if it is reactive and hyperplastic. Rarely, fragments of liver tissue may be present where the physician performing the aspiration had tried to enter the lung too far inferiorly on the chest wall.

Noncellular Inanimate Components

Many different nonliving structures may be present in specimens from the lower respiratory tract. Some may indicate specific problems; others may serve only to confuse and to produce incorrect diagnoses. Some structures may derive from the patient; others may contaminate the specimen after it has been taken from the patient. Curschmann's spirals, for example, are casts of small bronchioles formed from inspissated mucus. They are seen in any condition characterized by the chronic and excessive production of mucus. Occasionally, small inspissated masses of mucus will gather and adhere to one another, in a formation that is suggestive of nuclei. In extreme situations, these masses may mimic the nuclear hyperchromasia and molding of small cell undifferentiated carcinoma.

Ferruginous bodies have been noted in tissues and cellular specimens from the lungs for many years. They were formerly called asbestos bodies, reflecting the belief that they were all formed as a reaction to inhaled fibers of asbestos. Now it is recognized that inhalation of several different mineral fibers results in identical structures. These bodies are composed of various substances, including iron, that are encrusted on a thin needle-like fiber [❚*15.12*, left]. Increasing attention is being given to their relationship to bronchogenic carcinoma.

"Psammoma bodies" (calcospherites) and "corpora amylacea" are the names given to several varieties of dark-staining, rounded bodies with concentric rings and radial striations that appear in respiratory material. Corpora amylacea are composed of glycoproteins and do not calcify. Psammoma bodies are calcified and contain phosphates, iron, magnesium, and sudanophilic material. Corpora amylacea are seen in association with heart failure, pulmonary infarction, and chronic bronchitis. Psammoma bodies have been associated with the rare disease of pulmonary microlithiasis and with malignant neoplasms capable of producing these bodies.

As would be expected, any structure breathed into the respiratory passages or any particle of masticated food is capable of appearing in the respiratory specimen and producing great confusion if its identity is not recognized. Plant cells may be confused with cancer cells, and structures such as pollen and starch granules may be confused with infectious organisms [❚*15.12*, right].

Infectious Disease

Examination of cellular specimens from the respiratory tract is useful in the identification of a variety of different infectious organisms. The organisms most likely to be detected have a morphology specific enough to be distinguished by light microscopic methods or produce specific cellular changes. Infections caused by mycotic organisms, parasites, or certain viruses are those most likely to be detected in cytopathologic specimens.

Viral Infections

Changes in cells from the respiratory tract have been reported in association with a variety of viral infections including adenovirus, herpes simplex virus, measles, cytomegalovirus, parainfluenza, and respiratory syncytial virus. The cellular changes occurring in these patients can be divided into three general categories.

The first type is a cellular alteration. Papanicolaou observed and named ciliocytophthoria in 1956. This is a peculiar degeneration of the ciliated respiratory epithelium in which a pinching off occurs between the cilia-bearing cytoplasm and the nucleated cytoplasm, leaving an anucleated mass of cytoplasm-bearing cilia and a degenerating nucleus with a few fragments of adhering cytoplasm.

A second type of cellular alteration most frequently associated with viral pneumonia may occur and produce diagnostic problems in differentiation from cancer. This type of change is a form of regeneration and atypia of the respiratory epithelium that presents in sputum, bronchial material, and FNAs as tissue fragments composed of cells bearing enlarged hyperchromatic nuclei with prominent nucleoli. The tightly coherent features of the cells in the tissue fragments and the absence of atypical cells lying singly rule out the diagnosis of cancer.

The third type of cellular alteration is much more specific and may be diagnostic for specific viral infections. Of most practical importance are the changes seen in association with infection with herpes simplex and cytomegalovirus. The hallmarks of cellular alteration produced by herpes are multiple, molded nuclei that may either contain eosinophilic, irregular inclusion bodies (Cowdry type A inclusion bodies) or exhibit a peculiar type of nuclear degeneration that appears as slate gray, homogenized nuclear contents [❚15.13, left]. Cells infected by cytomegalovirus are larger and may show some multinucleation, but they have fewer nuclei and none of the molding seen in herpes simplex. Large, amphophilic, smooth intranuclear inclusions surrounded by prominent halos and marked margination of chromatin on the inner surface of the nuclear membranes are present. Cytoplasmic viral inclusions, also present in this disease, may be manifested by a textured appearance to the cytoplasm [❚15.13, right].

Bacterial Infections

Although the vast majority of lung infections produced by bacteria do not lend themselves to primary diagnosis by conventional cytologic methods, the cytologic specimen may be extremely helpful in a few instances.

Gram-Positive and Gram-Negative Bacteria

It is common for specimens of sputum to show bacillary and coccal forms of bacteria. These rarely indicate pulmonary infection, but rather are the result of bacterial overgrowth. *Actinomyces* organisms may be seen as contaminants from the tonsillar crypts. Similar observations are also usually true for bronchial material. In contrast, the presence of bacteria in a cytologic specimen from an FNA sample may be of extreme importance. Although the Papanicolaou stain will render bacteria visible, their red or blue staining has no connection to true gram-negative or gram-positive staining.

Opportunistic infections with *Legionella pneumophila* and *Legionella micdadei* appear to be increasing in frequency. *Legionella* is an extremely small gram-negative rod. Specimens of sputum, bronchial material, and particularly FNAs stained by the Dieterle method of silver impregnation may reveal the organisms; however, much greater sensitivity in detection of this organism is being achieved by immunofluorescence microscopy using anti-*Legionella* antisera, which are now commercially available.

The search for acid-fast organisms in a cytologic specimen is likely to be the most beneficial among those patients who have either suggestive morphologic evidence of granulomatous inflammation with necrosis or an extremely suggestive clinical history. Patients infected with *Mycobacterium avium-intracellulare* (the Battey bacillus) may show large alveolar macrophages that on acid-fast stain will reveal large numbers of branching acid-fast bacilli. Cell blocks prepared from FNA are useful for acid-fast staining when a tuberculous lesion is suspected to have been aspirated. Fluorescence microscopy with auramine-O may also reveal the organisms. Cytologic findings have been reported from patients with acquired immunodeficiency syndrome in whom mycobacteria were seen on the routine modified Wright-stained slides without special stains. The organisms appeared as negative images: unstained rod-shaped structures against the deep blue background of the stain.

Nocardiosis should be suspected when an FNA specimen reveals the presence of delicate branching filamentous rods with an inflammatory reaction consisting mainly of neutrophils. Positive acid-fast stains will further enforce this diagnosis.

Mycotic Infections

In mycotic infections, the etiologic agent is usually visible and in many cases has a morphology on which a specific diagnosis can be based. The detection of these organisms in a stained cytologic specimen may be the first clue to the nature of a patient's problems. The accuracy of observation depends on the ability of the cytotechnologist and the cytopathologist to appreciate the various forms that these organisms assume.

Blastomyces dermatitidis

In cytopathologic materials fixed in 95% alcohol and stained by the Papanicolaou technique, *Blastomyces dermatitidis* appears as single or budding yeast-like spherical cells, 8 to 15 µm in diameter, with thick refractile walls. The thickness of these walls along with some tendency for the cell mass to retract away from them may impart to these forms a double-contoured appearance. No hyphae are seen. Single budding is characteristic. The bud has a tendency to remain in close apposition to the mother cell so that a flattening of the two apposed surfaces occurs [❚15.14, left].

Cryptococcus neoformans

Cryptococcus neoformans is a single-budding, yeast-like organism. The budding is characterized by a tendency for the bud to pinch off, assuming a teardrop shape and leaving a markedly attenuated isthmus of attachment to the mother cell. Each cell is ovoid to spherical with a thickened wall and measures 5 to 20 µm in diameter. The cells are often surrounded by a mucoid capsule, which usually requires a special stain for visualization. On occasion, however, the capsule may stain with the Papanicolaou technique [❚15.14, right].

Coccidioides immitis

Coccidioides immitis can be seen frequently in the sputum of infected patients. Its spherules present a particularly dramatic appearance because of their capability to reach diameters in excess of 100 µm. The spherule may be empty or contain endospores. The endospores are round, nonbudding structures measuring 2 to 5 µm in diameter. Developing spherules may be confused with nonbudding forms of *B dermatitidis* [❚15.15, left].

Histoplasma capsulatum

Histoplasma capsulatum is an extremely small, budding yeast-like organism almost invariably found proliferating within the cytoplasm of macrophages. The organism is difficult to visualize on Papanicolaou stains [▮*15.15*, right] and is better identified using special stains such as methenamine silver [▮*15.16*, left].

Aspergillus *Species and Phycomycetes*

Aspergillus species and Phycomycetes are characterized as opportunistic fungi that may invade and produce infection in patients whose immune responses have been compromised. Among the opportunists, *Aspergillus* organisms are most frequently observed. The most characteristic presentation is that of thick, septate hyphae with brush-like branching at 45° angles. The presence of these hyphae in cytologic material is strong morphologic evidence of infection. *Aspergillus* species, along with several other organisms, have been implicated in the production of cellular atypias easily mistaken for squamous cell carcinoma [▮*15.16*, right].

Various members of the Phycomycetes group are capable of producing the disease now called phycomycosis (mucormycosis). The infecting fungus is characterized by ribbon-like, nonseptate, branching hyphae. They may vary widely in width from 6 to 60 µm. Culture is necessary to identify the fungus causing the infection, because multiple organisms with identical tissue morphology can produce the disease [▮*15.17*].

Candida *Species*

Species of *Candida* are the most frequently encountered fungi in cytologic specimens. Because of this frequency, their clinical significance may be discounted. All *Candida* species may appear as small, oval, 2- to 4-µm budding yeasts. Occasionally, they may elongate into pseudohyphal forms with additional budding at the points of constriction. Although their presence in pulmonary material is not usually significant, it may reflect an overwhelming candidiasis in the compromised host.

Parasites

Pneumocystis carinii

Pneumocystis carinii is capable of producing opportunistic infections in premature infants; in persons with immunologic disorders, immunoglobulin defects, and renal transplants; and in the presence of therapy with corticosteroids and chemotherapy. Currently, it is most frequently seen in patients with acquired immunodeficiency syndrome (AIDS). On Papanicolaou-stained material, the organisms may be difficult to identify because their staining is variable and faint, even in the most ideal of cases. Their most typical presentation is as a mass of partially eosinophilic or amorphous material. Within this mass may be a suggestion of small, superimposed circlets representing cyst outlines.

Although such masses are highly suggestive of *Pneumocystis* species, such a honeycombed, amorphous mass should be further evaluated by special stains [▮*15.18*, left]. In such a situation, the slide should be decolorized and restained with methenamine silver. This procedure immediately brings out the diagnostic features of these organisms. On methenamine silver staining, the organism is seen mainly as a spherical cyst measuring 6 to 8 µm in diameter with certain variations in form. It may be cup-shaped, crescent-shaped, or crinkled. Depending on the surface of the organism exposed to view, small globoid inner thickenings of the cyst wall can be seen [▮*15.18*, right]. Some laboratories prefer a Giemsa stain for identification. With this technique, up to eight round bodies, called trophozoites, can be identified within the cyst. These structures are about 0.5 to 1.0 µm in diameter and are difficult to visualize. The cyst wall does not stain.

Strongyloides stercoralis

Respiratory infection with *Strongyloides stercoralis* has been seen mostly in patients taking intensive steroid therapy for various clinical situations, including renal transplantation and severe asthmatic bronchitis. Pulmonary infection is produced when the filariform larvae migrate through the intestinal wall into the bloodstream and finally penetrate into the alveolar spaces. A hemorrhagic pneumonia is produced. The organisms are readily identified in the bloody sputum expectorated by these patients. The filariform larvae observed measure 400 to 500 µm in length and exhibit a closed gullet and a slightly notched tail [▮*15.19*].

CYTOPATHOLOGY OF LUNG CANCER

Bronchogenic carcinoma comprises a family of highly malignant neoplasms, all of which arise in the epithelia of the lower respiratory tract [**T***15.1*]. Diagnostic neoplastic cells are exfoliated from all these neoplasms and may be present in the various types of respiratory specimens examined. In the majority of cases, in addition to recognizing that cancer cells are present, the neoplasm can be classified from the cellular observations.

Squamous Cell Carcinoma

Squamous cell carcinoma of the lung shares with squamous cell carcinoma of the uterine cervix a demonstrable preinvasive stage of development. In the case of carcinoma of the lung, the epithelium of the tracheobronchial tree undergoes a series of alterations that can be morphologically classified as atypical metaplasia or as dysplasia and carcinoma in situ [▮*15.20*]. The invasive neoplasm is named squamous cell carcinoma because of the presence of various features of differentiation characteristic of squamous cells, such as individual cell keratinization, formation of pearly bodies, and presence of intracellular bridges. This tumor is more centrally located in the lung and is apt to exfoliate

Histologic Type	Frequency Distribution (%)
Squamous cell carcinoma	43
Adenocarcinoma	21
Acinar	18
Bronchoalveolar	3
Large cell undifferentiated carcinoma	23
Small cell undifferentiated carcinoma	12
Adenosquamous carcinoma	1

* This classification of bronchogenic carcinoma results from my experience in the laboratory over a 5-year period. This classification has been modified from that of the World Health Organization.

T *15.1*
*Classification of Bronchogenic Carcinoma**

large numbers of diagnostic neoplastic cells into the sputum, washing, brushing, or FNA. In sputum, the neoplastic cells occur singly and in loose clusters. Tissue fragments are rare. The cells are characterized by marked pleomorphism in size and shape. Classic forms are present, such as the tadpole cell, the fiber cell, and the third cell type similar in morphology to cells seen in squamous cell carcinoma of the cervix. The nuclei exhibit marked hyperchromasia with a tendency toward karyopyknosis. When chromatin pattern is preserved, it is arranged into irregular, sharp-bordered clumps with abnormal clearing of the parachromatin. Nucleoli, while not as common as in other malignant neoplasms, may be conspicuously large. Nuclear/cytoplasmic ratios may vary from extremely high to very low because of the extreme variability in the amount of cytoplasm produced by these cells.

Keratinization of this cytoplasm is reflected in an intense hyaline appearance of the cytoplasm with a bright orangeophilic staining most frequently seen. Keratinization may also be reflected in a hyaline appearance with more cyanophilic staining. Ectoendoplasmic ringing as described by Frost is another striking feature of abnormal keratinization in the cytoplasm [▮*15.21*-▮*15.23*].

As the differentiation of the squamous cell carcinoma becomes less apparent, nuclear/cytoplasmic features of differentiation are also less apparent. Cells from poorly differentiated squamous cell carcinomas are more apt to be present as tissue fragments in addition to single cells. The only clue to their differentiation may lie in the tendency of the cells to form a monolayer and for sharp cytoplasmic borders to be evident [▮*15.24*, ▮*15.25*]. Because of sampling, specimens of squamous cell carcinoma obtained by the techniques of bronchial brushing and FNA may exhibit less differentiation than sputum specimens from the same tumor of the same patient.

In FNAs from squamous cell carcinomas, the specimen will reflect the degree of differentiation and tissue preservation present at the site of the needle tip. When necrotic tumor with large masses of keratinized squamous ghosts dominate the cytologic picture, aspiration of a more peripheral portion of the tumor will increase the chance of obtaining diagnostic tumor cells.

Adenocarcinoma

Adenocarcinomas arise from the respiratory epithelium of the more peripherally situated bronchi, bronchioles, and alveolar epithelium. As a consequence, these neoplasms are much more likely to be found in the periphery of the lungs. Because of their growth pattern and their cells of origin, bronchogenic adenocarcinomas can conveniently be further divided into acinar adenocarcinomas and bronchoalveolar adenocarcinomas. Acinar adenocarcinomas arising from the bronchial epithelium are characterized by their tendency to form acinar structures and frequently to form mucus. Bronchoalveolar carcinoma comprises a group of neoplasms that arise from the terminal bronchiolar epithelium or from the type II alveolar cells of the alveolar epithelium. They produce a growth pattern that follows the anatomic outline of the alveolar spaces. Bronchoalveolar carcinomas may form single peripheral masses, or they may massively involve the entire lung. Depending on their location and size, they may exfoliate large numbers of diagnostic cells, few cells, or no cells at all.

While the cellular pattern reflective of the adenocarcinoma group is readily identified in specimens of respiratory material, attempts to further classify the adenocarcinoma into acinar and bronchoalveolar cell types are less successful. The works of Roger and associates, Smith and Frable, and Elson, Moore, and Johnston have explored the differences in cytologic presentation between these two types of adenocarcinoma. Most adenocarcinomas exfoliate large numbers of diagnostic cells into the respiratory specimen. The cells occur both singly and as tissue fragments. The nuclei of adenocarcinomas may be exceedingly bland in appearance. The chromatin may be finely granular to the extent of imparting a ground-glass appearance to the nuclei. The individual nucleus may be disarmingly round and regular. A striking nuclear feature of acinar adenocarcinoma may be the central placement of a macronucleus. The cytoplasm may vary from homogenous to extremely vacuolated. Foamy cytoplasm is frequently encountered. Many of the cells will exhibit extremely high nuclear/cytoplasmic ratios and be identified only as undifferentiated cancer cells. In well-differentiated acinar neoplasms, the cells may assume a columnar shape. Tissue fragments may be composed of ball-like clusters of cells or may demonstrate true acinar structures. As the differentiation of the neoplasm decreases, the regularity and uniformity of the cells also decrease, resulting in more hyperchromasia, more pleomorphism, and more bizarre cell forms [▮*15.26*, ▮*15.27*].

Because of their origin from at least three different cell lines and their ability to vary widely in degree of differentiation, the bronchoalveolar carcinomas may either be readily identified as distinct entities or recognized only as adenocarcinomas. In the former situation, the cytopathologic material will reveal large numbers of tissue fragments composed of extremely well-differentiated columnar epithelium that may produce mucus. These tissue fragments will occur in a population of large numbers of macrophages that have been attracted by the mucus. The presence of small ball-like clusters of cells that exhibit small nucleoli and show no molding between individual cells may be an important criterion for correct recognition of this neoplasm [▮*15.28*-▮*15.30*].

The cytologic appearance of bronchoalveolar carcinoma in FNAs is similar to that described in the previous paragraph, except that sheets of tumor cells may be prominent and tissue fragments containing alveolar septa may be present.

Large Cell Undifferentiated Carcinoma

Large cell undifferentiated carcinoma is a type of bronchogenic carcinoma composed of large neoplastic cells with no cellular or tissue evidence of differentiation at the level of examination by light microscopy. Most of these neoplasms, when examined ultrastructurally, reveal cytoplasmic evidence that they are adenocarcinomas or squamous cell carcinomas. Large cell undifferentiated carcinoma is more a designation for convenience in classification than one that represents a true biologic entity.

About half of these carcinomas arise in large bronchi. The neoplasms exfoliate large numbers of diagnostic cells into the respiratory specimen. The cells occur both as single cells and as tissue fragments. The single cells are large and possess multiple criteria for malignancy, including high nuclear/cytoplasmic ratios, marked aberrations in the chromatin patterns, and multiple, enlarged, irregular nucleoli. Cytoplasm may be wispy or homogeneous with a tendency toward cyanophilia. Large tissue fragments may be present without any recognizable architectural pattern being assumed by the cells [▮*15.31*]. Giant cell carcinomas, so named because of the presence of many multinucleated tumor giant cells, are occasionally seen.

All of the non–small cell carcinomas of the lung may exfoliate only large anaplastic malignant tumor cells into the cytologic specimens, so that the cytologic diagnosis of large cell undifferentiated carcinoma is made. Furthermore, sampling methods such as bronchial brushings or FNA may reach only undifferentiated portions of squamous carcinomas or adenocarcinomas. In my experience, FNAs obtained from poorly differentiated adenocarcinomas have been particularly difficult to classify correctly.

Small Cell Undifferentiated Carcinoma

Small cell undifferentiated carcinoma is the most malignant of the bronchogenic cancer group. It is composed of small, uniform cells with high nuclear/cytoplasmic ratios and hyperchromatic nuclei with occasional nucleoli. On ultrastructural examination, many of these tumors will be found to contain membrane-bound cytoplasmic granules referred to as neurosecretory granules. Some small cell undifferentiated carcinomas are capable of producing a variety of hormones such as adrenocorticotropic hormone (ACTH), antidiuretic hormone (ADH), serotonin, and calcitonin. Most of these neoplasms occur in major bronchi toward the central part of the lungs.

The individual cell from small cell undifferentiated carcinoma is approximately 1½ to 2 times the size of a lymphocyte. It is a rounded cell possessing a centrally placed nucleus with a uniform but deeply staining chromatin pattern. Micronucleoli are occasionally visible. The exfoliation pattern for this neoplasm may vary from large numbers of cells and tissue fragments to several cells present only on one slide out of many examined. In specimens of sputum, large numbers of tumor cells may be found entrapped in strands of mucus. A most characteristic presentation results with clusters of these small tumor cells exhibiting extreme molding superimposed on irregular nuclear outlines. Because this tumor is highly prone to necrosis, the cellular specimen will frequently exhibit karyopyknosis, disintegration of the cytoplasm, and formation of dense cyanophilic masses of necrotic debris [▮*15.32*, left; ▮*15.33*]. In specimens prepared from bronchial brushings, by FNA, and by the Saccomanno technique, nuclear molding may be much less evident because of greater dispersion of the cells [▮*15.32*, right].

The cytologic presentation of small cell undifferentiated carcinoma in bronchial brushings and FNAs can vary from one that is characteristic to one that produces a significant problem in differential diagnosis. In most cases, large numbers of tumor cells may be present. The finding of tissue fragments is of diagnostic importance to exclude lymphoma, but this differential may be more difficult than in sputum. A tumor diathesis is helpful in excluding carcinoid tumors, although the rarely encountered atypical carcinoids may cause exceptional difficulty in differential diagnosis. In my experience, the so-called intermediate cell variant of small cell undifferentiated carcinoma has caused the greatest interpretative difficulty, being at times suggestive of poorly differentiated squamous cell carcinoma.

Adenosquamous Carcinoma

Adenosquamous carcinoma is a type of bronchogenic carcinoma in which both squamous cell carcinoma and adenocarcinoma are present. This duality of differentiation may be reflected in the cytologic specimens. Most bronchogenic carcinomas are actually adenosquamous carcinoma, reflecting the biologic multipotentiality of the precursor cells. The true incidence of adenosquamous carcinoma, then, is most likely related to the diligence with which histopathologic sections, cytologic specimens, and electron microscopic preparations are examined [▮*15.34*].

Other Primary Neoplasms of the Lung

Other primary neoplasms of the lung may exfoliate diagnostic cells into cellular specimens from the respiratory tract, although less frequently than the bronchogenic carcinoma groups, or be obtained by FNA. These neoplasms include carcinoid, adenoid cystic carcinoma, mucoepidermoid tumor, leiomyosarcoma, pulmonary blastoma, and Hodgkin's and non-Hodgkin's lymphomas.

Although carcinoids typically present as exophytic endobronchial lesions, tumor cells are rarely observed in sputum because of the intact bronchial mucosa overlying the tumor.

When observed in bronchial brushing specimens and FNAs, the tumor cells occur singly as well as in sheets and three-dimensional ball-like clusters. The cells are characterized by small, round-to-oval, uniform nuclei with a stippled, granular chromatin pattern and small nucleoli. Cytoplasm is scant to moderate in amount and may vary from homogeneous to lace-like in appearance. Necrosis is absent unless the lesion has been traumatized or secondarily infected [▮*15.35*]. Peripheral carcinoids in FNA specimens may show the typical morphology but on occasion may exhibit a spindle cell pattern. When the tumor type in routine cytologic preparations is in question, additional studies, such as immunoperoxidase stains for chromogranin or electron microscopy for documenting neurosecretory granules, may be extremely helpful.

Atypical carcinoids constitute only about 10% of all carcinoid tumors. They may occur centrally, but they more commonly arise in the periphery of the lung. Histologically, they maintain the overall architecture of carcinoid tumor but cytologically are characterized by greater cellular pleomorphism, nuclear hyperchromasia, mitotic figures, necrosis, and even nuclear molding, so that the cytologic features begin to merge imperceptibly with those of small cell undifferentiated carcinoma. In general, they exhibit more cytoplasm and less nuclear atypia than the latter. Nevertheless, this differential diagnosis may be exceedingly difficult or impossible in cytologic material, just as it is in transbronchial biopsy specimens.

Metastatic Cancer

Although metastatic cancer to the lung is more common than bronchogenic cancer, cytologic evidence of its presence is not reported as frequently as that of the primary tumors. There are several reasons for this. First, cytopathologic techniques are not called on as frequently for suspected metastatic cancer to the lung as they are for suspected primary cancer. Second, unless the tumor has metastasized to the alveolar space, it must ulcerate through the bronchial mucosa to produce exfoliation of cells.

Various studies have shown that cells from metastatic tumors to the lung may be seen in respiratory material in 50% to 70% of cases. Patterns of malignant cells that deviate from those recognized for the primary lung tumors strongly suggest the presence of cancer metastatic to the lung. Metastatic tumors to the lung occurring as diffuse nodules or as single tumors involving a major bronchus present different cytologic patterns. In cases of diffuse metastases, tumor cells may occur in clusters simulating a pattern of bronchoalveolar carcinoma but with far fewer cells. Occasionally, a cell cluster may actually represent the cast of an alveolar space. The background of the smear is usually clean with virtually no macrophages. On occasion, it is possible to recognize the primary site of the neoplasm by noting cell characteristics and spatial arrangement. When large single metastases produce exfoliation through an ulcerated bronchus, the presentation of bronchogenic carcinoma may be mimicked. If prior surgical tissue is present for comparison with the cytologic specimen, then it may be possible to determine whether the tumor cells are consistent with the previous primary cancer [▮*15.36*-▮*15.40*]. Differences noted between the cytologic specimen and the tissue specimen may signal the presence of a second cancer that is either metastatic to the lung or a primary cancer of the lung.

The ability to study the cytologic characteristics of tumors metastatic to the lungs has been markedly enhanced by the use of FNA to sample the pulmonary nodules of metastatic disease. This technique has been unusually innovative in that it has resulted in a major modification of the diagnostic approach to the patient with suspected metastatic tumor. Before the advent of FNA, such patients would have been subjected either to thoracotomy or treated on the bases of radiologic and clinical findings. In these patients, the aspirate will usually reveal the answers to the critical questions of malignancy, differentiation, and organ of origin. In patients with multiple primary cancers, additional information may be provided regarding which primary cancer has metastasized.

In the diagnostic assessment with FNA of a patient with suspected cancer metastatic to the lung, the differential diagnosis should be approached in the same manner as if tissue from open biopsy were being evaluated. The patient's clinical history must be reviewed for either documentation or prior suspicion of a preexisting neoplasm. All previous histologic and cytologic specimens should be reviewed and the cellular changes in the FNA compared with the preexisting diagnostic material.

A marked difference exists between the cytologic presentation of neoplasms metastatic to the lung in FNAs and in specimens of sputum and bronchial material. This difference lies mainly in the amount of cellular material available for study. Most metastatic masses when aspirated yield large numbers of tumor cells and tissue fragments. Extensive necrosis and inflammation may also be present and partially obscure the tumor. Once a diagnosis of cancer is established, the major diagnostic decision is the determination of metastatic cancer vs primary lung cancer. In these patients, paraffin sections of cell blocks become useful when special stains and immunocytochemistry are needed for differential studies. Tissue fragments fixed in glutaraldehyde become extremely valuable for electron microscopy.

AUTHOR'S NOTE

The original chapter on cytology of the respiratory tract for this manual was written by the late John R. McDonald, MD. No serious and knowledgeable student of pathology of the lung would fail to remember his name and his pioneering contributions during the developmental years of clinical cytology. In acknowledgment of these accomplishments, the present chapter, retaining many of his thoughts, is respectfully dedicated to his memory.

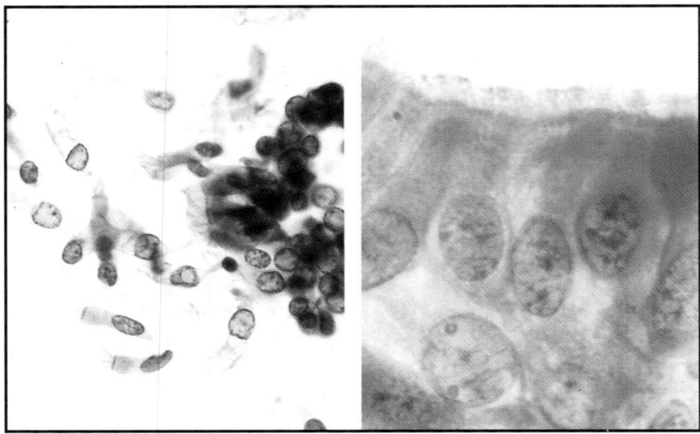

▮15.1

Left, Ciliated bronchial columnar cells; bronchial brushing (Papanicolaou, x400). Right, Ciliated bronchial columnar cells; bronchial brushing (Papanicolaou, x1000).

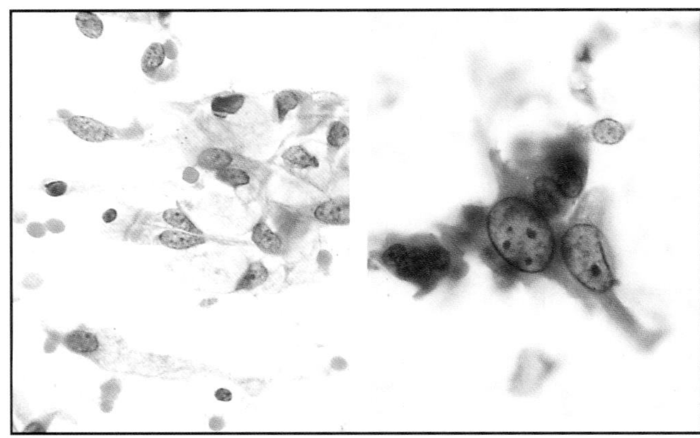

▮15.2

Left, Mucus-producing bronchial columnar cells; bronchial brushing (Papanicolaou, x400). Right, Reactive bronchial columnar cells, also called "irritation forms"; bronchial brushing (Papanicolaou, x400).

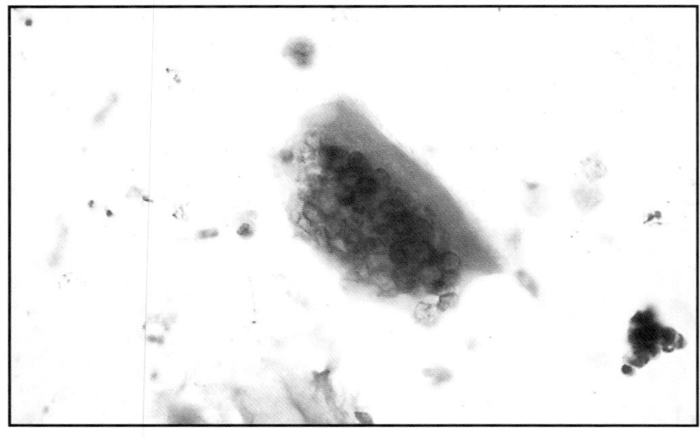

▮15.3

Multinucleated ciliated bronchial columnar cell; sputum (Papanicolaou, x400).

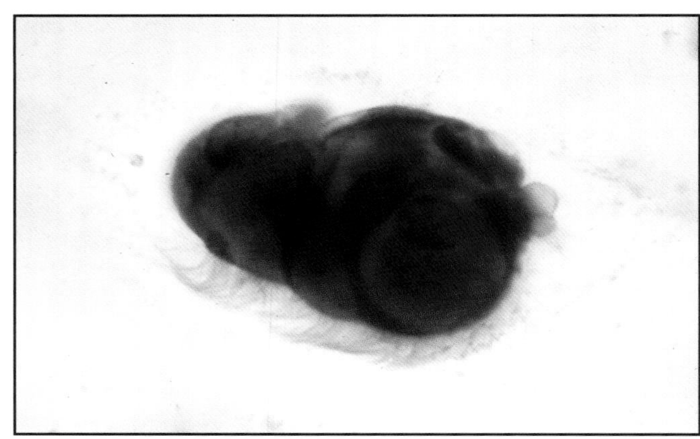

▮15.4

Papillary fragment of hyperplastic ciliated bronchial columnar epithelium; sputum (Papanicolaou, x1000).

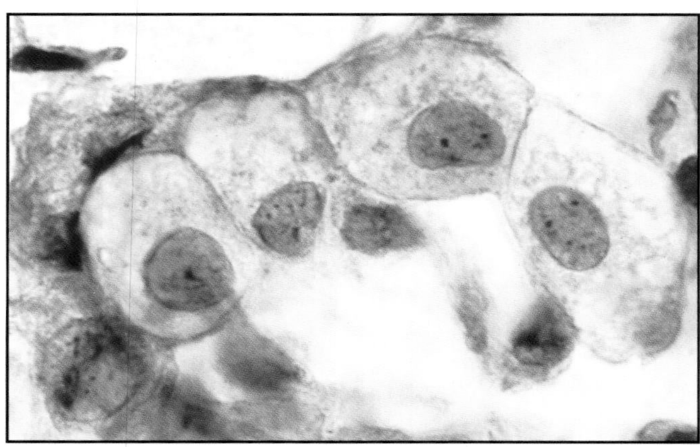

▮15.5

Fragment of bronchoalveolar epithelial cells. Polygonal cells in center are most likely derived from terminal bronchiolar epithelium; fine-needle aspirate (Papanicolaou, x400).

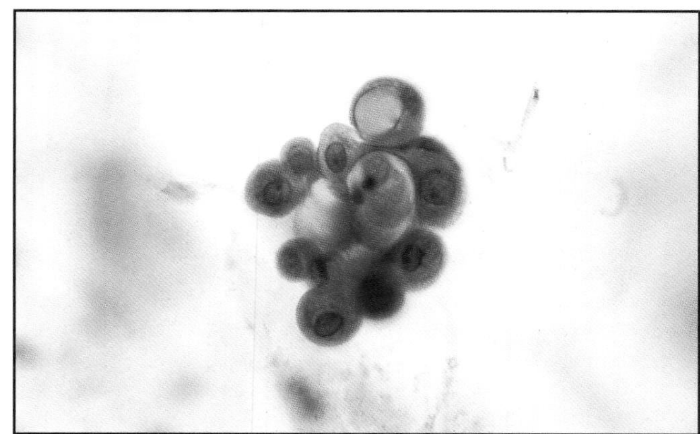

▮15.6

Reactive cells of bronchoalveolar origin in patient with pneumonia; sputum (Papanicolaou, x400).

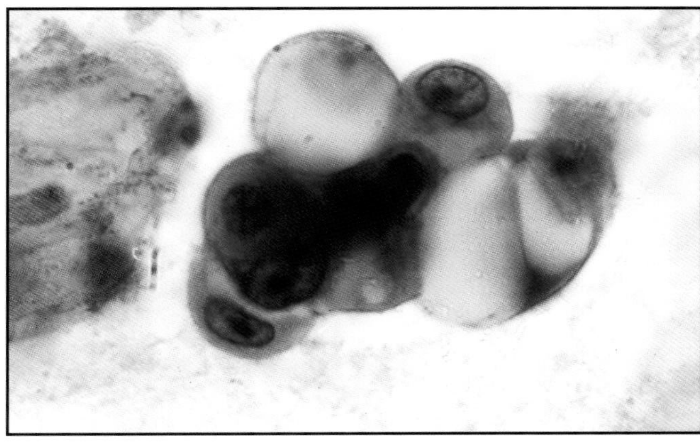

15.7

Reactive cells of bronchoalveolar origin in a patient with pneumonia. These cells were erroneously interpreted as adenocarcinoma; sputum (Papanicolaou, x400).

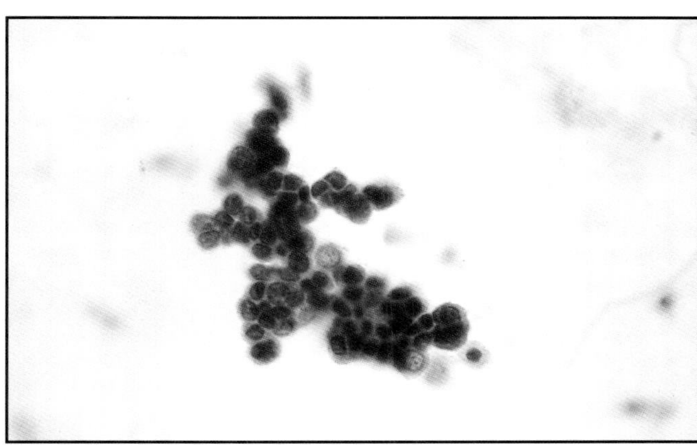

15.8

Reserve cell hyperplasia; bronchial brushing (Papanicolaou, x400).

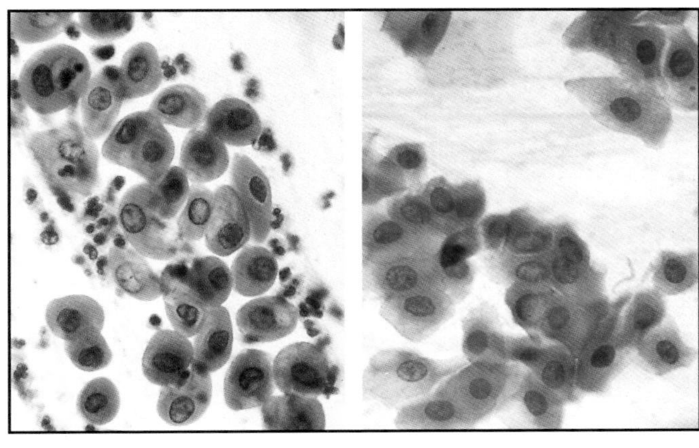

15.9

Left, Squamous metaplasia; sputum (Papanicolaou, x400). Right, Squamous metaplasia; sputum (Papanicolaou, x400).

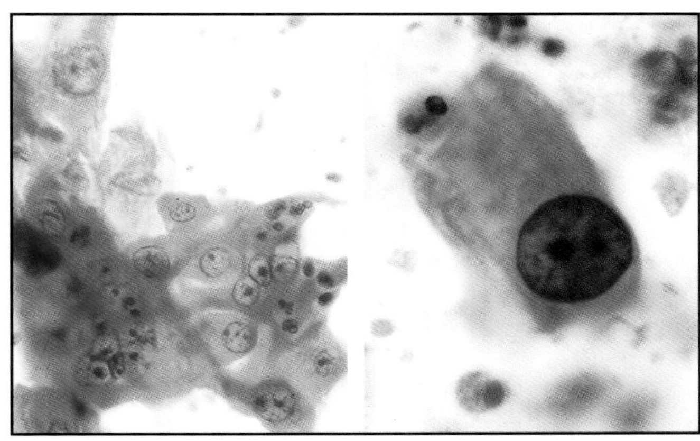

15.10

Left, Cellular changes induced by ionizing irradiation; bronchial brushing (Papanicolaou, x400). Right, Cellular changes induced by chemotherapy with busulfan; bronchial washing (Papanicolaou, x1000).

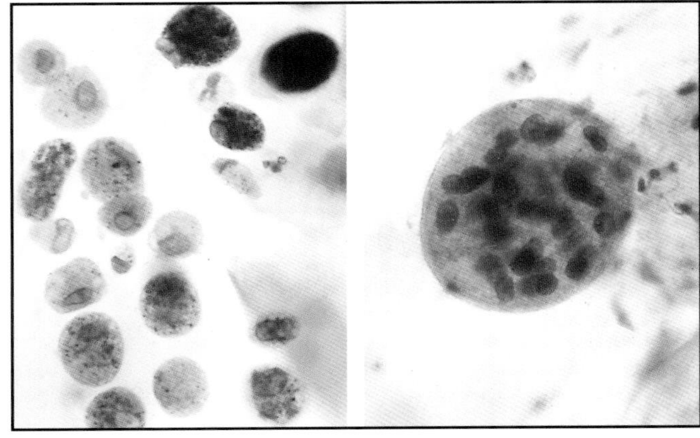

15.11

Left, Alveolar macrophages laden with carbon; sputum (Papanicolaou, x400). Right, Multinucleated giant macrophage; sputum (Papanicolaou, x400).

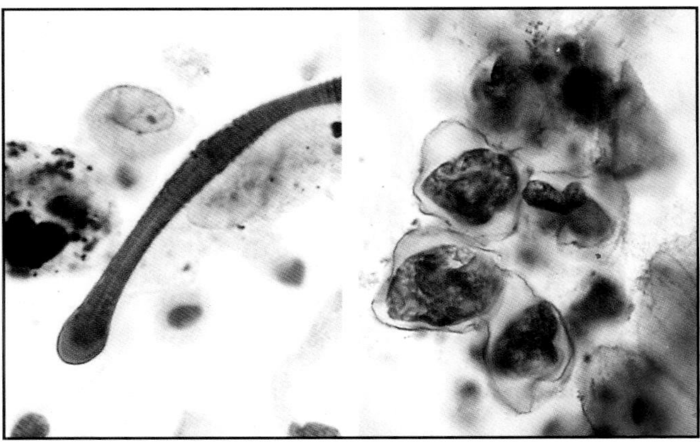

15.12

Left, Part of a ferruginous body; sputum (Papanicolaou, x400). Right, Plant cells simulating malignant neoplastic cells. Highly refractile cellulose walls are key to plant origin of these cells; sputum (Papanicolaou, x400).

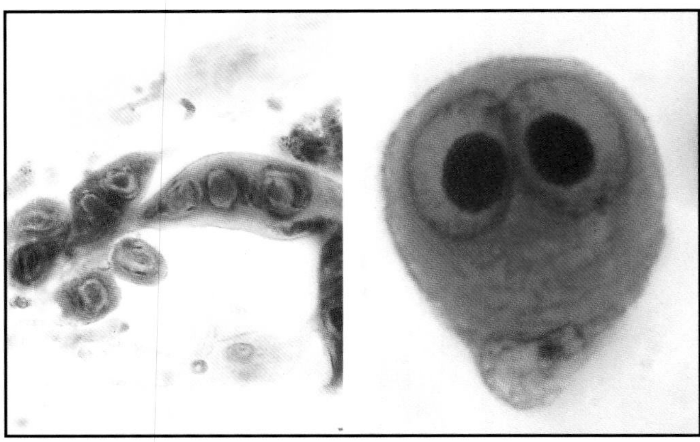

I15.13
Left, Herpes simplex virus infection; sputum (Papanicolaou, x400). Right, Cytomegalovirus infecting alveolar cells; bronchial brushing (Papanicolaou, x1000).

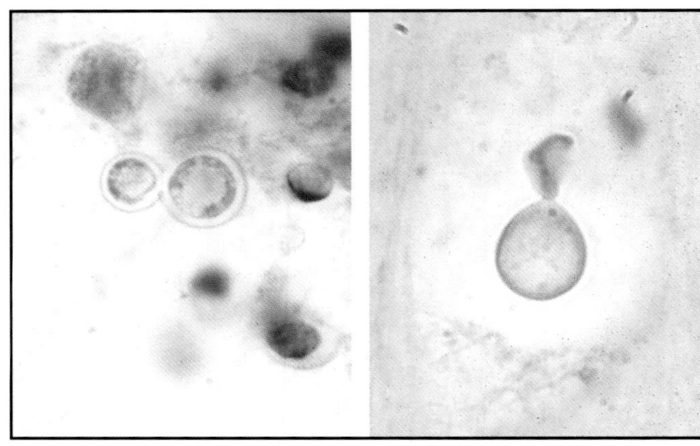

I15.14
Left, Blastomyces dermatitidis*; sputum (Papanicolaou, x1000). Right,* Cryptococcus neoformans*; sputum (Papanicolaou, x1000).*

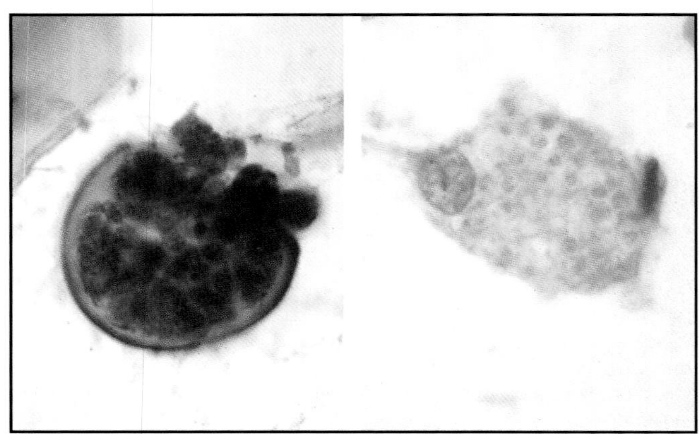

I15.15
Left, Coccidioides immitis. *Large spherule loaded with endospores and in process of rupturing; sputum (Papanicolaou, x1000). Right,* Histoplasma capsulatum. *Faintly staining yeast-like organisms are packing the cytoplasm of a macrophage (Papanicolaou, x1000).*

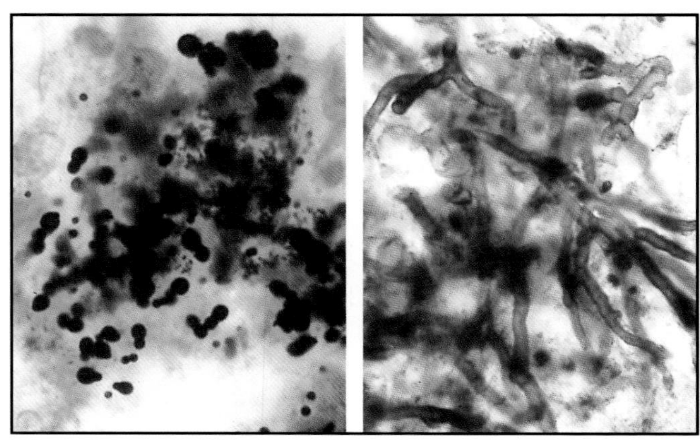

I15.16
Left, Histoplasma capsulatum*; tracheal aspirate (methenamine silver, x1000). Right,* Aspergillus *species; sputum (Papanicolaou, x400).*

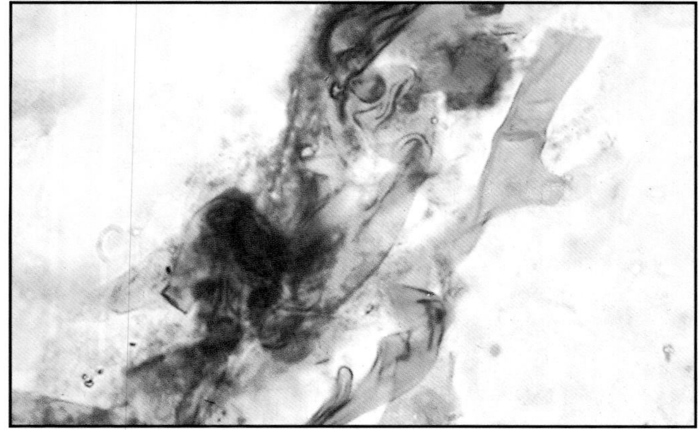

I15.17
Phycomycete-producing phycomycosis (mucormycosis); sputum (Papanicolaou, x1000).

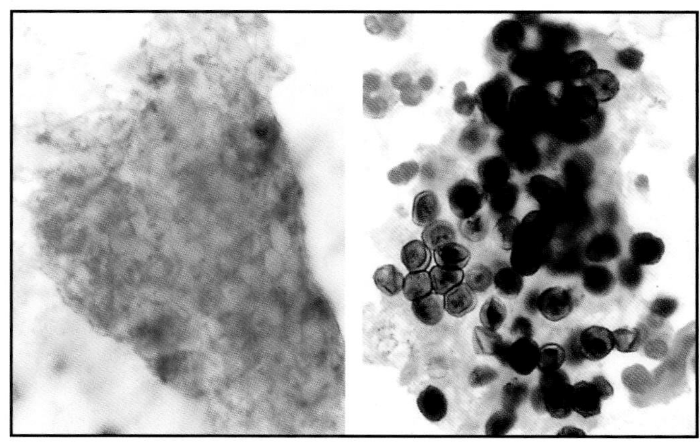

I15.18
Left, Pneumocystis carinii*; bronchial brushing (Papanicolaou, x1000). Right,* Pneumocystis carinii. *Same specimen as I15.16, right; (methenamine silver, x1000).*

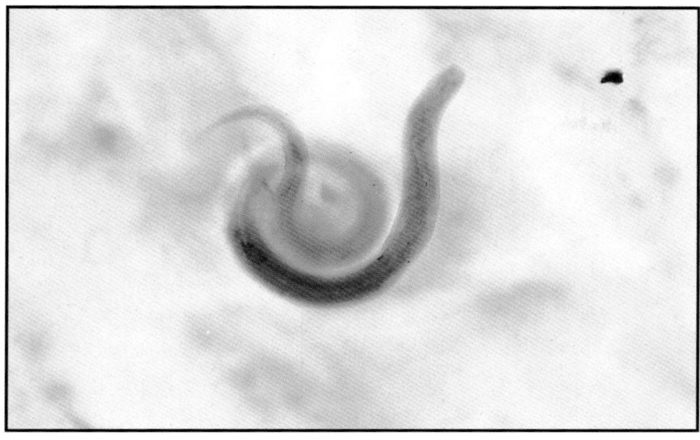

15.19
Strongyloides stercoralis; *sputum (methenamine silver, x400).*

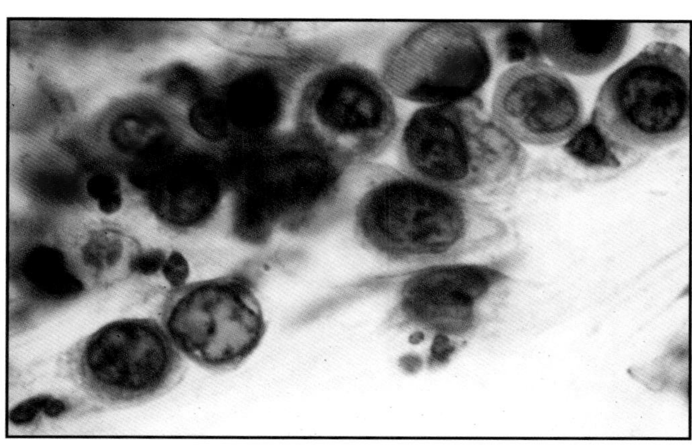

15.20
Squamous cell carcinoma in situ; sputum (Papanicolaou, x1000).

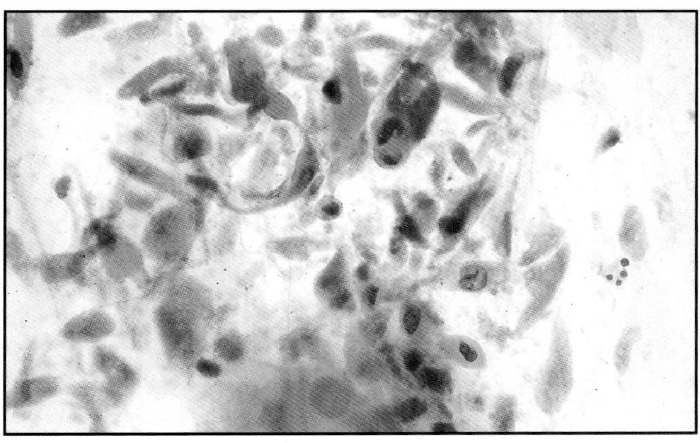

15.21
Keratinizing squamous cell carcinoma. Large amount of cytoplasm reflects marked keratinization; sputum (Papanicolaou, x400).

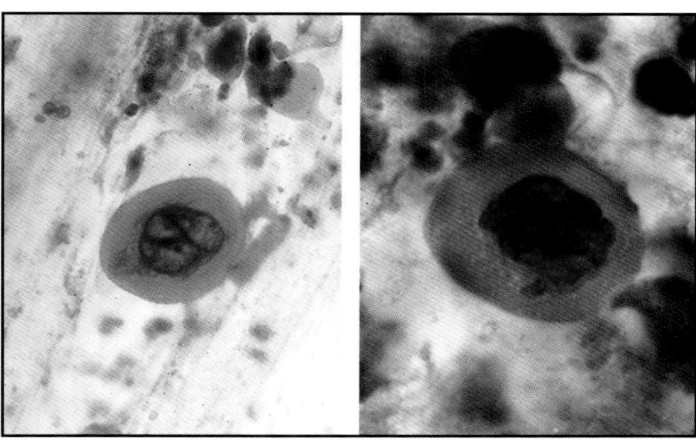

15.22
Left, Keratinizing squamous cell carcinoma; sputum (Papanicolaou, x400). Right, Keratinizing squamous cell carcinoma; sputum (Papanicolaou, x1000).

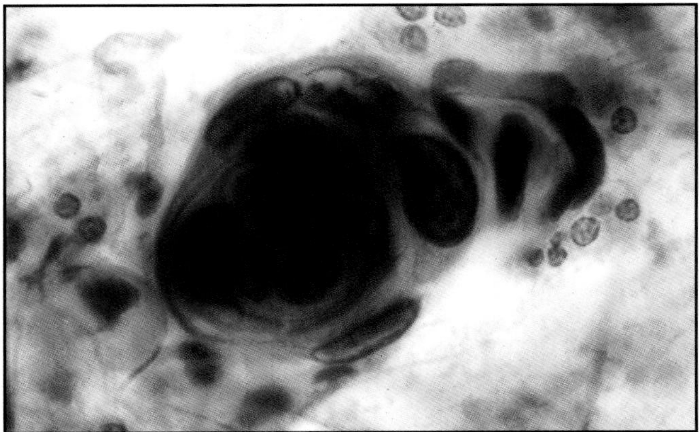

15.23
Keratinizing squamous cell carcinoma. The malignant pearly body shown is a manifestation of atypical differential in this squamous cell carcinoma; sputum (Papanicolaou, x1000).

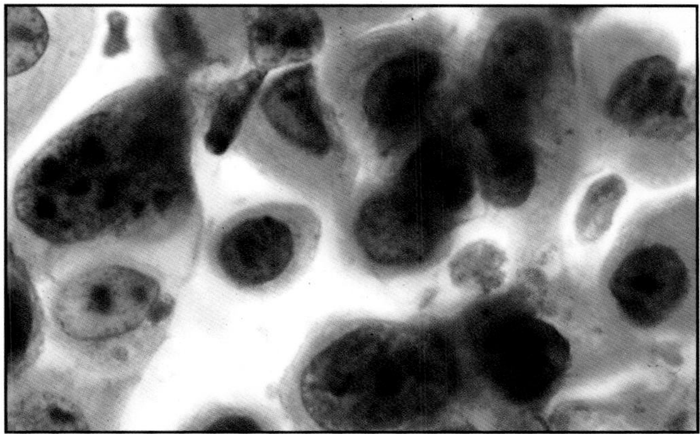

15.24
Poorly differentiated squamous cell carcinoma; sputum (Papanicolaou, x1000).

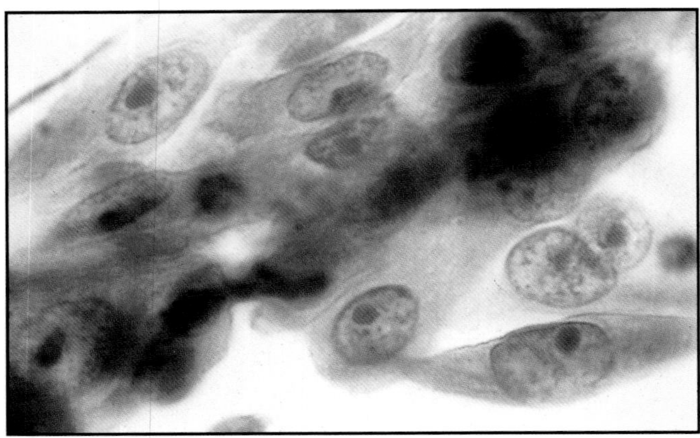

15.25
Poorly differentiated squamous cell carcinoma; sputum (Papanicolaou, x1000).

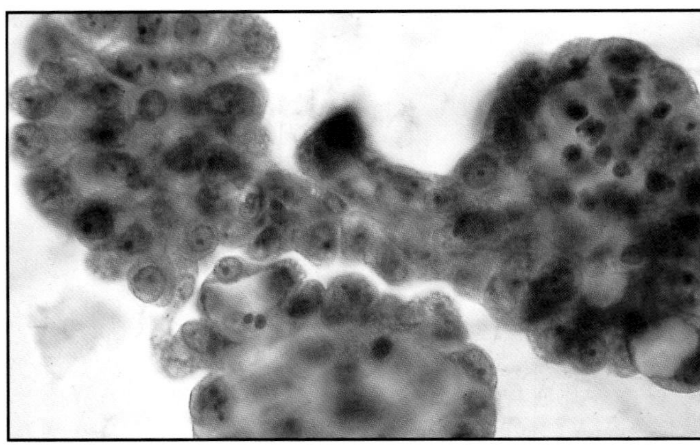

15.26
Acinar adenocarcinoma. Upper middle portion shows a hollow ball of tumor cells or acinus (Papanicolaou, x400).

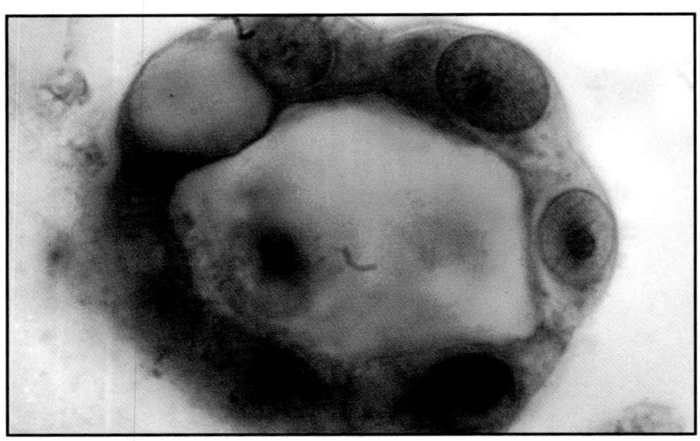

15.27
Acinar adenocarcinoma. Acinus composed of malignant cells has been brought into focus at midlevel to show in sharp outline the cavity of this hollow ball of cells; sputum (Papanicolaou, x1000).

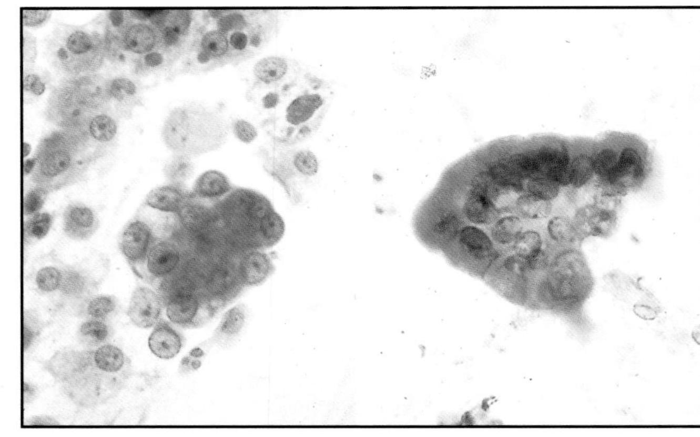

15.28
Left, Bronchoalveolar carcinoma. Three-dimensional ball-like cluster of tumor cells is depicted in center of field; sputum (Papanicolaou, x400). Right, Bronchoalveolar carcinoma. A papillary frond composed of well-differentiated cells is shown; FNA (Papanicolaou, x400).

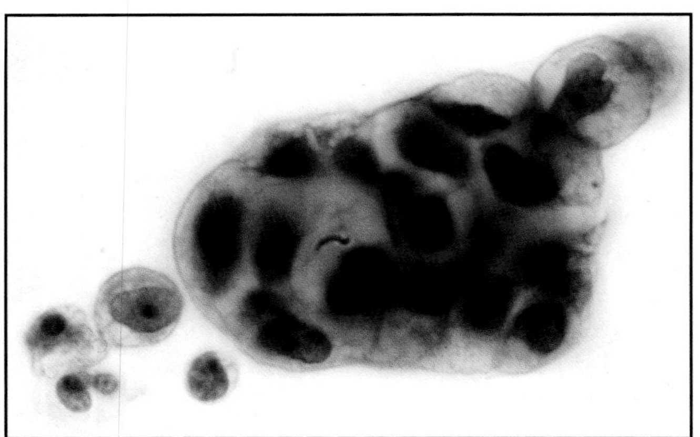

15.29
Bronchoalveolar carcinoma. Three-dimensional papillary cluster of cells is shown; sputum (Papanicolaou, x1000).

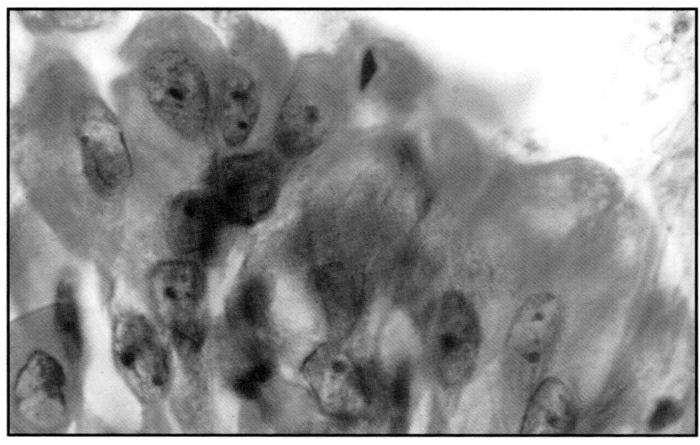

15.30
Bronchoalveolar carcinoma. Well-differentiated mucus-producing tumor cells are depicted; bronchial brushing (Papanicolaou, x1000).

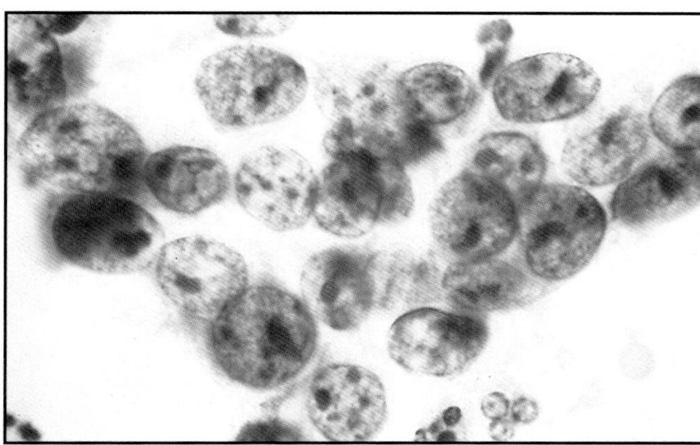

▮15.31
Large cell undifferentiated carcinoma; bronchial brushing (Papanicolaou, x1000).

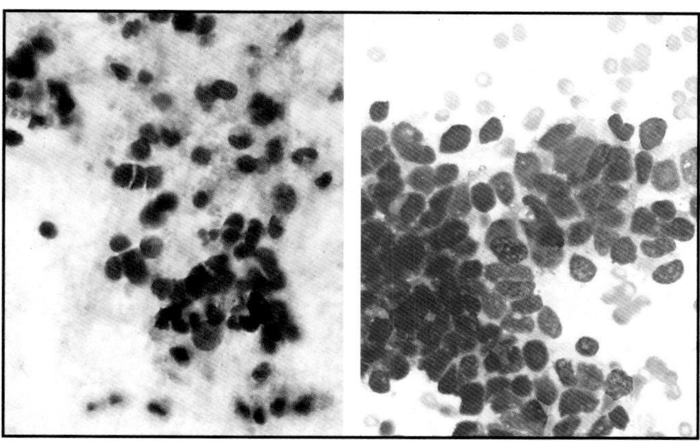

▮15.32
Left, Small cell undifferentiated carcinoma; sputum (Papanicolaou, x400). Right, Small cell undifferentiated carcinoma. Cells in this specimen are more scattered with less molding; fine needle aspirate (Wright-Giemsa, x400).

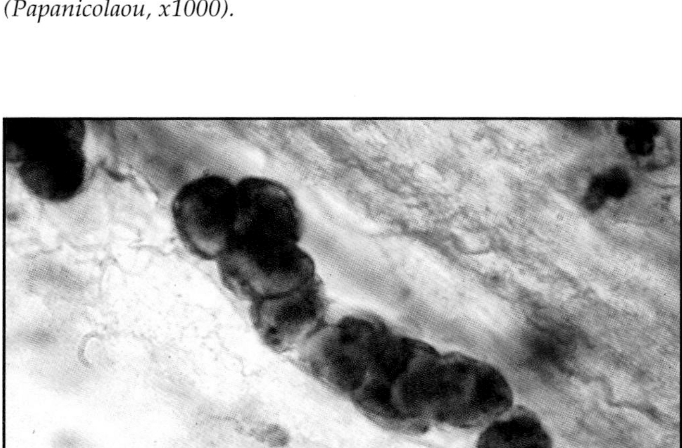

▮15.33
Small cell undifferentiated carcinoma. Although nuclei are poorly preserved, the specific nature of the molding supports an unmistakable diagnosis; sputum (Papanicolaou, x1000).

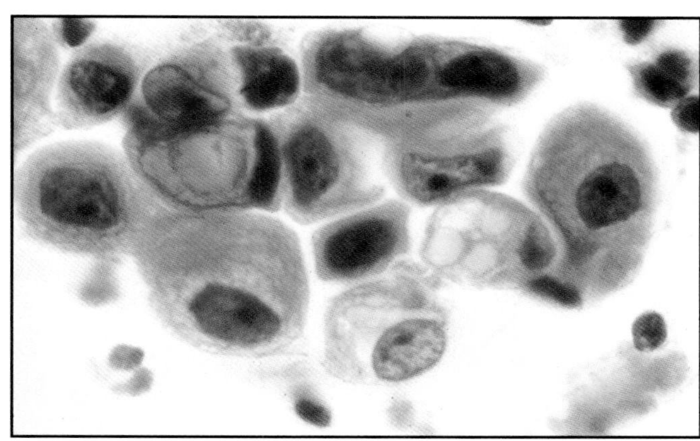

▮15.34
Adenosquamous carcinoma. Plate-like arrangement of cells and sharp cytoplasmic borders suggest squamous differentiation, but several cells also possess prominent secretory-type vacuoles; sputum (Papanicolaou, x1000).

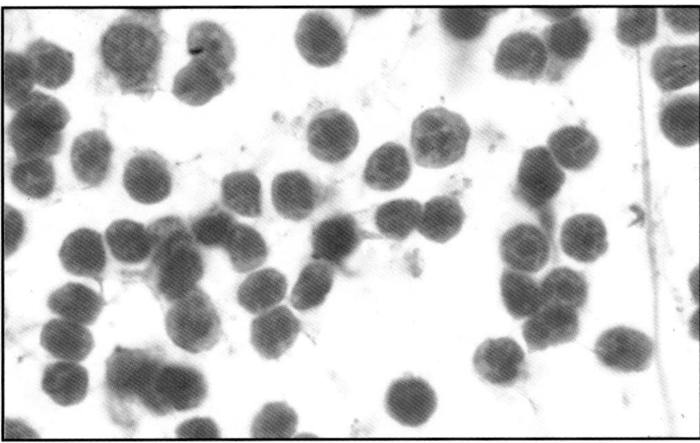

▮15.35
Bronchial carcinoid. Cells are forming interlacing ribbons and possess prominent nucleoli; fine needle aspirate (Papanicolaou, x1000).

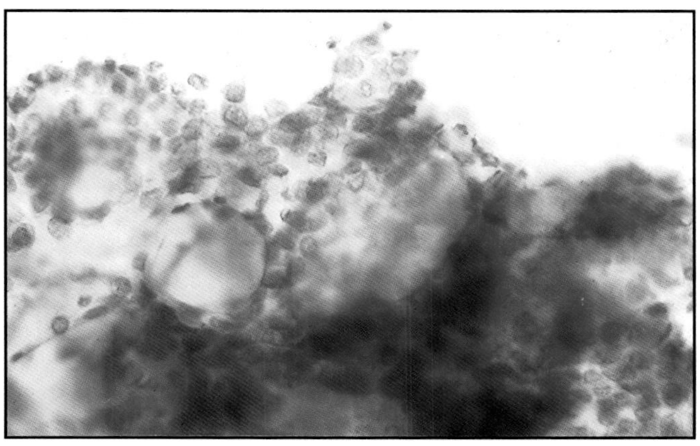

▮15.36
Adenoid cystic carcinoma metastatic from vulva. These large cell clusters within which multiple rounded structures are visible are characteristic; fine needle aspirate (Papanicolaou, x400).

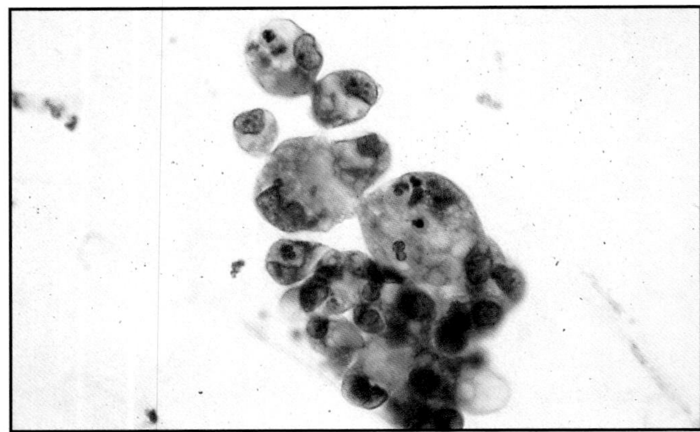

15.37

Adenocarcinoma, metastatic from colon; sputum (Papanicolaou, x400).

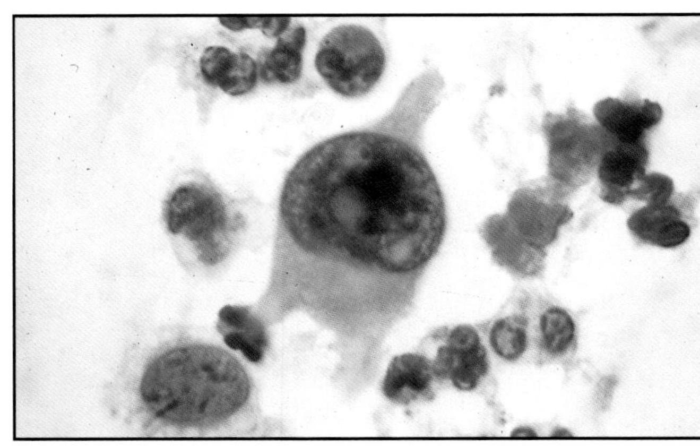

15.38

Malignant melanoma, metastatic from skin. Note intranuclear protrusions of cytoplasm, a helpful diagnostic feature; bronchial brushing (Papanicolaou, x1000).

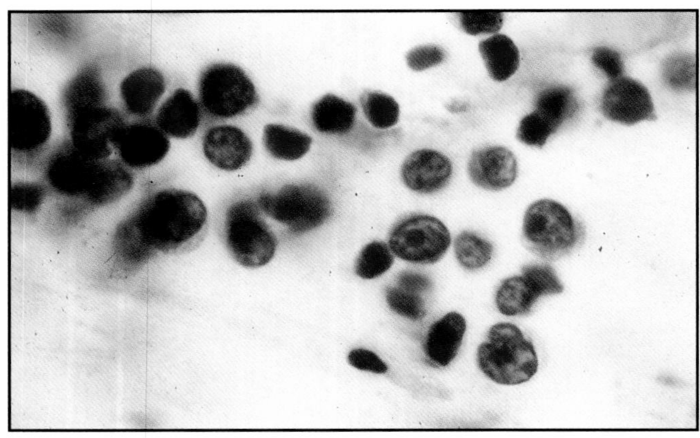

15.39

Histiocytic lymphoma. Note prominent nucleoli and irregular nuclear membranes; sputum (Papanicolaou, x1000).

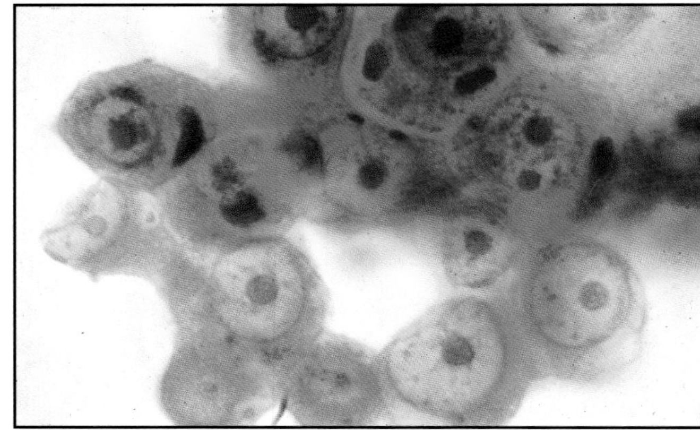

15.40

Hypernephroma, metastatic from kidney. Macronucleoli are characteristic; fine needle aspirate (Papanicolaou, x1000).

REVIEW EXERCISES

1. List and describe the salient cytologic features of epithelial cells from the respiratory tract exfoliating into cellular specimens.

2. What is sputum?

3. Define and discuss the significance of reserve cell hyperplasia and squamous metaplasia.

4. What are the possible cellular changes induced by irradiation therapy? What are the possible cellular changes induced by anticancer drug therapy?

5. Describe at least three ways in which the respiratory epithelium may respond to viral infection.

6. Compare and contrast the morphology of *Blastomyces dermatitidis*, *Cryptococcus neoformans*, and *Coccidioides immitis*.

7. Define bronchogenic carcinoma and discuss its subclassifications.

8. What is bronchoalveolar carcinoma, and what are the cytologic criteria for its diagnosis?

9. Describe the cytology of small cell undifferentiated carcinoma as found in sputum.

10. Discuss ways in which cytopathologic methods can be useful in the diagnosis of neoplasms metastatic to the lungs.

SELECTED READINGS

Bibbo M, Fennessy JJ, Lu C-T, Straus FH, Variakojis D, Wied GL. Bronchial brushing technique for the cytologic diagnosis of peripheral lung lesions. *Acta Cytol.* 1973;17:245-251.

Carter D, Eggleston J. *Tumors of the Lower Respiratory Tract.* Washington, DC: Armed Forces Institute of Pathology; 1980.

DeVita VT Jr, Hellman S, Rosenberg SA, eds. *Cancer: Principles and Practice of Oncology.* 3rd ed. Philadelphia, Pa: JB Lippincott; 1989.

Elson CE, Moore SP, Johnston WW. Morphologic and immunocytochemical studies of bronchioloalveolar carcinoma at Duke University Medical Center, 1968–1986. *Anal Quant Cytol Histol.* 1989;11:261-274.

Frable WJ, Johnston WW. *Respiratory Cytology Transparencies: Explanatory Text and Self-Evaluative Test.* International Cytology Slide Sets, XIX. Chicago, Ill: Tutorials of Cytology; 1974.

Frost JK. The cell in health and disease. In: Wied GL, ed. *Monographs in Clinical Cytology.* Basel, Switzerland: S Karger; 1969.

Grunze H, Spriggs AI. *History of Clinical Cytology.* Darmstadt, West Germany: GIT Verlag Ernst Giebeler; 1980.

Johnston WW. Cytologic correlations. In: Dail DH, Hammar SP, eds. *Pulmonary Pathology.* New York, NY: Springer Verlag; 1988.

Johnston WW. Cytologic diagnosis of lung cancer. *Pathol Res Pract.* 1986;181:1-36.

Johnston WW. Fine needle aspiration biopsy versus sputum and bronchial material in the diagnosis of lung cancer: a comparative study of 168 patients. *Acta Cytol.* 1988;32:641-646.

Johnston WW. Histologic and cytologic patterns of lung cancer in 2580 men and women over a 15-year period. *Acta Cytol.* 1988;32:163-168.

Johnston WW. Percutaneous FNAB of the lung. *Acta Cytol.* 1984;28:218-224.

Johnston WW. Pulmonary cytopathology in the compromised host. In: Greenberg SD, ed. *Lung Pathology for the Clinician.* New York, NY: Thieme-Stratton, Inc; 1982.

Johnston WW. Ten years of respiratory cytopathology at Duke University Medical Center, III: the significance of inconclusive cytopathologic diagnoses during the years 1970–1974. *Acta Cytol.* 1982;26:759-766.

Johnston WW, Amatulli J. The role of cytology in the primary diagnosis of North American blastomycosis. *Acta Cytol.* 1970;14:200-204.

Johnston WW, Bossen EH. Ten years of respiratory cytopathology at Duke University Medical Center, I: the cytopathologic diagnosis of lung cancer during the years 1970–1974 with a comparison between cytopathology and histopathology in the typing of lung cancer. *Acta Cytol.* 1981;25:103-107.

Johnston WW, Bossen EH. Ten years of respiratory cytopathology at Duke University Medical Center, II: the cytopathologic diagnosis of lung cancer during the years 1970–1974 with a comparison between cytopathology and histopathology in the typing of lung cancer. *Acta Cytol.* 1981;25:499-505.

Johnston WW, Elson CE. Respiratory tract. In: Bibbo M, ed. *Comprehensive Cytopathology.* Philadelphia, Pa: WB Saunders; 1991.

Johnston WW, Frable WJ. *Diagnostic Respiratory Cytopathology.* New York, NY: Masson Publishing Inc; 1979.

Kenney M, Webber CA. Diagnosis of strongyloidiasis in Papanicolaou-stained sputum smears. *Acta Cytol.* 1974;18:270-273.

Kern WH. Cytology of the hyperplastic and neoplastic lesions of terminal bronchioles and alveoli. *Acta Cytol.* 1965;9:372-379.

Kern WH, Schweizer C. Sputum cytology of metastatic carcinoma of the lung. *Acta Cytol.* 1976;20:514-520.

Koss LG. *Diagnostic Cytology and its Histopathologic Bases.* 3rd ed. Philadelphia, Pa: JB Lippincott Co; 1979.

Kreyburg L. *Histological Type of Lung Tumours.* Geneva, Switzerland; World Health Organization; 1981.

Linder J, Rennard SI. *Bronchoalveolar Lavage.* Chicago, Ill: ASCP Press; 1988.

Maygarden SJ, Flanders EL. Mycobacteria can be seen as "negative images" in cytology smears from patients with acquired immunodeficiency syndrome. *Mod Pathol.* 1989;2:239-243.

McDonald JR. Pulmonary cytology. *Am J Surg.* 1955;89:462-464.

Naib ZM, Stewart JA, Dowdle WR, Casey HL, Marine WW, Nahmias AJ. Cytological features of viral respiratory tract infections. *Acta Cytol.* 1968;12:162-171.

Naylor B, Railey C. A pitfall in the cytodiagnosis of sputum of asthmatics. *J Clin Pathol.* 1964;17:84-89.

Roger V, Nasiell M, Linden M, Engstad I. Cytologic differential diagnosis of bronchiolo-alveolar carcinoma and bronchogenic adenocarcinoma. *Acta Cytol.* 1976;20:303-307.

Rosenthal DL. Cytopathology: pulmonary disease. In: Wied GL, ed. *Monographs in Clinical Cytology.* Basel, Switzerland: S Karger; 1988.

Saccomanno G. *Diagnostic Pulmonary Pathology.* Chicago, Ill: ASCP Press; 1978.

Smith JH, Frable WJ. Adenocarcinoma of the lung: cytologic correlation with histologic type. *Acta Cytol.* 1974;18:316-320.

Woolner LB, McDonald JR. Bronchogenic carcinoma: diagnosis by microscopic examination of sputum and bronchial secretions, preliminary report. *Mayo Clin Proc.* 1947;22:369-381.

CHAPTER 16

Urinary Tract

William H. Kern, MD, FIAC

CONTENTS

The urinary tract comprises the kidneys, which excrete water and waste products in the form of urine; the ureters, which convey the urine to the urinary bladder where it is temporarily retained; and the urethra, through which urine is discharged from the body [**F** *16.1*]. Cells from the epithelial lining of the urinary tract desquamate readily into the urinary stream. On occasion, cells exfoliate from the renal tubules and, in men, from the prostate or seminal vesicles. Urinary specimens from women should be taken by using a catheter, since voided urine often contains cells from the female genital tract.

ANATOMY

The kidneys are paired bean-shaped organs situated in the upper dorsal part of the abdomen, one on each side of the vertebral column, and covered anteriorly by peritoneum. The hilum of the medial border expands into the renal sinus, which contains the renal pelvis with the major and minor calyces. This funnel-shaped structure continues into the ureters. The ureters are narrow, muscular, urothelium-lined tubes that empty into the urinary bladder near its base.

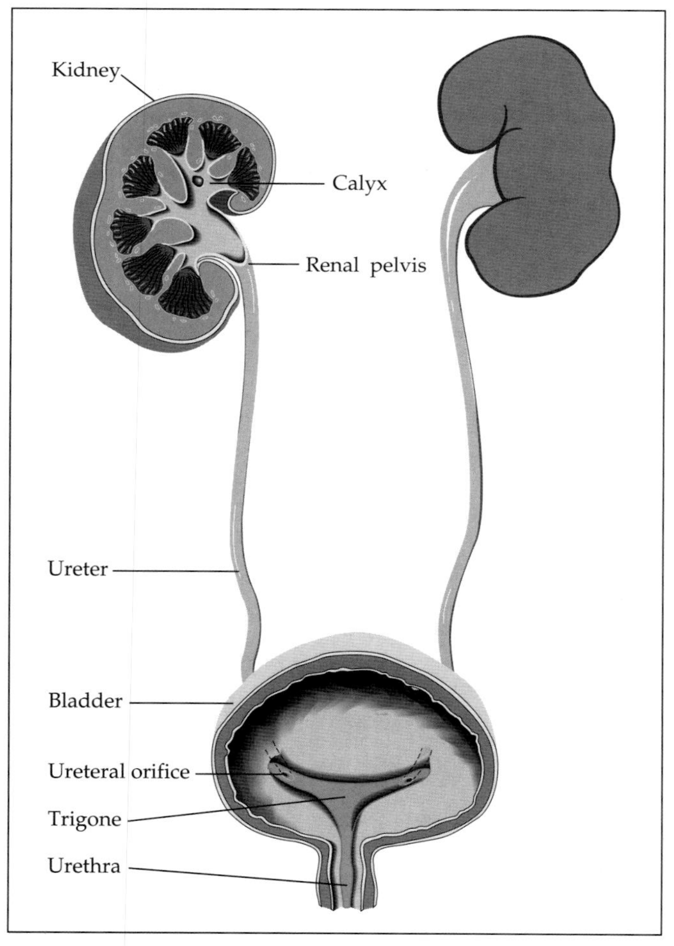

F *16.1*
Anatomy of the urinary tract.

The urinary bladder is a urothelium-lined sac with a muscular wall that acts as a reservoir for the urine. It is located behind the symphysis and anterior to the rectum. In women, it is positioned anterior and below the uterus. The size, position, and thickness of the bladder wall vary according to the amount of fluid it contains. It receives urine from both ureters and discharges it through the single urethra that joins the bladder at its lowermost point. The trigone is a triangle at the base of the bladder that is formed by the orifices of the urethra and the two ureters.

The male urethra is 18 to 20 cm long [**F** *16.2*]. The proximal prostatic portion is surrounded by the prostate gland and contains the openings of the two ejaculatory ducts. The next segment, the short membranous urethra, passes through the urogenital diaphragm. The cavernous urethra in the penis is the distal and longest portion and terminates at the external urethral orifice.

The female urethra is 3 to 4 cm long and extends from the bladder to the external orifice in the vestibule [**F** *16.3*]. It is embedded in the anterior wall of the vagina. Many small urethral glands open into both the female and the male urethral lumen.

The prostate is a firm, solid, partly glandular and partly muscular body that is located below the internal urethral orifice in males and surrounds the proximal portion of the urethra. It continuously produces secretions that drain into the urethra. The two seminal vesicles lie against the posterior surface of the bladder. The excretory duct of each joins with the ductus deferens of the same side to form one of the ejaculatory ducts.

HISTOLOGY

The excretory passages of the urinary tract, namely the renal pelves, ureters, bladder, and urethra, are principally lined by so-called transitional cell epithelium (urothelium). The epithelium is adaptable to the changing volume as urine passes into and out of the bladder. In the empty bladder, six to eight layers of rounded or even columnar or club-shaped cells are seen. In the distended state, the epithelium appears to be only two to three cells deep. The cells in the intermediate and basal portions of the epithelium have well-developed desmosomal connections and a plasma membrane that is folded in the empty bladder but may unfold in the dilated bladder. The superficial cells are larger, flat, and elongated. Their cytoplasm stretches over several of the underlying intermediate cells, and, therefore, they are also called umbrella or cap cells. Areas of the bladder in the dome as well as the trigone may be lined by single layers of columnar mucus-producing cells. A

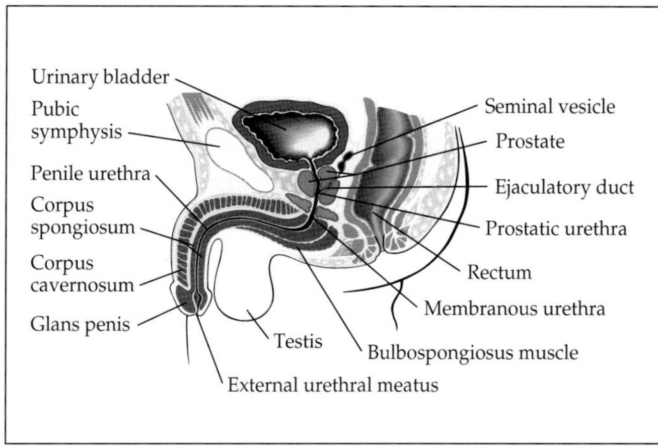

F *16.2*
Anatomy of the male urinary tract.

noncornifying squamous lining may be seen in small portions of the trigone of women.

The prostatic part of the male urethra is lined by transitional epithelium, but the short membranous and the long cavernous urethra are lined by stratified or pseudostratified columnar epithelium. Stratified squamous epithelium is found near the meatus. The urethral mucosa contains many recesses, the lacunae of Morgagni, which communicate with deeper branching tubules, and the glands of Littré.

The epithelium of the female urethra near the bladder is transitional, and that in the remaining portions is predominantly stratified squamous, often with interspersed areas of pseudostratified columnar epithelium. Epithelial invaginations are lined by mucus-producing cells similar to those found in the glands of Littré in the male urethra.

The walls of the excretory passageways contain well-developed coats of smooth muscle, the contractions of which move the urine forward.

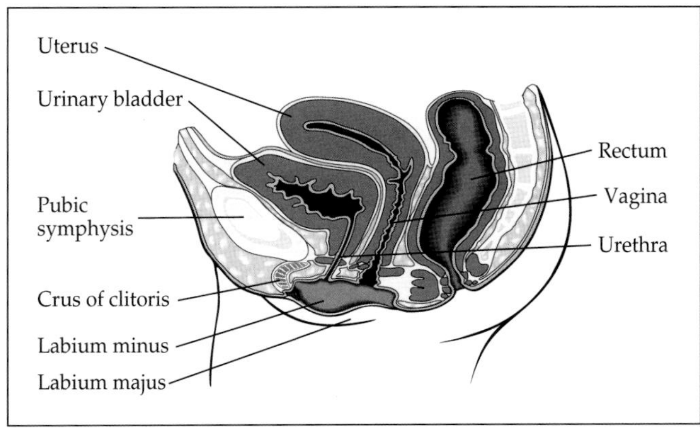

F *16.3*
Anatomy of the female urinary tract.

The prostate includes approximately 30 to 50 tortuous tubular alveolar glands, lined by simple or pseudostratified columnar cells, and in some areas by cuboidal epithelial cells. Some alveoli contain laminated waxy concretions, the corpora amylacea.

The epithelia of the seminal vesicles, ejaculatory ducts, deferent ducts, and bulbourethral glands also vary from simple cuboidal to columnar but may be pseudostratified. A yellow lipochrome pigment is frequently seen in the epithelial cells of the seminal vesicles and can be helpful in recognizing cells from this site.

The kidneys are histologically complex organs. The functioning microunits, the nephrons, consist of glomeruli and tubules. The latter are lined by single layers of epithelial cells that are of the same size or slightly larger than transitional cells and contain uniformly round nuclei that are also larger than those of normal transitional cells. These cells may exfoliate under pathologic conditions but are difficult to differentiate from transitional cells. The renal pelves are lined by transitional epithelium that closely resembles the epithelium of the ureters and bladder.

NORMAL CYTOLOGY

Transitional epithelial cells are present in all urine specimens, and squamous cells are present in many [❚*16.1*, ❚*16.2*]. Transitional cells are more numerous in urine specimens taken with a catheter and in the presence of inflammation or other pathologic changes.

Many of the transitional cells are relatively small, but nuclear and cell sizes vary considerably. The average nuclear diameter is 7.5 µm, and the cell diameter varies from 9 to 50 µm. Most cells occur singly, but some are arranged in clusters or sheets. The cytoplasm is opaque, granular, or vacuolated. The nucleus may be eccentric, particularly in vacuolated cells. Most nuclei are round, but some have an irregular or wrinkled outline. Few cells contain small nucleoli. The cell size depends on the site of origin. The usually more numerous intermediate and basal cells are smaller, cuboidal, and have generally small and round or wrinkled nuclei. The superficial cells (also often called umbrella or cap cells) are considerably larger and often binucleated or multinucleated [❚*16.3*, ❚*16.4*]. Nucleoli are more prominent than in the smaller cell types. The cytoplasm is abundant, and the nuclear/cytoplasmic ratio is considerably less than 50%.

Squamous cells of superficial or intermediate types are often seen, more commonly in women. They may represent vaginal contamination, or they may originate from the urethra or zones of squamous epithelium in the bladder.

Some columnar epithelial cells are transitional, but they may originate from areas of the bladder that occasionally are lined by columnar mucin-secreting epithelium or from nests of von Brunn. The latter are buds of transitional epithelium that extend from the surface into the lamina propria and may centrally become cystic and lined by columnar cells [▮*16.5*]. Columnar cells lining the tubules and ducts of the prostate may also exfoliate into the urine, particularly after prostatic massage. Prostatic cells are small, have homogeneous round nuclei, and contain a finely granular or clear cytoplasm. Small concentric, occasionally calcified, prostatic concretions (corpora amylacea) are rarely observed. Cells are occasionally shed from the lining of the lacunae of Morgagni and the glands of Littré. The morphologic appearance of these cells corresponds to the site of origin.

Epithelial cells with eosinophilic cytoplasmic inclusions are frequently observed in the urine. Most of the inclusions appear in cells with degenerated or absent nuclei and are not associated with a specific disease process.

Histiocytes are present in inflammatory conditions and resemble histiocytes found elsewhere. They have indistinct cell borders, a foamy cytoplasm, and eccentric, lobed, or bean-shaped nuclei. They are often difficult to differentiate from degenerated transitional epithelial cells.

Polymorphonuclear leukocytes and red blood cells are frequently seen, and bacteria, fungi, trichomonads, spermatozoa, various casts, and crystals are sometimes observed in urine. Their presence should be noted, since they may indicate a pathologic process.

PATHOLOGY AND CYTOLOGY OF NON-NEOPLASTIC CONDITIONS

Inflammatory conditions of the lower urinary tract are common and are often bacterial in origin. Obstruction of free urinary flow due to benign prostatic hyperplasia or adenocarcinoma of the prostate predisposes to inflammation. Kidney or bladder calculi, diverticula of the urinary bladder, strictures, and malformations are usually associated with inflammation and often with epithelial hyperplasia and degeneration. These inflammatory atypias can be marked but are rarely precursors of malignant changes. As a result of the inflammation, many red blood cells and leukocytes appear in the urine. Increased numbers of transitional cells are present but are often obscured by the heavy inflammatory exudate.

The degenerative changes associated with inflammation are prominent. Nuclei are enlarged, often have prominent cleared zones and chromatin bars, and undergo karyorrhexis [▮*16.6*]. The changes associated with renal and ureteral calculi may also produce hematuria and leukocyturia. More importantly, tight clusters of urothelial cells with slightly enlarged, irregular, and hyperchromatic nuclei may be seen [▮*16.7*]. This atypia may be incorrectly interpreted as malignancy, but the abnormal cells are relatively sparse, in contrast to the considerably increased cellularity seen in bladder cancers, and are often associated with the presence of many red blood cells. Inflammation may also be followed by increased numbers of clusters of large superficial cells in voided urine.

Diverticula of the bladder are often lined by metaplastic squamous epithelium, and metaplastic squamous cells are prominent in the urine of these patients. Squamous metaplasia and hyperkeratosis may also be associated with various forms of cystitis.

Cytomegalic inclusion disease is caused by cytomegalovirus (CMV), a member of the herpesvirus group. This condition usually occurs in childhood but is also seen in patients who receive chemotherapy for cancer, are immunosuppressed because of allografts, or have acquired immunodeficiency syndrome (AIDS). Renal tubular epithelium is frequently involved. The affected cells, as seen in the urine, contain large intranuclear, usually single, basophilic, or eosinophilic inclusions.

Polyomaviruses, along with papillomaviruses, belong to the papovavirus group. They also may infect the urinary tract if the host's immunity is impaired. The nuclear inclusions are even larger than those of CMV and are dense, homogeneous, and basophilic.

Malacoplakia is a granulomatous disease of the bladder or upper urinary tract that is characterized by the presence of soft umbilicated yellow plaques in the mucosa. The plaques consist of histiocytes, many of which contain homogeneous or concentrically laminated calcospherites, the Michaelis-Gutmann bodies. Cytologically, the urine contains histiocytes with multiple granules in an abundant foamy cytoplasm. Some of the histiocytes contain the characteristic spherical laminated calcospherites, which average 8 μm in diameter.

Decoy cells have characteristics of malignancy and contain fairly large, round, oval, or cup-shaped nuclei that may be markedly hyperchromatic or have a coarse chromatin pattern. A slight tag of cytoplasm attached to the nucleus has led to their classification as "comet" cells. They are occasionally found in otherwise normal urine and in association with inflammatory conditions or cancer, but they should not be confused with cancer cells.

When a cystectomy is performed for bladder cancer, ileal conduits are created by forming a bladder-like pouch from a segment of ileum. Ureters are implanted into the pouch and the ileal "bladder" empties through the abdominal wall. Urine obtained from the ileal conduit contains numerous often degenerated intestinal epithelial cells, many histiocytes, and leukocytes. Cells characteristic of transitional cell carcinoma can be identified when cancer develops in the ureters or renal pelves.

Irradiation changes are seen in both benign and malignant transitional cells after approximately 28 Gy (2800 rad) has been delivered. The transitional cells show the usual radiation effect and become enlarged with large, vesiculated but sometimes pyknotic nuclei. The cytoplasm becomes vacuolated and at times eosinophilic. The diagnosis of carcinoma should be reserved strictly for conditions in which transitional cells are shed, employing the usual cytologic criteria of malignancy. Chemotherapeutic agents (in particular, systemically given cyclophosphamides and agents such as thiotepa and mitomycin C given intravesically for superficial bladder cancer) also cause significant changes in neoplastic as well as non-neoplastic urothelium. The nuclei become enlarged, irregular, and hyperchromatic with a salt-and-pepper chromatin distribution. Nucleoli and multinucleation may be observed. This is often associated with karyorrhexis and significant degenerative changes. The distinction from viable, recurrent, or residual carcinoma may be difficult. The latter diagnosis should be made only if unequivocally viable malignant cells are present [▮*16.8*].

TUMORS OF THE URINARY TRACT

Tumors arising from the epithelium lining the urinary tract (urothelium) exfoliate readily into the urinary stream; tumors arising in deep tissues, such as in the kidney or prostate, are unlikely to exfoliate until they have become large and disrupt the normal urothelial lining. Urine cytology, therefore, is most useful in the diagnosis of carcinoma of the bladder, renal pelvis, ureters, and urethra. The cytotechnologist should be familiar with the cytologic characteristics of tumors that develop in these areas.

Tumors of transitional epithelium are often multicentric and may affect any part of the epithelial lining from the calyces to the external urethral meatus. Most of the tumors, however, occur in the urinary bladder. The tumors are classified according to four criteria: the pattern of growth [**F** *16.4*], cell type, grade of malignancy, and pathologic stage. The pattern may be papillary or nonpapillary and in situ (noninvasive) or invasive. The cell type is usually transitional but may be squamous or glandular. The stage indicates the extent of invasion and is closely related to the prognosis. Deep muscle invasion and extension into perivesical tissues are ominous and are seen in cytologically poorly differentiated tumors.

Papilloma

Transitional cell papillomas are uncommon small benign papillary tumors with a thin fibrovascular core and a covering of transitional epithelium less than seven layers in thickness.

The individual cells resemble normal transitional cells. They have a regular shape but are often columnar and somewhat elongated, and they appear at right angles to the basement membrane. Mitoses are absent. Papillomas may be multiple and may recur after resection. They do not invade or metastasize. Since the cells covering the papillary processes of a papilloma are morphologically similar to normal bladder epithelial cells, a cytologic diagnosis is usually not possible. A diagnosis of papilloma or very low-grade papillary carcinoma may be suggested if small papillary fronds or increased numbers of clusters composed of mildly atypical transitional cells are present [▮*16.9*]. A few clusters of cytologically normal-appearing transitional epithelial cells, however, should not be identified as being from a papilloma because they may become dislodged as a result of a cystoscopy, catheterization, or calculus and may not be true papillary processes.

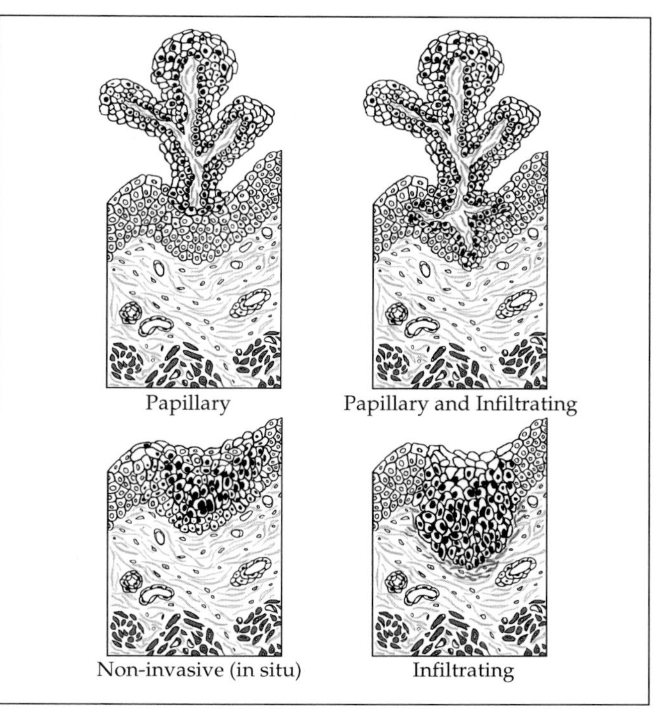

F *16.4*
Classification of tumor growth patterns.

Transitional Cell Carcinoma

Papillary transitional cell carcinomas also have papillary fronds covered by thickened (more than six cell layers) transitional cell epithelium. Only slight cytologic and architectural abnormalities may be noted, but increased cellularity, loss of polarity of the cells, cellular pleomorphism, nuclear hyperchromasia, and mitotic activity may be seen. Most papillary carcinomas are larger than papillomas and have broader, thicker villi. The epithelial and stromal proliferation is considerably less uniform. Depending on the degree of differentiation, the tumors are graded from I to III (or from I to IV by pathologists who consider transitional cell papillomas to be transitional cell carcinomas, grade I). Almost all grade I carcinomas are noninvasive, and the cytologic atypia is slight. Submucosal invasion or extension into the muscularis or to the serosa is common in the higher-grade, poorly differentiated tumors.

Nonpapillary infiltrating transitional cell carcinomas are flat, plaque-like, or ulcerated. They may arise in small or large fields of abnormal, atypical, transitional epithelium and often involve large regions of the urinary tract. They are usually less differentiated than the papillary carcinomas and may include areas of characteristic keratinizing squamous cell carcinoma. Invasive squamous cell carcinoma also occurs in a pure form, often arising in squamous metaplasia.

Carcinoma in situ may precede, accompany, or follow invasive cancer. It is a histologic abnormality of the transitional epithelium cytologically resembling carcinoma but without evidence of invasion. The lesion may exist for as long as 6 or 7 years before it becomes invasive. It may be asymptomatic or, because of exfoliation and erosion, it may produce symptoms of dysuria, frequency, and nocturia suggesting cystitis. Carcinoma in situ appears to evolve by progression from normal epithelium through stages of hyperplasia and progressively more severe dysplasia. Many of these intermediate stages as well as characteristic carcinoma in situ are often seen to involve large portions of bladder epithelium adjacent to invasive carcinoma.

Adenocarcinomas

Primary adenocarcinoma of the urinary tract is uncommon and is sometimes associated with cystitis cystica or glandularis, a condition in which nests of transitional epithelial cells that extend from normal mucosa into the submucosa become separated and eventually form mucus-secreting cysts. Some adenocarcinomas arise from urachal remnants in the dome of the bladder. Many of these tumors produce mucin.

Adenocarcinomas of the kidney in late stages invade the renal pelvis and then exfoliate into the urine. This invasion is associated with and usually preceded by hematuria, an important symptom. Adenocarcinomas of the kidney are often of the clear cell type. The nuclei are moderately enlarged and irregular, and the cytoplasm is abundant, well defined, and prominently vacuolated [▮*16.10*]. A cytologic diagnosis is possible only in late or advanced stages, and, thus, cytology is not a useful diagnostic tool for this condition.

Wilms' tumor or nephroblastoma of the kidney is one of the more common tumors found in young children. It consists of immature mesenchymal tissue and epithelium-lined tubular and glomerular structures.

Adenocarcinomas of the prostate are a common cancer of older men and are often well differentiated. They exfoliate infrequently into the urine, but tumor cells can be identified after a prostatic massage, although this is not recommended as a diagnostic procedure. Poorly differentiated, advanced, or recurrent adenocarcinomas of the prostate may invade the bladder neck and trigone. Large or pleomorphic malignant cells characteristic of carcinoma can be found [▮*16.11*], but may be difficult or impossible to differentiate from cells of high-grade transitional cell carcinoma.

The bladder is occasionally the site of metastases and, more frequently, is invaded by carcinomas from adjacent organs, such as the uterine cervix or the colon. Malignant squamous cells from a carcinoma of the cervix may be found; or, if an advanced rectal carcinoma has formed a rectovesical fistula, columnar elongate tumor cells with cigar-shaped hyperchromatic nuclei, typical of colonic carcinoma, may appear in the urine [▮*16.12*].

CYTOLOGY OF TRANSITIONAL CELL CARCINOMA

Most carcinomas of the urinary tract epithelium are transitional cell carcinomas. Since carcinomas of the bladder are approximately 20 times more frequent than carcinomas of the renal pelvis and ureter, carcinoma of the bladder is by far the most common source of cancer cells in the urine.

It is rare to see only a few malignant cells. In papillary and nonpapillary invasive carcinomas, the urine cellularity is always increased considerably. As many as 25% or more of the cells present may be malignant [▮*16.13*]. Red blood cells, leukocytes, and necrotic debris indicate that the lesion is probably ulcerating and invasive. In contrast, the backgrounds of most well-differentiated papillary carcinomas and of many transitional cell carcinomas in situ are clean. Some transitional cell carcinomas in situ are, however, associated with erosions and a "pseudocystitis." In these cases, an inflammatory reaction may be noted. Because of this usually considerable cellularity, screening of urine specimens is rarely required to the same extent as screening of cervical/vaginal and pulmonary specimens. The examination of urine specimens resembles more that of fluid specimens or even aspirates in that the identification of the nature of the cytologic abnormalities rather than the finding of few abnormal cells is critical.

Cells that exfoliate from urothelial carcinomas may be single or clustered. The more prominent the clustering, the more likely it is that the tumor is papillary in configuration [▮*16.13*-▮*16.16*]. As previously noted, if the cytologic abnormalities in well-differentiated papillary carcinomas are minor [▮*16.14*], a definite cytologic diagnosis may not be possible. The cytologic and particularly the nuclear features of the less-differentiated papillary tumors [▮*16.15*, ▮*16.16*] resemble those of the moderately and poorly differentiated nonpapillary carcinomas and permit a diagnosis of malignancy. The nuclei of these cancer cells are considerably enlarged, averaging 75 to 90 μm^2, more than twice the size of nuclei of normal transitional cells. The nuclear/cytoplasmic ratio is high. Most nuclei are irregular in outline [▮*16.17*], are hyperchromatic, and have an irregular, coarse chromatin pattern [▮*16.18*-▮*16.20*]. Nucleoli are prominent. These features, including the overall increase in nuclear size, ragged outlines, and the chromatin pattern, are characteristic of carcinoma and diagnostic in most cases. In my laboratory, the sensitivity of urine cytology for primary carcinoma of the bladder is 83%.

Of bladder cancers, 2% to 3% are squamous cell carcinomas, and many poorly differentiated and particularly recurrent transitional cell carcinomas contain a component of keratinizing squamous carcinoma. Keratinizing malignant epithelial cells may then be present in urine specimens [▮*16.21*].

The cellular examination of urine samples is particularly useful in the follow-up of patients known to have had surgical resection or transurethral fulguration of bladder tumors. These patients have a high rate of recurrence. Medium- or high-grade recurrent carcinomas can be reliably diagnosed during cytologic follow-up studies, sometimes before any demonstrable clinical or cystoscopic evidence of disease is noted. Conversely, well-differentiated grade I papillary transitional cell carcinomas are rarely diagnosable, either as primary or as recurrent tumors. Strict adherence to established nuclear criteria of malignancy is essential to avoid false-positive diagnoses, particularly in cases of nephrolithiasis, various inflammatory conditions, or ureteral catheterization specimens in which reactive changes are prominent and superficial cells are numerous. In the case of nephrolithiasis, a helpful clue is that the abnormal cells that may be present in this condition occur in small numbers.

Transitional cell carcinoma in situ is a flat, neoplastic, nonpapillary intraepithelial lesion and may precede invasive carcinoma by several years. During this time, it can be diagnosed by cytologic studies. The sensitivity is high because high-grade abnormalities, with nuclear features similar to those of invasive carcinoma, are noted cytologically. The high sensitivity of urine cytology in the diagnosis of transitional cell carcinoma in situ is important for industrial workers exposed to carcinogens and for patients with treated bladder carcinoma, who often develop multicentric carcinoma in situ before recurrence of additional invasive tumors. Unequivocal transitional cell carcinoma in situ is, in turn, preceded by transitional cell hyperplasia and dysplasia, characterized by increasing nuclear size and hyperchromasia [▮*16.22*, ▮*16.23*]. If cells of this type are found in the urine of patients who had undergone treatment for well-differentiated papillary tumors of the urinary bladder, it is likely that they have borderline lesions or transitional cell carcinoma in situ associated with the low-grade papillary tumors. The in situ carcinoma is clinically much more significant, because of the probability of progression to invasive and potentially lethal bladder cancer. The cytotechnologist and cytopathologist must carefully note and report these findings. In cases of more extensive transitional cell carcinoma in situ, and in those associated with erosion or "pseudocystitis," abnormal cells are numerous. Because of this, it may be difficult or impossible to cytologically distinguish these lesions from invasive carcinoma [▮*16.23*, ▮*16.24*].

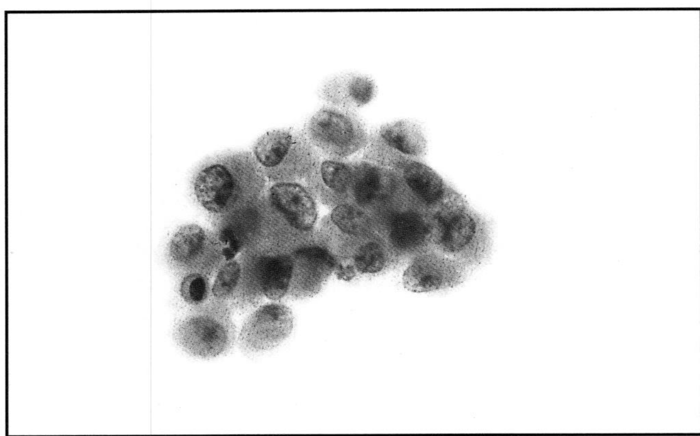

16.1

Transitional (urothelial) cells of the intermediate-pyramidal type and squamous cells (x500).

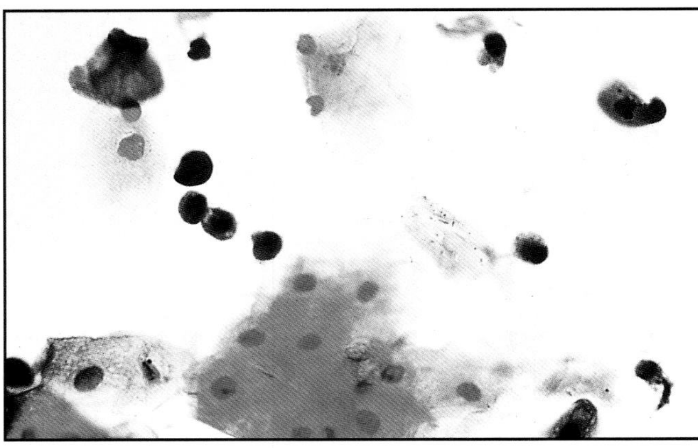

16.2

Normal squamous and small (intermediate or basal type) transitional cells, normal transitional epithelial cells, intermediate and superficial type (x500).

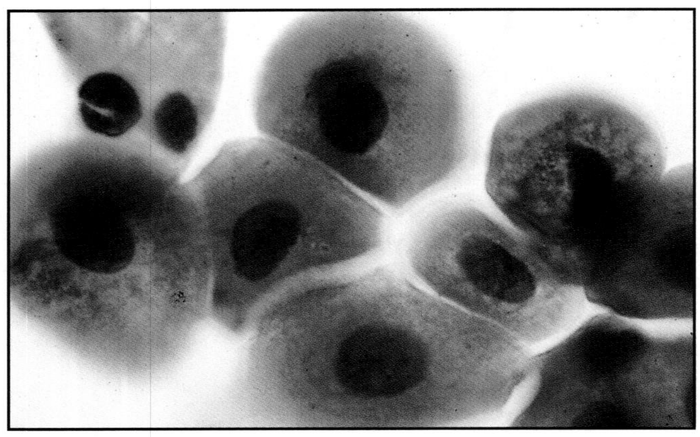

16.3

Transitional cells of intermediate and superficial type (x750).

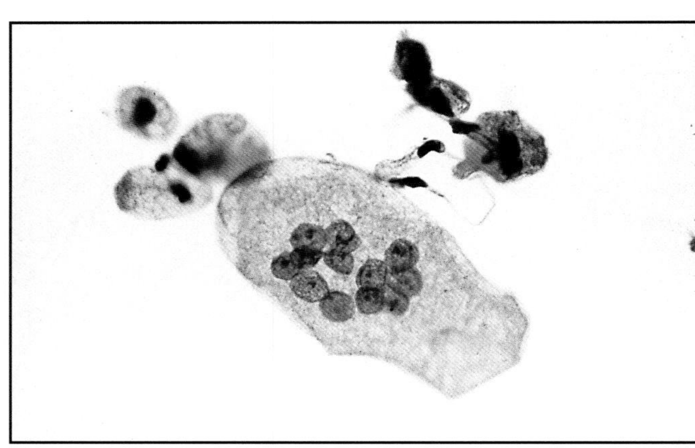

16.4

Multinucleated, superficial-type, transitional epithelial cells from urethral catheterization specimen (x500).

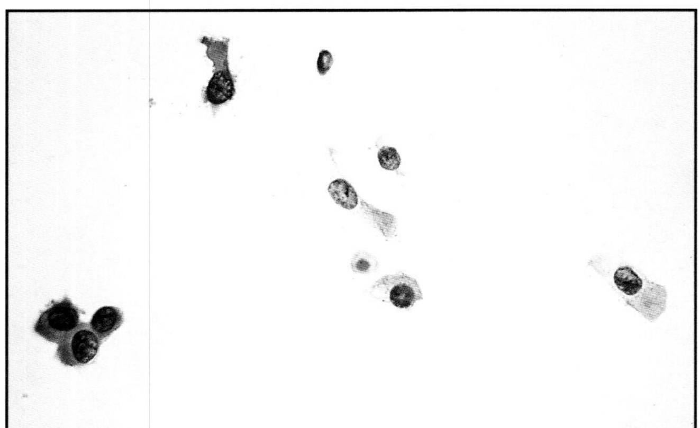

16.5

Columnar and normal transitional epithelial cells (x500).

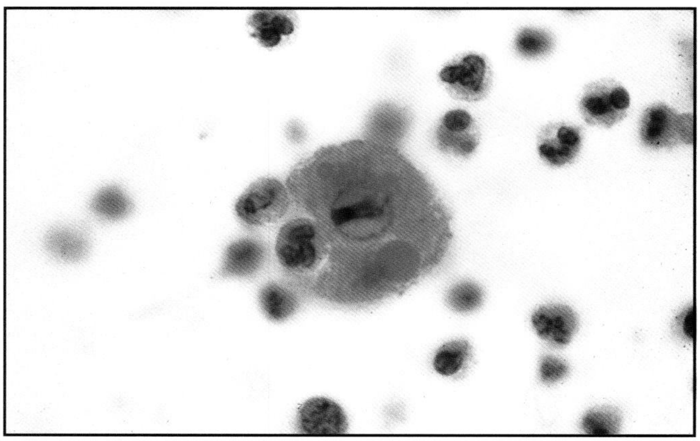

16.6

Acute inflammation; polymorphonuclear leukocytes and degenerating urothelial cells with partially cleared nucleus containing "chromatin bar" and eosinophilic intracytoplasmic inclusion body (x500).

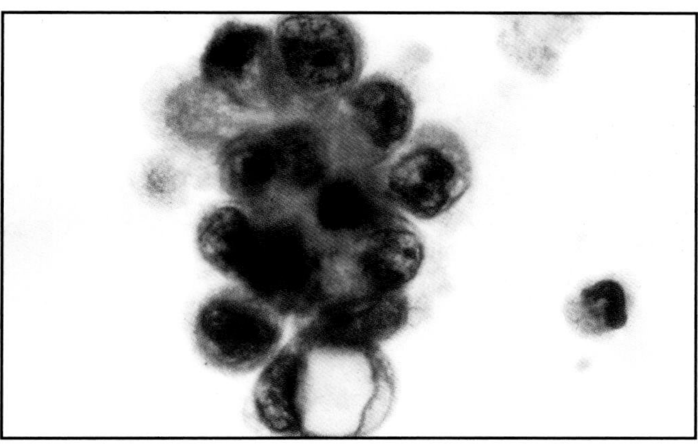

16.7

Cluster of atypical, reactive urothelial cells. This type of change may be associated with calculi or inflammation; in contrast to bladder cancer, cellularity is sparse (x500).

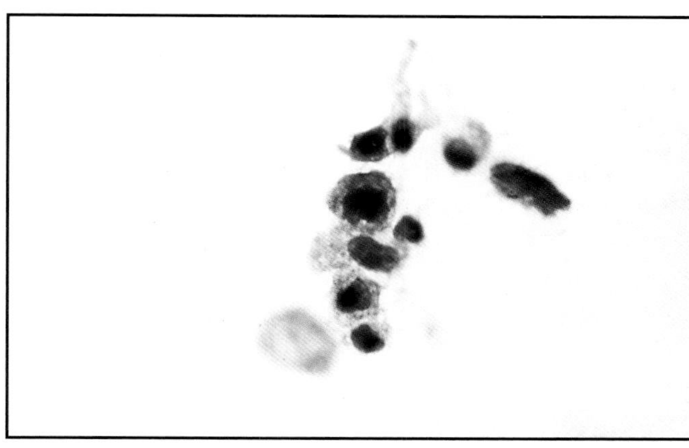

16.8

Marked degenerative changes, with nuclear hyperchromasia and irregularity, secondary to cyclophosphamide treatment (x500).

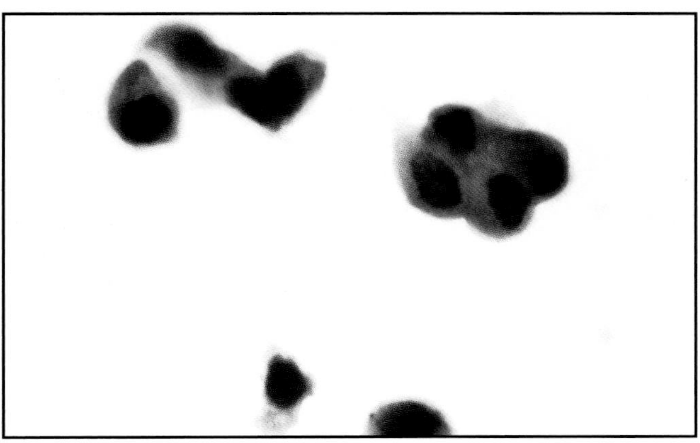

16.9

Clusters of mildly atypical urothelial cells, with slightly elongated nuclei in voided urine, in low-grade, well-differentiated papillary carcinoma (x500).

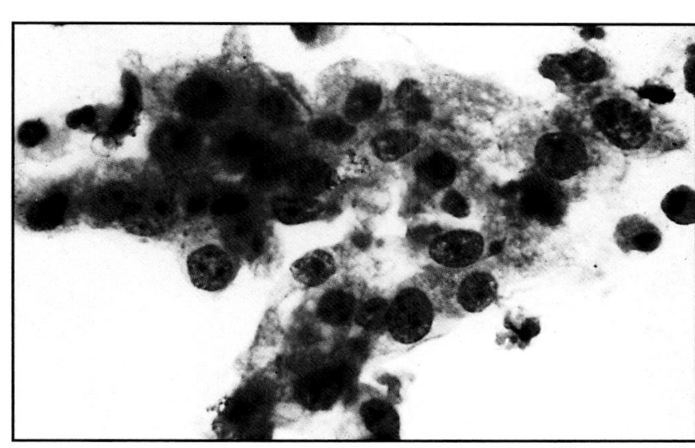

16.10

Clear cell adenocarcinoma of kidney. The nuclei contains small nucleoli; the cytoplasm is faintly vacuolated or granular (x500).

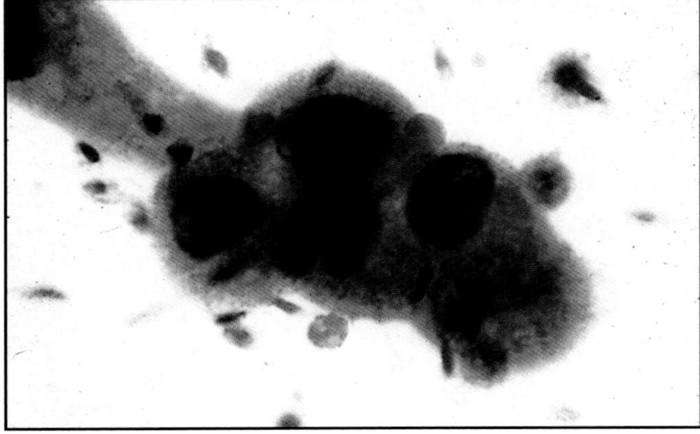

16.11

Cluster of malignant cells exfoliated from poorly differentiated adenocarcinoma of prostate (invading bladder neck and bladder floor) (x750).

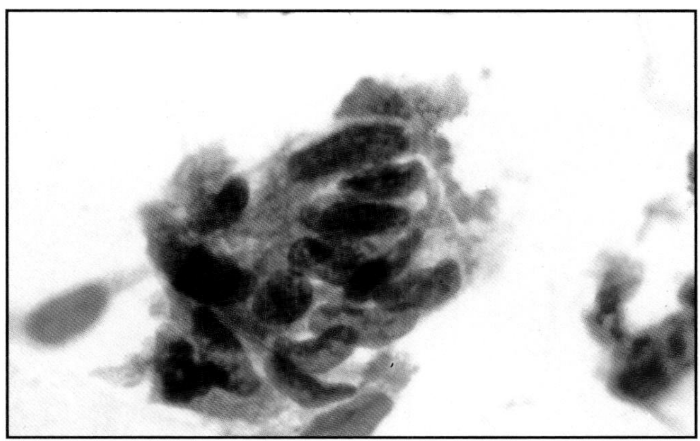

16.12

Adenocarcinoma of the rectum, with rectovesical fistula and exfoliation of malignant cells in urine. The nuclei are characteristically elongated or cigar shaped (x500).

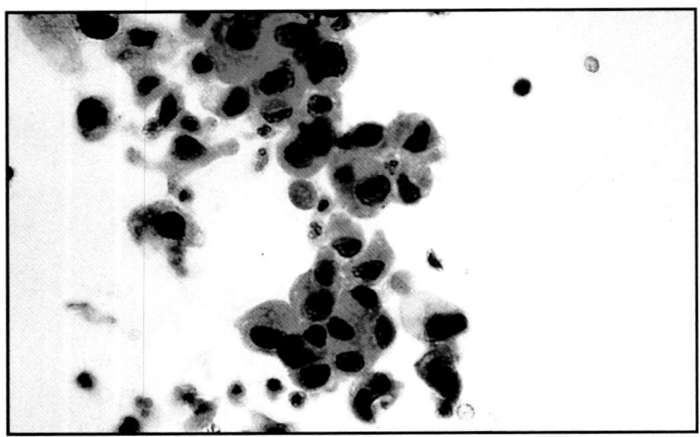

16.13
Numerous clustered and single malignant cells in urine in a patient with moderately differentiated invasive transitional cell carcinoma (x500).

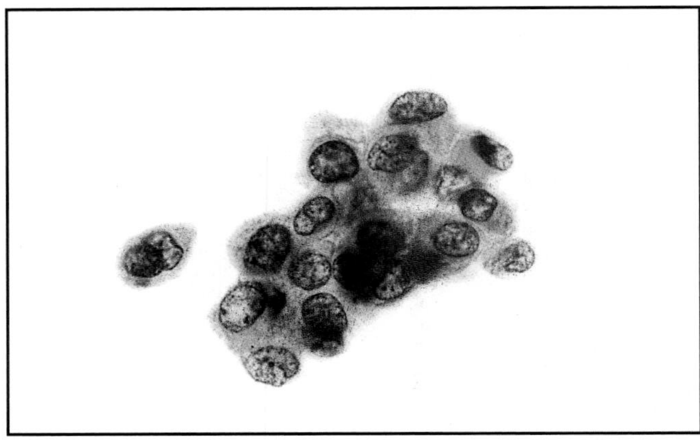

16.14
Papillary transitional cell carcinoma, grade I. Increased numbers of clusters of cells with slightly enlarged often elongated hyperchromatic nuclei present. Background is clean (x500).

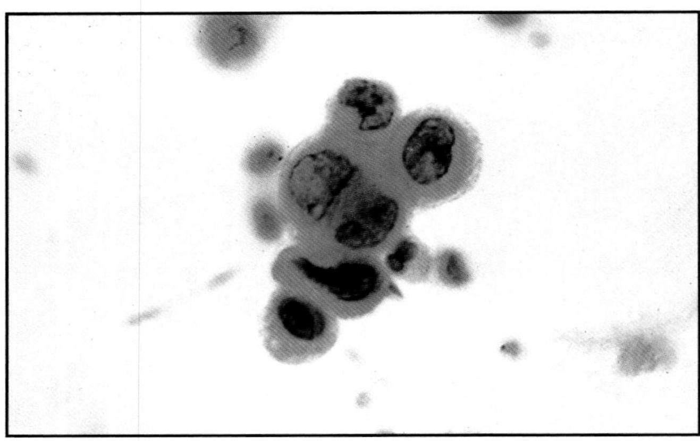

16.15
Papillary transitional cell carcinoma, moderately differentiated. The more striking nuclear irregularities and hyperchromasia permit a definite diagnosis of carcinoma (x500).

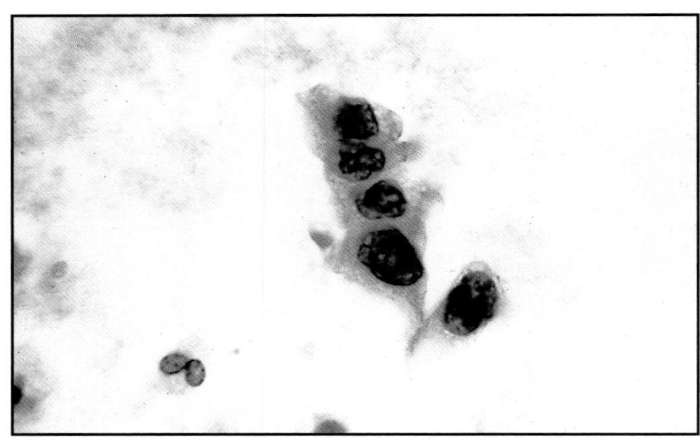

16.16
Papillary transitional cell carcinoma, moderately differentiated. The cells are clustered, and the nuclei are markedly hyperchromatic and pleomorphic (x500).

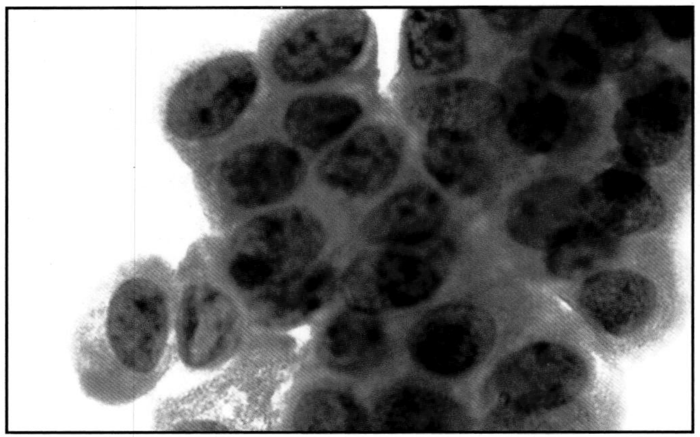

16.17
Loosely cohesive neoplastic cells, with irregularly outlined nuclei and a coarse chromatin pattern, in moderately differentiated transitional cell carcinoma (x970).

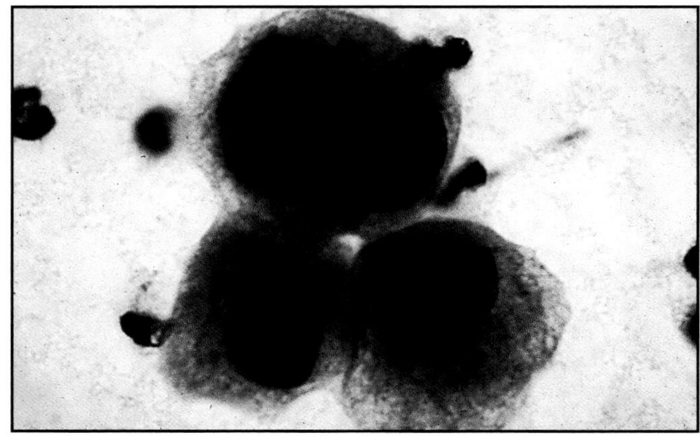

16.18
Transitional cell carcinoma of bladder, high grade. The nuclei are large and markedly hyperchromatic (x750).

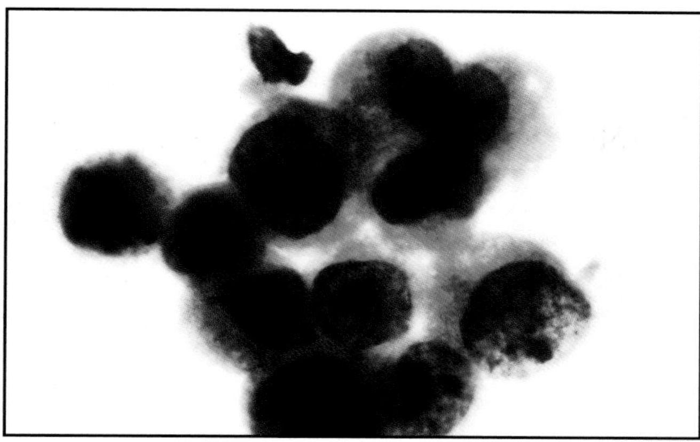

▮16.19
Transitional cell carcinoma, grade III. The nuclei are large and hyperchromatic with an irregular coarse chromatin pattern (x750).

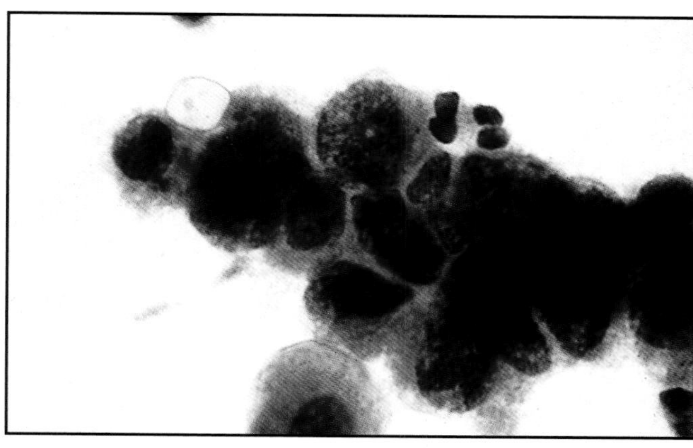

▮16.20
Transitional cell carcinoma, grade III. The nuclei are markedly enlarged, hyperchromatic, and pleomorphic. The nuclear/cytoplasmic ratio is high (x750).

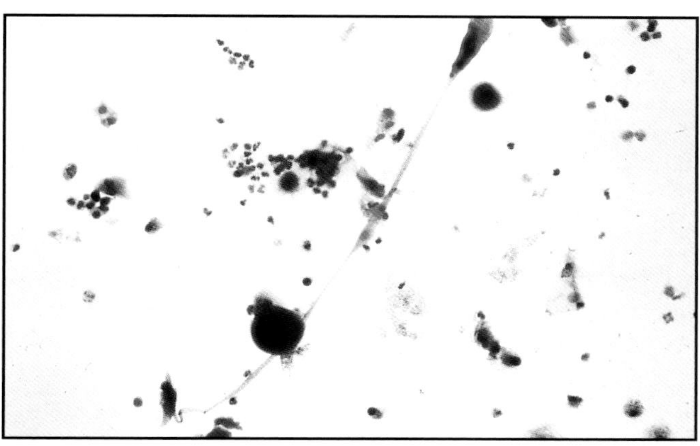

▮16.21
Keratinizing squamous cell carcinoma of the bladder showing tadpole cells with very long tails (x250).

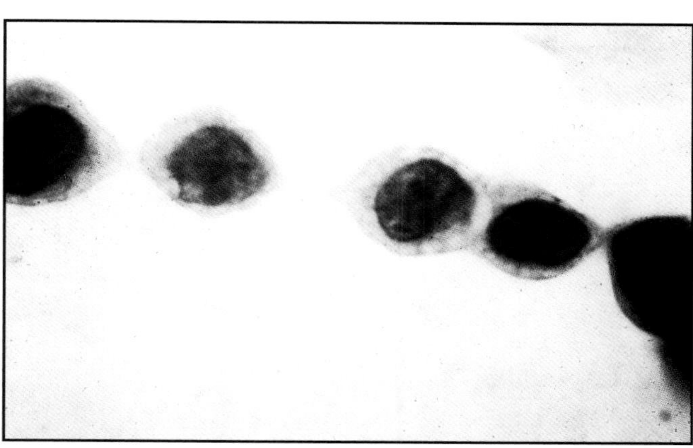

▮16.22
Transitional cell carcinoma in situ vs severe urothelial dysplasia (borderline lesion). The background is clean. This lesion preceded invasive, high-grade transitional cell carcinoma by 3 years (x750).

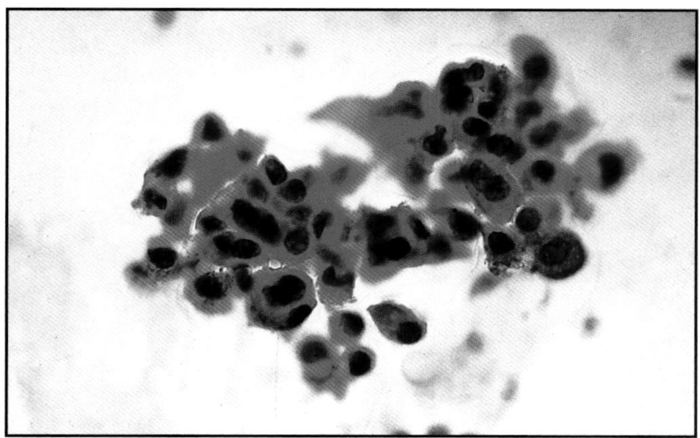

▮16.23
Loose cluster of malignant urothelial cells in transitional cell carcinoma in situ (x500).

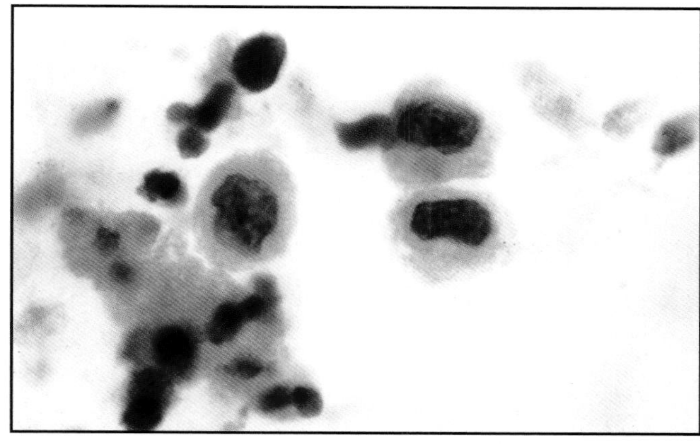

▮16.24
Single malignant cells, with pleomorphic hyperchromatic nuclei, in transitional cell carcinoma in situ. The necrotic debris in the background suggests erosion and pseudocystitis (x500).

REVIEW EXERCISES

1. Briefly describe the epithelial lining of the urinary tract from the renal calyces to the urethral meatus, in males and females.

2. What non-neoplastic diseases of the urinary tract are associated with reactive or inflammatory epithelial atypia?

3. What is the significance of eosinophilic cytoplasmic inclusions?

4. Describe the morphology of a transitional cell papilloma of the urinary bladder. What if any cytologic abnormalities may be observed?

5. What are the cytologic features of transitional cell carcinoma in situ?

6. What cytologic findings are useful in distinguishing atypia associated with nephrolithiasis from changes characteristic of carcinoma of the bladder?

7. In what type of patient or clinical situation are cytologic studies of the urine particularly important?

SELECTED READINGS

Badalement RA, Hermansen DK, Kimmel M, et al. The sensitivity of bladder wash flow cytometry, bladder wash cytology, and voided cytology in the detection of bladder carcinoma. *Cancer.* 1987;60:1423-1427.

Boon ME, Blomjois CEM, Zwartendijk J, et al. Carcinoma in situ of the urinary bladder: clinical presentation, cytologic pattern and stromal changes. *Acta Cytol.* 1986;30:360-366.

Cant JD, Murphy WM, Soloway MS. Prognostic significance of urine cytology in initial follow-up after intravesical mitomycin C for superficial bladder cancer. *Cancer.* 1986;57:2119-2122.

Crabbe JGS. "Comet" or "decoy" cells found in urinary sediment smears. *Acta Cytol.* 1971;15:303-305.

de Vere White RW, Deitch AD, West B, et al. The predictive value of flow cytometric information in the clinical management of stage O (Ta) bladder cancer. *J Urol.* 1988;139:279-282.

Droller MJ, Erozan YS. Thiotepa effects on urinary cytology in the interpretation of transitional cell cancer. *J Urol.* 1985;134:671-674.

Eggensperger D, Schweitzer S, Ferriol E, et al. The utility of cytodiagnostic urinalysis for monitoring renal allograft injury. *Am J Nephrol.* 1988;8:27-34.

El-Bolkainy MN. Cytology of bladder carcinoma. *J Urol.* 1980;124:20-22.

Eldidi MM, Patten SF Jr. New cytologic classification of normal urothelial cells: an analytical and morphometric study. *Acta Cytol.* 1982;26:725. Abstact.

Eriksson O, Johansson S. Urothelial neoplasms of the upper urinary tract: a correlation between cytologic and histologic findings in 43 patients with urothelial neoplasms of the renal pelvis or ureter. *Acta Cytol.* 1976;20:20-25.

Esposti P, Moberger G, Zajicek J. The cytological diagnosis of transitional cell tumors of the urinary bladder and its histologic basis: a study of 562 cases of urinary tract disorders including 170 untreated and 182 irradiate bladder tumors. *Acta Cytol.* 1970;14:145-155.

Friedell GH, Parija GC, Nagy GK, et al. The pathology of human bladder cancer. *Cancer.* 1980;45:1823-1830.

Highman W, Wilson E. Urine cytology in patients with calculi. *J Clin Pathol.* 1982;35:350-356.

Highman WJ. Transitional carcinoma of the upper urinary tract: a histological and cytopathological study. *J Clin Pathol.* 1986;39:297-306.

Holmquist ND. Detection of urinary tract cancer in urinalysis specimens in an outpatient population. *Am J Clin Pathol.* 1988;89:499-504.

Johnston WW, Bossen E, Amatulli J, et al. Exfoliative cytopathologic studies in organ transplantation, II: factors in the diagnosis of cytomegalic inclusion disease in urine or renal allograft recipients. *Acta Cytol.* 1969;13:605-610.

Kern WH. The cytology of transitional cell carcinoma of the urinary bladder. *Acta Cytol.* 1975;19:420-428.

Kern WH. The diagnostic accuracy of sputum and urine cytology. *Acta Cytol.* 1988;32:651-654.

Kern WH. The grade and pathologic stage of bladder cancer. *Cancer.* 1984;53:1185-1189.

Kern WH. Screening tests for bladder cancer. In: Miller AB, ed. *Screening for Cancer.* Orlando, Fla: Academic Press; 1985:121-140.

Kern WH. Urinary tract. In: Bibbo M, ed. *Comprehensive Cytopathology.* Philadelphia, Pa: WB Saunders Co; 1991:433-467.

Koss LG, Deitch D, Ramanathan R, Sherman AB. Diagnostic value of cytology of voided urine. *Acta Cytol.* 1985;29:810-816.

Koss LG, Nakanishi T, Freed SZ. Nonpapillary carcinoma in situ and atypical hyperplasia in cancerous bladder: further study of surgically removed bladders by mapping. *Urology.* 1977;9:442-455.

Koss LG, Tamson RM, Robbins MA. Mapping cancerous and precancerous bladder changes. *JAMA.* 1974;227:281-286.

Loveless KJ. The effects of radiation on the cytology of benign and malignant bladder epithelia. *Acta Cytol.* 1973;17:355-360.

Melamed MR, Koss LG, Ricci A, et al. Cytohistological observations on developing carcinoma of the urinary bladder in man. *Cancer.* 1960;13:67-74.

Murphy WM, Nagy GK, Rao MK, et al. "Normal" urothelium in patients with bladder cancer: a preliminary report from the National Bladder Cancer Collaborative Group A. *Cancer.* 1979;44:1050-1058.

Murphy WM, Soloway MS, Jukkola AF, et al. Urinary cytology and bladder cancer: the cellular features of transitional cell neoplasms. *Cancer.* 1984;53:1555-1565.

Piscioli F, Detassis C, Polja E, et al. Cytologic presentation of renal adenocarcinoma in urinary sediment. *Acta Cytol.* 1983;27:383-390.

Rosvanis TK, Rohner TJ, Abt AB. Transitional cell carcinoma in an ileal conduit. *Cancer.* 1989;63:1233-1236.

Schumann GB. Cytodifferentiation of urinary epithelial fragments: papillary transitional cell carcinoma in a renal allograft recipient. *Acta Cytol.* 1981;25:302-306.

Suprun H, Bitterman W. A correlative cytohistologic study on the interrelationship between exfoliated urinary bladder carcinoma cell types and the staging and grading of these tumors. *Acta Cytol.* 1975;19:265-273.

Trillo AA, Kuchler LL, Wood AC, et al. Adenocarcinoma of the urinary bladder: histologic, cytologic and ultrastructural features in a case. *Acta Cytol.* 1981;25:285-290.

Wolinska WH, Melamed MR. Urinary conduit cytology. *Cancer.* 1973;32:1000-1006.

Wolinska WH, Melamed MR, Klein FA. Urethral cytology following cystectomy for bladder carcinoma. *Am J Surg Pathol.* 1977;1:225-234.

Wolinska WH, Melamed MR, Klein FA. Cytology of bladder papilloma. *Acta Cytol.* 1985;29:817-822.

CHAPTER 17

Gastrointestinal Tract

Philip M. Dvoretsky, MD

CONTENTS

Examination of cellular material from the esophagus, stomach, duodenum, and colon by visually guided endoscopic brushings has been an accurate diagnostic modality for many years, and is complementary to tissue biopsy in terms of diagnostic sensitivity. There are many reasons that cytologic examination increases diagnostic sensitivity in the gastrointestinal tract. In some disease processes, there is narrowing of the lumen of the esophagus or the colon; the biopsy forceps may not be able to reach such lesions and obtain a diagnostic sample, whereas the brush may be guided into such areas to obtain a cellular sample. A greater surface area can be sampled by the brush than by the biopsy forceps, and the cellular sample does not suffer from the "crush" artifact that often detracts from small tissue specimens. Finally, some disease processes have a nonspecific appearance; the endoscopist may not be able to visualize and select the precise region for biopsy but may use a brush to sample several locations with comparative ease.

Cytologic evaluation of endoscopic brushings is superior to examination of cells from blind saline lavage for two reasons: (1) the brushing is obtained by direct visual observation of the lesion; and (2) it is much less cumbersome to process than the lavage specimen. As soon as the brush is removed from the endoscope, a cytotechnologist should be present to quickly rotate it on a slide. The slide is immediately placed in 95% ethanol. Such rapid smear preparation and fixation produces well-fixed cellular material and helps to avoid air-drying. However, when a malignant lymphoma is being considered, some of the slides should be air-dried and stained by one of the Romanowski stains. The cytotechnologist should also obtain information such as the precise site of each specimen, relevant clinical history, and the clinical differential diagnosis.

It is helpful for a brush sample to be taken before a biopsy specimen to minimize contamination of the former by blood. In the instance the cellular sample is bloody, the slide can be placed in 1% glacial acetic acid for 2 to 3 minutes, which will allow for hemolysis of the red blood cells. The slides can then be transferred to 95% ethanol.

In this chapter, the cytologic features of neoplastic, inflammatory, and infectious processes from the esophagus, stomach, duodenum, and colon are described, and the diagnostic sensitivity and specificity of cytologic sampling from endoscopic brushings are discussed.

ESOPHAGUS

Normal Cytologic Features

The esophageal mucosal epithelium is nonkeratinizing, stratified squamous in type. Thus, intermediate and superficial squamous cells are observed following esophageal brushing similar to those seen in samples from the uterine cervix. The cells contain uniform, round to oval nuclei, low nuclear/cytoplasmic ratio, and abundant cytoplasm. The nuclei have finely granular, evenly distributed chromatin and lack discernible nucleoli. If the brushing involves the esophagogastric junction, sheets of glandular epithelium are observed that have a central honeycombed appearance and palisaded columnar epithelial cells at the periphery. The nuclei of these glandular cells are uniform and round, and contain micronucleoli and finely granular, evenly distributed chromatin. At times, ciliated tracheobronchial epithelial cells and pigment-laden macrophages swallowed from the respiratory tract, or partially digested food may be observed.

Malignant Neoplasms

Practically all of the malignant neoplasms of the esophagus are either squamous cell carcinomas or adenocarcinomas. Although the majority of these are squamous cell carcinomas, there has been a recent relative increase in adenocarcinomas, most of which occur in the distal one third of the esophagus. The majority of esophageal carcinomas occur in the middle and distal thirds of it.

Squamous Cell Carcinomas

These carcinomas of the esophagus usually have a mixed keratinizing and nonkeratinizing character. In the keratinizing type, both two-dimensional aggregates and isolated neoplastic cells with distinct cell boundaries are observed. Cellular and nuclear pleomorphism are pronounced. The cell nucleus is often opaque, with chromatin distribution difficult to discern. In some hyperchromatic nuclei, irregular coarsely granular chromatin may be seen but nucleoli are inconspicuous. The cell cytoplasm is abundant and dense with fibrillar material present in parallel arrays [▮*17.1*]. In the nonkeratinizing type of squamous cell carcinoma, the cells are present in syncytia and individually. The cells have a high nuclear/cytoplasmic ratio, scant and poorly defined cytoplasm, and nuclei containing prominent nucleoli as well as irregularly distributed, coarsely granular chromatin [▮*17.2*].

Adenocarcinoma

In contrast, the cells derived from adenocarcinoma of the esophagus are observed singly and in two-dimensional aggregates with prominent cellular overlap. Neoplastic cell nuclei have single or multiple macronucleoli superimposed on finely granular chromatin that is evenly or irregularly distributed. The cytoplasm is granular and vacuolated [▮*17.3*]. As the neoplasm becomes more poorly differentiated, there are a greater number of single cells, nuclear enlargement and pleomorphism become more pronounced, and irregularity of nuclear chromatin distribution is easier to see.

Reactive Processes

Barrett's Metaplasia

Barrett's metaplasia of the esophageal epithelium usually results from chronic esophageal reflux by gastric contents, and is felt to precede esophageal adenocarcinoma in approximately 10% to 15% of cases. The metaplastic epithelium may be of the intestinal type, the gastric type, or a mixture of these two types. The cytologic features of the intestinal type of Barrett's metaplasia are tightly cohesive sheets of uniform glandular cells in which "cell windows" or clear cytoplasmic spaces represent intestinal goblet cell differentiation [▮*17.4*]. Since gastric glandular epithelium is observed irregularly in the distal 3 cm of the esophagus, the finding of gastric-type glandular cells in this location may be normal. The diagnosis of Barrett's metaplasia, gastric type, can be made with confidence only when a sheet of gastric-type glandular cells is observed proximal to this location. This represents an instance in which location of the brushing specimen has diagnostic importance.

Repair/Regeneration

The cellular features of repair/regeneration in the esophagus are not different from those in the uterine cervix. The cells are present in two-dimensional sheets, and atypical single cells are absent. Although the cell nuclei are enlarged, they are relatively evenly spaced within the sheet of cells, there is abundant cytoplasm, and cell boundaries are distinctly seen. The nuclear/cytoplasmic ratio is increased and nuclei have one or more macronucleoli; however, irregularity of chromatin distribution is not observed [▮*17.5*]. In some repair reactions, the nuclei may overlap and compress each other. Combined with the nuclear enlargement and presence of macronucleoli previously described, these features may be suggestive of squamous cell carcinoma. In such difficult and worrisome situations, the absence of abnormal single cells and the presence of evenly distributed chromatin particles should preclude an outright diagnosis of carcinoma. It is reasonable to report that atypical cells of squamous type are present due to repair; however, a more serious process cannot be excluded.

Two infectious organisms that result in esophageal epithelial atypia are the *Candida albicans* fungus and herpesvirus. Both organisms are observed in immunosuppressed patients in several organs; they may be observed in the same lesion. In candidal infections, pseudohyphae and budding yeast forms are seen within inflammatory as well as necrotic debris. It is diagnostically helpful to see the fungus within such an exudate since *Candida* may represent a contaminant from the oral cavity. The cytologic features of herpetic esophagitis are similar to those seen in other locations and include multinucleation, nuclear molding, dispersion of the chromatin particles imparting a "ground-glass" appearance, and Cowdry type A intranuclear viral inclusions. The latter feature may not be present in all cases.

Two noninfectious causes of esophageal squamous atypia are folate deficiency and irradiation effect, both of which have similar abnormalities. These morphologic changes include nuclear as well as cellular enlargement with preservation of a low nuclear/cytoplasmic ratio, multinucleation, cytoplasmic polychromasia, and cytoplasmic inclusions. Patients who are malnourished and those with megaloblastic anemias constitute the patient populations susceptible for folate deficiency.

Sensitivity and Specificity

The sensitivity of esophageal brush cytology, defined as

$$\frac{\text{true-positive diagnoses}}{\text{true-positive diagnoses + false-negative diagnoses}}$$

varies from 82% to 96%. Thus, the disease is detected by cytologic examination in a high percentage of cases wherein it is actually present. In addition, several studies have demonstrated that cytologic examination correctly diagnosed esophageal carcinoma in 6% to 30% of cases that had normal findings on tissue biopsy specimens. It appears, therefore, that cytologic brushings are complementary to tissue biopsy, particularly in patients with narrowing of the esophageal lumen or with endoscopically undetectable lesions.

The specificity of esophageal brush cytology, defined as

$$\frac{\text{true-negative diagnoses}}{\text{true-negative diagnoses + false-positive diagnoses}}$$

varies from 93% to 100%. Thus, false-positive diagnoses occur in less than 10% of cases and usually result from misinterpretation of atypical reparative reactions.

STOMACH

Normal Cytologic Features

Cohesive sheets of uniform glandular cells are present in a honeycombed pattern centrally associated with columnar cells at the periphery of the aggregate. The cells have uniform, round to oval nuclei containing regular, finely granular chromatin, small nucleoli, and granular to vacuolated cytoplasm. Strips of parietal and chief cells may be seen, the former containing large, dense eosinophilic granules in the cytoplasm.

Malignant Neoplasms

Most of the gastric cancers are adenocarcinomas, but sarcomas, lymphomas, and metastatic carcinomas also occur in the stomach and are seen in gastric brushings when they replace or ulcerate the gastric mucosal epithelium.

Adenocarcinoma

Adenocarcinoma of the stomach can be divided into the intestinal type and the diffuse or gastric type. The intestinal type is often preceded and accompanied by chronic gastritis as well as intestinal metaplasia of the gastric mucosal epithelium. Histologically, this type of adenocarcinoma is composed of discrete as well as anastomosing glandular structures in its well-differentiated state. On the other hand, the diffuse or gastric type of adenocarcinoma is believed to arise from native gastric epithelium and is not associated with chronic gastritis or intestinal metaplasia. Histologically, sheets of cells rich in cytoplasmic mucin and including signet ring cells infiltrate and replace the gastric wall.

Cytologically, although most of the cells in well-differentiated adenocarcinoma of the intestinal type are observed in two-dimensional aggregates, isolated neoplastic cells are seen and their presence is important in establishing the diagnosis. The cells have eccentric, uniformly enlarged nuclei that contain prominent nucleoli as well as finely granular chromatin with focal irregularity of distribution. The cytoplasm is finely granular and abundant [❚*17.6*]. Cellular and nuclear overlap as well as nuclear molding by adjacent cell membranes may occur but are more typically observed in more poorly differentiated adenocarcinomas of this type. As the neoplasms become more poorly differentiated, a greater number of syncytial aggregates as well as isolated cells, increased nuclear/cytoplasmic ratio, nuclear pleomorphism, nucleoli, and abnormal chromatin distribution all become more pronounced.

In the gastric or diffuse type of adenocarcinoma, the cells are more frequently isolated or appear in smaller, two-dimensional aggregates. The nuclei are often eccentric and hyperchromatic due to coarsely granular chromatin. Nucleoli are usually prominent. There may be marked variation in both nuclear size and nuclear/cytoplasmic ratio. The cytoplasm has microvacuoles and macrovacuoles, the latter pushing the nucleus into an eccentric position and creating a "signet ring" cell [❚*17.7*].

Malignant Lymphoma

The cytologic features of malignant lymphoma consist of a monomorphous population of isolated lymphoid cells. Although clumping of these cells may be seen, no true cellular aggregates occur. Necrotic debris may be present as a result of gastric mucosal ulceration and may partially obscure the abnormal neoplastic lymphoid cells. The morphologic features of the lymphomatous cells differ depending on their cell type. The cells of the large cell type of malignant lymphoma have a high nuclear/cytoplasmic ratio, scant and delicate cytoplasm, hyperchromatic nuclei with either round or cleaved contour, and nucleoli near the nuclear membrane [❚*17.8*].

In the morphologic differential diagnosis of malignant lymphoma is an entity known as pseudolymphoma, which may form a mass in the stomach and ulcerate the gastric mucosa. The cellular features of pseudolymphoma are a polymorphous population of lymphoid cells, immunoblasts, tingible-body macrophages, plasma cells, and eosinophils [❚*17.9*]. Essentially, this process represents a mixed inflammatory response that includes lymphoid hyperplasia. It should be noted that a lymphoid hyperplasia may be observed adjacent to a true malignant lymphoma. However, one should be cautious about diagnosing malignant lymphoma with a polymorphous lymphoid population without first conducting special immunophenotypic studies.

Smooth Muscle Neoplasms

Endoscopic brushings of gastric smooth muscle neoplasms yield isolated cells and syncytial cell aggregates. The cells are spindle-shaped to polygonal and have elongated cytoplasmic processes. The nuclei are usually elongated with blunt ends but have considerable pleomorphism. Nuclear chromatin varies from finely granular and evenly distributed to coarsely granular and irregular in distribution. Similarly, nucleoli may be inconspicuous or prominent [❚*17.10*]. Multinucleation is observed. It is known that both the size of the neoplasm and the mitotic count in histologic sections are important features for predicting the likelihood of malignancy. Unfortunately, no data are available from analysis of gastric brushings that can predict the biologic behavior of smooth muscle tumors based solely on cytologic features. Thus, while it is possible to cytologically classify a tumor as stromal or smooth muscle in type, it may not be possible to state whether such a tumor is benign or malignant.

Metastatic Malignant Neoplasm

A metastatic malignant neoplasm is occasionally observed in gastrointestinal brushings. Such an observation creates a problem when the clinician either does not know that there is a malignancy at another site or neglects to share this information with the cytopathology laboratory. If the cytologist is alert for either atypical or frankly malignant cells in an area of the gastrointestinal tract that is not native to such cells, then the possibility of a metastasis should be considered. For example, brushing of an ulcerated gastric tumor yielded two-dimensional aggregates of cells with a low nuclear/cytoplasmic ratio, uniformly small, round nuclei with regular, finely granular chromatin as well as inconspicuous nucleoli, and abundant granular to clear cytoplasm [❚*17.11*]. The first step in this case was to recognize that these cells do not resemble benign or malignant gastric epithelial cells. On perceiving and reporting that the cellular features were suggestive of a renal cell carcinoma metastatic to the stomach, it was learned that the patient had hematuria. Subsequent evaluation revealed a renal neoplasm, and a well-differentiated renal cell carcinoma was resected. Thus, the cytologic features of the metastasis may suggest the origin of a previously unknown primary neoplasm.

Reactive Processes

The cytologic features of repair/regeneration in the stomach are similar to those previously described in the esophagus and will not be repeated here. The most common source of reparative atypia is gastric peptic ulceration. The other processes that contain reactive glandular atypia are acute and chronic gastritis and pernicious anemia.

Sensitivity and Specificity

The sensitivity of gastric brush cytology varies from 64% to 100%, which is similar to that of tissue biopsy in the same region. Even so, it has been reported that, in patients with gastric cancer, gastric brushings were diagnostic for cancer in 15% of cases that were negative on evaluation of biopsy specimens. Thus, as in the esophagus, the diagnostic usefulness of cytologic brush specimens is confirmed.

The specificity of gastric brushings is 96% to 99%. When false-positive interpretations occur, they are usually due to misinterpretation of regenerating glandular epithelium at the margin of an ulcer or due to active granulation tissue in the ulcer base.

DUODENUM

Normal Cytologic Features

Duodenal epithelial cells are observed in sheets in which the glandular cells are arranged in a honeycomb pattern centrally with cytoplasmic "cell windows" reflective of goblet cell differentiation. There are columnar cells at the periphery of the sheet containing round nuclei and abundant apical cytoplasm with a distinctive luminal brush border.

Malignant Neoplasms

Adenocarcinoma

The cellular features of duodenal adenocarcinoma are similar to those of gastric adenocarcinoma of intestinal type, and their description does not require repetition. A neoplasm that is important to recognize is the villous adenoma, since up to 89% of small intestinal adenocarcinomas arise in association with adenomas. In addition, about 33% to 50% of duodenal villous adenomas contain foci of adenocarcinoma. The cellular features of villous adenoma include cohesive two-dimensional aggregates of columnar cells with or without nuclear overlap, nuclear palisading, eccentric nuclear position, uniformly slender nuclei containing finely granular evenly distributed chromatin, and apical granular cytoplasm [▮*17.12*]. Nucleoli may either be inconspicuous or prominent.

Carcinoid Tumor

The cytologic features of duodenal carcinoid tumor are cohesive two-dimensional cell aggregates, cells with uniform round to oval nuclei containing finely granular, evenly distributed chromatin without discernible nucleoli, and abundant, densely granular cytoplasm [▮*17.13*]. This neoplasm is uncommon in the duodenum and, even when it occurs, does not often extend to the mucosal surface to be observed on duodenal brushings.

Reactive Processes

In the duodenum, there are distinct differences in the morphologic features of repair/regeneration. As is the case elsewhere in the gastrointestinal tract, abnormal isolated cells are rare or absent, the cells are present in sheets, and the enlarged nuclei contain prominent nucleoli as well as evenly distributed chromatin. However, the distinctive presence of multiple cytoplasmic vacuoles of variable size results in nuclear eccentricity as well as nuclei at different levels within the cell. If there is any nuclear pleomorphism in addition, it is possible to mistake the reparative process for adenocarcinoma. Hence, the absence of abnormal isolated cells as well as nuclear chromatin clearing become especially important in diagnosing a repair reaction in this location.

In patients with steatorrhea, the diagnosis of *Giardia lamblia* infection can be easily established by brushings because the number of organisms that are obtained is large, far exceeding that which can be seen on a histologic biopsy specimen. These protozoan organisms have paired nuclei and flagella with karyosomes seen within each nucleus [▮*17.14*].

COLON

Normal Cytologic Features

There are sheets of uniform epithelial cells exhibiting a honeycomb arrangement centrally associated with a columnar cell shape peripherally. The cells have uniform, round to oval nuclei containing finely granular chromatin, inconspicuous nucleoli, and pale-staining cytoplasm.

Malignant Neoplasm

On cytologic examination, the cells of well-differentiated adenocarcinoma are present in two-dimensional aggregates. Isolated cells are unusual but should be observed before making the diagnosis of adenocarcinoma. The cells have a columnar shape and exhibit nuclear palisading. The nuclei are enlarged and contain finely granular chromatin as well as one or more nucleoli. Focal irregularity of chromatin distribution is usually present. The cell cytoplasm is abundant and granular. As the neoplasm becomes more poorly differentiated, isolated neoplastic cells, nuclear overlapping, nuclear compression by adjacent cells, nucleoli, and chromatin clearing are more readily observed [❚*17.15*], which is the case with adenocarcinomas elsewhere in the gastrointestinal tract.

Tubulovillous or villous adenomas are much more common in the colon than in the duodenum. However, the cellular features are similar, consisting of cohesive sheets of pseudostratified columnar cells. The nuclei are slender and elongated, and are eccentrically arranged in a palisaded configuration with abundant granular cytoplasm at the other end of the cell. The nuclei usually have finely granular, evenly distributed chromatin associated with inconspicuous or small nucleoli [❚*17.16*]. As increasing degrees of cytologic atypia occur within villous adenomas, the nuclei become larger, nucleoli increase in size and in number, and the chromatin distribution may be focally irregular. In some cases, it may not be possible to distinguish between well-differentiated adenocarcinoma and atypical villous adenoma solely on a cytologic basis. This is hardly surprising because the majority of adenocarcinomas arise from adenomas containing cytologic atypia.

Reactive Processes

The most common reactive process in which cellular material is observed from colonic brushings is ulcerative colitis. In ulcerative colitis, the background of the smear contains a large number of inflammatory cells. Colonic epithelial cells are present in cohesive sheets and contain enlarged nuclei that have prominent nucleoli as well as finely granular evenly distributed chromatin. The cell cytoplasm is abundant and granular to vacuolated. The greater the duration of disease, the greater the risk of colonic adenocarcinoma arising in the setting of ulcerative colitis. As the degree of cytologic abnormality becomes more severe, the cells may be isolated or present in three-dimensional clusters, the nuclear/cytoplasmic ratio is increased, and the nuclear chromatin may be more coarsely granular as well as irregularly distributed. In such a setting, it may not be possible to distinguish between a severe cytologic atypia in ulcerative colitis and adenocarcinoma.

Sensitivity and Specificity

The sensitivity of colonic brushings varies from 50% to 86%. The causes of cytologic false-negative diagnosis include colonic luminal narrowing with associated poor accessibility of the endoscope, necrotic debris covering the lesion with failure of the brush to pick up viable diagnostic cells, and the presence of only a small focus of adenocarcinoma arising within a larger villous adenoma or within widespread inflammatory bowel disease. Even so, the cytologic brush specimen was positive in 32% of cancer cases in which the biopsy specimen was negative. Thus, although colonic cytology has limitations in its diagnostic value, it is still complementary to the histologic biopsy specimen. The combined sensitivity of the brush and biopsy specimens is 92% to 100%.

The specificity of colonic cytologic evaluation is 100% in several studies. However, the diseases that may cause false-positive diagnoses are ulcerative colitis and villous adenomas, in which the glandular epithelial cells contain marked cytologic atypia and mimic adenocarcinoma.

SUMMARY

It is clear that cytologic examination of endoscopic brush specimens in neoplastic as well as in infectious or inflammatory processes is complementary to tissue biopsy specimens because it increases diagnostic sensitivity. However, for cytologic examination to be useful, it is crucial to practice optimal technique in smear preparation, fixation, and staining; to obtain pertinent clinical history and endoscopic impressions; and to compare the cytologic case material with available current or previous histologic specimens so that diagnostic pitfalls can be avoided.

ACKNOWLEDGMENT

I thank Douglas King, Senior Cytologist, Diagnostic Cytology Laboratory Inc, Indianapolis, Ind, for photographing many of the images in this chapter.

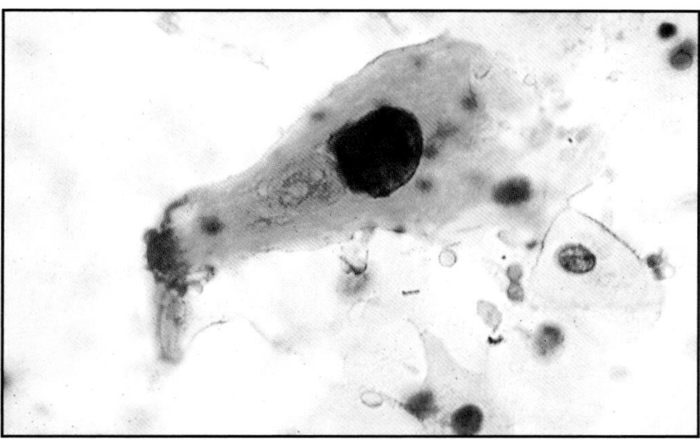

▌17.1

Esophageal squamous cell carcinoma, keratinizing type. There is marked nuclear enlargement, hyperchromasia, and abundant, dense cytoplasm containing parallel arrays of fibrillar material.

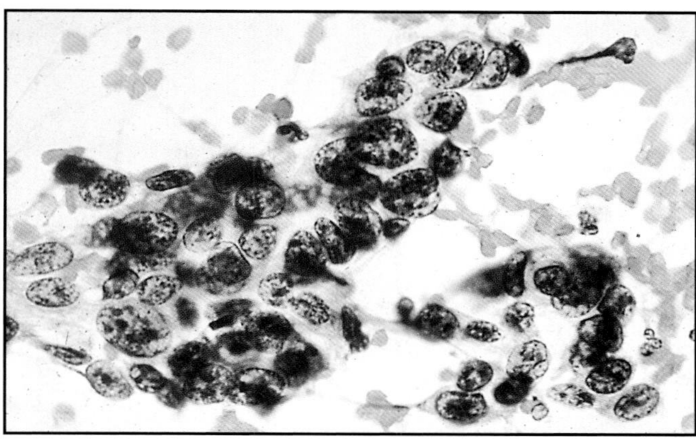

▌17.2

Esophageal squamous cell carcinoma, nonkeratinizing type. This syncytial aggregate contains cells that have irregular, coarsely granular chromatin, prominent nucleoli in their nuclei, and scant cytoplasm.

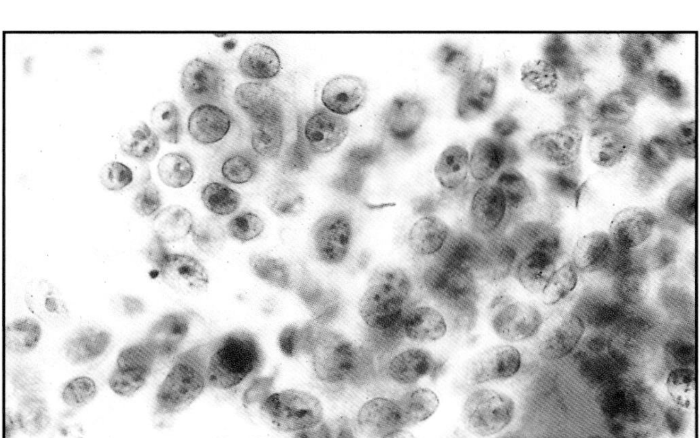

▌17.3

Esophageal adenocarcinoma. This is a three-dimensional aggregate of cells in which cell nuclei have macronucleoli superimposed on a finely granular chromatin pattern, with pale granular to vacuolated cytoplasm.

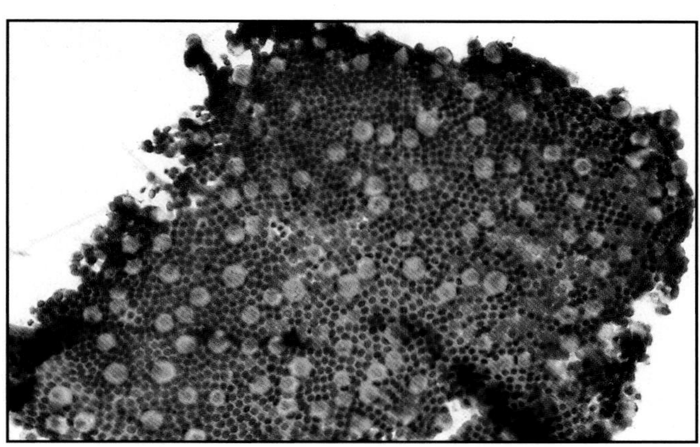

▌17.4

Esophageal Barrett's metaplasia, intestinal type. The cytoplasmic "cell windows" reflect goblet cell differentiation, diagnostic of this entity.

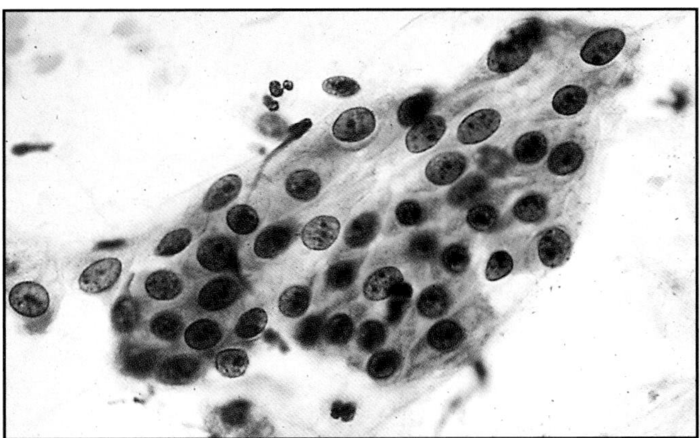

▌17.5

Esophageal repair reaction. The cells are present in a sheet. Cell nuclei are enlarged and evenly spaced. Nucleoli are seen in each nucleus, which contain finely granular and evenly distributed chromatin.

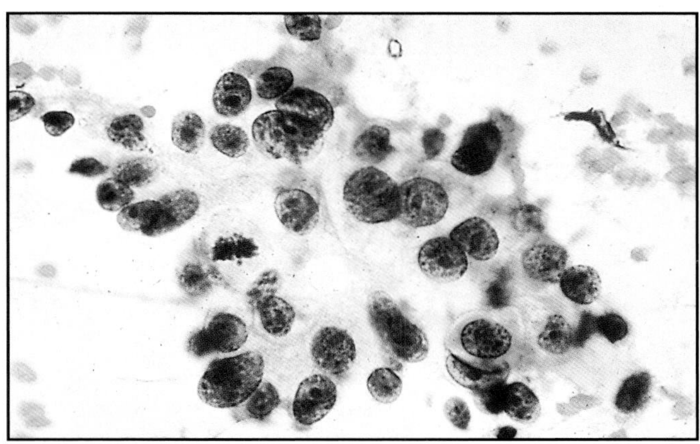

▌17.6

Well-differentiated gastric adenocarcinoma, intestinal type. Nucleoli and chromatin clearing are observed in many nuclei. In addition, nuclear molding by adjacent cell membranes is helpful in establishing the diagnosis.

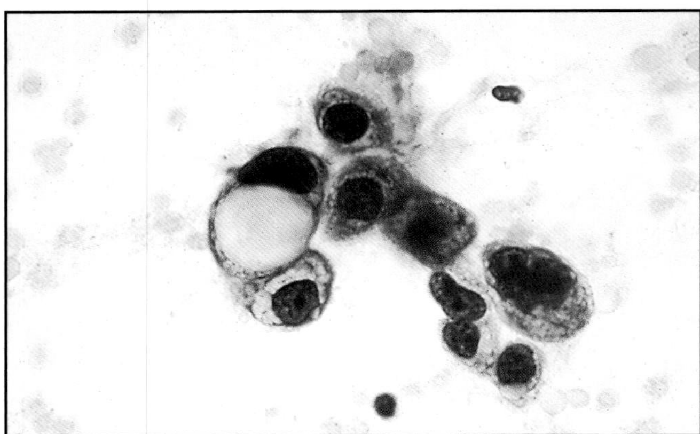

17.7

Gastric adenocarcinoma, diffuse type. Although nuclear size and nuclear/cytoplasmic ratio may vary, nucleoli and coarsely granular chromatin with focal irregularity of distribution remain prominent. Cytoplasmic vacuolization and signet ring cells are characteristic.

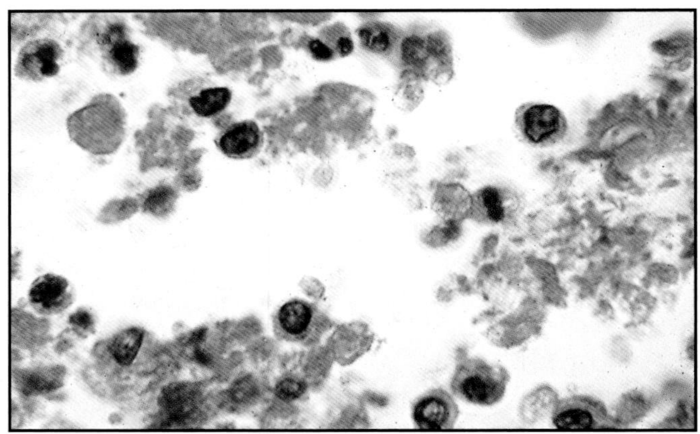

17.8

Gastric malignant lymphoma, large cell type. Isolated lymphoid cells are seen, which have a high nuclear/cytoplasmic ratio, nuclei with irregular borders, paramembranous nucleoli, and scant cytoplasm.

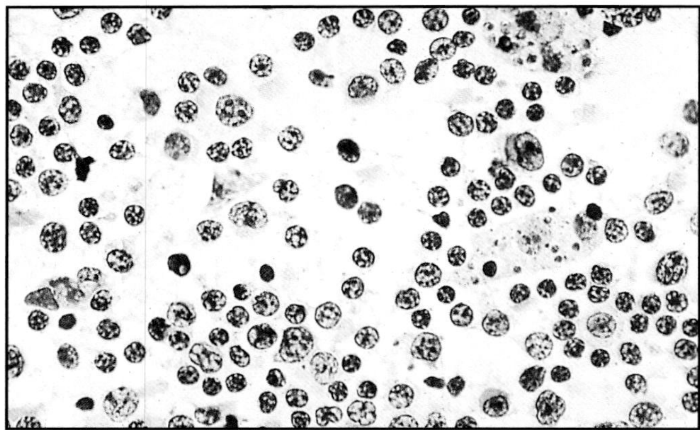

17.9

Gastric pseudolymphoma. Note the polymorphous cellular population, which includes large lymphoid cells, immunoblasts, small mature lymphoid cells, and tingible-body macrophages.

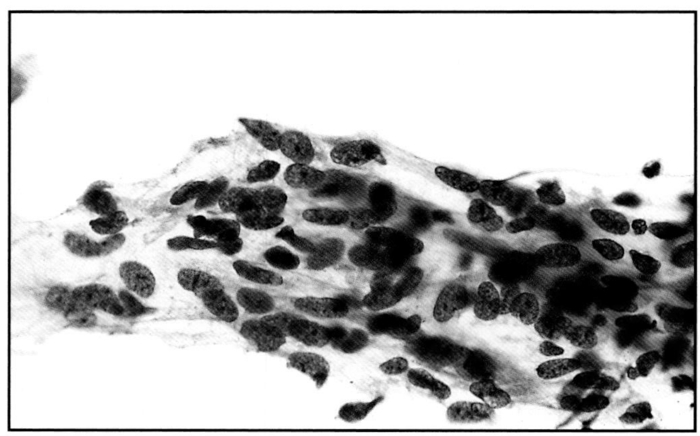

17.10

Gastric leiomyosarcoma. Spindled cells are present in an aggregate with cellular overlap. The cell nuclei contain finely granular, regular chromatin, and small nucleoli focally. There is abundant, bipolar cytoplasm.

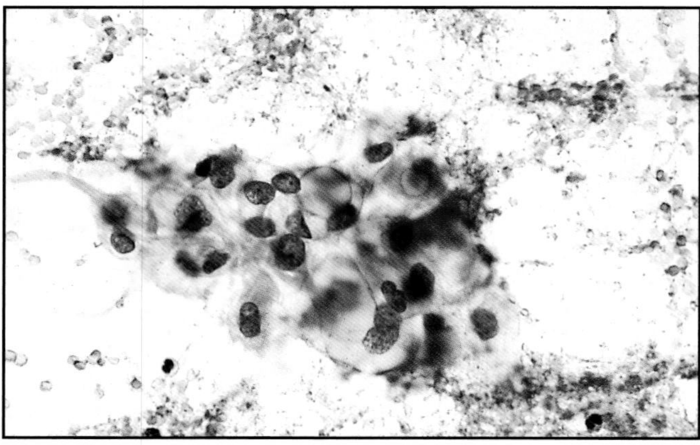

17.11

Metastatic renal cell carcinoma involving the stomach. The low nuclear/cytoplasmic ratio, abundant cytoplasm, and small nuclei that lack nucleoli are suggestive of a renal cell primary site.

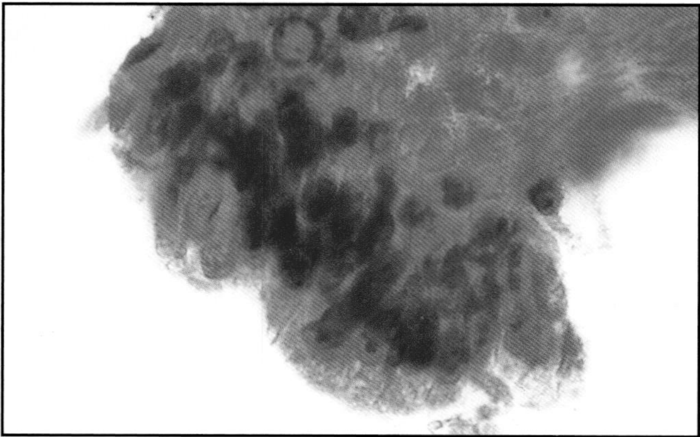

17.12

Duodenal villous adenoma. The elongated nuclei are palisaded and overlap one another, containing finely granular evenly distributed chromatin. (Photograph is courtesy of Barbara Ducatman, MD, Beth Israel Hospital, Boston, Mass.)

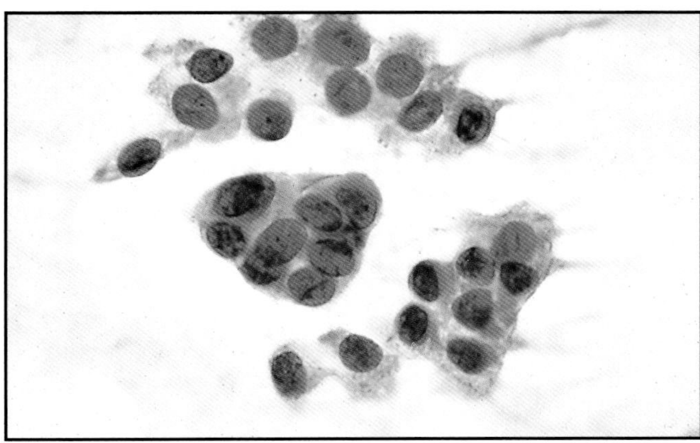

▮*17.13*

Duodenal carcinoid. The cell nuclei are uniform, contain finely granular, regular chromatin, and lack nucleoli. The cytoplasm is abundant and granular.

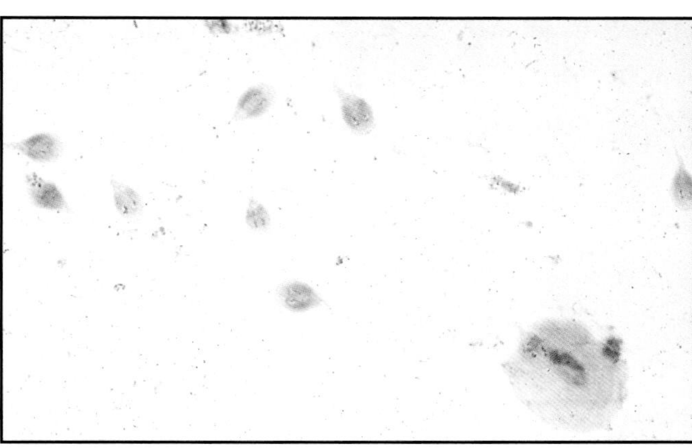

▮*17.14*

Duodenal Giardia lamblia. *The organisms are binucleated, contain a teardrop shape, and have observable flagella.*

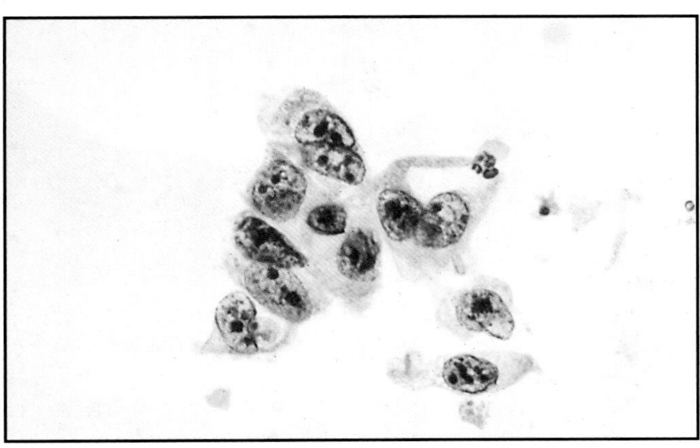

▮*17.15*

Colonic moderately differentiated adenocarcinoma. Isolated neoplastic cells, focal nuclear compression by adjacent cell membranes, macronucleoli, and chromatin clearing are all pronounced.

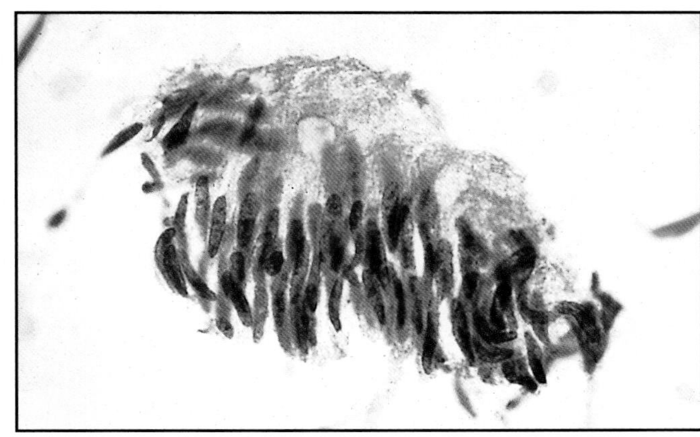

▮*17.16*

Colonic villous adenoma. The slender nuclei are eccentrically arranged and palisaded, containing finely granular chromatin. Abundant granular cytoplasm is observed in the apical portion of the cell.

REVIEW EXERCISES

1. Why is gastrointestinal endoscopic brushing helpful in increasing diagnostic sensitivity?
   a) The brush may reach lesions that are inaccessible to the biopsy forceps.
   b) The brush may sample poorly defined lesions more extensively than the biopsy forceps.
   c) The crush artifact present in biopsy specimens does not hinder the evaluation of brushings.
   d) All of the above

2. What is done to an especially bloody smear?
   a) Throw it away because it is messy.
   b) Allow it to air-dry.
   c) Place it in glacial acetic acid before placing it in 95% ethanol.
   d) Ask the clinician for more history.

3. In keratinizing squamous cell carcinoma of the esophagus, the cell cytoplasm is finely granular and vacuolated. True or false?

4. In the typical repair reaction, isolated abnormal cells are absent or rarely seen and the nuclear chromatin distribution is evenly distributed. True or false?

5. In diagnosing well-differentiated gastric adenocarcinomas of the intestinal type, what observation is most helpful?
   a) The presence of abnormal isolated glandular cells
   b) The presence of a tumor diathesis
   c) The presence of spindled cells
   d) Prominent nucleoli within nuclei

6. What are two characteristic features in the cell cytoplasm of the diffuse type of gastric adenocarcinoma?

7. The cytologic features of malignant lymphomas include a monomorphous population of isolated abnormal lymphoid cells. True or false?

8. What is the key cytologic feature of duodenal or colonic adenoma?
   a) Abundant granular to vacuolated cytoplasm
   b) Occasional isolated signet ring cells
   c) Large nucleoli within every nucleus
   d) Columnar epithelial cells that contain palisaded, elongated nuclei

SELECTED READINGS

Bardawil RG, D'Ambrosio FG, Hajdu SI. Colonic cytology: a retrospective study with histopathologic correlation. *Acta Cytol.* 1990;34:620-626.

Bemvenuti GA, Prolla JC, Kirsner JB, Reilly RW. Direct vision brushing cytology in the diagnosis of colo-rectal malignancy. *Acta Cytol.* 1974;18:477-481.

Berry AV, Baskind AF, Hamilton DG. Cytologic screening for esophageal cancer. *Acta Cytol.* 1981;25:135-141.

Cabre-Fiol V, Vilardell F. Progress in the cytological diagnosis of gastric lymphoma: a report of 32 cases. *Cancer.* 1978;41:1456-1461.

Cabre-Fiol V, Vilardell F, Sala-Cladera E, Perez-Mota A. Preoperative cytological diagnosis of gastric leiomyosarcoma: a report of three cases. *Gastroenterology.* 1975;68:563-566.

Chambers LA, Clark WE. The endoscopic diagnosis of gastroesophageal malignancy: a cytologic review. *Acta Cytol.* 1986;30:110-114.

Festa VI, Hajdu SI, Winawer SJ. Colorectal cytology in chronic ulcerative colitis. *Acta Cytol.* 1985;29:262-268.

Rilke F, Pilotti S, Clemente C. Cytology of non-Hodgkin's malignant lymphomas involving the stomach. *Acta Cytol.* 1978;22:71-79.

Robey SS, Hamilton ST, Gupta PK, Erozan YS. Diagnostic value of cytopathology in Barrett esophagus and associated carcinoma. *Am J Clin Pathol.* 1988;89:493-498.

Shu YJ. Detection of esophageal carcinoma by the balloon technique in the People's Republic of China. In: Koss, Coleman, eds. *Advances in Clinical Cytology, Vol 2.* New York, NY: Masson Publishing USA Inc; 1984:67-102.

Shurbagi MS, Erozan TS. The cytopathologic diagnosis of esophageal adenocarcinoma. *Acta Cytol.* 1991;35:189-194.

Takeda M. *Atlas of Diagnostic Gastrointestinal Cytology.* New York, NY: Igaku-Shoin Medical Publishers Inc; 1983.

Takeda M. Gastric cytology: recent developments. In: Koss, Coleman, eds. *Advances in Clinical Cytology, Vol 2.* New York, NY: Masson Publishing USA Inc; 1984:49-66.

Wang HH, Ducatman BS, Thebault BS. Cytologic features of premalignant glandular lesions in the upper gastrointestinal tract. *Acta Cytol.* 1991;35:199-203.

Wang HH, Jonasson JG, Ducatman BS. Brushing cytology of the upper gastrointestinal tract: obsolete or not? *Acta Cytol.* 1991;35:195-198.

CHAPTER 18

Central Nervous System

Dorothy L. Rosenthal, MD, FIAC
Diane B. Mandell, CT(ASCP), CFIAC

CONTENTS

The pathology of the central nervous system (CNS) is often bewildering to the novice, and the apparent difficulty in mastering the subject is compounded by the mystique surrounding it. Much of the terminology and many of the lesions and their cytologic presentation are unique to the CNS, and most pathologists receive inadequate training in neuropathology. Patients for whom CNS cytology is performed either have symptoms relating to a CNS disease or are candidates for CNS involvement by a metastatic neoplasm. Examination of the cytology specimen may provide the only definitive diagnosis for the patient. Consequently, treatment may be initiated that could ultimately affect the patient's thought processes, psychomotor abilities, or disease progression, which is a significant responsibility for the cytologist.

Exposure to cerebrospinal fluid (CSF) specimens in the daily cytology work load is infrequent. Tissue verification of spinal fluid cellular findings is rare, as brain biopsies are infrequent, and often comes long after the initial cytologic diagnosis. Only by constantly reviewing previous cases (or by autopsy) when tissue or follow-up becomes available is it possible to become proficient in the cytologic interpretation of CSF.

A final problem for the student is terminology. Much controversy exists in the literature about the source of the cells seen, especially in reactive processes; different terms for the same cells only add to the confusion. The best ways, then, to acquire proficiency are as follows: to review basic neuroanatomy; to appreciate the major histologic patterns of the more common primary brain tumors; to be alert for the common metastatic tumors to the CNS; and to learn the cellular characteristics of the cells of the leukemias and the lymphomas.

The aim of this chapter is to provide the student with a guide to cytologic diagnosis. A pragmatic approach to any specimen is the most realistic way to proceed, especially with cytologic specimens from the CNS. Diagnostic categories utilize the cytologic pattern, the patient's age and history, and test results to eliminate or indicate certain diseases. The diagnostic choices thus are divided into the following categories: "normal" or negative; inflammatory conditions; reactive conditions; primary tumors; metastatic tumors; and leukemias/lymphomas. Each of these categories has its characteristic patterns and cellular components.

Physicians benefit from a meaningful interpretation of the cells, rather than simply a "positive" or "negative" diagnosis. By communicating carefully and closely with clinicians, the cytologist not only gains pertinent medical history but can determine that the specimen is fresh (processed within 30 minutes if at all possible). Perhaps the greatest asset to accurate diagnosis is a well-prepared specimen with good cellular detail. The techniques section at the end of this chapter contains the specific Cytospin preparation used at the University of California at Los Angeles. The air-dried cytocentrifuge preparation, which is stained with a modified Diff-Quik Giemsa method, and the wet-fixed sample, which is stained by the Papanicolaou method, provide two views of the cell. Contamination of the CSF by peripheral blood can often be determined better in the Cytospin air-dried preparation because red blood cells are frequently lysed by wet fixation.

Finally, a single specimen will not always provide a definitive answer, and a simple "equivocal" is sometimes the most appropriate response. A spinal tap, when performed by an experienced physician, is minimally traumatic, and a repeated tap in 7 to 10 days (allowing the reaction to the initial tap to subside) will provide material for another evaluation, often the conclusive one.

SPECIMEN REQUIREMENTS

Clinical History

Accurate patient information is vital to reaching a valid diagnosis. Such data are best gathered by close communication between the clinician and the laboratory. Of greatest import are (1) clinical impression; (2) symptoms and physical findings; (3) results from tests done within recent months that involve the CNS, including invasive procedures (myelogram and arteriogram) and noninvasive procedures (computed tomography [CT scan] and magnetic resonance imaging [MRI]); (4) previous therapy, including intrathecal medication and irradiation to brain or cord; (5) surgical history, including presence or insertion of shunts, fine needle aspiration (FNA), brain biopsy, or cyst drainage; (6) source of CSF, such as lumbar space, cisterna, ventricle, shunt, or parenchymal cyst; and (7) temporal relationship of specimen to therapy, surgical intervention, invasive diagnostic procedures, or previous tap, all of which will provoke reactive cellular responses additional to the cytopathology of the disease itself.

Specimen Collection

The collector of CSF should be expert enough to avoid a bloody tap or aspiration of solid material. Aspiration of the nucleus pulposus or bone marrow can lead to a false-positive diagnosis. Quick delivery to the laboratory and immediate processing are imperative, since spinal fluid is not a good environment for these fragile cells; diagnostic material may disintegrate in less than 1 hour and yield a false-negative assessment. Addition of alcohol is less than ideal because it causes the cells to shrink. If fixation is needed, the Saccomanno method is the better option.

FNA of solid brain tissue should be performed by an experienced neurosurgeon, utilizing controlled localizing techniques (eg, CT scan or MRI). Smears must be made more rapidly than those made from FNAs from other sites because of the accelerated clotting time of brain tissue. Immediate microscopic assessment for adequacy and preliminary diagnosis, using a rapid stain, should be provided to the clinician whenever possible, in the same way that a frozen section is performed.

Specimen Preparation

Total cell recovery and good cellular detail are two prime requisites for any method; budgetary requirements and ease of handling should also be considered. Specimen preparation methods available include the various filtration methods (eg, Nuclepore and Millipore); sedimentation or centrifugation directly onto a glass slide; and centrifugation with smear transfer of the sediment onto a glass slide. At UCLA, the cytocentrifuge is currently considered the optimal method. Two chambers are prepared: one air-dried, stained with modified Diff-Quik Giemsa stain; the other alcohol-fixed, stained with Papanicolaou stain. Both methods complement each other, and the air-dried sample can be used for discussion of contentious cases with hematologists, who are familiar with the Giemsa stain.

Special Studies

With the current availability of immunochemical procedures, extra slides should be prepared whenever possible to allow such tests to be performed. Glial fibrillary acidic protein, neuron-specific enolase, and common leukocyte antigen are frequently helpful in identifying the cell line, especially when faced with a small cell neoplasm. The epithelial membrane markers (carcinoembryonic antigen, epithelial membrane antigen, milk fat globule) are useful to distinguish carcinomas from high-grade astrocytomas. Occasionally, tumor-specific antibodies, such as prostate-specific antigen and alpha-fetoprotein (liver), will indicate the primary tumor. Simultaneous staining of available tissue from the suspected parent neoplasm is important to assure that the original tumor is also antigen positive. A separate aliquot should be taken for flow cytometry if the cellular sample is sufficient and the disease warrants the test.

PHYSIOLOGY OF CEREBROSPINAL FLUID

CSF, an ultrafiltrate of plasma, is produced by the choroid plexus. It flows from the ventricles to the subarachnoid space; both areas comprise the so-called CSF compartment [**F** *18.1*]. Reabsorption occurs through arachnoidal villi into venous sinuses [**F** *18.2*]. The blood-brain barrier, located at the capillary level, prohibits certain substances from entering the CSF compartment. This is an important factor

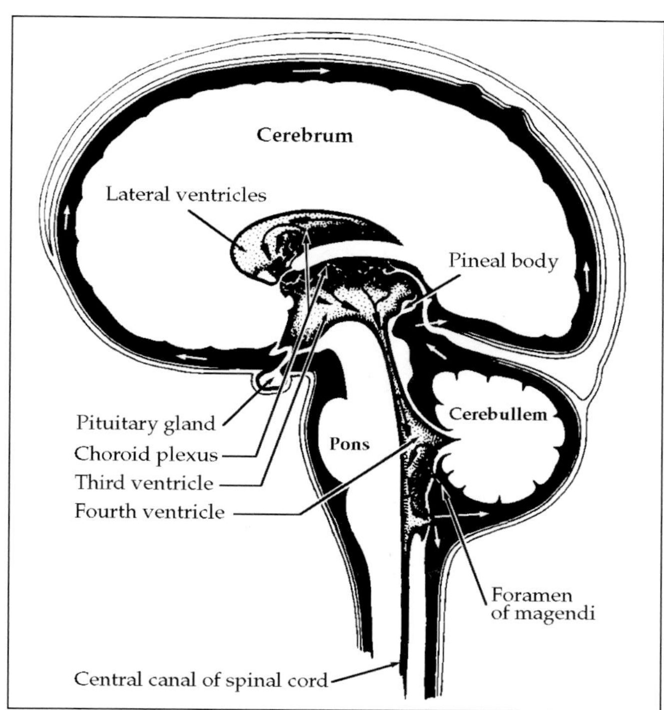

F *18.1*

Profile of brain and cord showing flow of CSF and location of major structures.

in chemotherapy and necessitates intrathecal medication for effective treatment. The total fluid contained in the CSF compartment is 150 mL; 500 mL is produced in a 24-hour period, a turnover rate of approximately 14%.

FACTORS INFLUENCING CELL EXFOLIATION

Contact of tumor with the CSF compartment will increase cell recovery. Therefore, if the anatomic location is considered, the most likely tumors to shed cells are meningioma, metastatic carcinoma, medulloblastoma, ependymoma, and sarcoma. However, meningioma, which occurs in the subarachnoid space, rarely exfoliates spontaneously. The ability of a tumor to shed depends on the cohesiveness of the tumor. Metastatic squamous cell carcinoma and adenocarcinoma appear in the CNS in about equal numbers. However, malignant squamous cells are rare in spinal fluids.

In deep-seated tumors, cells probably enter the CSF by direct extension or via a perivascular cuff of tumor cells in Virchow-Robin space with migration along the meninges. Secondary tumors may be found in the subarachnoid space by erosion of a metastatic nodule or by way of meningeal metastases. Usually, very few diagnostic cells are recovered in the CSF sample. If many neoplastic cells

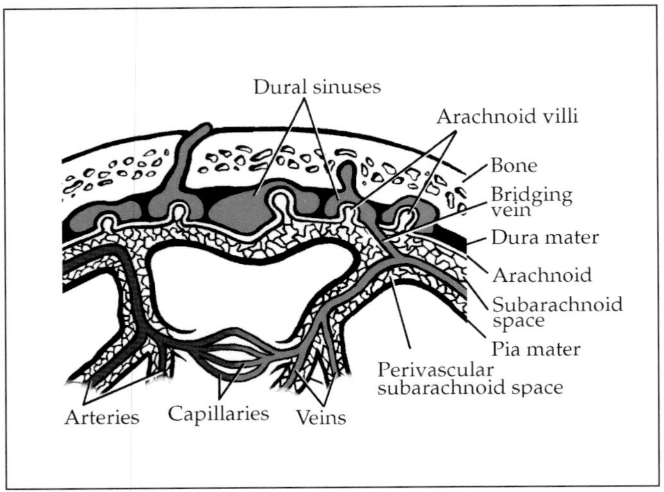

F *18.2*
Relationship of meninges, brain, and blood vessels.

are found, then extensive leptomeningeal involvement ("meningeal carcinomatosis," "carcinomatous meningitis") is probably present.

CELL PATTERNS

As in histopathologic specimens and other types of cytologic specimens, CNS cell samples present in a variety of cell patterns. Although a choice of "positive" or "negative" is sometimes considered adequate, more significant information can be gleaned from most cellular samples. Consider the importance of distinguishing between an inflammatory/infectious process and a reactive one. The difference between obstetric head trauma and an infectious meningitis in the neonate is critical to the care of the patient and is readily reflected in the cytologic interpretation of the CSF.

Cytologic differences between FNA smears and CSF specimens are similar to differences between aspirates and other body fluids or spontaneously exfoliated cells. Cells in FNA smears do not have a chance to "round up," and thus, cell relationships will more closely resemble histologic patterns. Nuclear characteristics, however, will be maintained. With a background in neuropathology and with clinical information, the cytologist can provide meaningful information.

The diseases encountered during cytopathologic examination will depend on the clinical emphasis and population of patients seen in a particular hospital or clinic. A schema that correlates cell identification and clinical setting to arrive at a differential diagnosis is shown [**T** *18.1*].

TUMORS OF THE CENTRAL NERVOUS SYSTEM

Since general experience with cytologic samples containing neoplastic cells is limited, certain guidelines are helpful. If the cell population is mixed, the lesion will usually be benign; if the cells are monomorphous, a neoplasm is probably present. However, lymphocytes frequently accompany tumor cells as a host response, so their presence should not suggest that the "mixture of cells" is a benign process.

The likelihood of a CNS neoplasm shedding cells into CSF varies with the type of lesion. For example, approximately 33% of the primary brain tumors shed cells into CSF, 50% of metastatic tumors shed cells, and 66% of CNS leukemias shed cells. The sensitivity also depends on the location of the tumor and its accessibility to the CSF compartment. Multiple taps to collect CSF increase the chances of recovering diagnostic cells.

PRIMARY BRAIN TUMORS

Primary brain tumors account for 1% of all deaths and 9% of all neoplasms of the CNS. In the child 70% are infratentorial, and in the adult 70% are supratentorial. Primary tumors have less tendency to exfoliate than metastatic tumors; therefore, the number of cells in a cytologic sample is usually small. Gliomas are by far the most common primary brain tumors in both adults and children. Anatomic site of the primary tumor is important to cell recovery in the CSF. Medulloblastomas, ependymomas, and lymphomas tend to shed the greatest amount of material. The question of benign vs malignant is usually replaced by low grade vs high grade since anatomic location and age of the patient are equally significant predictors of morbidity and survival.

Gliomas

Astrocytoma is the most common primary brain tumor in children and adults. It may be of low or high grade (glioblastoma multiforme). The anatomic location is important to operability and therefore survival. Cell presentation varies depending on the grade of the tumor. Cells from a low-grade tumor often look epithelial and benign. Nuclei are round to oval. Nucleoli are indistinct with bland chromatin. There is more hyperchromasia and multinucleation the higher the grade of the tumor [**I** *18.4*]. The high-grade neoplasm shows severe nuclear hyperchromasia and variation in cytoplasmic shape. The cytoplasm may be opaque or lacy; cell borders may be distinct or hazy. Glial fibrils (cytoplasmic extensions) are apparent in Papanicolaou-stained smears of needle aspirates and touch preparations; immunochemistry for glial fibrillary

Normal Population
- Lymphocytes: only a few; the only cells observed in a "negative" fluid
- Monocytes: infrequent
- Leptomeningeal cells: very infrequent
- Ependymal cells: expected in a ventricular tap, otherwise rare

Inflammatory Conditions
- Neutrophils: acute conditions (eg, acute bacterial meningitis), also early tuberculosis and early viral meningitis
- Lymphocytes: viral meningitis, late bacterial meningitis, tuberculosis
- Plasma cells: syphilis, tuberculosis, other immune responses
- Eosinophils: sometimes with parasites, allergic conditions, subacute meningitis
- Inflammatory histiocytes, including multinucleated histiocytes: tuberculosis, fungi; also seen postoperatively after placement of shunts and Ommaya reservoir

Reactive Conditions (eg, after CNS investigative procedure)
- Normal cells: increased number, especially of leptomeningeal cells and monocytes [▮*18.1*]
- Ependymal or choroid plexus cells [▮*18.2*]
- Astrocytes: rare
- Neurons: rare
- Macrophages (may contain ingested material listed)
  - Fat: following oil myelogram, trauma, infarct [▮*18.3*], parenchymatous destructive disease
  - Blood pigment: after intracranial hemorrhage (not fresh blood, as in a bloody tap)
  - Melanin: not pathognomonic of melanoma; observed in melanosis cerebrei, a rare benign condition

Contaminants
- Cartilage
- Bone marrow elements
- Debris (eg, albumin, starch crystals, skin squames)
- Tumor cells from other samples

Organisms
- Bacteria: rarely are rods or cocci identified; these may be contaminants
- Fungi: stain pale pink or purple with the Papanicolaou stain and purple with May-Grünwald-Giemsa; do India ink preparation if *Cryptococcus* is suspected; periodic acid-Schiff or silver stain for other fungi
- Tuberculosis and treponemes (syphilis): need special stains; will not be seen with routine morphologic stains
- Parasites: rare but can be identified; usually provoke a mixed reactive inflammatory pattern with variable eosinophilia

T *18.1*
Sources of Benign Cells in Cerebrospinal Fluids

acidic protein (GFAP) can be used to confirm the glial nature of the cells. Cell aggregates are common, especially in cystic lesions, and may be confused with cell balls of a metastatic adenocarcinoma.

Ependymomas and choroid plexus papillomas originate in the lining of the ventricular system. These tumors are easily recovered in CSF because of the accessibility of the cells to the CSF compartment. Ependymoma is the most common tumor of the spinal cord. These cells bear a striking resemblance to columnar epithelial cells of benign lesions or, when atypical, they resemble cells from an adenocarcinoma. Nucleoli are inconspicuous, and chromatin is usually fine. Rosettes can occasionally be recognized, but they should not be confused with those of neural crest tumors.

Oligodendrogliomas are rare tumors of adults. The cells are monotonous with delicate cytoplasm that suspends the round nuclei in a transparent syncytial "wash." Chromatin is finely granular, and nucleoli are indistinct [▮*18.5*].

Neural Crest Tumors

Medulloblastomas, retinoblastomas, and neuroblastomas occur in children and young adults. The cells are small, hyperchromatic, and usually exfoliate in clusters (an essential criterion for diagnosis) [▮*18.6*, ▮*18.7*]. Cytoplasm is very scant, and nuclei mold against each other. Chromatin is dark and smudged, and nucleoli are inconspicuous. Rosettes are rare. It is impossible to cytologically separate these lesions [▮*18.8*]. Careful attention to criteria, especially cell clusters, will help distinguish these cells from those of leukemia.

Midline Tumors

Pinealoma, found in both children and adults, is located at the end of the third ventricle under the corpus callosum. Neoplasms at this site are locally destructive.

Over half of these tumors cytologically resemble germinomas of the gonads, complete with accompanying lymphocytes. Tumor cells are monomorphous with round nuclei, moderate amounts of lacy cytoplasm, and prominent nucleoli. The cells of pinealoma are easily confused with those of oligodendroglioma or metastatic seminoma.

Pituitary adenomas comprise 10% of all intracranial growths in adults. They often produce abnormal endocrine activity. The cytomorphology usually appears benign. A honeycomb or papillary pattern is frequently present. The nuclei are small and uniformly round, and the chromatin is bland. Nucleoli are small but can be prominent.

Meningiomas

Meningiomas are tumors of young adults. They arise from the coverings of the brain and rarely exfoliate but are easily approached by image-guided FNA. They are usually surgically resectable. The cells resemble small fibroblasts with oval nuclei and inconspicuous nucleoli, and they grow in tight whorls. Psammoma bodies may be present [▮*18.9*]. Most cytologic samples are needle aspirates. If cells exfoliate spontaneously and appear in CSF, a meningiosarcoma should be considered.

Metastatic Tumors

Metastatic tumors account for 50% of all intracranial neoplasms; lung [▮*18.10*] and breast [▮*18.11*] predominate among the common adenocarcinomas metastatic to the brain. Melanomas [▮*18.12*] and choriocarcinomas, while uncommon tumors, metastasize to brain frequently. More than 80% of patients with metastases to the brain have multiple lesions. Secondary tumors of the CNS usually shed more cells than do primary tumors. Clusters are infrequent in contrast to exfoliative patterns in other body fluids. One must know the clinical history, for it is rare that the CSF is the first "positive" specimen (oat cell carcinoma of the lung and gastric adenocarcinoma are exceptions). It is helpful if one compares the cytomorphology in cerebrospinal fluid with the histology of the primary tumor. "Second" primary tumors are becoming more the rule than the exception with increasingly successful therapy of patients' "first" tumors. Infections also can present clinically and radiographically as tumor masses.

Leukemias/Lymphomas

Leukemic involvement of the CNS is common, especially if only systemic chemotherapy has been given. Lymphomas as a rule shed greater numbers of cells than do the leukemias. The cell type is usually difficult to identify in CSF. However, the diagnosis is already established by the clinical history and bone marrow sample or lymph node biopsy specimen, which may be available for comparison. The role of the cytologist is to decide the presence or absence of blasts in the CSF. Close collaboration of the cytologist with the hematology technologists and pathologists enhances the accuracy of the diagnosis.

Since leukemias will have a clinically established diagnosis of cell type, the appropriate "positive" CSF diagnosis is "blasts present, consistent with history." The number of blasts is sometimes small. Unless peripheral blood contamination is present, thus invalidating any diagnosis, even a few blasts should be reported. Their rarity, however, should be emphasized. The decision to change therapy will be made by the clinician.

The cytologic features of blasts are best appreciated in very fresh, well-fixed, and properly stained preparations. If any time has elapsed (30 minutes or more) between collection and processing, the chromatin quality will deteriorate, impeding interpretation. The prototypic blast is that of acute lymphocytic leukemia [▮*18.13*, ▮*18.14*]. Chromatin is even, with little clumping or clearing. Nucleoli are prominent and often multiple. Nuclear membranes are irregular, with notches or noses and clefts. Cytoplasm is scant, appearing absent. The overall cell size is approximately twice that of mature lymphocytes.

The other leukemias and lymphomas vary somewhat from this description of primitive lymphoid cells [▮*18.15*]. Cytoplasm may be more abundant with granules or vacuoles depending on the intended cell line. Aberrant cytoplasmic shapes are common in the lymphomas. Nuclei may be more convoluted and cerebroid, especially in the poorly differentiated large-cell lymphomas. If the image in the microscope does not fit the clinical diagnosis, comparison with the diagnostic bone marrow or conference with the hematopathologist/oncologist is advised. Some unexpected changes may be attributable to therapy, but occasionally the cell line transforms or was originally misdiagnosed. The newest cytologic challenge results from human immunodeficiency virus–infected patients with primary CNS lymphoma.

The CNS is a vulnerable site for leukemic involvement without intrathecal therapy, and the chances of CNS involvement increase with survival. Therefore, many serial samples can be expected from a patient as treatment proceeds and the disease waxes and wanes. The cytologist should be cautious of intercurrent infection, manifested either by numerous neutrophils (acute meningitis) or by reactive lymphocytes with plasma cells (viral meningitis, fungal infection, tuberculosis).

One must also be aware of reactive changes to intrathecal therapy [▮*18.16*]. Nucleoli in lymphocytes and monocytes are common following chemical or radiation therapy. Persistent blasts are difficult to identify among reactive elements. Careful inspection and tedious identification of all cells in the preparation are necessary to alert the clinician to the effectiveness of the intrathecal medication. Well-preserved blasts, distinct from reactive lymphocytes, should be present in order to diagnose a specimen as "positive." If blasts appear degenerated (ie, show breaks in the chromatin pattern or nuclear membrane), these should be reported as degenerative blasts, distinguishing them from viable-appearing blasts. A repeated tap in 7 to 10 days will frequently clarify the issue. Close consultation with the clinicians and hematologists is vital to decide on treatment alterations based on cellular findings in a CSF specimen.

In all samples, contamination of the CSF by peripheral blood precludes the certain identification of the location of blasts (ie, CSF vs circulating blood). Repeated tap is always recommended.

CEREBROSPINAL FLUID CYTOLOGIC PROCEDURES

Cerebrospinal Fluid Parameters

Although the following parameters usually are not measured in the cytology laboratory, their deviation from normal is often a helpful clue to the possible presence of abnormal cells.

Opening pressure	Less than 180 mm H_2O
Protein	0.15–0.45 g/L (15-45 mg/dL)
Glucose	2.4-4.1 mmol/L (43–73 mg/dL)
Cell count	Less than 5 cells/mm^3
Specific gravity	1.005–1.008

CNS tumors are commonly accompanied by elevated CSF protein and decreased CSF glucose. An elevated cell count should, of course, be considered suspect, but a normal count does not necessarily mean an absence of neoplastic cells, especially in cases of leukemia, nor does an increased white blood cell count always imply "leukemia." Here, the cytomorphology of any cells present is far more important than a quantitative cell count.

Cytospin Preparation of Cerebrospinal Fluid

1. Assemble Cytospin apparatus (Shandon-Cytocentrifuge, Shandon Southern Instruments, Sewickley, Pa).
   a) Two precircled Shandon frosted end-labeled slides
   b) Two white filter cards
   c) Two cytocentrifuge chambers

   Always check to make sure that the holes in the filter paper and cytocentrifuge chamber are properly aligned.
2. Balance the specimen with an equal setup at the other pole.
3. With the chambers in place, add 1 drop of 22% bovine albumin and then quickly add 7 drops of CSF.
4. Cytospin I or II: Quickly cover the head with the stainless steel shield. Lock the lid. Follow manufacturer's instructions.
5. Set the time for 5 minutes and set the speed to 850 rpm.
6. As soon as the machine stops running and the shield unlocks, carefully remove the chamber.
7. Separate the filter card from the chamber. Be careful not to drag the filter card across the slide.
8. The air-dried slide is stained with either Wright's stain, Diff-Quik stain, or Giemsa stain. The alcohol-fixed slide is stained by the Papanicolaou method.
9. Put the chambers in 10% chlorine solution for disinfection.

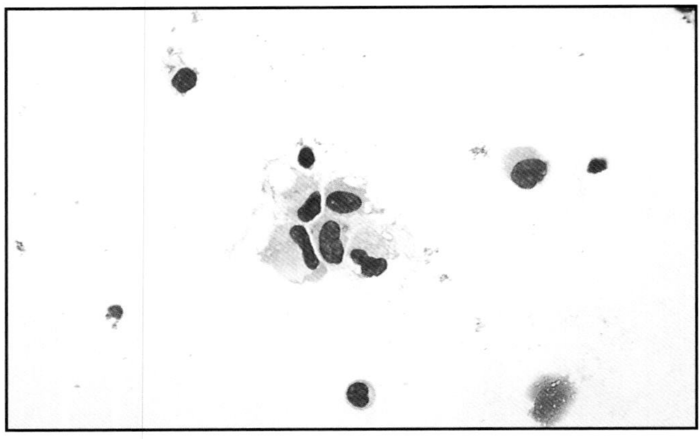

I *18.1*

Reactive pleocytosis. Monocytes and lymphocytes are shown (lumbar puncture, modified May-Grünwald-Giemsa stain, x400).

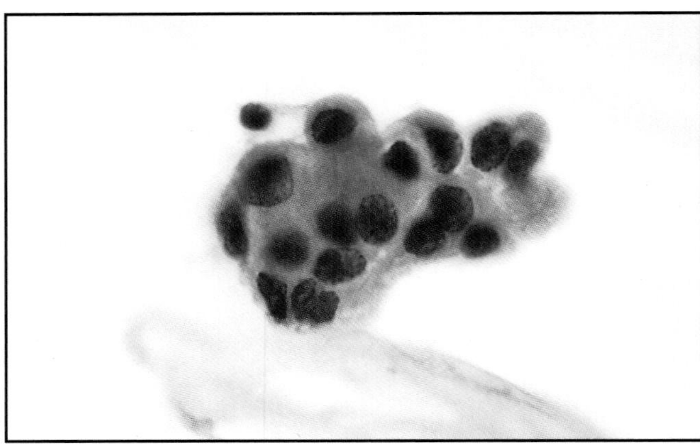

I *18.2*

Choroid plexus cells in a child with leukemia who has had numerous treatments with intrathecal therapy (lumbar puncture, Papanicolaou stain, x1000).

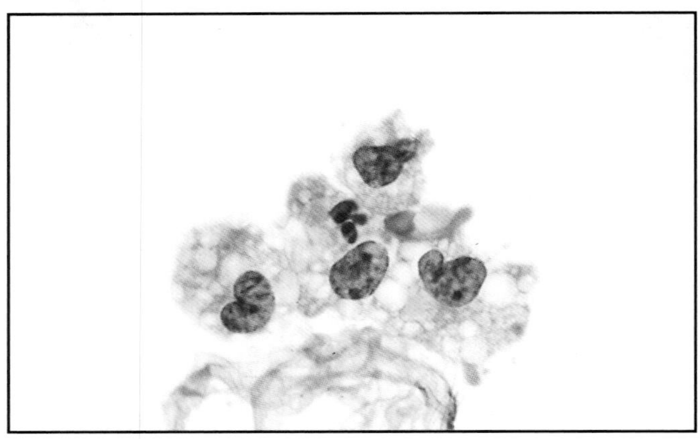

I *18.3*

Macrophages. Vacuolated cytoplasm probably represents fat released from destroyed white matter following a stroke (lumbar tap, Papanicolaou stain, x1000).

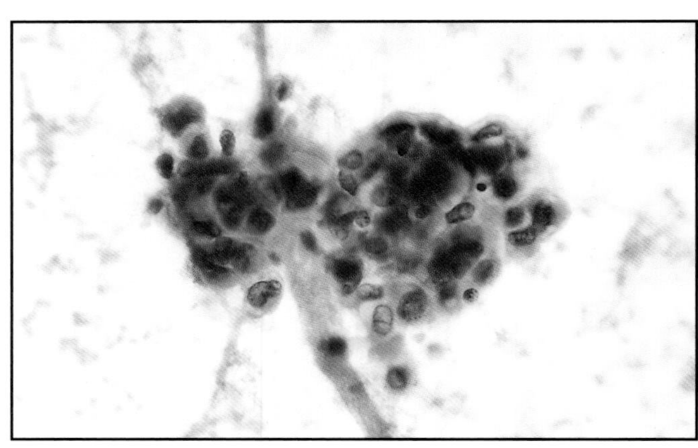

I *18.4*

Astrocytoma, grade III (intraoperative cyst fluid, Papanicolaou stain, x400).

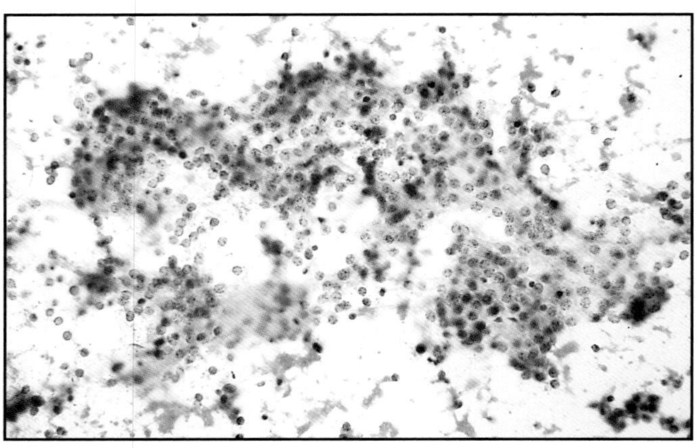

I *18.5*

Oligodendroglioma (FNA, Papanicolaou stain, x200).

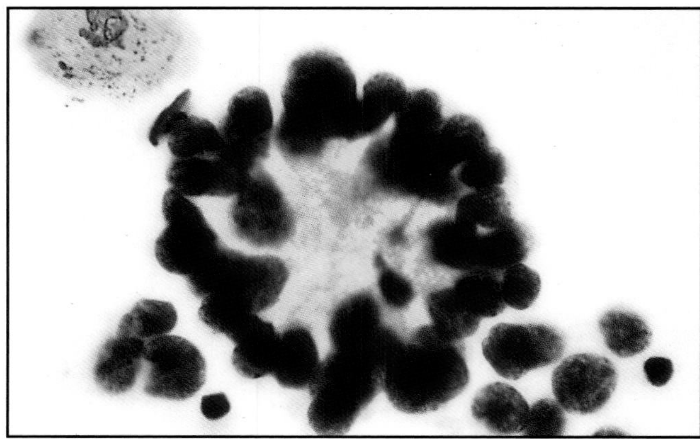

I *18.6*

Medulloblastoma. A rarely encountered rosette is depicted (lumbar puncture, Papanicolaou stain, x1000).

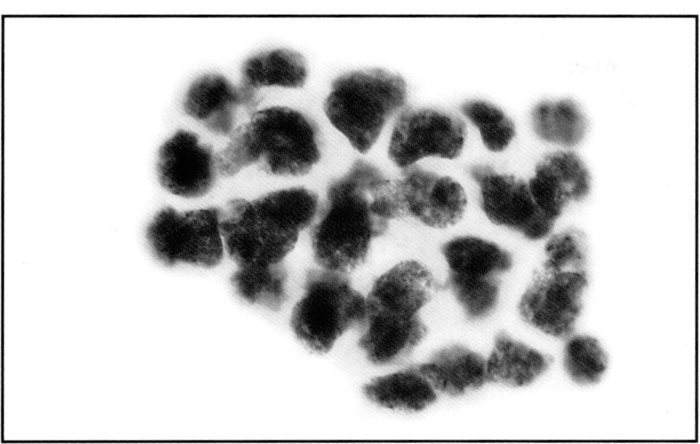

▮18.7
Medulloblastoma. This is a more typical presentation (lumbar puncture, Papanicolaou stain, x1000).

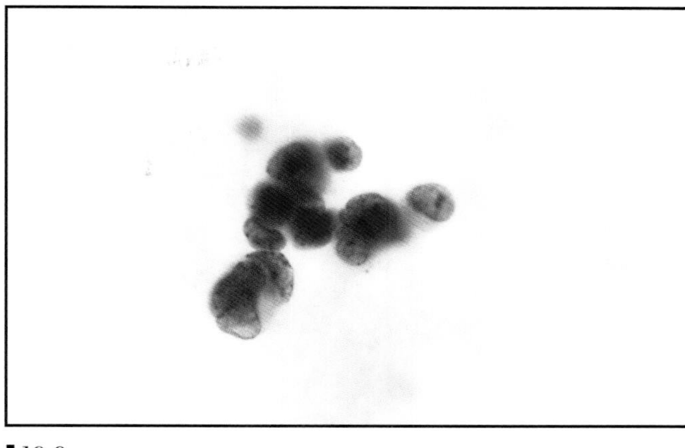

▮18.8
Retinoblastoma. Note the similarity of the cytologic features to those of medulloblastoma (lumbar puncture, Papanicolaou stain, x1000).

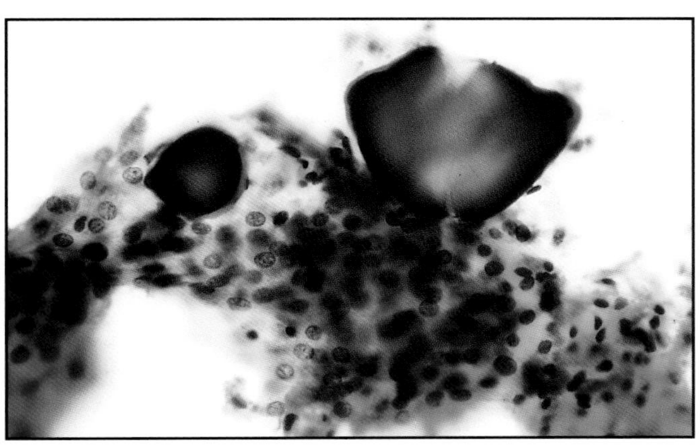

▮18.9
Meningioma. Small cells grow in three-dimensional whorls, often accompanied by psammoma bodies (FNA, Papanicolaou stain, x400).

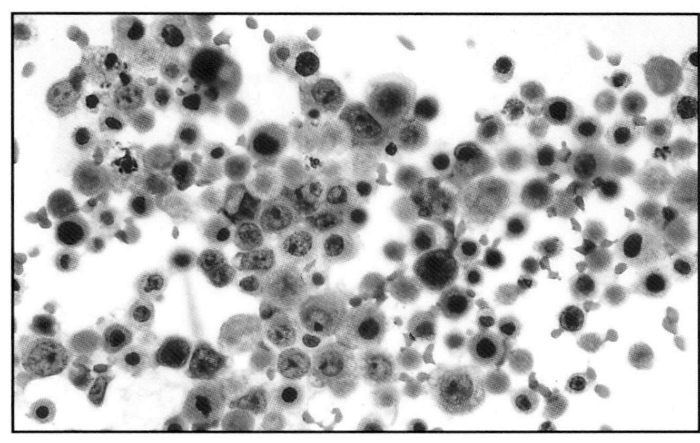

▮18.10
Meningeal carcinomatosis. Cells have typical features of an adenocarcinoma and are consistent with the patient's history of lung cancer (lumbar puncture, modified May-Grünwald-Giemsa stain, x400).

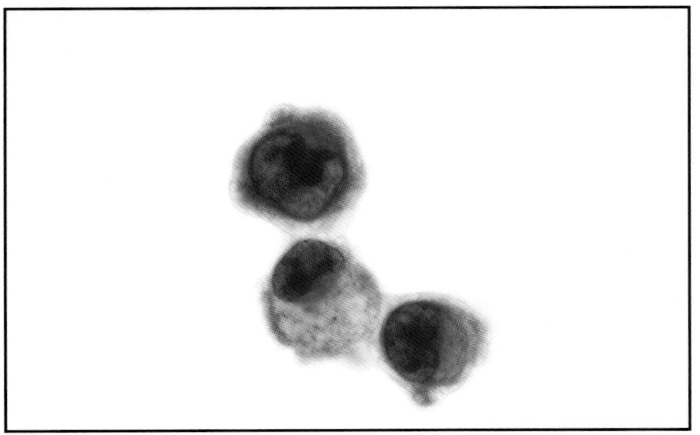

▮18.11
Breast adenocarcinoma. Glandular neoplasms usually shed cells singly rather than in cell balls as in other body fluids (lumbar puncture, Papanicolaou stain, x1000).

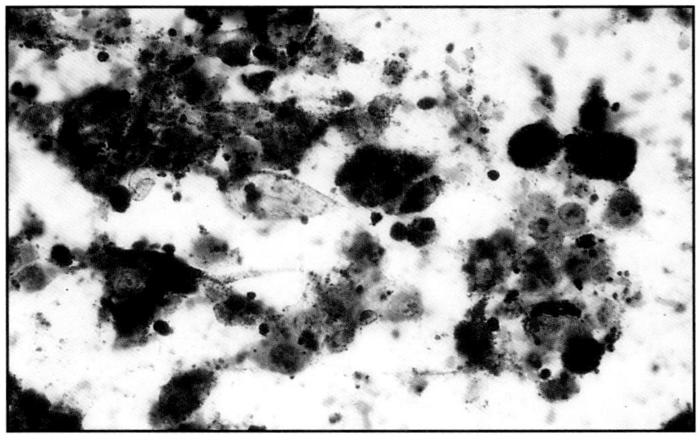

▮18.12
Melanoma. Pigment frequently separates from the tumor cells and may be engulfed by macrophages (FNA, Papanicolaou stain, x400).

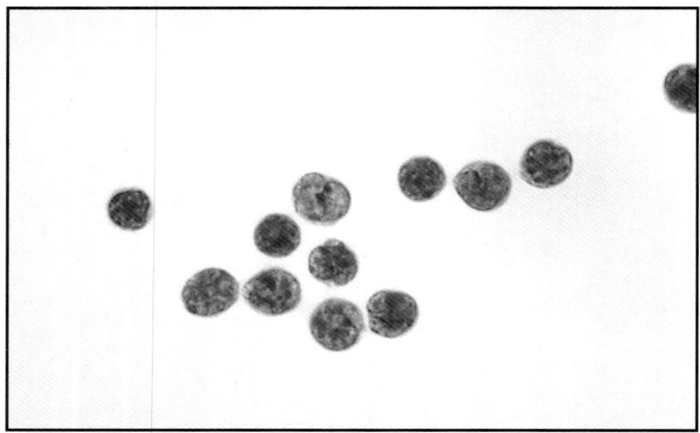

18.13
Blasts of acute lymphoblastic leukemia (lumbar puncture, modified May-Grünwald-Giemsa stain, x1000).

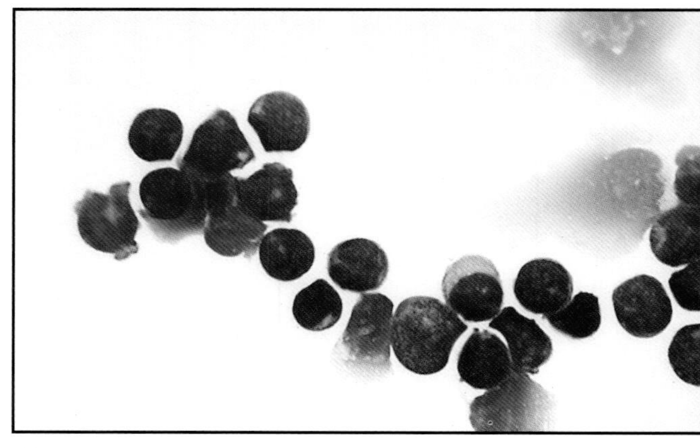

18.14
Blasts of acute lymphoblastic leukemia. Note the difference in nuclear features and cell size, dependent on the fixation and stain (lumbar puncture, Papanicolaou stain, x1000).

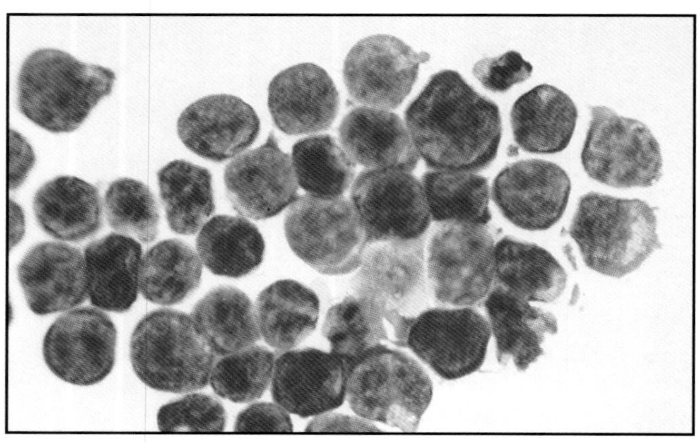

18.15
Burkitt's lymphoma. Cells of a lymphoma are usually more variable in size and nuclear shape than leukemic blasts (lumbar puncture, modified May-Grünwald-Giemsa stain, x1000).

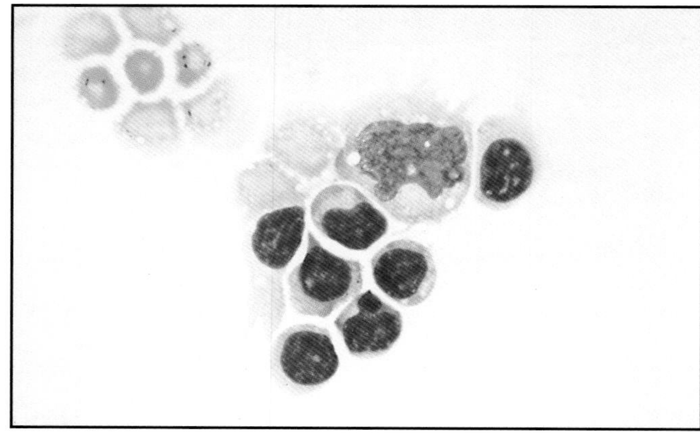

18.16
Reactive pleocytosis following intrathecal chemotherapy for acute lymphoblastic leukemia (lumbar puncture, modified May-Grünwald-Giemsa stain, x1000).

REVIEW EXERCISES

1. Name the major distinguishing cytologic features that characterize the neural crest tumors.

2. What are two factors that determine whether cells from a tumor will appear in the CSF?

3. Name three of the cells one would expect to find in a reactive process.

4. The microscopic findings on a CSF specimen include the following cells: reactive lymphocytes, plasma cells, and monocytes. Choose among the following answers the most likely disease process in the patient.
   a) Metastatic breast cancer
   b) Multiple myeloma
   c) Multiple sclerosis
   d) Viral meningitis
   e) Tuberculosis

5. Name the glial tumors that are most likely to be confused with a metastatic adenocarcinoma on a CSF specimen.

SELECTED READINGS

Adams JH, Graham DI, Doyle D. *Brain Biopsy: The Smear Technique for Neurosurgical Biopsies.* London, England: Chapman and Hall Ltd; 1981.

Bigner SH. Central nervous system. In: Bibbo M, ed. *Comprehensive Cytopathology.* Philadelphia, Pa: WB Saunders Co; 1991:468-483.

Bigner SH, Johnston WW. *Cytopathology of the Central Nervous System.* New York, NY: Masson Publishing USA Inc; 1983.

Burger PC, Vogel FS. *Surgical Pathology of the Nervous System and Its Coverings.* 3rd ed. New York, NY: John Wiley & Sons; 1991.

Chandrasoma P. *Stereotactic Brain Biopsy.* New York, NY: Igaku-Shoin Medical Publishers Inc; 1989.

Gondos B, King EB. Cerebrospinal fluid cytology: diagnostic accuracy and comparison of different techniques. *Acta Cytol.* 1976;20:542-547.

Hajdu SI, Hajdu EO. *Cytopathology of Sarcomas.* Philadelphia, Pa: WB Saunders; 1976:323-356.

Koelmel HW. *Atlas of Cerebrospinal Fluid Cells.* 2nd ed. New York, NY: Springer-Verlag NY Inc; 1977.

Mathios AJ, Nielsen SL, Barrett D, King EB. Cerebrospinal fluid cytomorphology identification of benign cells originating in the central nervous system. *Acta Cytol.* 1977;21:403-412.

Naylor B. The cytologic diagnosis of cerebrospinal fluids. *Acta Cytol.* 1964;8:141-149.

Netter FM. *The CIBA Collection of Medical Illustration.* Summit, NY: RR Donnelley and Sons Co; 1980.

Oehmichen M. *Cerebrospinal Fluid Cytology: An Introduction and Atlas.* Philadelphia, Pa: WB Saunders; 1976.

Rosenthal DL. *Cytology of the Central Nervous System.* Basel, Switzerland: S Karger; 1984;8. Monographs in Clinical Cytology.

Rosenthal DL. Cytology of the central nervous system. In: *Compendium of Diagnostic Cytology.* 7th ed. Chicago, Ill: Tutorials of Cytology; 1992:324-329.

Rosenthal DL. Cytology of the central nervous system. In: Astarita RW, ed. *Practical Cytopathology.* New York, NY: Churchill Livingstone, Inc; 1990.

CHAPTER 19

Pleural, Peritoneal, and Pericardial Fluids

BERNARD NAYLOR, MB, CHB, FIAC

CONTENTS

The human body contains four major serous cavities: right and left pleural cavities, peritoneal cavity, and pericardial cavity. Under normal circumstances each cavity is only a potential cavity, comparable to the potential cavity of a balloon that is completely collapsed. Each of the collapsed cavities, or sacs, partly surrounds certain organs, again reminiscent of a collapsed balloon draped over a solid object. Each pleural sac surrounds a lung and lines one half of the thoracic cavity; the peritoneal sac covers the abdominal viscera and lines the abdominal wall; and the pericardial sac surrounds the heart. Two minor serous cavities, one surrounding each testis, are formed from embryologic extensions of the peritoneal cavity.

Each cavity is lined by mesothelium, a monolayer of cells that is morphologically the same in each cavity. The outer layer of mesothelium is referred to as the parietal layer; the inner layer, partly investing one or more organs, is referred to as the visceral layer. Therefore, the visceral layer of pleura forms the surface of the lungs, the visceral layer of peritoneum covers the stomach and intestines, and that of the pericardium surrounds the heart. As an organ enveloped by a serous cavity moves, such as when a lung expands and contracts, the two apposing mesothelial surfaces glide over each other, a movement facilitated by the lubricating effect of the small amount of fluid in each cavity. Because this fluid is similar to serum, these cavities are frequently referred to as serous cavities.

TYPES OF EFFUSION

Spontaneous accumulation of fluid in a serous cavity above the normal small amount is referred to as a serous effusion, which is then designated according to its location: pleural, peritoneal, or pericardial. Of these three types, pleural effusions are the most common, pericardial effusions the least. A peritoneal effusion is frequently referred to as ascites, and the fluid as ascitic fluid. Under a variety of circumstances, air may be introduced into a serous cavity, producing the condition of pneumothorax, pneumoperitoneum, or pneumopericardium. If the condition is also accompanied by an effusion, the terms are expanded to pneumohydrothorax, pneumohydroperitonium, and pneumohydropericardium. An effusion in the serous cavity surrounding a testis is referred to as a hydrocele; such specimens are rarely received in a cytopathology laboratory and will not be further considered.

Serous effusions are sometime referred to as "body cavity fluids," a deplorably vague term that has no place in the vocabulary of clinical cytology.

SAMPLING TECHNIQUE

A serous effusion is almost always removed by inserting a wide-bore needle through the body wall into the cavity. Pleural fluid is removed by thoracentesis, peritoneal fluid by abdominal paracentesis, and pericardial fluid by pericardiocentesis. Cytologic specimens are frequently obtained by "washing" the peritoneal cavity with physiologic saline solution at the time of abdominal surgery for neoplasm of the female genital tract, then aspirating the fluid. Peritoneal dialysate, from patients undergoing long-term peritoneal dialysis, is occasionally submitted for cytologic examination.

COLLECTING SEROUS FLUIDS

Fluid should be collected into a clean, dry container, which need not be sterile, and sent to the laboratory as soon as possible. If the fluid cannot be sent to the laboratory immediately, it should be kept in a refrigerator (but not allowed to freeze). When refrigerated, cells remain well preserved for many days. It is not necessary to add alcohol, formalin, or any other kind of preservative to a serous fluid. Furthermore, it is not necessary to add anticoagulant to the fluid if the cell block technique is to be used. If it is desirable to prevent the fluid from clotting, heparin should be used since it does not interfere with the staining reaction of the cells, unlike oxalate.

GROSS APPEARANCE OF SEROUS FLUIDS

The gross appearance of a serous fluid may reveal clues to the cause of the effusion. Therefore, the following features should be noted: volume, color, and clarity, and any other unusual features such as opalescence, high viscosity, or malodor. Physical features of serous fluids are listed that may give definite clues to the cause of an effusion and the nature of its cellular contents [**T** *19.1*].

Contrary to popular belief, heavily blood-stained fluids are not likely to contain cancer cells; only about 20% of such fluids contain them. Furthermore, of the fluids that contain cancer cells, about 50% show to the naked eye some degree of blood staining and 50% do not.

PREPARATION OF SEROUS FLUIDS

There are three widely used techniques to prepare serous fluids: a toluidine blue–stained wet film, wet-fixed smears stained by the Papanicolaou method, and a cell block stained with hematoxylin-eosin. Details of each of these methods are given in the chapter on cytopreparatory techniques (Chapter 35).

Feature	Possible Cause
Chocolate brown	Metastatic melanoma
Light brown	Hemosiderin (old hemorrhage)
Orange brown or greenish	Jaundice
Greenish-yellow, "fruit juice" appearance	Rheumatoid pleuritis or pericarditis
Heavy whitish flocculent sediment	Rheumatoid pleuritis or pericarditis
Visible spheroids or ellipsoids	Metastatic carcinoma
Shimmering, "gold-paint" appearance	Cholesterol crystals
Milky (chylous)	High content of emulsified lipid
High viscosity	Mesothelioma
Cloudy yellow	Neutrophils
Mucoid	Pseudomyxoma peritonei
Malodor	High bacterial content

T *19.1*
Physical Characteristics of Serous Fluids

Stained wet films are simple and quick to prepare and are ready to be examined immediately, after which they are discarded. The advantages of using wet films are as follows:

1. They frequently reveal a diagnostic cytologic picture, enabling a report to be issued rapidly.
2. They enable one to identify serous fluids that contain myriad neoplastic cells, the "super positive" specimens. It is then possible to remove such specimens from the routine staining circuit, thereby avoiding their cross-contamination of other specimens.
3. They may enable one to immediately identify interesting or unusual cytologic specimens, thus providing an opportunity to prepare more smears before the sediment is solidified for preparation of the cell block.
4. They may reveal certain constituents that are not seen in permanent smears, such as cholesterol crystals, psammoma bodies, and the cellular fragments known as detached ciliary tufts.

Cell blocks have enhanced our yield of positive results, especially when any spontaneously formed clot in a serous fluid has been routinely sectioned. Clot may form rapidly after a fluid is aspirated and in doing so entrap neoplastic cells, leaving smears prepared from the unclotted fluid devoid of such cells. Furthermore, cell block preparations demonstrate psammoma bodies extremely well and they also reveal certain histologic aspects of neoplasms, such as papillary, acinar, or duct-like formations.

CAUSES OF SEROUS EFFUSION

Three broad classes of disease may cause an accumulation of fluid in a serous cavity: inflammatory disease, circulatory disturbances, and malignant neoplasm. Inflammatory processes damage the capillary walls that ramify in the submesothelial connective tissue, thus allowing escape of protein and various cellular constituents of the blood into the serous cavity. This results in a fluid that contains leukocytes of various types as well as mesothelial cells. Such an effusion, which is called an exudate, is rich in protein and its specific gravity is in excess of 1.020.

If the disturbance is primarily circulatory, the outflow of fluid through a serous membrane exceeds the normal reabsorptive process. This may be the result of increased venous pressure, as in congestive heart failure or cirrhosis of the liver, or the result of hypoproteinemia in renal failure. Such an effusion, which is called a transudate, contains less protein and fewer cells than an exudate, and its specific gravity is usually below 1.015.

Serous effusions caused by neoplasm are transudates in cases where the neoplasm causes mechanical interference in the absorption of fluid; or they are exudates in cases where the neoplasm damages the capillaries of the serous membrane.

CYTOLOGY OF SEROUS FLUIDS

Various types of normal and abnormal cells may be found in any serous cavity, with one exception: the cytologic picture of rheumatoid pleuritis and pericarditis has not been described in peritoneal fluid.

Every serous fluid contains cells, often numerous, occasionally scanty. Non-neoplastic cells commonly found in serous fluids are derived from blood (erythrocytes and leukocytes) and mesothelial cells come from the serosal lining. The proportions of different types of cells vary considerably, depending on the cause and duration of the effusion and the presence or absence of inflammation. Examples of normal cells that are only rarely found in serous fluids are megakaryocytes, hepatocytes, cells detached from the fimbriated end of the fallopian tube, and cells derived from the alimentary or respiratory tract via a fistula.

It is difficult to ascertain what exactly is a normal range of cells in serous fluids because the serous cavities normally contain only a small amount of fluid, which is clinically undetectable. Only when there is an excess of such fluid, an abnormal situation, is it possible to aspirate it.

Red Blood Cells

Almost all serous fluids, even those that appear to the naked eye not to be blood stained, contain some red blood cells, easily recognized in wet films and permanent preparations. In wet-fixed smears red blood cells frequently undergo lysis, leaving residual empty cell membranes with a slightly cyanophilic staining reaction. Intact red blood cells may be phagocytosed by macrophages. When red blood cells disintegrate, their hemoglobin is converted into hematoidin or hemosiderin, which may impart a distinctly yellow appearance to the supernatant. In Papanicolaou-stained smears, hemosiderin appears as golden brown to olive-green granules, whereas hematoidin appears as sheaves of elongated yellow-brown crystals or as canary-yellow amorphous material.

Rarely is it possible to discern an abnormality of red blood cells in serous fluids. They may acquire a sickle shape [▮*19.1*] in persons with sickle cell anemia or the sickle cell trait. The phenomenon of rouleau formation, in which the red blood cells are stacked on each other like a stack of coins, may be seen in stained wet films of serous fluid from patients with certain dysproteinemias.

Neutrophil Leukocytes

Almost every serous fluid contains neutrophil leukocytes, varying in number from just the occasional cells to purulent fluids in which virtually every cell is a neutrophil. Purulent fluids have a cloudy yellow appearance and if infected may be malodorous. Inflammation in particular and necrosis of an underlying organ are the most frequent causes of a serous effusion containing numerous neutrophils. In fluids that are not infected, the neutrophils are usually well preserved. In infected fluids, however, many neutrophils become necrotic to form light gray to gray-blue particles without any visible nucleus [▮*19.2*]. The nucleus of a necrotic neutrophil may condense into a round, solitary, cyanophilic mass.

In stained wet films, neutrophils may contain light yellow, glistening cytoplasmic granules of lipid, so numerous as to crowd the cytoplasm. Cytoplasmic lipid granules are seen only in stained wet films and may be seen in a wide variety of other cells, including neoplastic cells. They are a nonspecific finding.

Eosinophil Leukocytes

Most serous fluids contain at least the occasional eosinophil leukocyte, which is recognizable in toluidine blue–stained wet films and Papanicolaou-stained preparations [▮*19.3*]. They are slightly larger than neutrophils and their nuclei are usually bilobed. In wet films their cytoplasmic granules are almost colorless. In Papanicolaou-stained smears the cytoplasmic granules are much less obvious, being manifested only by a fine eosinophilic granularity. Eosinophils should, however, be readily recognizable as such by their size and the bilobation of their nuclei.

A serous fluid in which 10% or more of its cells are eosinophils may be regarded as "eosinophilic." Eosinophilic pleural effusions may occur in a wide variety of conditions. A high proportion is associated with thoracic trauma, eg, accidents, thoracotomy, therapeutic pneumothorax, and repeated aspiration of pleural fluid. Perhaps air introduced into the pleural cavity (pneumothorax) by such events contains allergens that stimulate an eosinophilic reaction in the pleura. When pneumothorax can be excluded, the most common causes of eosinophilic pleural effusion appear to be pulmonary infarct, pneumonia, and neoplasm. Only a minority of cases can be attributed to recognizable hypersensitivity states, which include parasitic infections. The cause of a substantial residue of eosinophilic pleural effusions cannot be identified. These are termed idiopathic eosinophilic pleural effusions and, given time, they spontaneously disappear.

Eosinophilic pericardial and peritoneal effusions are rare and they, too, may be associated with a wide variety of underlying conditions. An eosinophilic peritoneal dialysate may be attributable to a hypersensitivity reaction caused by one or more agents used for peritoneal dialysis, such as antiseptics and particles of tubing.

Lymphoid Cells

Almost all serous fluids contains at least a few lymphoid cells, readily recognizable in wet films and Papanicolaou-stained preparations [▮*19.4*]. The nuclei of mature lymphocytes are neatly round, although some may be slightly indented or notched. Nucleoli may be impossible to find in Papanicolaou-stained smears, although they are readily found in wet films. A fluid containing large numbers of mature lymphocytes is also likely to contain a few larger, less mature forms in which the chromatin is more pale and the nucleoli are more visible. Lymphocytes seem to possess little or no cytoplasm in routine preparations. Plasma cells may also be found in fluids containing lymphocytes.

An important property of lymphoid cells is their tendency to remain separated from each other. Lymphocytes may touch each other, but the contact, reminiscent of a kiss, involves only a small segment of the periphery of each cell. Unlike a fluid that contains numerous neutrophils, it is difficult to find a necrotic lymphocyte in a fluid that contains numerous benign lymphoid cells. (In contrast, neoplastic lymphoid cells in serous effusions frequently exhibit necrosis.) Most lymphoid cells in benign effusions are of T cell origin. T and B lymphocytes cannot be distinguished in routine preparations, but can be identified by immunologic methods.

An effusion dominated by benign lymphoid cells is a manifestation of chronic inflammation, which may be secondary to a variety of underlying conditions. Most lymphocytic effusions are pleural, and the underlying cause is usually pneumonia or neoplasm (which stimulates a chronic inflammatory reaction of the overlying pleura). Tuberculous pneumonia is a well recognized cause of lymphocytic pleural effusion; other types of pneumonia may also stimulate a lymphocytic inflammatory reaction of the overlying pleura, resulting in effusion. Apart from lymphocytic effusions associated with a miscellany of underlying conditions, a certain number have no recognizable cause.

Macrophages

Macrophages (histiocytes) are found in various proportions in almost every serous fluid. Their diameter ranges from about 15 to 100 μm, with most within the range of 20 to 40 μm. In wet films and smears the typical macrophage is identified by its size, eccentric bean-shaped or round nucleus, and lightly stained "lacy" cytoplasm bound by a delicate cell membrane [❚*19.5*]. The cytoplasm may contain phagocytosed leukocytes, nuclear particles, red blood cells, melanin, or hemosiderin. Macrophages tend to be discrete, although they may coalesce because of their long microvilli becoming entangled.

Macrophages may contain large solitary or multiple cytoplasmic vacuoles that seem to displace the nucleus to the periphery of the cell; such cells simulate adenocarcinoma cells with mucin-distended cytoplasm.

Most macrophages in serous effusions have a single nucleus, although binucleation is not uncommon. The presence of giant multinucleated macrophages is a rarity, virtually confined to effusions caused by rheumatoid pleuritis or rheumatoid pericarditis. Giant multinucleated mesothelial cells are far more common and may be mistaken for macrophages. The presence of large numbers of macrophages in the serous effusion is a nonspecific finding. Usually they are one of the cellular components of a mixed inflammatory picture.

Mesothelial Cells

Under normal circumstances, mesothelial cells form a flat monolayer. However, when an effusion develops they exfoliate, often in large numbers, as single cells and as clusters of cells. Exfoliated mesothelial cells continue to proliferate, since they are in a natural medium. In fact, in cytologic practice the benign cell most likely to contain a mitotic figure is the mesothelial cell.

The prototypical mesothelial cell is round, about 25 μm in diameter, and has a single central or slightly eccentric nucleus. The cytoplasm is dense and with the Papanicolaou stain exhibits various shades of blue-green, greenish-gray, and red-orange, depending on the type and timing of the EA stain and the thickness of the smear. It tends to fade at the periphery, imparting a slightly foamy appearance to the cell membrane. The nucleus is round or oval and possesses a well-defined, smoothly contoured membrane. The chromatin is uniformly granular and the nucleolus is readily identified [❚*19.6*-❚*19.8*].

Mesothelial cells vary considerably in size, from about 10 to 70 μm in diameter. The smallest mesothelial cells have scanty cytoplasm, whereas the giant forms have abundant cytoplasm and many nuclei [❚*19.9*]. They may be mistaken for giant multinucleated macrophages; however, the density and staining reaction of their cytoplasm denote their mesothelial nature.

Mesothelial cells may show cytoplasmic vacuolization, which may take several forms: a large solitary vacuole that seems to displace the nucleus, one or more tiny inconspicuous vacuoles scattered throughout the cytoplasm but more likely to be near the nucleus, and a small perinuclear vacuole that curves around the nucleus.

Mesothelial cells articulate with each other in a characteristic manner. One form of articulation consists of cells joined to each other at apposing surfaces. Between the conjoined cells, clefts or "windows" may develop, suggesting that the cells are about to become detached from each other [❚*19.8*]. Mesothelial cells may also form large flat mosaic sheets, a type of articulation much more readily seen in peritoneal washings than in spontaneously occurring effusions. Another type of articulation is illustrated [❚*19.7*], where the cytoplasm of one cell appears to be grasping an adjacent cell. This picture is carried to the extreme when one mesothelial cell seems to completely embrace another mesothelial cell.

Mesothelial cells readily undergo hypertrophy and hyperplasia in response to a wide variety of stimuli, such as inflammation of a serous membrane, inflammation or necrosis of an underlying organ, or the presence of a foreign substance in the serous cavity such as blood or air. Any long-standing, noninfected effusion, such as may occur in the peritoneal cavity in hepatic cirrhosis, may contain hypertrophic and hyperplastic mesothelial cells. It is not possible to tell from microscopic examination of such cells what the stimulus was that gave rise to their hypertrophy and hyperplasia. The clinical background may provide such information.

Mesothelial cells are frequently referred to as being "atypical" or "reactive," inappropriate designations for cells that are merely hypertrophic and usually hyperplastic. Furthermore, mesothelial cells in smears that are not well spread and well stained, especially when the fluid is bloody, may appear dark, thereby creating diagnostic uncertainty; hence the use of the term "atypical." This term is misleading since clinicians may interpret it as signifying a stage in the development of mesothelial neoplasia.

Specimens obtained by peritoneal washing or culdocentesis frequently contain large, flat mosaic sheets of mesothelium [❚*19.10*]. The size alone of these mesothelial fragments indicates that they are benign and detached either by surgical trauma or the washing procedure. Furthermore, the absence of nuclear features of malignancy indicates their benignity. Such specimens may contain spheroids, ellipsoids, or papillations composed of light green homogeneous acellular collagen surrounded by a group of mesothelial cells [▮*19.11*]. Such a formation, termed a "collagen ball," may be mistaken for a fragment of adenocarcinoma containing mucin-distended cytoplasm.

Megakaryocytes

Megakaryocytes are rarely seen in serous fluids. Their presence is usually a consequence of bone marrow being replaced by fibrous connective tissue or neoplasm, resulting in the formation of foci of extramedullary hematopoiesis in various organs, including the subserosal connective tissue. Should an effusion develop in a patient with extramedullary hematopoiesis, the fluid may contain megakaryocytes.

Detached Ciliary Tufts

Fluid obtained from the peritoneal cavity of females by laparotomy, laparoscopy, or culdocentesis or by a peritoneal catheter may contain tiny ciliated fragments of cytoplasm exfoliated from the fimbriated end of a fallopian tube. These fragments, referred to as detached ciliary tufts (DCTs), are extremely difficult to find in Papanicolaou-stained smears; they are however, easily recognized in stained wet films [▮*19.12*]. When the fluid is fresh, DCTs may exhibit a jerky rotatory and linear movement. Because of this, they have been mistaken for parasites. DCT formation is a physiologic phenomenon, quite different from ciliocytophthoria, which is a degenerative phenomenon. Cells exhibiting ciliocytophthoria frequently contain eosinophilic cytoplasmic granules and a nucleus; DCTs contain neither.

NON-NEOPLASTIC EFFUSIONS

Nonspecific Inflammation

Inflammation of a serous membrane is frequently a complication of a lesion in an underlying organ. For example, carcinoma of the lung may induce inflammation of the surrounding pulmonary parenchyma, which, in turn, may result in inflammation of the overlying pleura, the condition of pleurisy. This may result in the formation of a pleural effusion. Effusions that develop because of circulatory disturbances, such as congestive heart failure, may be sterile at their inception; in time, however, they may become infected, resulting in a fluid showing an inflammatory cytologic picture. Such inflammatory pictures are nonspecific in that it is not possible to discern from them what causes the inflammation. To determine this may require full knowledge of the clinical background.

Inflammation of serous membranes presents as two extremes: one cytologic picture consists entirely of neutrophilic leukocytes and the other consists of lymphoid cells—acute and chronic inflammation, respectively. Between these two extremes are cytologic pictures containing a mixture of the two types of cells, with or without modification by macrophages.

Furthermore, inflammation of a serous membrane may cause mesothelial cells to undergo hypertrophy and hyperplasia and to exfoliate in large numbers; such altered mesothelial cells may, therefore, accompany the inflammatory picture. On the other hand, inflammation of a serous membrane frequently results in exudation of fibrin, visible in smears as long, thin, cyanophilic strands. Fibrin may become so widely deposited over the mesothelium that it prevents mesothelial cells from exfoliating.

Specific Inflammatory Pictures

Rheumatoid Disease

Patients with rheumatoid arthritis develop granulomatous inflammation of the synovium lining their joints, characterized by a palisade of elongated macrophages, which may be accompanied by giant multinucleated macrophages. Patients with rheumatoid arthritis occasionally develop inflammation of the pleura or pericardium, characterized by the same type of inflammatory picture. In any resultant effusion the cytologic picture is that of elongated multinucleated macrophages [▮*19.13*], multinucleated giant round or oval macrophages, and a background of orangeophilic or cyanophilic (depending on the stain) granular particles [▮*19.14*], the product of the disintegration of macrophages that have undergone necrosis.

This triad of elongated spindle-shaped macrophages, multinucleated giant macrophages, and necrotic granular background material is pathognomonic of rheumatoid pleuritis or pericarditis. The picture has not been described in peritoneal fluid. The complete cytologic triad may not be present in every diagnosable specimen. For example, some specimens are dominated by the granular necrotic material and may contain few or none of the other two elements. However, even without the incomplete cytologic picture it may be possible to make a definite diagnosis of a rheumatoid effusion. It is important to diagnose rheumatoid pleuritis or pericarditis cytologically; otherwise, the patient may undergo extensive further investigation, including thoracotomy, to find out the cause of the effusion, or may be subjected to useless therapy, such as therapy against tuberculosis.

Systemic Lupus Erythematosus

Systemic lupus erythematosus (SLE), an autoimmune disease, is characterized by an excess of circulating antinuclear antibody. This causes the nuclei of some neutrophilic leukocytes to become swollen and homogenized to form a dense, smooth cyanophilic particle about the size of a leukocyte. Such particles when found in tissue or in serous fluids are referred to as hematoxylin bodies. A neutrophilic leukocyte that has phagocytosed a hematoxylin body is known as a lupus erythematosus (LE) cell [▮*19.15*]. Frequently the patient with SLE is young and female. Therefore, when examining a fluid from such a patient where the cause of the effusion is not obvious, careful search should be carried out for LE cells. It should be noted that LE cells will not be found in fluids that are devoid or almost devoid of neutrophilic leukocytes, although they need not dominate the cytologic picture for LE cells to be present.

In many serous fluids it is possible to find small macrophages that have phagocytosed a nucleus. Such cells, termed "tart cells" after the name of a patient in whom they were first observed, should not be mistaken for LE cells. In tart cells the phagocytosed nuclei are far from being perfectly homogeneous, whereas in LE cells they are homogeneous or almost completely homogeneous.

Miscellaneous Conditions

Congestive heart failure is frequently accompanied by a serous effusion, especially pleural effusion. Initially, such effusions are typically transudates, although if inflammatory complications set in, the fluid becomes an exudate. Consequently, the cellularity of such effusions varies considerably, ranging from effusions with few cells that are mainly mesothelial cells and macrophages to those that exhibit numerous neutrophilic leukocytes or lymphocytes. This cytologic picture is nonspecific.

Pneumonia may be accompanied by pleural effusion, and if the pneumonia is caused by bacteria the effusion is likely to contain numerous neutrophils. As the inflammation becomes chronic the cytologic picture may change to one of lymphocytes. Viral pneumonias are characterized by effusions containing numerous lymphoid cells.

Infarct implies necrosis of tissue owing to its blood supply being cut off. When infarcted tissue is covered by mesothelium, the mesothelial surface usually becomes inflamed, resulting in effusion. Depending on the degree of inflammatory reaction that takes place on the overlying mesothelium, the cytologic picture in any resultant effusion is variable, ranging from that of acute inflammation (neutrophils) to that of chronic inflammation (lymphoid cells), with or without the accompaniment of numerous hypertrophic and hyperplastic mesothelial cells.

Pneumothorax, the condition of air in the pleural cavity, may be accompanied by pleural effusion, the condition of hydropneumothorax. The presence of air in the pleural cavity may be the cause of the eosinophilia that is often seen in such effusions.

Tuberculosis of the lung typically produces a pleural effusion in which virtually all cells are lymphoid, with very few or no mesothelial cells. The scarcity or absence of mesothelial cells may be attributed to the deposition of fibrin on the pleural surface, which forms a barrier to exfoliation. In fact, the presence of mesothelial cells in a pleural effusion should be regarded as evidence against a tuberculous causation. Tuberculous effusions may become secondarily infected, in which case the cytologic picture may become dominated by neutrophils.

In tuberculous pericarditis the cytologic picture is similar to that of tuberculous pleuritis. In tuberculous peritonitis, lymphoid cells are likely to predominate, although they may be mixed with macrophages, neutrophils, and mesothelial cells. In this situation, the presence of mesothelial cells does not exclude peritoneal tuberculosis.

Patients with hepatic cirrhosis frequently develop a long-standing sterile transudative peritoneal effusion. Because of the long-standing nature of the effusion, it may contain numerous hypertrophied and hyperplastic mesothelial cells. A general attitude prevails that cytologic interpretation of such fluids is unusually difficult. This should not be the case since mesothelial cells in these fluids are no different morphologically from mesothelial cells elsewhere. Careful attention to their morphologic features will reveal that the cells are truly mesothelial rather than those of a metastatic neoplasm.

Parasitic, Fungal, and Viral Infections

Although parasitic infections are widespread throughout the world, seldom do we see evidence of such infection in serous fluids in a North American practice. In 35 years of operation, we have seen the following parasites in pleural or peritoneal fluid: *Echinococcus granulosus*, *Paragonimus westermani*, *Strongyloides stercoralis*, and *Trichomonas* species. Parasitic infection of a serous fluid is especially well displayed by the use of toluidine blue–stained wet films.

Disseminated fungal disease is virtually confined to immunosuppressed patients, patients with indwelling venous or peritoneal catheters, or patients with artificial heart valves. In view of the large number of patients who are now immunosuppressed, it is surprising that fungi are not seen in serous fluids more frequently. In our laboratory, we have seen examples of candidiasis, cryptococcosis, coccidioidomycosis, aspergillosis, and North American blastomycosis manifested in serous effusions.

While viral infections, especially of the lung, undoubtedly may stimulate the formation of a serous effusion, the finding of cells in an effusion that show clear morphologic evidence of viral infection is a rarity. We have seen only two convincing examples, both of which were pleural specimens containing classic herpetic virocytes.

Fistula

Fistulas are abnormal connections between surfaces lined by epithelium or mesothelium, or by epithelium and mesothelium. Consequently, when one end of a fistula is connected to a serous cavity that contains an effusion, a bizarre cytologic picture may result because of the presence of cells that normally have no access to the serous cavity. The most striking of the cytologic pictures is one that contains vegetable cells, as, for example, in a patient with a gastropleural fistula [▮*19.16*].

Endometriosis

Endometriosis, the presence of endometrium-like tissue outside the uterine cavity, is frequently found in ovaries and, to a lesser extent, on the pelvic peritoneum. Consequently, peritoneal washings may be submitted to the laboratory with a request that they be examined for endometrial cells. The diagnosis of endometriosis from such specimens is fraught with difficulty because individual endometrial stromal cells may resemble macrophages or lymphocytes and endometrial epithelial cells may resemble mesothelium. The most convincing cytologic evidence of pelvic endometriosis lies in a cell block specimen containing tissue fragments composed of epithelial and stromal cells like those found in endometrium.

Curschmann's Spirals

Curschmann's spirals have rarely been found in spontaneously occurring serous effusion and peritoneal washings. Their presence could be attributed to epithelial mucus secreted by neoplastic cells in the fluid or to connective tissue mucin that leaked from the submesothelial connective tissue into the serous effusion.

Ferruginous Bodies

Rare examples of ferruginous bodies, typical of true asbestos bodies, have been described in pleural fluid. The only way they could get into the pleural fluid would be by a fistulous connection between the respiratory tract and the pleural cavity or by a thoracentesis needle inadvertently penetrating pulmonary parenchyma.

Radiation Reaction

Well-documented and convincing accounts of radiation reaction in mesothelial cells in serous fluids do not exist. Anecdotal cases have been recorded, although in these examples the enlargement of mesothelial cells that was illustrated could have resulted from a variety of stimuli known to cause hypertrophy of mesothelial cells.

NEOPLASTIC EFFUSIONS

Generally, the identification of neoplastic cells in serous effusions is not too difficult. Their identification depends on knowing the range of deviation of cells that would be considered normal to the specimen. With the exception of mesotheliomas and a few ovarian carcinomas, neoplastic cells have a totally different appearance from the benign cells that accompany them.

Not all malignant cells in serous effusions display the classic morphologic features of malignancy, such as large size, high nuclear/cytoplasmic ratio, large, hyperchromatic, and irregularly shaped nuclei, prominent nucleoli, and abnormal mitotic figures. For example, the cells of oat cell carcinomas and some adenocarcinoma are small; frequently mesotheliomas and adenocarcinomas have a low nuclear/cytoplasmic ratio; and the nuclei of mesotheliomas and some adenocarcinomas are not hyperchromatic or irregular in shape. The diagnosis of neoplasm in a serous fluid depends on a constellation of morphologic features that allows one to determine that the cells are alien to the type of specimen, an observation that, with few exceptions, denotes that the cells are cancerous.

Supplementary methods can be applied to neoplastic cells in serous effusions, such as electron microscopy and histochemical stains; seldom, however, are they of any practical value. The supplementary technique most widely applied to cells in serous effusions, especially in cell block preparations, is immunocytochemistry. This has proven especially useful in discriminating between cells of mesothelioma and adenocarcinoma and in deciding whether nonpigmented neoplastic cells are those of an amelanotic melanoma.

Most neoplasms in serous fluids can be classified by type, such as adenocarcinoma, lymphoma, oat cell carcinoma, squamous cell carcinoma, and melanoma. However, trying to determine from which organ they arose is a much less successful exercise. With experience it is sometimes possible to deduce the origin of an adenocarcinoma from cells exfoliated into an effusion, especially when given the age and sex of a patient, but there are always cases where the deduction turns out to be wrong. From a practical point of view this is largely a redundant exercise, since the clinical background usually provides the best evidence as to the primary site of the neoplasm.

Adenocarcinoma

Most adenocarcinoma cells in serous fluids originate from neoplasms of breast, lung, or ovary. They may show the classic features of adenocarcinoma: a tendency to form large, smoothly contoured clusters composed of cells with eccentric, malignant-appearing nuclei, prominent nucleoli, and vacuolated cytoplasm. However, adenocarcinomas in serous effusion exhibit great morphologic variation, not only in the size of the cells but also in their degree of organization, with some represented by large clusters whereas others are almost entirely isolated with little or no contact with each other.

Adenocarcinoma cells may be solitary, they may form clusters composed of only a few cells, or they may form large papillary fragments or spheroids composed of hundreds of cells. Well-circumscribed spheroids of adenocarcinoma composed of fairly uniform cells have been dubbed "proliferation spheres." They are most likely to be derived from metastatic carcinoma of breast. Proliferation spheres may be solid or hollow, as revealed by cell block preparations. If hollow, it is possible in smears to discern an emptiness when focusing up and down on the sphere, with the cells in the center being in two different focal planes.

Adenocarcinoma cells frequently are vacuolated, although in some specimens very few or none contain cytoplasmic vacuoles. Extensive cytoplasmic vacuolization is particularly common in carcinomas of the ovary and lung.

With some adenocarcinomas, the cytologic picture consists almost entirely of isolated cells, with only the occasional cluster. This is especially likely to be true with carcinoma of the stomach and some carcinomas of the breast, especially those of lobular type. Many gastric adenocarcinomas are characterized by cells of signet ring type, with a large cytoplasmic vacuole and an eccentric nucleus. Some adenocarcinoma cells may contain a tiny cytoplasmic vacuole with a central dense spot, like the bull's eye of a target. The vacuoles are lined by microvilli and the spot is mucus. Such cells are most frequently seen with adenocarcinomas of the breast, especially those of lobular type.

Squamous Cell Carcinoma

It is uncommon to find squamous carcinoma cells in a serous fluid. They are most likely to be found in pleural fluids and to have originated in primary neoplasms of the lung or upper respiratory tract. The most frequently found type of squamous carcinoma cell is a round cell with one or more central nuclei and nonkeratinizing cytoplasm [▮*19.17*], the malignant counterpart of a parabasal cell. The whole range of neoplastic squamous carcinoma cells may, however, be found in fluids, such as polygonal keratinizing carcinoma cells [▮*19.18*], fragments of keratin with or without barely visible nuclei, malignant pearls, and cells that exhibit no evidence of squamous differentiation. Occasional vacuolated squamous carcinoma cells may be found. If squamous carcinoma cells do not show clear evidence of keratinization, it is easy to overlook their squamous origin. One should expect, however, that in every example of metastatic squamous cell carcinoma in a serous fluid the patient will be known to have or have had squamous cell carcinoma.

Anaplastic Carcinoma

Anaplastic carcinomas in serous fluids are best exemplified by metastatic small cell anaplastic carcinoma (oat cell carcinoma) of lung. In smears stained by the Papanicolaou method, the cells appear discretely or in small clusters. The cells are small, about twice the size of lymphocytes; they show, however, a degree of nuclear angulation not seen in lymphoid cells [▮*19.19*]. Like lymphoid cells, they possess very little cytoplasm and many of the cells may seem to be composed entirely of hyperchromatic nuclei. An important distinction between these cells and those of non-neoplastic or neoplastic lymphoid cells is that oat cells exhibit genuine cohesion whereas lymphoid cells do not. Oat cells frequently form tiny chains with side arms coming off at various angles. Such a chain may resemble the silhouette of a vertebral column or a stack of coins. Oat cells also exhibit a characteristic type of articulation where one cell seems to be capping another, causing its nucleus to acquire a quarter moon shape. These configurations and the cells composing them are virtually diagnostic of metastatic bronchogenic oat cell carcinoma.

Other small cell anaplastic nonlymphomatous neoplasms, such as Wilms' tumor and neuroblastoma, may give a similar appearance, but the clinical background of these cases is entirely different. In general, the more anaplastic a carcinoma, the more likely are its cells to be devoid of cytoplasm and the configuration of the cells to resemble those of metastatic oat cell carcinoma.

Urothelial Carcinoma

Urothelial (transitional cell) carcinomas rarely produce an effusion containing carcinoma cells. The carcinoma cells in such effusions do not have any distinctive characteristics and, to some extent, may resemble mesothelial cells except that their nuclei show features of malignancy.

Melanoma

Patients with advanced melanomas frequently develop a serous effusion containing recognizable melanoma cells. Classically, melanoma cells in serous fluids are round, about the size or a little larger than mesothelial cells, and tend to be discrete, although clusters may be present. The cytoplasm is abundant and contains brown pigment. Nuclei are central or eccentric and may contain large nucleoli [▮*19.20*]. Some nuclei may contain a vacuole, which is an invagination of the cytoplasm.

A fluid containing numerous heavily pigmented melanoma cells may be chocolate brown, with a clear light yellow supernatant. Heavily pigmented melanoma cells are, however, the exception. Usually, melanoma cells contain just a light dusting of brown cytoplasmic pigment or no pigment at all. In some specimens of fluid all of the melanoma cells are amelanotic, although macrophages in the fluid specimen may contain melanin. In such cases the melanomatous nature of the neoplastic cells may be demonstrated by the use of immunocytochemistry, with the melanoma cells giving a positive reaction for S-100 and HMB-45. In addition, transmission electron microscopy may reveal melanosomes.

Diffuse Malignant Mesothelioma

Diffuse malignant mesothelioma is a rare neoplasm, but it has assumed considerable importance because of its relationship to the inhalation of asbestos. The neoplasm may develop in any serous cavity, with pleural mesotheliomas being by far the most common. Mesotheliomas develop simultaneously on both layers of mesothelium, first as tiny nodules that grow and later fuse to form a thick rind that obliterates the serous cavity. Diffuse malignant mesotheliomas are of two histologic types: epithelial and sarcomatous. When a mesothelioma consists of both types it is said to be biphasic. From the point of view of cytology, only the epithelial type of mesothelioma can be recognized as such in serous effusions. The sarcomatous type may exfoliate spindle-shaped neoplastic cells, but their mesothelial lineage is not obvious.

The diagnosis of mesothelioma in a serous effusion is a two-step process. First, the neoplastic cells have to be recognized as having a mesothelial lineage, which is usually not difficult to do since they faithfully reproduce the morphologic features of non-neoplastic mesothelial cells. Deciding that these cells are those of malignant neoplasm is more difficult, however, because cells exfoliated from mesotheliomas typically do not exhibit obvious nuclear features of malignancy. Instead, one has to rely on other cytologic features to make the diagnosis.

Mesothelioma cells in a serous fluid typically present as a large number of exfoliated cells that look mesothelial. Many cells are discrete but clusters of the cells are numerous. The individual cells are large, and their nuclear/cytoplasmic ratio may be quite low. Nuclei are round or oval with smooth contours and the chromatin is finely stippled. Nucleoli are prominent [❚*19.21*].

The diagnosis of malignant mesothelioma may not be immediately apparent; however, the profusion of cells, the large number of cell clusters, and the large average size of the cells is more than one would expect with mesothelial hypertrophy and hyperplasia. With experience, in most cases of mesothelioma the diagnosis of mesothelioma can be correctly made by cytology, which is most desirable because a cytologic diagnosis may eliminate the need for thoracotomy or laparotomy. This is especially important since malignant mesotheliomas have an unpleasant tendency to grow into thoracotomy or laparotomy scars.

Occasionally, it may be desirable to demonstrate that the cells of a mesothelioma in a serous fluid are not, in reality, the cells of metastatic adenocarcinoma. It is possible to apply immunocytochemistry to cell block material to discriminate between the two types of neoplasm. Typically, adenocarcinoma and mesothelioma give a positive reaction for cytokeratin. Adenocarcinomas give positive reactions for carcinoembryonic antigen, B72.3, and Leu M1, whereas mesotheliomas give negative reactions.

A serous effusion caused by mesothelioma may contain a high concentration of hyaluronic acid, which may increase the viscosity of the fluid so much that it has a honey-like consistency. Usually, the viscosity of such effusions is not so pronounced, but the discerning eye may recognize that the viscosity is increased by just agitating the fluid in a centrifuge tube and noticing how quickly it settles once the tube is held still.

Carcinoma of Lung

In a high proportion of pleural fluids containing cancer cells, the cells are derived from a primary carcinoma of the lung. In most cases they are adenocarcinomas, with the remainder being small cell anaplastic carcinomas or, less commonly, squamous cell carcinoma, both of which are discussed above. Some carcinomas of the lung defy precise histologic typing; nevertheless, when these carcinomas exfoliate into a serous fluid their morphologic features are essentially those of adenocarcinoma, and the neoplasms are thus classified. Consequently, the morphologic range of adenocarcinomas in serous fluids is quite broad, with one extreme represented by well-differentiated bronchioloalveolar cell carcinoma and the other by pleomorphic giant carcinoma.

The typical adenocarcinoma of the lung is characterized by large, obviously malignant cells that exhibit the classic features of adenocarcinoma. Many of the cells occur singly and are accompanied by large clusters, which may be papillary. The cells show various degrees of vacuolization. The most differentiated examples, those derived from bronchioloalveolar cell carcinomas, are composed of cells with a low nuclear/cytoplasmic ratio and vacuolated mucin-containing cytoplasm. At the other extreme are pleomorphic giant cell carcinomas, which exhibit morphologic features of adenocarcinoma when exfoliated into a serous fluid, such as a tendency of their cells to cluster and their nuclei to be eccentric, although cytoplasmic vacuolization may be absent.

Carcinoma of the Breast

In many cases of recurrent carcinoma of the breast, the first manifestation is a pleural effusion containing carcinoma cells. Such an effusion may not develop until a decade or more after treatment of the primary neoplasm. Breast carcinoma cells in the serous fluid are usually of medium to small size. One classic presentation consists of large, compact spheroids composed of hundreds of cells that are fairly uniform in shape and size [▮*19.22*]. Because of the compactness of these spheroids, it is usually impossible to discern the cytologic features of malignancy of individual cells, although careful inspection usually reveals isolated adenocarcinoma cells in the background between the spheres.

Cell block preparations reveal many of these so-called "proliferation spheres" to be hollow, a feature that can be discerned in smears by the rather empty appearance of the center of the sphere. Careful focusing reveals the cells in the center of a sphere to be in two different focal planes. These proliferation spheres are characteristic of duct cell carcinoma of the breast.

Lobular carcinomas are typically manifested by numerous small isolated cells that could be mistaken for small mesothelial cells or macrophages, especially the former. Apart from the great number of such cells, which are of uniform shape and size, careful examination of individual nuclei will reveal irregularity of shape, heavy nuclear membranes, and prominent nucleoli. Cells of lobular carcinomas frequently display a tiny cytoplasmic vacuole containing a dark spot [▮*19.23*]. The vacuole is lined by microvilli and the spot consists of mucus. Cells of lobular carcinomas also have a tendency to form small caterpillar-like chains similar to those seen with oat cell carcinoma [▮*19.24*]. The cells of lobular carcinoma of breast are quite different, however, in that they are larger and possess visible cytoplasm and visible nucleoli.

Carcinoma of the Ovary

Ovarian carcinoma is a frequent cause of ascites, which is often the first manifestation of the disease. The cytologic appearance of metastatic ovarian carcinoma in a serous fluid depends, to a large extent, on the histologic appearance of the carcinoma. Many examples consist of large, hypervacuolated carcinoma cells occurring singly [▮*19.25*] and in large papillary tissue fragments. Another common type consists of papillary tissue fragments [▮*19.26*] composed of smaller, more uniform, nonvacuolated cells, which may contain psammoma bodies. Psammoma bodies are usually difficult to find in Papanicolaou-stained smears, in which their staining reaction ranges from deep blue to red-orange. They are readily found in cell block preparations and stained wet films. In the latter they are seen as concentric laminated bodies that do not take up the toluidine blue stain [▮*19.27*]. One variant of ovarian adenocarcinoma consists of cells that are similar to mesothelial cells [▮*19.28*], a reflection of their origin from the mesothelium that invests the ovary.

Pseudomyxoma Peritonei

This is the condition of massive, mucoid ascites caused by disseminated, well-differentiated, mucin-secreting adenocarcinoma that originated in an ovary or the large intestine, particularly the appendix. Such fluids are extremely difficult to smear, and the carcinoma cells they contain are usually very sparse and difficult to identify as malignant because they are so well differentiated.

Carcinomas of the Gastrointestinal Tract

Advanced adenocarcinoma of the stomach frequently causes ascites in which the fluid contains numerous carcinoma cells, some with a large cytoplasmic vacuole that seems to displace the nucleus to the periphery of the cell, giving a so-called signet ring appearance [▮*19.29*].

Colonic adenocarcinomas may also cause ascites, although the fluid usually contains far fewer cells. In both gastric and colonic carcinomas, the background of the smears may contain streaks of mucus secreted by the carcinoma cells.

Miscellaneous Carcinomas

Apart from the types of carcinoma listed above, carcinoma cells arising from neoplasms in other organs are seen much less frequently in serous fluids, partly because of less frequent occurrence of these carcinomas and partly because their mode of spread does not include a serous cavity. Those that present as adenocarcinomas (as most do) seldom produce cells that can be said to be characteristic of a particular primary neoplasm.

Lymphoma and Leukemia

Serous effusion is a common complication of lymphoma and leukemia, especially the former. In almost every case, the patient is known to have the disease, although on a rare occasion the finding of lymphoma cells in a serous effusion may be the first morphologic manifestation of the condition.

An important aspect of lymphoma and leukemia cells in serous fluids is that they do not exhibit genuine attachment to each other. If such attachment can be found, the cells are neither lymphomatous nor leukemic. Another striking feature is that a high proportion of these cells frequently exhibit necrosis, a phenomenon rarely seen with carcinomas. The entire cell may appear as a faint, cyanophilic blob or the nucleus may become pyknotic or undergo fragmentation to form tiny round cyanophilic particles reminiscent of a dispersed drop of mercury, so-called mercury drop karyorrhexis.

Smears stained by the Papanicolaou method seem to achieve the same reliability in the identification of cells as lymphomatous or leukemic as smears stained by one of the routinely used hematologic (Romanowsky) stains. However, for the typing of leukemias and lymphomas in serous effusions, the latter method is superior. In reality, not being able to precisely type lymphoma or leukemia in a serous fluid is not of importance since the type is usually already known.

Cells of non-Hodgkin's lymphoma in a serous fluid frequently dominate the cytologic picture. The cells of low-grade (well-differentiated) lymphomas are exemplified by cells that are morphologically indistinguishable from benign lymphocytes; such cells may also be seen with chronic lymphocytic leukemia. Demonstrating their neoplastic nature may require flow cytometry to reveal their monoclonality.

Lymphoma cells of higher grades are generally not difficult to recognize. The cells are larger, as are their nuclei, which show various degrees of polymorphism, and their nucleoli are more prominent [▮*19.30*]. Necrosis of individual cells is more likely to occur and may dominate the cytologic picture. The cytologic extreme of high-grade lymphoma is manifested by large-cell immunoblastic lymphoma of the polymorphous type [▮*19.31*].

Myelomatosis is a low-grade lymphoma. Its cells are seldom seen in serous fluids. When present, they are numerous and they possess the morphologic features of plasma cells [▮*19.32*] but are larger, more often multinucleate, and possess prominent nucleoli.

The cells of all types of leukemia may be found in serous fluids. Morphologically they are similar to those of lymphomas, although they do not reach the size of the large cell high-grade lymphomas. Like lymphoma cells they are frequently necrotic.

Hodgkin's Disease

Generally, the cytologic picture is nonspecific. The only diagnostic feature of Hodgkin's disease in an effusion is the multinucleated Reed-Sternberg cell, which may be accompanied by the mononuclear variant known as a "Hodgkin's cell." However, effusions due to Hodgkin's disease usually do not contain either type of cell and when present they are in small numbers. Careful scrutiny of several smears may be required before finding one convincing example. The typical Reed-Sternberg cell is binucleate with the nuclei facing each other, like a mirror image, and nucleoli are prominent.

Neoplasms Rarely Seen in Serous Fluids

Almost every other type of malignant neoplasm may metastasize to a serous cavity, resulting in an effusion containing malignant cells. Since the incidence of these neoplasms is much less than those discussed above, the finding of their cells in a serous effusion is a rare event. Neoplasms of this category include nonlymphomatous sarcomas, neuroendocrine tumors, thymoma, nephroblastoma, neuroblastoma, and germ cell neoplasms. The cytomorphology of these neoplasms in serous fluids corresponds closely to that seen in histologic sections.

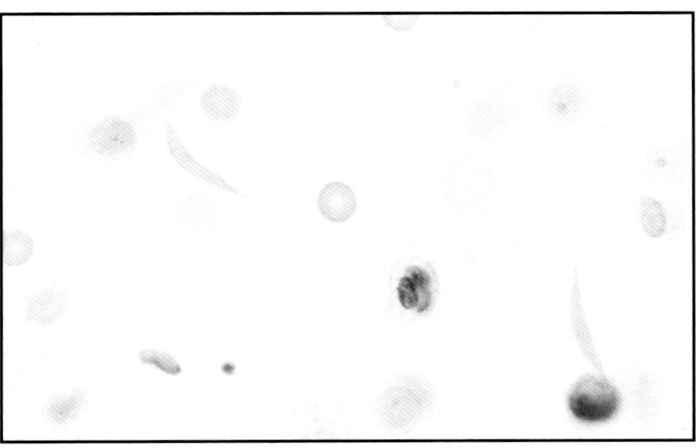

19.1
Pleural fluid. Sickled red blood cells. The patient did not have sickle cell anemia but had the sickle cell trait (Papanicolaou).

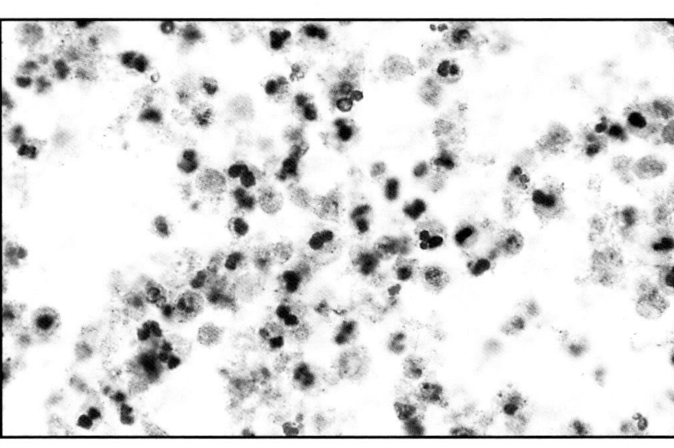

19.2
Pleural fluid. Viable and necrotic neutrophil leukocytes. The patient had empyema (Papanicolaou).

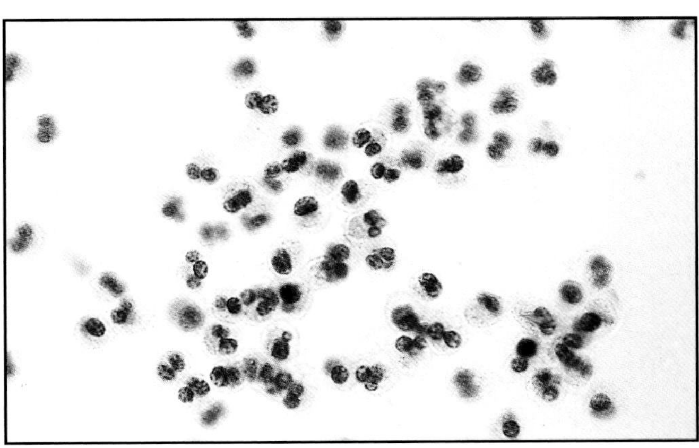

19.3
Pleural fluid. Most of the cells in this effusion are eosinophil leukocytes. The patient had bronchial asthma (Papanicolaou).

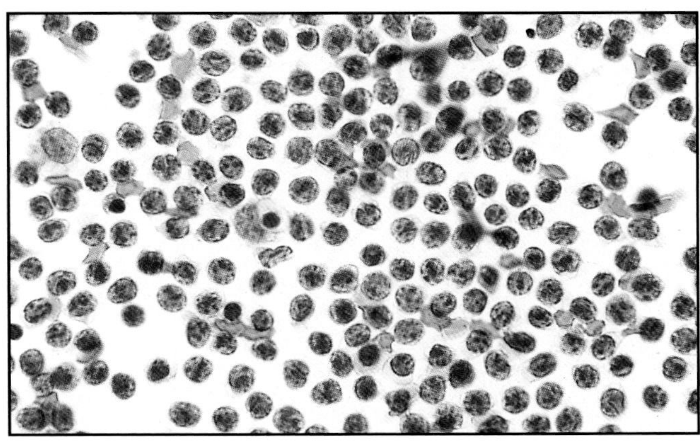

19.4
Pleural fluid. Lymphocytic effusion due to pulmonary tuberculosis. Virtually every cell in this field is a lymphocyte. The cells of chronic lymphocytic leukemia or well-differentiated lymphocytic lymphoma could look like these benign lymphoid cells (Papanicolaou).

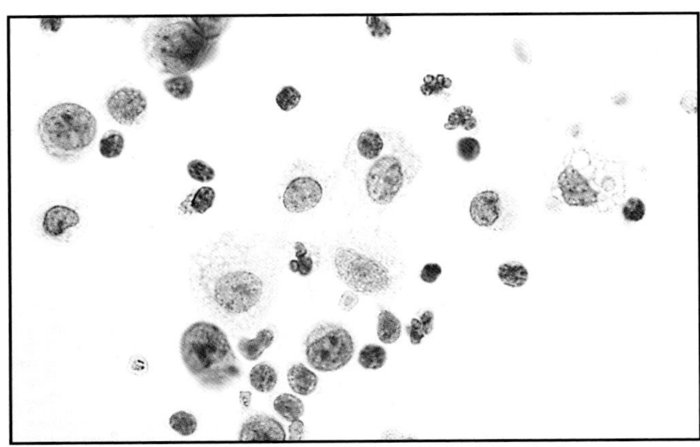

19.5
Peritoneal fluid. The larger cells with delicate, lacy cytoplasm are macrophages (Papanicolaou).

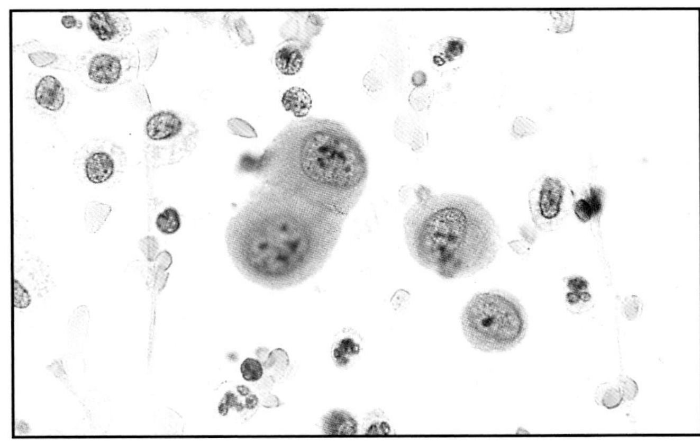

19.6
Pleural fluid. The large cells are mesothelial. The conjoined pair shows the characteristic articulation at flattened apposing surfaces (Papanicolaou).

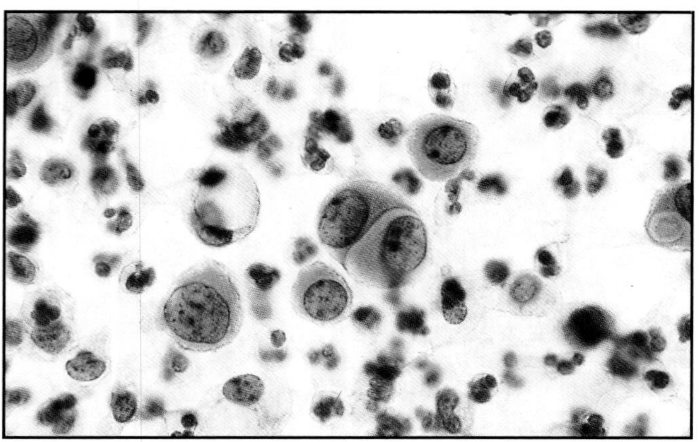

▌19.7

Pleural fluid. Mesothelial cells in an inflammatory background. The pair in the center shows the characteristic clasping type of articulation (Papanicolaou).

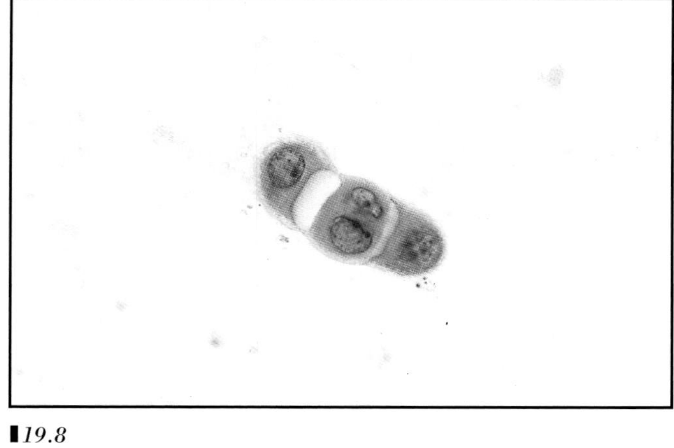

▌19.8

Pleural fluid. A chain of mesothelial cells illustrating intercellular "windows" (Papanicolaou). (From Comprehensive Cytopathology. *© 1991, WB Saunders Co.)*

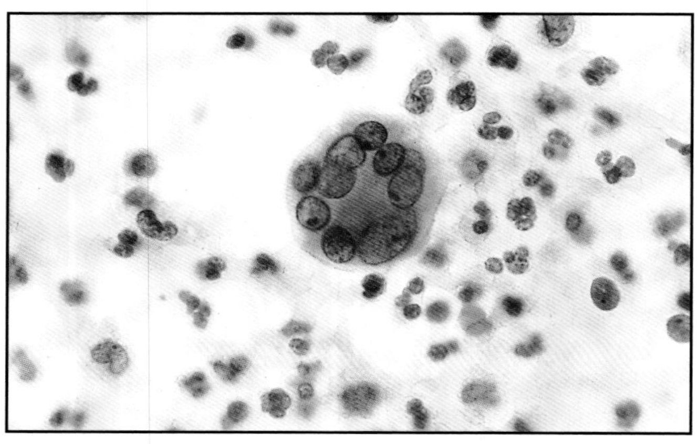

▌19.9

Pleural fluid. A giant multinucleated mesothelial cell. Focusing revealed this cell to have a least 15 nuclei (Papanicolaou).

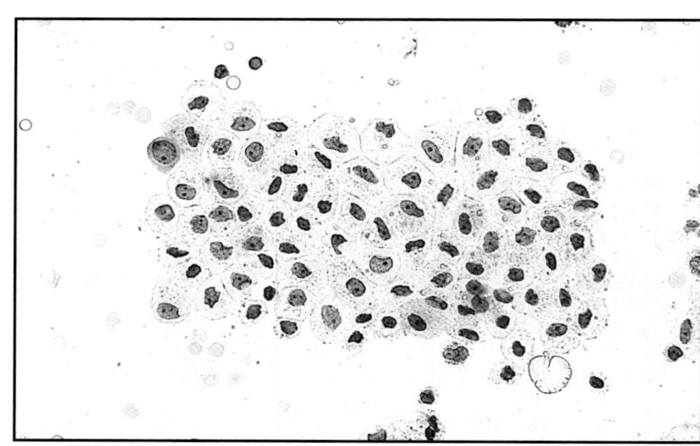

▌19.10

Peritoneal washing. A flat mosaic of mesothelial cells. Such a formation is commonly seen in peritoneal washings (toluidine blue–stained wet film).

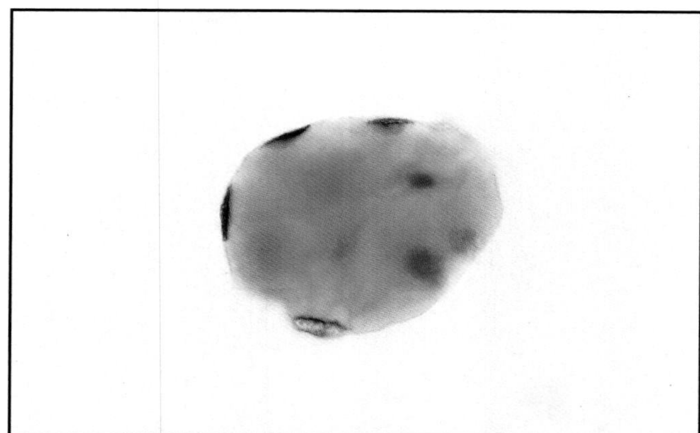

▌19.11

Peritoneal washing. A collagen ball, consisting of collagen covered by mesothelial cells. Such a formation may be detached from the surface of an ovary (Papanicolaou).

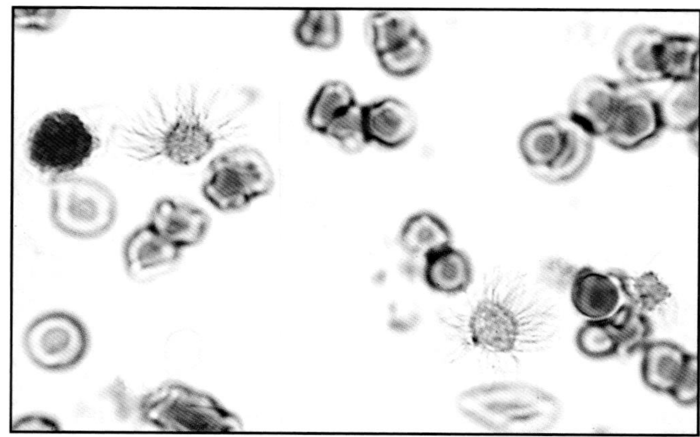

▌19.12

Peritoneal washing. Two detached ciliary tufts, consisting of particles derived from ciliated cells lining the fallopian tube (toluidine blue–stained wet film). (From Practical Guide to Surgical Pathology With Cytologic Correlations. *© 1992, Springer-Verlag NY Inc.)*

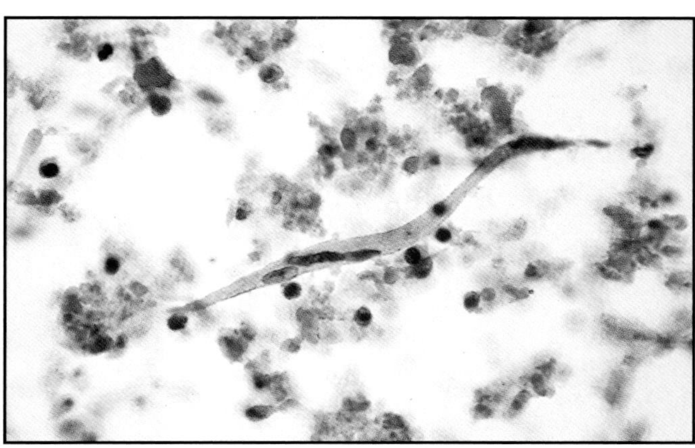

I19.13

Pleural fluid. Rheumatoid pleuritis. An elongated multinucleated macrophage in a background of granular material (Papanicolaou). (From Nosanchuk and Naylor. © 1968, Williams and Wilkins.)

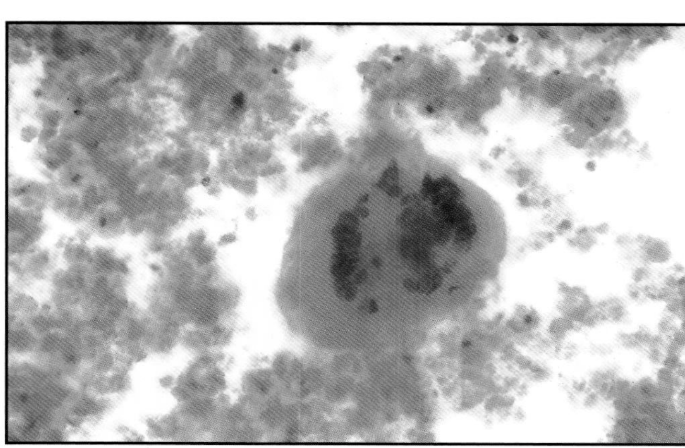

I19.14

Pleural fluid. Rheumatoid pleuritis. An oval multinucleated giant macrophage in a background of granular material (Papanicolaou).

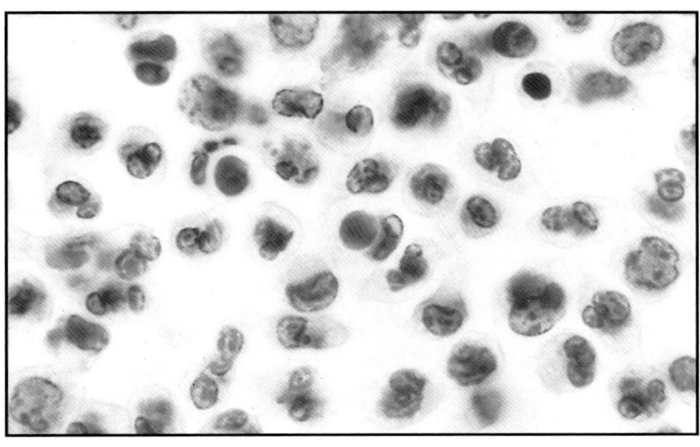

I19.15

Pericardial fluid. Lupus erythematosus cells (center and upper left). The phagocytosed material in the center cell is the more homogenized (Papanicolaou).

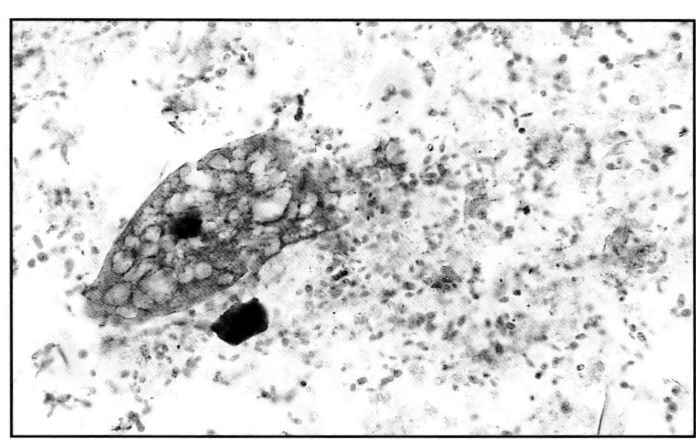

I19.16

Pleural fluid. A vegetable cell, a squamous epithelial cell, unidentified fungus, and amorphous granular material. The patient had a gastropleural fistula (Papanicolaou).

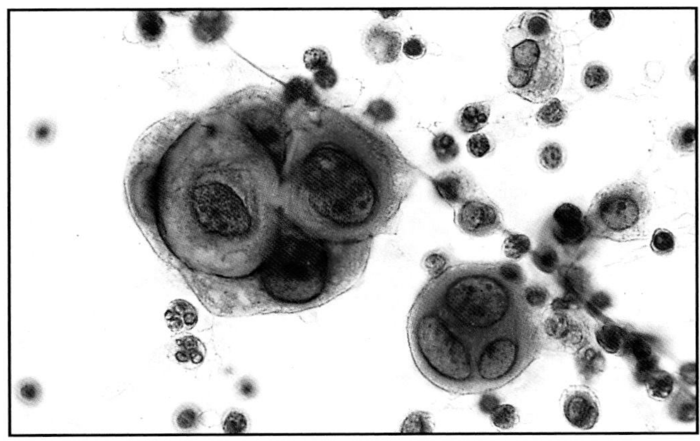

I19.17

Pleural fluid. Same specimen as I19.18. A tissue fragment composed of nonkeratinizing squamous carcinoma cells. The cells resemble a malignant form of parabasal squamous cell (Papanicolaou).

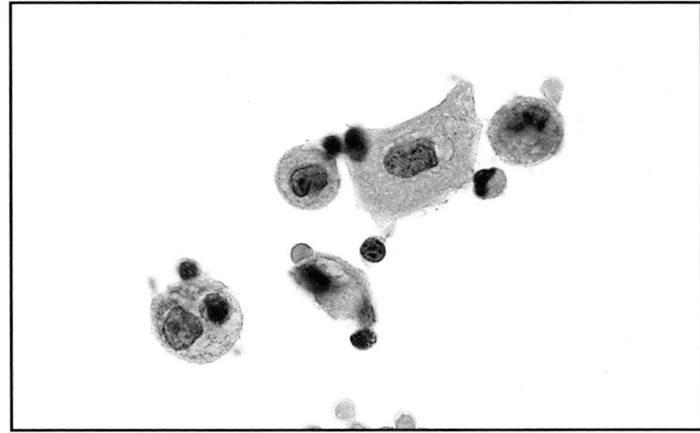

I19.18

Pleural fluid. A keratinizing polygonal squamous carcinoma cell. The patient had squamous cell carcinoma of the lung (Papanicolaou).

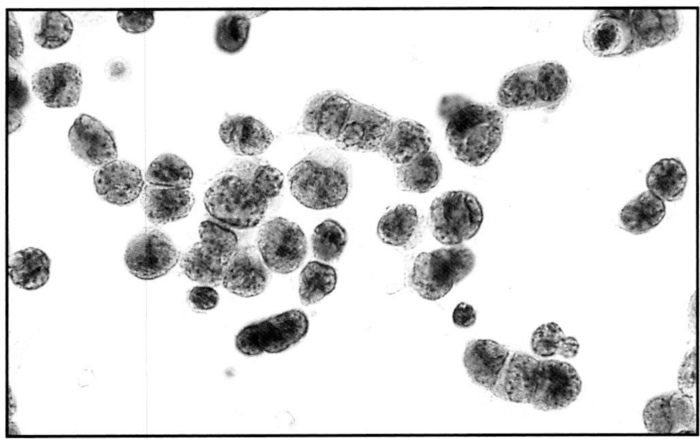

19.19

Pleural fluid. Small cell anaplastic (oat cell) carcinoma. The cells are small and possess little cytoplasm. They show the characteristic molding with formation of tiny chains (Papanicolaou).

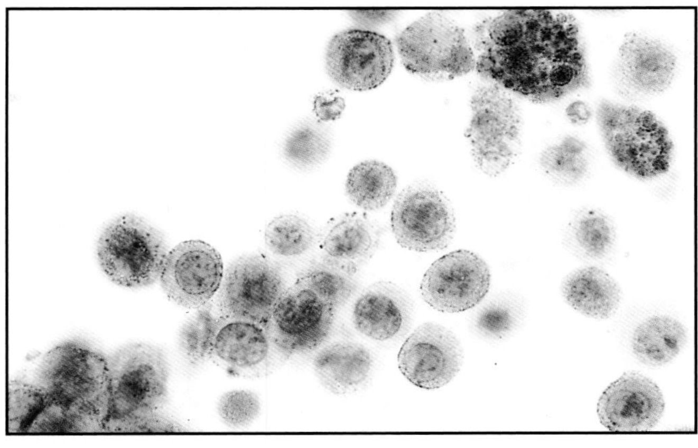

19.20

Peritoneal fluid. Pigmented cells of malignant melanoma. The primary neoplasm was in the skin. The heavily pigmented cells in the top right corner are probably melanin-containing macrophages (melanophages) (Papanicolaou).

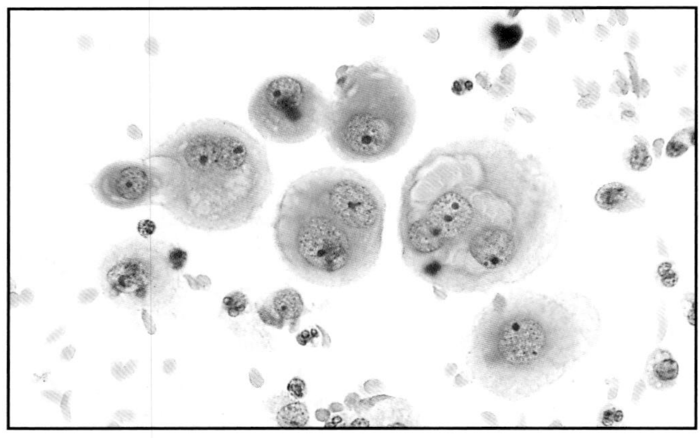

19.21

Pleural fluid. Diffuse malignant mesothelioma of epithelial type. These large cells show morphologic features of mesothelial cells. They are, however, much larger than benign mesothelial cells. The yellow cytoplasmic material in one of the cells is glycogen.

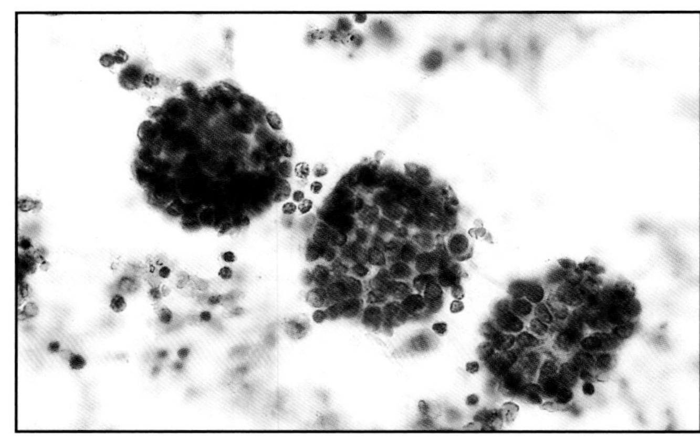

19.22

Pleural fluid. "Proliferation spheres" of metastatic carcinoma of the breast. Such formations are typical of some breast carcinomas, especially of ductal type. Focusing gives the impression of hollowness at the center of the balls of cells (Papanicolaou).

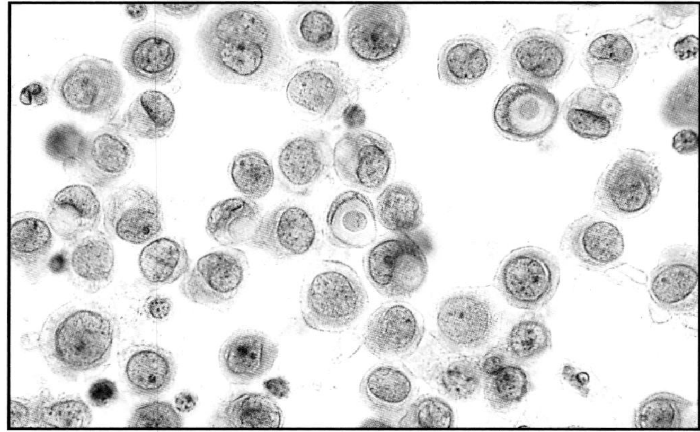

19.23

Peritoneal fluid. Virtually every cell in this field is metastatic lobular carcinoma of breast. The cells are small and mainly discrete. Several contain one or more cytoplasmic vacuoles in which there is a central globule of mucus (Papanicolaou).

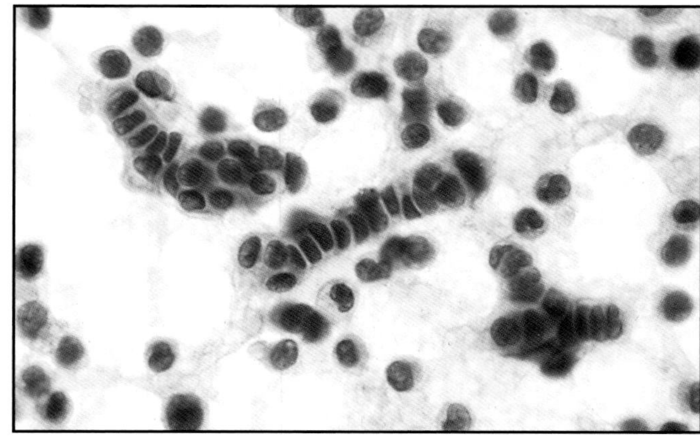

19.24

Pericardial fluid. A chain-like group of small adenocarcinoma cells. The patient had lobular carcinoma of the breast (Papanicolaou).

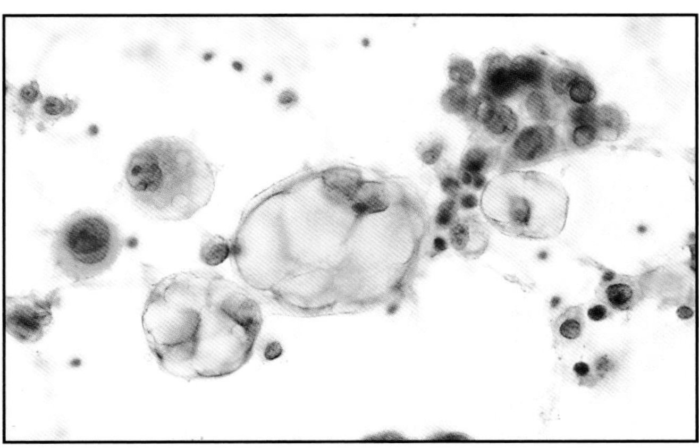

I19.25

Peritoneal fluid. Ovarian adenocarcinoma. These carcinoma cells vary considerably in size and degree of vacuolization. Elsewhere in the smear were large papillary fragments of carcinoma, many of them vacuolated (Papanicolaou).

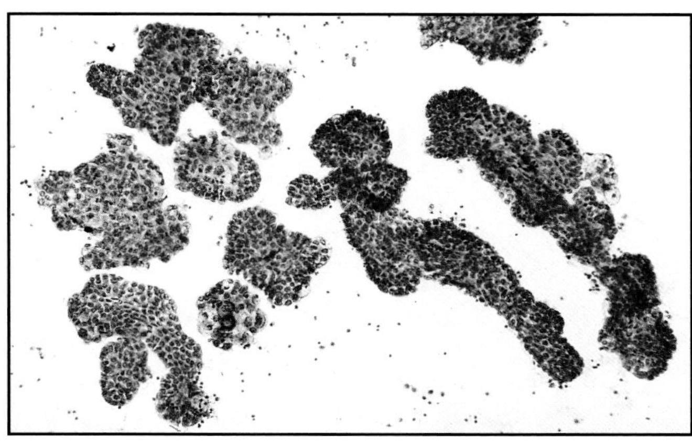

I19.26

Peritoneal fluid. Papillary fragments of serous cystadenocarcinoma of the ovary. These cells are much smaller and more uniform in size than those in I19.25 and very few are vacuolated (Papanicolaou).

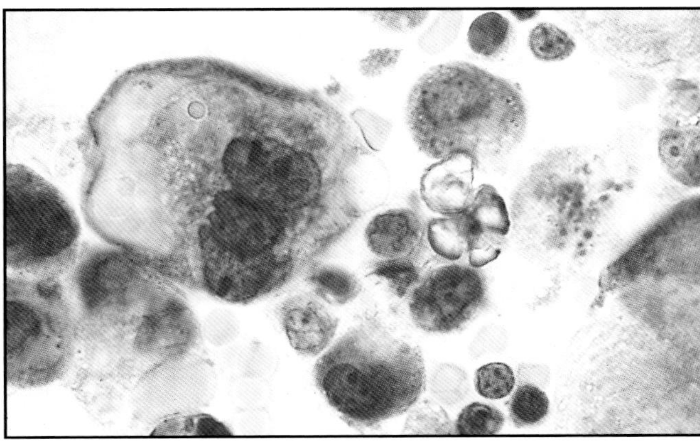

I19.27

Peritoneal fluid. Adenocarcinoma of ovary. One psammoma body in the field is revealed by its not taking up the stain. This psammoma body is fractured by the coverslip being pressed onto the slide (toluidine blue–stained wet film).

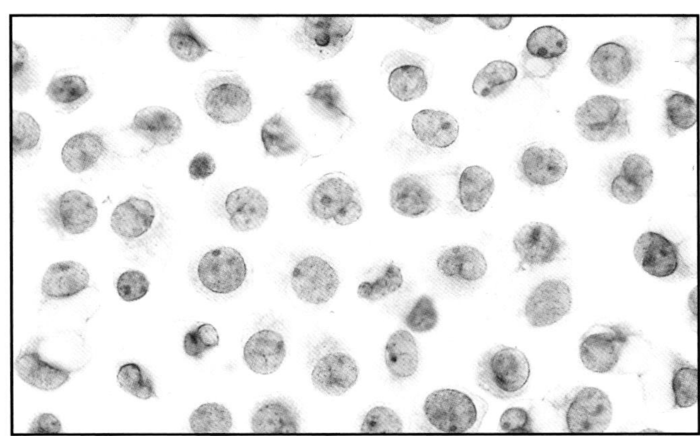

I19.28

Peritoneal fluid. Adenocarcinoma of the ovary. Virtually every cell in this field is an adenocarcinoma cell. They are fairly uniform in shape and size. The pronounced vacuolization of some of these cells reveals they are not mesothelial (Papanicolaou).

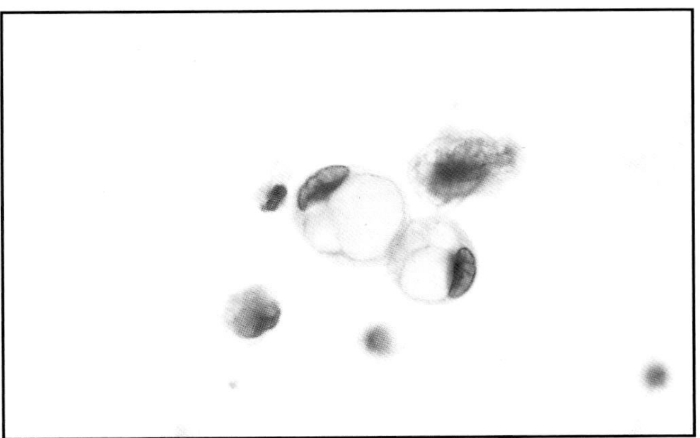

I19.29

Peritoneal fluid. Metastatic adenocarcinoma of the stomach. A pair of adenocarcinoma cells of signet ring type (Papanicolaou).

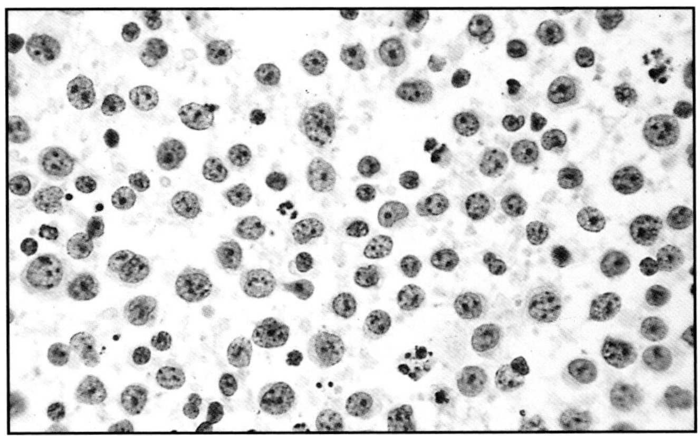

I19.30

Pleural fluid. Large cell lymphoma, intermediate grade. All the cells are discrete. Some are necrotic, as evidenced by nuclear fragmentation. The background consists of light gray particles, produced by disintegration of lymphoma cells (Papanicolaou).

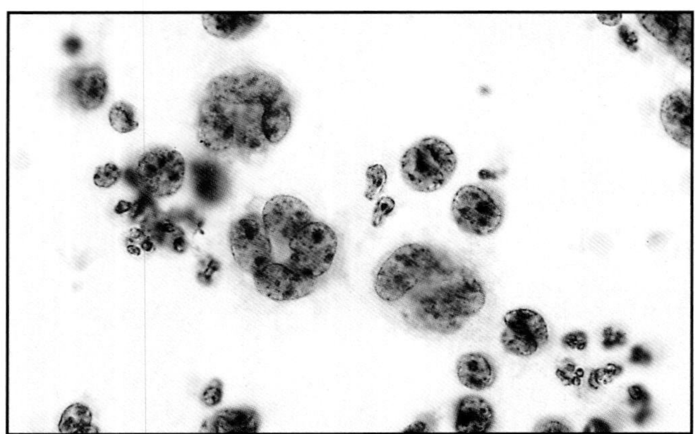

▌19.31

Pleural fluid. High-grade large cell immunoblastic lymphoma of the polymorphous type (Papanicolaou).

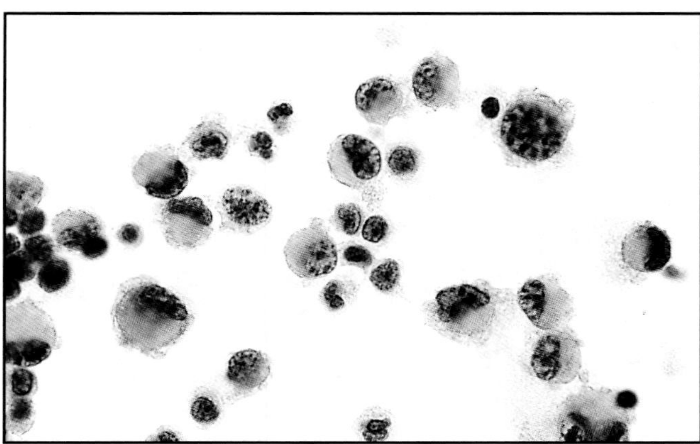

▌19.32

Pleural fluid. Plasmacytoma. These cells resemble plasma cells in that their nuclei are eccentric and exhibit tiny clumps of chromatin (Papanicolaou).

REVIEW EXERCISES

1. Which morphologic feature are the cells of diffuse malignant mesothelioma in a serous fluid likely to exhibit?
   a) Vacuolated cytoplasm
   b) Discreteness
   c) Finely stippled chromatin
   d) Multinucleation

2. Which of the following is least likely to exhibit widespread necrosis of cells in a serous effusion?
   a) Metastatic adenocarcinoma
   b) Pleural empyema
   c) Malignant lymphoma
   d) Rheumatoid pericarditis

3. The neoplasm most likely to be manifested as papillary tissue fragments in a serous fluid is metastatic
   a) carcinoma of breast.
   b) malignant lymphoma.
   c) melanoma of skin.
   d) carcinoma of ovary.

4. A specimen of peritoneal fluid that has a distinctly mucoid consistency is likely to be from a patient with
   a) peritoneal mesothelioma.
   b) pseudomyxoma peritonei.
   c) purulent peritonitis.
   d) metastatic carcinoma of breast.

5. Pleural fluid that contains giant multinucleated macrophages in a background of granular material is characteristic of
   a) rheumatoid pleuritis.
   b) tuberculous pneumonia.
   c) large cell lymphoma.
   d) esophagopleural fistula.

SELECTED READINGS

Ashton PR, Hollingsworth AS, Johnston WW. The cytopathology of metastatic breast cancer. *Acta Cytol.* 1975;19:1-6.

Johnston WW. The malignant pleural effusion: a review of cytopathologic diagnosis of 584 specimens from 472 consecutive patients. *Cancer.* 1985;56:905-909.

Kim K, Naylor B. *Practical Guide to Surgical Pathology With Cytologic Correlations: A Text and Color Atlas.* New York, NY: Springer-Verlag NY Inc; 1992.

Kumar NB, Naylor B. Megakaryocytes in pleural and peritoneal fluids: prevalence, significance, morphology, and cytohistological correlation. *J Clin Pathol.* 1980;33:1153-1159.

Naylor B. The pathognomonic cytologic picture of rheumatoid pleuritis. *Acta Cytol.* 1990;34:465-473.

Naylor B. Pleural peritoneal and pericardial fluids. In: Bibbo M, ed. *Comprehensive Cytopathology.* Philadelphia, Pa: WB Saunders Co; 1991:541-614.

Naylor B. Cytological aspects of pleural, peritoneal and pericardial fluids in patients with systemic lupus erythematosus. *Cytopathology.* 1992;3:1-8.

Nosanchuk JS, Naylor B. A unique cytologic picture in pleural fluid from patients with rheumatoid arthritis. *Am J Clin Pathol.* 1968;50:330-335.

Sidawy MK, Chandra P, Oertel YC. Detached ciliary tufts in female peritoneal washings: a common finding. Acta *Cytol.* 1987;31:841-844.

Smith-Purslow MJ, Kini SR, Naylor B. Cells of squamous cell carcinoma in pleural, peritoneal, and pericardial fluids: origin and morphology. *Acta Cytol.* 1989;33:245-253.

Spriggs AI, Boddington MM. *Atlas of Serous Fluid Cytopathology: A Guide to the Cells of Pleural, Pericardial, Peritoneal and Hydrocele Fluids.* In: Gresham GA, ed. Current Histopathology Series, vol 14. Dordrecht, the Netherlands: Kluwer Academic Publishers; 1989.

Veress JF, Koss LG, Schreiber K. Eosinophilic pleural effusions. *Acta Cytol.* 1979;23:40-44.

Whitaker D, Shilkin KB. Diagnosis of pleural malignant mesothelioma in life: a practical approach. *J Pathol.* 1984;143:147-175.

Wojcik EM, Naylor B. Collagen balls in peritoneal washings: prevalence, morphology, origin and significance. *Acta Cytol.* 1992;36:466-470.

CHAPTER 20

Aspiration Cytology

William J. Frable, MD, FIAC

CONTENTS

Aspiration cytology (aspiration biopsy, or fine needle aspiration biopsy) is now established in many parts of the United States. It is contributing significantly to timely diagnosis of both neoplastic and non-neoplastic disease and reducing the need for open surgical biopsy for many patients. The method of aspirating a cell sample from a tumor through a narrow-gauge needle was first described in the United States by Martin and Ellis in 1930. As Webb has documented, however, the history of this type of biopsy extends back to the mid-19th century, predating the invention of the rotary microtome for cutting tissue sections. Fueled by the experience of a group of Swedish clinicians trained chiefly in hematology and oncology, aspiration cytology has gained renewed recognition—in postwar Europe and throughout the next two decades within the United States. Contributing to the utility of this procedure has been its cost-effectiveness; the increased availability of well-trained cytopathologists; and major advances in radiologic imaging, namely, computed tomography, ultrasonography, and image-intensified fluoroscopy.

Since aspiration biopsy may be performed on any visible tumor mass or within any organ, the physician utilizing this procedure must be familiar with general anatomy, while both the cytotechnologist and cytopathologist are required to have a good knowledge of normal cell elements from a variety of organs and tissues as they appear in smears. This latter experience is best acquired by making touch imprints or studying aspiration samples from normal tissues submitted as routine surgical specimens or obtained during postmortem examinations.

Aspiration biopsy can be applied to practically all benign and malignant tumor types encountered in surgical pathology. A reference file of smear preparations is useful, whether obtained from touch imprints or from smears of neoplasms found at the surgical cutting table; cytotechnologists can profit from this reference file by increasing their knowledge of the variety of tumor cell types that are either not seen or only rarely found in exfoliative cytologic samples. Particular emphasis in this filing system should be placed on specimens of tumors from breast, lymph nodes, thyroid, salivary glands, lung, and liver since these are the common sites for fine needle aspiration biopsy.

FINE NEEDLE METHOD

I employ an aspiration biopsy method that uses a fine needle (22 and 23 gauge) with an external diameter of 0.6 to 1.0 mm. There have been recent variations in needle design: the Franseen type has a notched tip and stylus, and the side port needles have a slot in the side. The Franseen needle has a tendency to procure small microcores, while the slotted-side needles seem to result in a greater volume of aspirate when applied to hard solid tumors as may occur in the breast. The Chiba needle (21 and 22 gauge) is frequently used by radiologists for transthoracic and transabdominal aspirations. For bone lesions with an intact cortex, either a hole must be drilled through the cortex prior to aspiration or a bone marrow core biopsy needle must be employed. The larger the external diameter of the needle, the greater the likelihood of complications. The fine needle technique described here presents virtually no problems, except for transthoracic and, rarely, transabdominal aspiration.

Training and Planning

Prior to attempting aspiration biopsy a good knowledge of anatomy and some physical examination skills are necessary. Most "lumps and bumps" are superficially located, or at least in such a position that they are not directly in relation to potentially hazardous sites for biopsy. The aspiration should be planned in such a way that subsequent treatment is not compromised. When primary malignant tumors are aspirated the needle tract should be placed in a location that will be included in a subsequent excision.

Knowledge of the clinical problem of any patient undergoing needle aspiration biopsy is important. The surgical pathologist-cytopathologist is uniquely trained to perform needle aspiration biopsy because of his or her general interest in biopsy interpretation. The surgical pathologist-cytopathologist with a special interest in oncology should find the technique a useful and rewarding contribution to the care of patients with tumors. Pathologists should not be reluctant to consult with and examine patients, as this is the best way to obtain specific clinical information to help formulate an accurate biopsy diagnosis.

Basic Equipment

The following equipment is required for rapid and efficient performance of fine needle aspiration biopsy:

1. Cameco Syringe Pistol (Precision Dynamics Corp, San Fernando, Calif), Aspir-Gun (Everst Co, Linden, NJ), or other type aspiration handle
2. 10- or 20-mL disposable plastic syringe with Luer Lok Tip (Becton Dickinson and Co, Rutherford, NJ), depending on aspiration gun handle size
3. 22- to 23-gauge, 0.6- to 1.0-mm external diameter disposable needles, 3.8 cm and 8.8 cm, 15 and 20 cm long, with or without stylus
4. Alcohol prep sponges; Betadiene sponges for deeper aspirations of transabdominal, transthoracic, bone, or deep soft tissue
5. Sterile gauze pads
6. Microscopic glass slides with frosted ends
7. Small vial of balanced salt solution and/or RPMI tissue culture transport media

8. Vial of 50% alcohol for sample of aspirate for flow cytometry if needed
9. Suitable alcohol spray fixatives for immediate fixation of wet smears
10. Vial of local anesthesia, 1% to 2% lidocaine, is optional; topical spray anesthesia for aspirates in children or intraoral aspirates
11. Small vial of buffered glutaraldehyde for fixing aspirate for electron microscopy if required

A small plastic tray easily holds all the equipment. Local anesthesia is usually required for needle aspiration of transthoracic or transabdominal masses but is rarely necessary for other clinically palpable lumps. Aspiration biopsy is virtually nontraumatic. It may be repeated frequently enough to procure amounts of material for diagnostic purposes, special tests, flow cytometry, and immunohistochemistry for tumor markers.

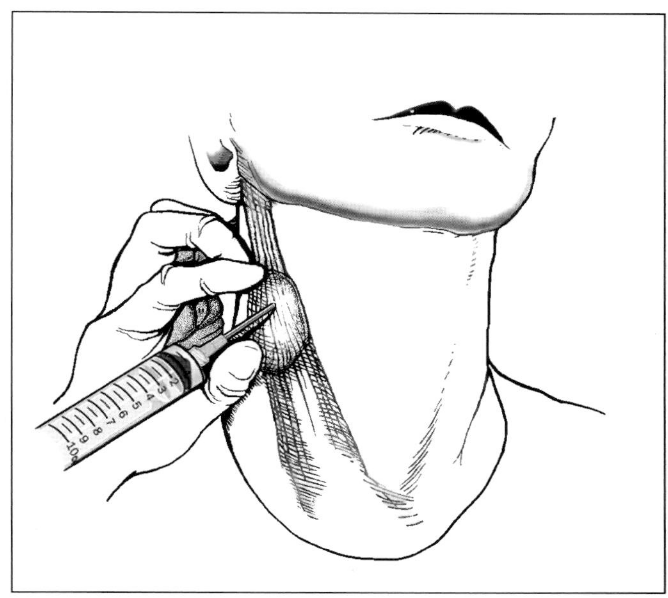

F *20.1*

Aspiration biopsy, enlarged cervical lymph node. With the needle in node, vacuum pressure is applied to the syringe by retracting the pistol trigger.

ASPIRATION TECHNIQUE

These preliminary steps need to be followed for successful aspiration biopsy:

1. Review the medical history of the patient and determine the clinical problem in relation to the lesion on which the biopsy is to be performed.
2. Decide whether the biopsy is justified.
3. Attempt to determine by palpation the location of the lesion for biopsy in relation to surrounding structures. Estimate its depth. Assess the optimal approach to accomplish the aspiration biopsy. Deeply seated lesions are usually best approached directly and perpendicularly to the skin surface. Superficial lying and very small tumors may best be approached by penetrating the skin at a nearly horizontal plane, subsequently feeling for the mass with the tip of the needle.
4. Place the patient in a comfortable position for aspiration biopsy but with the mass readily palpable and easily grasped during the biopsy. This is most important in head and neck lesions, where the prominence of an enlarged lymph node, or lump, may depend on whether the patient is lying down or sitting up. The prominence of the sternocleidomastoid muscle and its relationship to the cervical lymph nodes mandate positioning the patient so that a minimum of soft tissue is traversed before reaching the target [**F** *20.1*]. When aspirating thyroid lesions, place a small pillow under the patient's upper back and extend the neck and tilt the head back. Aspirate thyroid nodules only in a plane perpendicular to the transverse vertebral process, which may act as a reference point for deep-lying thyroid nodules.
5. Take time to examine the patient's lesion thoroughly while describing the technique and what is to be accomplished with it.

Although the aspiration is considered a type of biopsy, we do not usually obtain written legal consent from patients prior to performing this procedure except for children. The radiology department obtains consent for deep aspirations that are image guided. Obtaining biopsy permission is a matter of personal choice and clinic and hospital policy.

Performing the Aspiration

1. Grasp the lesion with one gloved hand, usually with two fingers, or push it into a position where it seems fixed and stable.
2. Prepare the skin with an alcohol sponge as for a venipuncture.
3. Determine puncture site and lay the syringe pistol with attached needle against the skin at that site.
4. Insert the needle through the skin with a quick motion.
5. Advance the needle into the mass.
6. Puncture of the target may be tested by differences in resistance, feeling that a capsule was penetrated, or slight lateral motion of the syringe pistol.
7. Apply suction to the aspirating syringe. (The amount of suction varies with the lesion aspirated: eg, thyroid, very little; scirrhous breast cancer, maximum.)

8. Move the needle back and forth within the tumor with short, quick strokes in nearly the same line as the original puncture. (Varying the direction of the needle does not aid in procuring good aspirates. Making multiple separate passes is a better technique for obtaining an adequate specimen.)
9. Note at all times the junction of the needle and the hub of the syringe for the appearance of any specimen. It is critical to the procurement of high-quality aspirates to keep the material within the needle and not aspirate excessive blood or fluid, which dilutes the cellular composition of the specimen.
10. Release the trigger of the syringe pistol at the first appearance of any sample at the junction of the syringe and the needle, and let the vacuum in the syringe equate to normal. A specimen may not appear in the hub of the syringe during 10 or 12 passes within the lesion, but this does not indicate an unsuccessful aspiration. After this number of passes, if no sample is seen, the aspiration is stopped by allowing the air pressure in the syringe to return to normal.
11. Withdraw the needle from the mass when air pressure in the syringe equalizes.
12. Apply pressure to the puncture site with a sterile gauze pad.

Never withdraw the needle from the mass with any vacuum in the syringe pistol. With residual vacuum the small aspirate biopsy will be pulled into the syringe. It is difficult to recover from the barrel of the syringe and begins to dry immediately. The specimen could be irretrievably lost. If a cyst is detected, it should be evacuated as completely as possible. After aspiration of any cyst, it is essential that any residual mass detected be reaspirated.

The basic aspiration technique for deep lesions is the same following the administration of local anesthesia through the chest or abdominal wall to the pleura or peritoneum. Many radiologists prefer to place a guide needle, usually 18 gauge, to the surface of the target, check its position by imaging, and then place the actual aspiration needles through the guide needle, again checking position by imaging.

Becoming adept at needle aspiration biopsy takes practice. This is possible using both cadavers and surgical specimens, from which a collection of biopsies from normal tissues as well as tumors may be procured. Practice enables one to acquire skills in the technical aspects of aspiration biopsy and in preparation of smears.

SMEAR PREPARATION

1. Detach the needle from the syringe and fill the syringe with air immediately following completion of the aspiration.
2. Reattach the needle and place the needle in the center and on the surface of a plain glass slide.
3. Advance the plunger of the syringe to express a small drop of aspirate, 2 to 3 mm in diameter, onto the slide [**F***20.2*].
4. Carry out this procedure over a series of slides as quickly as possible.
5. Invert a second plain glass slide over the drop, and as it spreads gently pull the two slides apart horizontally [**F***20.2*].
6. Alternatively, as the drop spreads, pull the two slides apart vertically.
7. Repeat this procedure for all slides, immediately fixing some slides with alcohol spray while the slide surface is still wet.
8. Allow unfixed smears on plain slides to air-dry.

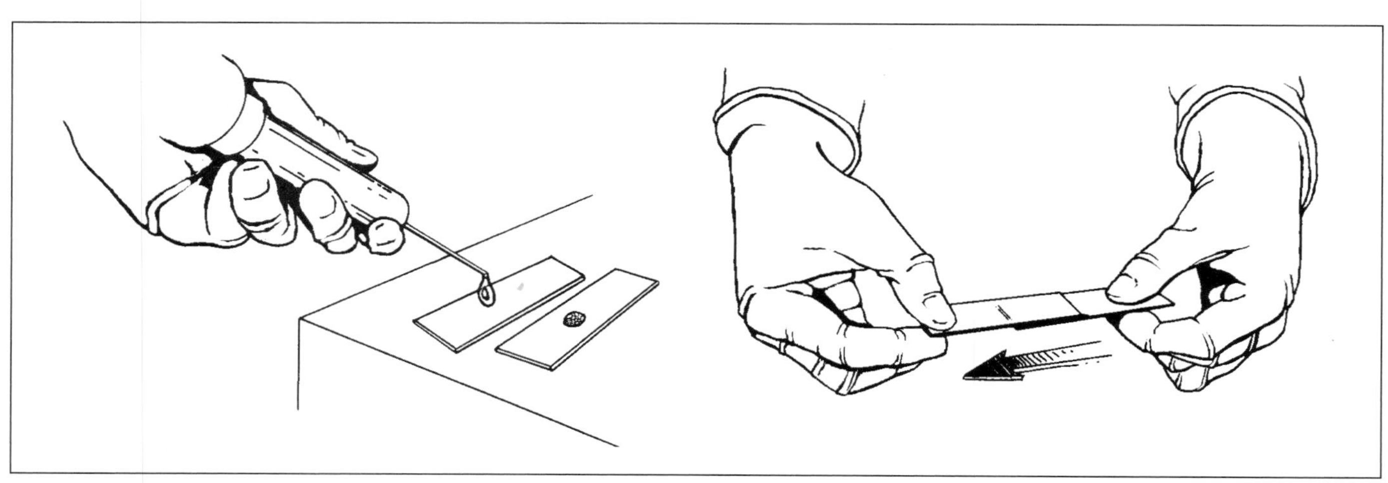

F*20.2*

Smear preparation. Left, A small drop of the specimen is expressed on the glass slide. Right, the drop spreads as a second slide is inverted over it; the slides are then drawn apart, sliding one against the other.

Care must be taken to place the bevel of the needle against the slide while expressing the biopsy sample so that there is no intervening air gap. This prevents splattering or excessive air-drying prior to fixation in alcohol. Some cytopathologists prefer to express all of the sample onto a single slide and then make a number of smears by spreading this large drop of specimen over a series of slides, noting particularly the presence of small tissue fragments to be concentrated on the edge of a glass slide and compressed in the same area of the smear. This should be done quickly but gently to avoid crushing artifacts. The important point is that smears should occupy only a small area of the slide. This creates a tissue-like pattern to the smear and reduces the area of the smears that must be screened for diagnostic features.

Aspiration biopsies that are diluted by fluid or blood do not provide good smears. They occupy large areas of the slide. Diagnostic cells, if present, are usually found at the edges of these smears and consist principally of single cells. The following steps can be used in dealing with bloody or diluted smears:

1. Place one drop (usually 5-10 mm in diameter) of biopsy sample on the slide as above.
2. Hold the slide with the drop in one hand.
3. Hold a second slide with the other hand and bring the edge up to the drop [**F***20.3*, top left].
4. The drop will spread along the edge of the slide. As it does push the edge of the slide to the end farthest from the drop in the manner of making a blood smear and about halfway down the slide [**F***20.3*, top right].
5. At that point lift the spreader slide straight up [**F***20.3*, center left].
6. Immediately tilt the smear slide away from the leading edge of the smear so that the blood runs back toward the original point of the drop [**F***20.3*, center right].
7. Continue smear preparation with the clean edge of the spreader slide, beginning at the edge of the smear slide where the spreader slide was lifted from the smear [**F***20.3*, bottom left].
8. The majority of tissue particles will be found in the portion of smear just prepared from the leading edge [**F***20.3*, bottom right].

The method of smear preparation just described is not easy and requires practice and dexterity. For specimens that are largely fluid, use standard cytologic technique, Cytospin, or filter preparation after centrifugation. Both techniques are extremely useful for examining cyst fluid encountered in aspiration, particularly that obtained from breast and thyroid.

Deep aspirations performed by the inexperienced may result in largely bloody samples. Blood pulled into the syringe should be processed entirely as a cell block. Smears should be made only from the sample left within the needle. Even a few milliliters of blood may result in quick clotting, which interferes with good smear preparation. Cells become entrapped within the clotted blood, distorting the picture of the smear and resulting in heavy and uneven staining.

Samples for cell blocks are handled by either the plasma thrombin clot method, or with the new Cytoblock system (see appendix this chapter). The Cytoblock method has recently been introduced into our laboratory with great success. Notched tip needles have a tendency to provide microcores. These usually need to be dislodged by inserting the stylus into the needle and pushing them out onto a plain glass slide. One should not attempt to smear these small cores. They can be rolled gently over a small area of the slide to make a smear, but the core should then be quickly placed in fixative for small biopsy tissue processing.

Fixatives and Stains

1. Air-dried smears are stained by the Romanowsky method.
2. Smears spray fixed in 95% ethanol, 95% methanol, or 95% isopropanol are for Papanicolaou staining.
3. Spray-fixed smears should dry at least 1 hour prior to staining.
4. When using aerosol-spray fixatives, do not hold the can closer than 30 cm from the slide, to prevent freezing artifacts.
5. Smears for staining by rapid hematoxylin-eosin benefit from immersion for a few seconds in equal parts of 50% ethanol and 10% neutral-buffered formalin. This treatment also improves staining of frozen sections. In the quick hematoxylin-eosin stain procedure for aspiration smears, use of hot (tap, not boiling) water in the rinsing steps improves the overall quality of the slides.
6. Cytospin preparations for immunohistochemistry should be prepared from a rinse of the aspirate in balanced salt solution. Cytospin preparations are air-dried for the most consistent results. The largest number of antibodies are available for use with immunohistochemistry methods.
7. Air-dried slides for immunohistochemistry may be stored frozen (at least –25°C) for up to 4 weeks.

Experience and personal preference seem to dictate what stains are used on aspiration biopsy smears. Surgical pathologists may prefer hematoxylin-eosin. Cytopathologists may prefer the Papanicolaou stain. Hematologists may prefer the Romanowsky stains, Diff-Quik, May-Grünwald-Giemsa, Giemsa, or Wright's stain. Use of the Romanowsky group can lead to an immediate diagnosis following the aspiration biopsy. The quality of the aspirate and the smear can be checked. Repeat aspiration can be obtained for both diagnosis and special studies if needed.

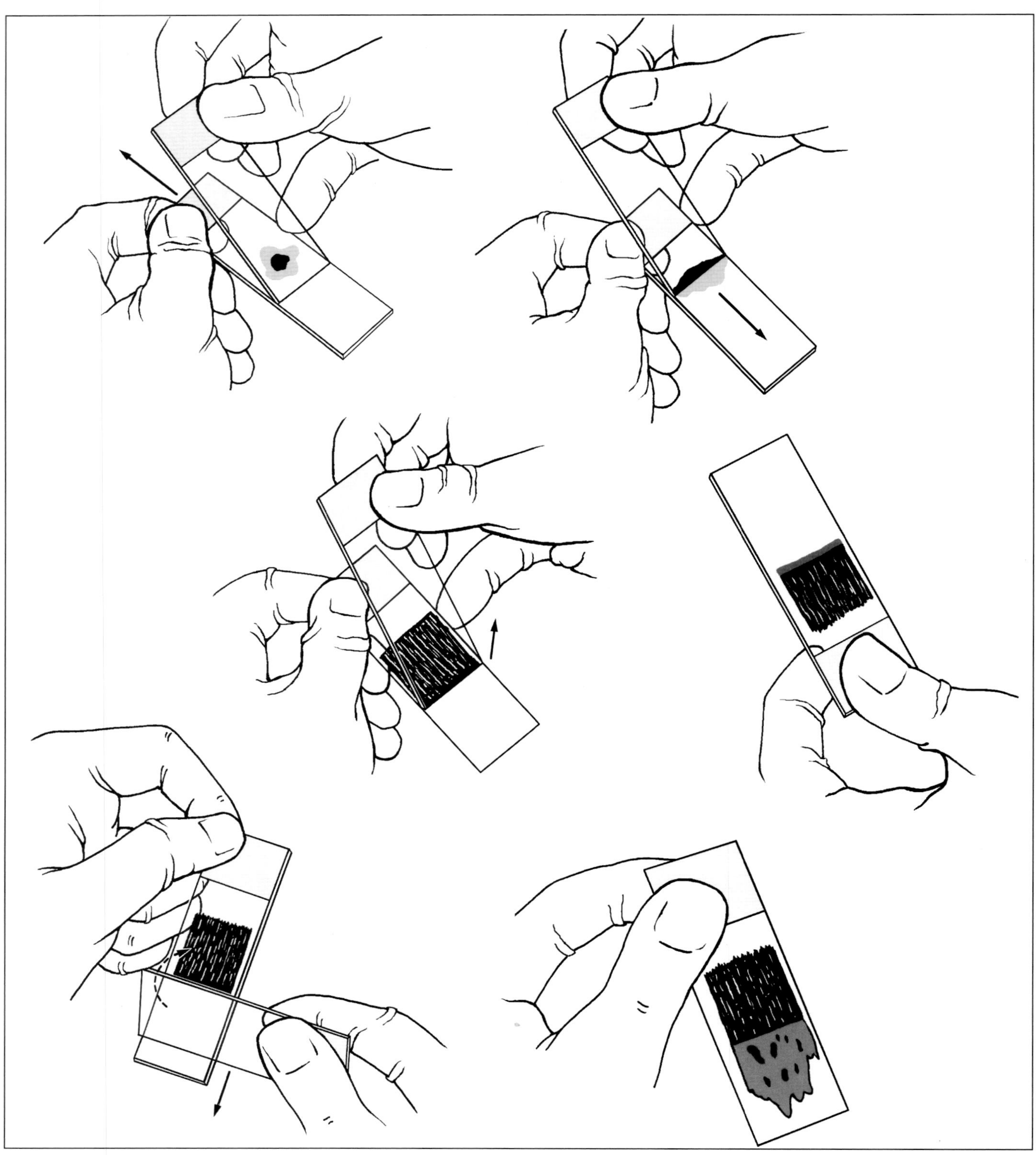

F20.3

Smear preparation for bloody or diluted smears. Top left, Hold the slide with the drop; bring the edge of a second slide up to the drop. Top right, As the drop spreads along the edge of the slide, push the edge to the end farthest from the drop in the manner of making a blood smear (about halfway down the slide). Center left, Lift the spreader slide straight up. Center right, Immediately tilt the smear slide away from the leading edge of the smear so that the blood runs back toward the original point of the drop. Bottom left, Continue smear preparation with the clean edge of the spreader slide. Bottom right, The majority of tissue particles are found in the portion of smear just prepared from the leading edge. (Figure adapted from Grohs.)

Diff-Quick stain is a three-step procedure that takes less than 20 seconds to perform. A comparison of the general properties of air-dried vs wet-fixed smears and the features emphasized by Romanowsky stains and Papanicolaou stain are presented [T*20.1*, T*20.2*] from the monograph on aspiration biopsy by Orell and colleagues.

The cytologic overview of aspiration biopsy is virtually limitless. In the chapters that follow, consideration will be given the aspiration biopsy diagnosis in a number of important organs, tissues, and body sites. Aspiration biopsy may stimulate further understanding of neoplasms presenting in a variety of cytologic samples.

APPENDIX

Equipment

Cameco Syringe Pistol, 20.0 and 10.0 mL size. Available from Precision Dynamics Corporation, 13880 Del Sur St, San Fernando, CA 91340-3490. (800) 847-0670.

Aspir-Gun. Available from Everst Company, 5 Sherman St, Linden, NJ 07036.

Inrad Aspiration Biopsy Syringe Gun. Available from INRAD Inc, 620 Watson SW, Grand Rapids, MI 49504. (800) 253-1540.

20.0 and 10.0 mL disposable plastic syringe with Luer Lok Tip. Available from Becton Dickinson, Division of Becton Dickinson & Co, Rutherford, NJ 07070.

22-, 23-, and 25-gauge 0.6 to 1.0 mm external diameter disposable needles, 3.8 cm and 8.8 cm long, with or without mandrin. (Used for most aspirations of palpable lumps.) Available from Becton Dickinson.

21- and 22-gauge aspiration biopsy needles, 15 cm and 20 cm long, with or without mandrin. (For biopsy of lung, transabdominal, and pelvic masses, and prostate.) Available from Cook Co Inc, P.O. Box 227, Spencer, IN 47460. Both Chiba style and Franseen type needles are available.

Franseen type needle, 22 gauge, 8.8 cm with mandrin available from Manan Mfg Co Inc, Skokie, IL 60076. Distributed by First Medical Supply Inc, P.O. Box 634, Baltimore, MD 21203. (301) 377-1519.

ROTEX II needle 0.55 mm, 15.0 and 20.0 cm length (used primarily for hamartomas), available from Ursus Konsult AB, Grev Turegatan 2, S- 114 35, Stockholm Sweden.

Staining Techniques

Papanicolaou Stain

Any of the modifications available in most laboratories are satisfactory. Gill's hematoxylin is available from Polysciences Inc, Paul Valley Industrial Park, Warrington, PA 18976. (215) 343-6484. Staining times may need to be adjusted for variations in thickness of smears. Gill's modified OG-6 and EA for Papanicolaou stain are also available from Polysciences Inc.

Diff-Quik Stain Set

This commercial stain kit, a modified Wright stain, is a three-solution, three-step method that is both fast and practical. It provides good cell detail and identifies stromal

Property	Air-Dried Smear, Romanowsky Stain	Wet-Fixed Smear, Papanicolaou Stain
Dependence on smear technique	Strong	Moderate
Dry smear	Good fixation	Drying artifacts common
Wet smear	Artifacts common	Good fixation
Tissue fragments	Cells poorly seen, heavy ground substance staining	Individual cells seen clearly
Cell and nuclear area	Exaggerated, differences enhanced	Comparable with tissue sections
Cytoplasmic detail	Well demonstrated	Poorly demonstrated
Nuclear detail	Different pattern from Papanicolaou-stained sample	Excellently demonstrated
Nucleoli	Not always discernible	Well demonstrated
Stromal components	Well demonstrated and often differentially stained	Poorly demonstrated
Partially necrotic tissue	Poor definition of cell detail	Good definition of single intact cells

*Adapted from Orell et al.

T*20.1*
*General Properties of Air-Dried vs Wet-Fixed Smears**

Romanowsky Stain
- Epithelial
  - Mucin, intracellular, or extracellular, colloid (thyroid)
  - Secretory granules (prostate, lipofuscin granules [seminal vesicles])
  - Lipid vacuoles
  - Fire flares (thyroid)
  - Bare bipolar nuclei (benign breast)
  - Bile plugs
  - Basement membrane globules (adenoid cystic carcinoma)
  - Amyloid
- Lymphoid
  - Cytoplasmic basophilia
- Lymphoglandular bodies
- Hematopoietic cells
- Lipid vacuoles

Papanicolaou Stain
- Epithelial
  - Squamous differentiation/keratinization
  - Oncocytes (salivary gland tumors)
  - Psammoma bodies
- Lymphoid
  - Nuclear outline
  - Nuclear chromatin pattern
  - Nucleoli

*Adapted from Orell et al.

T *20.2*
*Features Emphasized by Romanowsky and Papanicolaou Stains**

fragments by metachromasia. This stain is comparable to the May-Grünwald-Giemsa and Wright-Giemsa, but it is much quicker. Fixation is with methanol containing 1.8 mg/L triarylmethane dye, 100% pure dye content. Solution I is buffered eosin Y. Solution II is a buffered solution of thiazine dyes, methylene blue, and azure A. Azure A undergoes slow constant oxidation to azure B, which is the actual staining solution of the original Romanowsky method. Available from American Scientific Products, division of American Hospital Supply Corporation, McGaw Park, IL 60085.

Staining procedure: The air-dried smears are dipped for 5 seconds (five dips) in the fixative solution followed by five 1-second dips in solutions I and II. The excess stain is drained from the slides between solutions. Following the last staining (solution II), the slide is rinsed with water and either allowed to dry or examined wet. When the smear completely dries, it may be made permanent by immersing it in xylene for several seconds and mounting it with a permanent histologic mounting medium and a coverslip. Staining times may need modification depending on the thickness of the smear and the age of the stain. Examination of the finished stain should have a gross purple-blue color, not brown or orange. If the latter color is seen, the slide is understained. It is quite difficult to overstain with Diff-Quik.

Modified May-Grünwald-Giemsa Stain

May-Grünwald stock stain: 1.0 g eosin-methyl blue, 1000 mL methanol.

Giemsa stock stain: Add 1.0 g Giemsa powder to 66.0 mL glycerin. Incubate at 37°C for 3 hours, mixing occasionally. Add 66.0 mL methanol to the incubated stain. Store in the refrigerator.

May-Grünwald working stain: To 40 mL of stock stain add 20 mL methanol in a Coplin jar.

Giemsa working stain: Add 45 mL of Giemsa stock stain to 45 mL of distilled water in a Coplin jar.

Staining procedure: Immerse the air-dried aspiration smears in May-Grünwald working stain for 15 minutes. Rinse gently in tap water. Immerse the smears in Giemsa working stain for 15 minutes. Rinse gently with tap water. Allow to air-dry. Dip in xylene for 10 seconds and mount with a permanent histologic mounting medium and a coverslip.

Prepare May-Grünwald working stain fresh once per week. Prepare Giemsa stain fresh daily. The stock Giemsa stain is good for 6 months if refrigerated. The stock May-Grünwald stain is good indefinitely and does not require refrigeration.

Modified Wright-Giemsa Stain

Wright stain: Any formula in standard laboratory use is satisfactory.

Giemsa stain: See Giemsa stock stain.

Buffer solution pH 6.4 and pH 6.8

Giemsa working stain: Dilute 1 part Giemsa stock stain with 9 parts of buffer pH 6.8. Prepare fresh daily.

Staining procedure: Flood the air-dried aspiration smears with methanol and allow the alcohol to evaporate completely. Then flood the smears with Wright's stain for 3 minutes. Add buffer solution of pH 6.4 drop by drop to the Wright's stain, blowing on the slide to mix stain and buffer. The stain develops a green sheen when enough buffer has been added. Allow to stand for 4 minutes. Wash in tap water and dry completely. Stain in working Giemsa 3 minutes. Wash with tap water and dry completely. Dip in xylene for 10 seconds and mount with a permanent histologic mounting medium and a coverslip.

Hematoxylin-Eosin Stain

Eosin Y solution

Harris hematoxylin

Dilute ammonium hydroxide: Add one drop of concentrated ammonium hydroxide to 100.0 mL of distilled water.

Staining procedure: Use on air-dried aspiration smears.

Absolute ethyl alcohol	1 minute
95% ethanol	1 minute
Tap water	Several dips
Harris hematoxylin	2 minutes

Tap water	Several dips
Dilute ammonium hydroxide	1 to 2 dips
Eosin Y	30 seconds
Tap water	Several dips
Tap water	Several dips
95% ethanol	Several dips
95% ethanol	Several dips
Absolute ethanol	Several dips
Acetone	Several dips
Xylene	1 minute

Mount with a permanent histologic mounting medium and a coverslip.

Cell Block Preparation

Cytoblock Cell Block Preparation System. Available from Shandon Inc, 171 Industry Dr, Pittsburgh, PA 15275. (800) 245-6212. Kit includes Cytoblock cassettes, Cytoblock Reagent 1 (clear fluid), and Cytoblock Reagent 2 (colored fluid).

Directions:

1. Record patient information on the Cytoblock.
2. Use samples previously fixed in neutral-buffered formalin.
3. Concentrate the fixed cells by centrifuging the sample for several minutes. Pour off the excess fluid and drain the tube on a paper towel.
4. Estimate the amount of sample present. If the total amount of sample is two drops or less, add four drops of Reagent 2 to the specimen pellet and mix by vortexing.
5. If the sample is more than two drops, divide into several cell blocks based on two drops per block. For example if there are four drops of sample (enough for two Cytoblocks), add eight drops of Reagent 2 and vortex.
6. Assemble Cytoblock cassettes into Cytoclip (Cytospin standard equipment) and keep horizontal. The locating peg on the back of the Cytoblock cassette fits into the hole in the Cytoclip to be properly oriented.
7. Add three drops of Reagent 1 into the center of the well in the board insert. Reagent 1 should coat the entire circumference of the well in the board insert. Use care and avoid getting any Reagent 1 on the top surface of the board insert.
8. With the backing paper projecting toward the top of the Cytoclip, place a Cytofunnel (Cytospin equipment) disposable chamber over the prepared Cytoblock and secure the metal clip holder in the usual manner. (See Cytospin operating instructions.)
9. Place the assembled Cytoclip into the Cytospin rotor.
10. Place the mixed cell suspension in each Cytofunnel.
11. Close the Cytospin and set for 5 minutes at 1500 rpm. Use the low acceleration setting. Start the Cytospin
12. When the Cytospin stops, remove the Cytofunnel assemblies and place horizontally. Release the clip and remove the funnels. Removal may require rocking the funnel to the side to separate the funnel assembly from the underlying board insert. Be certain the cell button is in the well and has not adhered to the funnel. Then discard the funnel.
13. Place one drop of Reagent 1 in the center of the insert board well, on top of the cell button. Close the Cytoblock cassette and place in fixative to await tissue processing.
14. After processing in the standard tissue processor open the Cytoblock cassette. Fold back paper and remove the board insert. Use fine forceps inserted through holes under the board insert.
15. Dislodge the cell button into the base mold and embed flat. Discard the board insert and backing paper.
16. Reclose the Cytoblock cassette and place flat side up (round peg side down) on top of base mold. Fill with paraffin.
17. Handle as any paraffin block but trim carefully since cell buttons may be quite thin.

Preparation of Cytospins for Tumor Markers

1. Aspirates for Cytospin preparation and tumor markers are received as a needle rinse into balanced salt solution. Enough sample should be present so that the fluid is slightly cloudy. If grossly bloody, saponization should be performed (see below). If the sample is grossly cloudy, it should be diluted with balanced salt solution until slightly cloudy before being used for Cytospin preparations.
2. Follow the manufacturer's directions to set up the Shandon Cytospin.
3. Samples that are blood tinged or have required saponization should be washed in balanced salt solution and centrifuged for 15 minutes at 1500 rpm. Restore the original volume.
4. Break Cytospin filter seal by scraping your finger nail around the edge of the circle on the filter a couple of times. This allows for better absorption of fluid.
5. Load Cytospin with sample chamber, filter, and slides so the chamber is balanced.
6. Using a disposable pipette, add specimen to the specimen chamber one drop at a time—usually two to five drops, depending on cellularity of the sample.
7. Cellularity can be checked initially by using one drop of sample on a slide and one drop of supravital stain. Mix thoroughly with an applicator stick and coverslip. Examine under the microscope with high power field (x400). If every other field has 5 to 10 cells, then one drop of sample provides an adequate

cytospin sample. If the cell estimate is higher than this, dilute with balanced salt solution to at least this distribution of cells or lower.

8. Follow addition of sample drops to Cytospin chamber with two drops of 20% fetal calf serum in RPMI (tissue culture transport media).
9. Spin for approximately 5 minutes at speed of 500 rpm.
10. When cytospin stops, remove slides and filters. Discard filters.
11. Allow slides to air-dry.
12. Determine Cytospin quality again by using a representative slide and staining it with Diff-Quik. Examine for adequate cellularity under the microscope.
13. If necessary add or decrease the number of sample drops used. Cells should not overlap, as this causes confusing staining patterns and edge effects.
14. Prepare an adequate number of quality slides to process the immunohistochemistry tests ordered.
15. Wash sample chambers in bleach, rinse with water, and allow to dry after use.

Saponization

This procedure may be applied to visibly bloody fluids and may be used in small amounts on samples that exhibit traces of blood.

Materials:

1% saponin (wt/vol)
1.0 g saponin
0.2 g sodium *p*-hydroxybenzoate (preservative)
99.0 mL distilled water

3% calcium gluconate (wt/vol)
3.0 g calcium gluconate
0.2 g sodium *p*-hydroxybenzoate (preservative)
97.0 mL distilled water

Prepare solutions above in beakers. Mix thoroughly. Filter into clear brown bottles, date, and label. Expiration for these solutions is 2 weeks.

Methods:

1. Pour sample into designated centrifuge tube, leaving sufficient space for addition of saponization solutions (see steps 2-4).
2. If specimen is grossly bloody, add two disposable pipettes full of 1% saponin and vortex for 30 seconds. Let sit for an additional 30 seconds. Coloration and/or transparency of the sample should change noticeably.
3. Add three disposable pipettes full of 3% calcium gluconate and vortex for 30 seconds.
4. The saponin and calcium gluconate must always be used in a 2:3 ratio. The actual amounts may be varied according to the amount of blood present in each specimen. It is feasible to use only a ratio of two drops to three drops, if blood is present only in minute amounts.
5. Prepare for centrifugation and Cytospin.
6. If the presence of blood is detected only after initial centrifugation, saponin may still be used. Decant supranatant, vortex suspension, and add the solutions in a ratio of two drops to three drops. Prepare for Cytospin.

Supravital Stain

Materials:

Toluidine blue
0.5 g toluidine blue
20 mL 95% ethanol
80 mL distilled water

Dissolve toluidine blue in alcohol, add distilled water, filter, and store in dark bottle in the refrigerator. Date solution, but its refrigerator life is unlimited.

Immunostaining of Cytospins: Three-Step Avidin-Biotin Complex (ABC) Method

1. Etch circle around Cytospin area with a diamond etching pencil. Brush lightly to remove glass particles. Also label slide with patient identification.
2. Fix in cold acetone (4°C) for 10 minutes.
3. Allow to air dry for 5 minutes or more on a flat surface.
4. Rehydrate by placing in modified phosphate-buffered saline (PBS) for 10 minutes.
5. Wipe off excess PBS. Cytospins must be kept wet at all times.
6. Serum blocking, if necessary, should be carried out at this point. Place slides in humidified chamber and incubate with serum for approximately 15 minutes. Wash with PBS for 5 minutes.
7. Place in humidified chamber and apply primary antibody (mouse monoclonal is preferred to rabbit polyclonal). Incubate for 1 hour at room temperature.
8. Rinse gently with PBS. Wash by placing in PBS (fresh) for 5 minutes.
9. Wipe off excess PBS.
10. Place in humidified chamber and apply biotinylated secondary antibody (anti-mouse IgG or anti-rabbit IgG). Incubate for 45 minutes. Note: Preparation of secondary antibody using Vectastain kit (Vector Laboratories Inc, Burlingame, Calif):
    a) For 10 mL of PBS add one drop of secondary antibody.
    b) For less volume of secondary antibody, 10 µL of antibody to 2.0 mL of PBS may be used.
11. Rinse gently with PBS. Wash by placing in PBS (fresh) for 5 minutes.

12. Methanol–hydrogen peroxide blocking may be done at this point. Add 200 mL of absolute methanol to 50 mL of 3% hydrogen peroxide. Block for approximately 20 minutes and wash in two changes of PBS (10 minutes each). Note: Deionized water may be used in place of absolute methanol. This gives a less violent reaction, resulting in less damage to cellular morphology.
13. Wipe off excess PBS.
14. Place in humidified chamber and apply Vectastain ABC Reagent. Incubate for approximately 45 minutes. Note: Preparation for Vectastain ABC Reagent:
    a) Add one drop of Reagent A to 5 mL of PBS; mix.
    b) Add one drop of Reagent B; mix.
    c) Allow to stand for 30 minutes before use.
15. Rinse gently with PBS. Wash by placing in PBS (fresh) for 5 minutes.
16. Wipe off excess PBS.
17. Place in humidified chamber and apply DAB solution (d,d-diaminobenzidine). Incubate for 5 minutes. Note: DAB solution must be prepared immediately before use:
    a) Add 10 mL of TRIS buffer (0.5 mol/L, pH 7.6) to a 10-mg bottle of DAB (Polysciences Inc); mix.
    b) Add 0.16 mL of 3% PBS-H202 prepared by dissolving 1 tablet of urea-H202 in 100 mL of distilled water immediately before use.
18. Rinse gently with PBS. Wash by placing in PBS (fresh) for 5 minutes.
19. Slides are now ready to counterstain. Rack slides and dip in each of the following solutions approximately 10 times (with the exception of hematoxylin):
    PBS
    Distilled water
    Hematoxylin (3-4 minutes)
    Distilled water
    PBS
    Distilled water
    80% ethanol
    95% ethanol
    100% ethanol
    Xylene
    Xylene
    Xylene

Note: Lillie-Meyer hematoxylin may provide better nuclear staining with immunohistochemical procedures than Harris hematoxylin.

20. Mount slides with a permanent histologic mounting media and a coverslip.

Immunohistochemical Detection of Estrogen and Progesterone Receptor on Fine Needle Aspirates From Breast Tumors

Instructions for Preparation of Microscopic Slides:

1. Add 3.0 mL of tissue adhesive from the Abbott-ER-ICA Monoclonal kit (Abbott Laboratories, North Chicago, Ill) to 300 mL of distilled deionized water in a staining jar. Mix thoroughly by stirring.
2. Place clean microscope slides in a slide rack and immerse in the tissue adhesive solution for 5 minutes.
3. Rinse the treated slides in a distilled or deionized water bath for 1 minute. Repeat this step one time using fresh distilled deionized water.
4. Air-dry the slides at room temperature.
5. Store the slides in a clean slide container.

Note: The tissue adhesive solution prepared in step 1 may be stored at 2°C to 8°C and reused for up to 1 month.

Use these prepared slides for making the aspiration smears from breast tumors for receptor studies as follows:

1. Collect fresh fine needle breast aspirates and prepare smears immediately. Place smears while still wet in Coplin jar of 3.7% formaldehyde in PBS for 10 to 15 minutes. Make a minimum of six smears that contain tumor cells. Do not allow Cytospin slides to dry at any time. Aspirates are preferable to Cytospin preparations from fine needle aspirates of breast tumors, which have given inconsistent results and are usually low in cellularity. Touch preparations or scrapes from small tumors prepared as smears can also be used.
2. After fixation, place slides in PBS for 4 to 6 minutes.
3. Transfer slides to cold methanol at –10°C to –25°C for 3 to 5 minutes, then transfer to cold acetone at –10°C to –25°C for 1 to 3 minutes. Rinse in PBS at room temperature for 4 to 6 minutes.
4. Transfer slides to a container of fresh PBS and rinse for an additional 4 to 6 minutes.
5. Using a diamond-tip pen, make a circle around the sample area on the slide.
6. Return slides to PBS.
7. Proceed to the staining procedure within 2 hours of completing fixation, or immediately after preparation remove specimen from PBS and place in –10°C to –25°C specimen storage medium. Store at –10°C to –25°C for up to 4 weeks.

Materials Required but not Provided:

3.7% Formaldehyde-PBS Solution
1 volume formaldehyde (37%)
9 volumes PBS

Specimen Storage Medium:

To make 500 mL of specimen storage medium, dissolve 42.8 g sucrose and 0.33 g magnesium chloride (anhydrous) in PBS. Adjust final volume to 250 mL. Add 250 mL glycerol and mix by stirring. Store at –10°C to –20°C.

Storage Instructions for the Kit

1. Open and remove the box containing the control slides. This box must be stored frozen (–10°C or colder).
2. Store box of control slides at –10°C or colder. Store other kit reagents at 2°C to 8°C.

3. Bring all kit reagents except control slides to room temperature for use and return to storage conditions indicated above immediately after use.

Immunocytochemical Staining Procedure

Note: Careful control of the timing of all steps is critical for reproducible results.

Prior to Performing the Assay:

1. Refer to instructions for use of prepared slides for making aspiration smears from breast tumors.
2. If fixed specimens have been stored at –10°C to –20°C, place them in PBS bath for 5 minutes. Repeat using fresh PBS bath.
3. Prepare a humidified chamber by placing moistened paper towels in a container with a lid. The chamber should contain a rack on which slides can be positioned horizontally.
4. Bring all reagents except control slides to room temperature for use.

Procedural Notes:

1. Apply kit reagents one drop at a time in sufficient quantity to cover the circled aspirate smear; usually two drops are sufficient.
2. Perform all incubation steps in the humidified chamber at room temperature.
3. Drain excess buffer or reagent from a slide onto a paper towel and then wipe the area around the etched circle of the smear with an absorbent wipe or equivalent. Note: Do not touch the smear or the estrogen-positive cells (control slide) within the circle. Touching will destroy the smear or the cells.
4. When adding primary antibody and control antibody to the control slide, do not allow reagents to mix.
5. During the PBS washes following the incubation with peroxidase- antiperoxidase complex, prepare the chromogen substrate solution.

Assay Procedure:

1. Remove excess PBS from fixed smear and control slide.
2. Add blocking reagent one drop at a time to each circle containing sample (specimen or control).
3. Incubate for 15 to 20 minutes in humidified chamber.
4. Remove excess blocking reagent.
5. Add primary antibody one drop at a time to one slide of each specimen and control antibody to a second slide from the same specimen. Add the primary antibody to one circle on the control slide and control antibody to the other circle. Incubate 30 minutes in humidified chamber.
6. Place slides in PBS bath for 5 minutes. Repeat using fresh PBS.
7. Remove excess PBS.
8. Add bridging antibody one drop at a time to each sample. Incubate 20 minutes in humidified chamber.
9. Place slides in PBS bath for 5 minutes. Repeat using fresh PBS.
10. Remove excess PBS.
11. Add peroxidase-antiperoxidase complex one drop at a time to each sample. Incubate 30 minutes in humidified chamber.
12. Place slides in PBS bath for 5 minutes. Repeat using fresh PBS.
13. Remove excess PBS.
14. Slides are now ready to counterstain. Rack slides and dip in each of the following solutions approximately 10 times (with the exception of hematoxylin):
    - PBS
    - Distilled water
    - Hematoxylin (1 minute)
    - Distilled water
    - PBS
    - Distilled water
    - 80% ethanol
    - 95% ethanol
    - 100% ethanol
    - Xylene
    - Xylene
    - Xylene
15. Coverslip slides with a permanent histologic mounting media.

Specimen Results:

If estrogen receptor is detected in the specimen, the immunocytochemical staining will be located in the nuclei of the cells treated with the primary antibody and will appear reddish-brown. The nuclei of the cells that do not contain significant amounts of estrogen receptor will be blue. Other brown staining that might occur in the cytoplasm, leukocytes, erythrocytes, or necrotic cells, will also be apparent in the specimen treated with control antibody and should be considered nonspecific.

The same specimen treated with control antibody, in place of the primary antibody, should not demonstrate significant nuclear staining. Staining observed in the control antibody section is considered nonspecific.

SELECTED READINGS

Cardoza PL. *Atlas of Clinical Cytology.* Leiden, the Netherlands: Targa b.v.'s-Hertogenbosch; 1979.

Deeley TJ. *Needle Biopsy.* London, England: Butterworth & Co Publishers; 1974.

Frable WJ. Thin-needle aspiration biopsy. In: Bennington J, ed. *Major Problems in Pathology.* Philadelphia, Pa: WB Saunders Co; 1983;14.

Gill GW. The Shandon Cytospin 2 in diagnostic cytology: techniques, tips, and troubleshooting. In: *Cytospin 2 Handbook.* Sewickley, Pa: Shandon Southern Instruments Inc; 1982:1-73.

Grohs HK. *Principles of Aspiration Technique and Smear Preparation: An Illustrative Guide*. Dept of Pathology, Salem Hospital, Salem, MA 01970.

Harris MJ. Cell block preparation: three-percent bacterial agar and plasma-thrombin clot methods. *Cytotech Bull.* 1974;11:6-7.

Holmquist MD. The effect of distance in aerosol fixative of cytologic specimens. *Cytotech Bull.* 1979;15:25-27.

Kline RS. *Handbook of Fine Needle Aspiration Biopsy Cytology.* 2nd ed. New York, NY: Churchill Livingstone Inc; 1992.

Koss LG, Woyke S, Olszewski W. *Aspiration Biopsy: Cytologic Interpretation and Its Histologic Basis.* 2nd ed. New York, NY: Igaku-Shoin Medical Publishers Inc; 1992.

Linsk JA, Franzen S. *Clinical Aspiration Cytology.* 2nd ed. Philadelphia, Pa: JB Lippincott Co; 1989.

Orell SR, Sterrett GF, Walters MN-I, et al. *Manual and Atlas of Fine Needle Aspiration Cytology.* 2nd ed. New York, NY: Churchill Livingstone Inc; 1992.

Soderstrom N. *Fine Needle Aspiration Biopsy.* Stockholm, Sweden: Almqvist & Wiksell; 1966:13-18.

Zajicek J. *Aspiration Biopsy Cytology, Part I: Cytology of Supradiaphragmatic Organs.* New York, NY: S. Karger; 1974:1-15,20-26. Monographs in Clinical Cytology, vol 4.

Zajicek J. *Aspiration Biopsy Cytology, Part II: Cytology of Infradiaphragmatic Organs.* New York, NY: S. Karger; 1979.

C H A P T E R 21

Breast

Yolanda C. Oertel, MD

CONTENTS

ANATOMY

In the sexually mature woman, the mammary gland consists of 15 to 20 lobes radiating from the nipple, separated by connective tissue and surrounded by abundant adipose tissue. Each lobe has multiple lobules. Each lobule consists of secretory acini, terminal ducts, and intralobular connective tissue.

GENERAL CONSIDERATIONS

Cellular material may be obtained by scraping the nipple, by sampling nipple secretions or discharge, and, more frequently, by fine needle aspiration (FNA) of palpable breast masses.

Lesions of the nipple are rare. Hence, samples from nipple scrapings are not common. Paget's disease (described by Sir James Paget in 1874), a crusted lesion of the nipple with an underlying (in situ or infiltrating) ductal adenocarcinoma, is one of the few instances in which such samples are taken. Herpesvirus infection mimicking Paget's disease can be encountered.

Nipple discharge may result from systemic neuroendocrine disorders, lesions within the breast (such as intraductal papillomas), or lactational changes induced by tranquilizing drugs or oral contraceptives. If the nipple discharge is serous or milky, the smear shows many foamy histiocytes, some of which may be multinucleated. If the nipple discharge is blood-tinged, usually it is related to an intraductal papilloma. The smear contains hemosiderin-laden macrophages and a few epithelial clusters. These cellular clusters have clear cytoplasm with scalloped borders. In general, the cytologic examination of a nipple discharge does not contribute substantially to the diagnosis.

The most common sample (from breast lesions) received in the laboratory may be fluid removed or "aspirated" from a cyst. The processing of such fluids is unnecessary and expensive, because it is extremely rare to find malignant cells. Only when the fluid is hemorrhagic should it be sent for cytologic examination. Even then, more diagnostic help may be obtained by aspirating residual lesions after the fluid has been evacuated. Smears from the sediment of cyst fluids typically show amorphous debris, leukocytes, macrophages, a few clusters of ductal cells with small regular nuclei and scanty cytoplasm, and some groups of ductal cells with apocrine metaplasia.

The use of FNA of palpable breast lesions is becoming more widespread in the United States. The following points must be emphasized:

1. Great attention should be paid to the technique of obtaining the sample. It is deceptively simple, but must be performed carefully.
2. The preparation and staining of smears depends on the pathologist's preference and the availability of reagents. Some pathologists prefer hematologic stains on air-dried smears. However, excellent results can be obtained with hematoxylin-eosin or Papanicolaou stains.
3. If a patient has a palpable mass and the aspirate shows only benign cells, the referring physician should be aware that the next step is to decide whether to perform an excisional biopsy, or to monitor the patient and reevaluate her at a later date. FNA is an aid to clinical judgment, but it does not substitute for it.

COMMON FEATURES

The following cellular elements are found frequently in breast aspirates:

1. Ductal cells [▮*21.1*, ▮*21.2*] are arranged in small, tightly cohesive groups. They have regular, round to oval nuclei, no visible nucleoli, and scanty cytoplasm.
2. Apocrine metaplastic cells [▮*21.2*, ▮*21.3*] are large, round, or polygonal cells with round nuclei, prominent nucleoli, and abundant grayish-pink cytoplasm with hematologic stains (cytoplasm stains green to orange with the Papanicolaou stain).
3. Stripped "bipolar nuclei" are single ovoid nuclei without visible nucleoli and without visible cytoplasm. They may represent the naked nuclei of fibroblasts or myoepithelial cells.
4. Myoepithelial cells appear as small, dark, ovoid nuclei scattered within clumps of ductal cells.
5. Histiocytes with small vesicular nuclei and foamy cytoplasm are a common finding.
6. Fibroadipose tissue must be present for a sample to be considered adequate. The mature adipocytes have eccentric nuclei and delicate cell membranes.

NON-NEOPLASTIC DISEASES

Fibrocystic Changes (Fibrocystic Mastopathy)

The aspirated material is usually thin and colorless. The smears show fragments of mature adipose tissue [▮*21.4*] or fibroadipose tissue, some tight clusters of essentially normal ductal cells [▮*21.1*, ▮*21.2*] with small regular nuclei and scanty cytoplasm, and groups of apocrine metaplastic cells [▮*21.2*, ▮*21.3*] with abundant cytoplasm and enlarged round nuclei with prominent nucleoli. Finding these elements is essential for this cytologic diagnosis. Foamy histiocytes and red blood cells are seen in the background. Sometimes squamous metaplastic cells are observed. Oleic acid crystals (as a result of trauma to fat cells) may also be present.

Ductal Hyperplasia (Papillomatosis)

The aspirated material is unremarkable. Smears exhibit sheets (monolayers), often folded, composed of regular ductal cells and occasional myoepithelial cells. Also present are clumps of ductal cells with glandular lumina in their centers and irregular borders with finger-like projections. Stripped nuclei may be present in the background.

Fibrous Mastopathy

Such lesions are moderately firm on palpation and rubbery on aspiration. Smears usually show scant cellularity with a mixture of adipose tissue, some ductal cells, and fibrocollagenous tissue fragments.

Fatty Replacement

No discrete lesion will be found clinically. On aspiration it feels soft, and the smears show abundant, mature fibroadipose tissue.

Mastitis

During the acute phase, the smears show many polymorphonuclear leukocytes and fibrin strands. The process may be sterile or secondary to an infection. The aspirated material may be sent for bacterial culture. As the process becomes chronic, lymphocytes, plasma cells, and macrophages become more numerous.

Rarely will mastitis be secondary to tuberculosis. In such instances caseating and/or noncaseating granulomata are seen with clusters of epithelioid histiocytes, lymphocytes, and some multinucleated giant cells.

Fat Necrosis

A common cause of fat necrosis is jogging and aerobic exercise without wearing appropriate support. Clinically, the resulting lesions may resemble mammary carcinomas (a firm mass with skin retraction, or "peau d'orange"). In some instances axillary lymph nodes are palpable because of the presence of lipogranulomas. Thick, yellow, paste-like material is aspirated. Smears have a "bubbly" appearance, due to innumerable vacuoles of various sizes. Many polymorphonuclear leukocytes, foamy and hemosiderin-laden macrophages, and some multinucleated histiocytes are seen. Some clusters of ductal epithelial cells may show some nuclear atypia [▮*21.5*], which may be a source of false-positive diagnosis. Cellular atypia in an inflammatory background should be interpreted with caution.

Fat necrosis may also be a source of false-negative diagnosis, particularly in older women with large breasts. In such patients, a $1\frac{1}{2}$-in needle may not reach an underlying carcinoma. If a diagnosis of fat necrosis is made and the lesion does not resolve in 2 to 3 weeks, the patient should be aspirated again using longer needles, or the lesion should be excised.

Subareolar Abscess

Clinically these lesions may mimic mammary carcinoma (a mass with overlying "peau d'orange"). The aspirate is yellow and paste-like. The smears show many anucleated squames and squamous cells in an acute and chronic inflammatory background [▮*21.6*]. The squamous cells may have well-preserved nuclei or nuclear "ghosts." Multinucleated histiocytes and newly formed capillaries may be seen. Sometimes the lesion disappears after the aspiration; in such cases the procedure is not only diagnostic but also therapeutic.

Gynecomastia

The aspirations are usually painful. The smears are moderately cellular. The epithelial cells are arranged in small to fairly large sheets and cellular clusters with some variation in nuclear size. The cytoplasm is scanty to moderate in amount and occasionally markedly vacuolated. Myoepithelial cells are easily observed among the epithelial cells as small, ovoid, dark nuclei. Some atypical single epithelial cells may be seen.

Intramammary Lymph Nodes

On routine physical examination these small nodes may be mistaken for a neoplasm. The patient may be sent for an excisional biopsy or for an FNA, and a diagnosis of "benign lymphoid tissue" is made. The smears show a varied population of mature lymphocytes, immunoblasts, plasma cells, histiocytes (some with tingible bodies in the cytoplasm), and lymphoid tangles.

BENIGN NEOPLASMS

Fibroadenoma

Fibroadenoma is the most common benign mammary neoplasm. It usually occurs in young women as a discrete nodule. On aspiration it is rubbery. However, we have aspirated a calcified fibroadenoma in an elderly patient; the gritty consistency was indistinguishable from that of a scirrhous carcinoma. The smears are extremely cellular [▮*21.7*]. The epithelial cells are arranged in sheets with a "honeycomb" appearance and in irregular clumps and clusters with blunt branching [▮*21.7*, ▮*21.8*]. The small hyperchromatic nuclei of myoepithelial cells are scattered through the sheets and clusters of epithelial cells. Large fragments of bright pink fibrocollagenous tissue are conspicuous at low magnification if hematologic stains are used [▮21.9]. Many naked "bipolar" nuclei are seen in the background [▮21.7]. These ovoid nuclei are thought to derive from either fibroblasts or myoepithelial cells. Small groups of ductal cells with apocrine metaplasia and some foamy histiocytes may be observed. Sometimes single atypical cells are noted; this finding may lead to an erroneous diagnosis of carcinoma if the pathologist loses sight of the overall appearance of the smears.

Papilloma

Clinically, findings may include nipple discharge or a subareolar nodule. The aspirated material is blood-tinged or grossly hemorrhagic. The smears are sparsely cellular and feature a proteinaceous background with erythrocytes. Large numbers of hemosiderin-laden macrophages (mononucleated and multinucleated) are present. There are a few small clusters of ductal cells with slightly enlarged nuclei. The cytoplasm of the cells at the periphery of these clusters appears clear.

Lipoma

Discrete, soft masses are detected on palpation and aspiration. Cytologic findings are identical to those of fatty replacement.

MALIGNANT EPITHELIAL NEOPLASMS

Mammary Adenocarcinoma

Mammary adenocarcinoma is the most frequent malignancy in women in the United States and the second leading cause of death due to carcinoma (following lung).

Unlike mammography, FNA is not a screening method to detect early mammary carcinoma. FNA is used to establish the diagnosis of carcinoma. The cytologic diagnostic criteria for the variants of ductal and lobular carcinoma of the breast follow:

1. Presence of "tumor cellularity" (markedly cellular smears). This is an essential criterion, with one exception: infiltrating lobular carcinoma of the breast, which is hypocellular.
2. Neoplastic cells arranged in clusters and as single cells.
3. Nuclear pleomorphism in the neoplastic cells, with one exception: adenoid cystic carcinoma of the breast.

It cannot be overemphasized that an accurate diagnosis depends largely on an adequate sample. The pathologist is only as good as the sample obtained or received. Hence, mastery of the aspiration technique is essential to obtain adequate samples.

Ductal Adenocarcinoma Not Otherwise Specified

Infiltrating ductal adenocarcinoma not otherwise specified (NOS) represents the largest proportion of mammary carcinomas. Clinically, it presents as a single or dominant firm mass fixed to the overlying skin. There may be skin dimpling and nipple retraction. On aspiration it feels gritty (as if aspirating an apple) and bleeds easily. The smears display "tumor cellularity" [▮21.10]. The neoplastic cells have nuclear pleomorphism and are arranged in sheets or clusters and singly. This is evident both on alcohol-fixed, Papanicolaou-stained ▮21.11, ▮21.12] and on air-dried, hematologic-stained [▮21.13, ▮21.14] material. The nuclear detail (irregular nuclear membranes, clumping of the chromatin, prominent nucleoli, etc) is better observed when Papanicolaou's stain is used [▮21.12]. These nuclear criteria are not needed with hematologic stains; only "tumor cellularity," nuclear pleomorphism, and the cellular arrangements are noted [▮21.13, ▮21.14].

Comedocarcinoma

The aspirate is thick, yellow, paste-like, and difficult to smear. Abundant necrotic debris is present in the smears, in addition to the many clusters and single neoplastic cells. Frequently, bizarre epithelial cells are seen.

Colloid Carcinoma

Clinically, the lesion presents as a soft mass that bleeds easily on aspiration. The smears are thick and show abundant, pale, pink mucoid material (brownish with Papanicolaou stain) traversed by branching capillaries [▮21.15, ▮21.16]. The neoplastic cells may be arranged in tight clusters lacking nuclear atypia. They may also be arranged in sheets or singly with cytoplasmic vacuoles of varied sizes, and slight to moderate variation in nuclear size and shape.

Papillary Carcinoma

Dark brown, thick fluid is usually aspirated. The smears are very cellular with large tissue fragments, some of which have a dense fibrovascular core. The epithelial cells are moderately enlarged and have regular nuclei and well-defined cytoplasm. Intracellular lumina are seen frequently.

Medullary Carcinoma

Clinically, the lesion presents as a large soft mass that bleeds easily on aspiration. In some cases enlarged, irregular, naked nuclei with prominent nucleoli are the predominant feature. These cells have to be differentiated from those of malignant lymphoma, as the treatment will be different. Additional samples showing the atypical epithelial cell clusters may solve this problem. If more samples are not diagnostic, an excisional biopsy or a frozen section are necessary prior to definitive surgical treatment. Many lymphocytes, histiocytes, and plasma cells are observed surrounding the epithelial cell clusters and in the background of the smears. In atypical medullary carcinomas, bizarre neoplastic cells are seen as well as abnormal mitotic figures [▮*21.17*].

Less-Common Ductal Adenocarcinomas

Among these variants are apocrine carcinoma, adenoid cystic carcinoma, and tubular carcinoma.

Apocrine carcinomas show large cellular clusters with grayish-pink (greenish to orange with Papanicolaou's stain) granular cytoplasm, "apocrine snouts," round nuclei (with marked variation in size), and prominent nucleoli. Microcalcifications are seen frequently. The differential diagnosis includes exuberant apocrine metaplasia of fibrocystic disease, particularly in older women. If all the diagnostic criteria are not present, then it is wise to request an excisional biopsy.

Adenoid cystic carcinoma yields very cellular smears. The epithelial cells are relatively small, and have scanty cytoplasm and round regular nuclei with occasionally visible nucleoli. The background of the smears is pale pink and mucoid, with a scattering of bright pink, dense, homogeneous globules that are the hallmark of this entity [▮*21.18*]. The globules are inconspicuous with Papanicolaou's stain.

Tubular carcinoma also yields markedly cellular smears with a pattern reminiscent of fibroadenoma. The irregular groups of epithelial cells are not as complex as in fibroadenoma, and they also have a central lumen. At higher magnification some of the epithelial cells in these tubular structures show small nuclei with visible nucleoli, while others have enlarged nuclei. Loose cells are present in the background.

Lobular Carcinoma

On aspiration lobular carcinoma feels gritty and yields a few drops of thin, colorless fluid. The most frequent pattern has scanty cellularity, and the smears may be interpreted as unsatisfactory by the inexperienced pathologist. Rare small groups of cells may be seen, sometimes attached to pale pink fibrocollagenous tissue. At higher magnification these cells are loosely cohesive and have scanty cytoplasm. Enlarged and somewhat irregular nuclei are present with or without visible nucleoli. Also, single epithelial cells are observed that are easily overlooked at low magnification. These cells are larger than monocytes; most have delicate cytoplasm, and some may show a single, large cytoplasmic vacuole (signet-ring cells). Other patterns consist of epithelial cells reminiscent of those seen in ductal hyperplasia, but the patient is postmenopausal.

Metastatic Tumors in the Breast

Metastases to the breast are rare. In our experience the most frequent metastases have been from malignant melanomas. The smears are very cellular. Usually, both round cells and spindled cells are present, arranged singly or in clusters. They have enlarged nuclei with prominent nucleoli and a moderate amount of cytoplasm. Mitotic figures are common as well as intranuclear cytoplasmic inclusions. Most of our cases of metastatic melanoma (whether to the breast or other organs) do not show conspicuous cytoplasmic pigment.

Axillary Lymph Node Metastases

Any patient with a breast lesion should have an examination of the axillae and supraclavicular areas. If a mass is palpable, it should be aspirated. Metastatic adenocarcinomas of the breast to axillary lymph nodes are easily diagnosed on aspirated material. The smears are very cellular. Atypical epithelial cells, singly or in clusters, are seen in a lymphoid background. However, lymphocytes will not be observed if the metastatic carcinoma has replaced the lymph node.

MALIGNANT NONEPITHELIAL NEOPLASMS

Leukemia and Lymphoma

There is nearly always a clinical history of lymphoma or leukemia. The palpable mass is soft and bleeds easily on aspiration. The specimen is bright red and the smears are extremely cellular. Marked cellular fragility is evident. Most often, the process is a non-Hodgkin's lymphoma; the atypical lymphoid cells have irregular nuclear outlines and prominent nucleoli. In leukemia a varied cell population may be evident.

Cystosarcoma Phyllodes

This is an uncommon cause of a firm mass in the breast. The smears show sheets of epithelial cells similar to those from fibroadenoma. Fragments of loose but cellular connective tissue, traversed by capillaries, are evident.

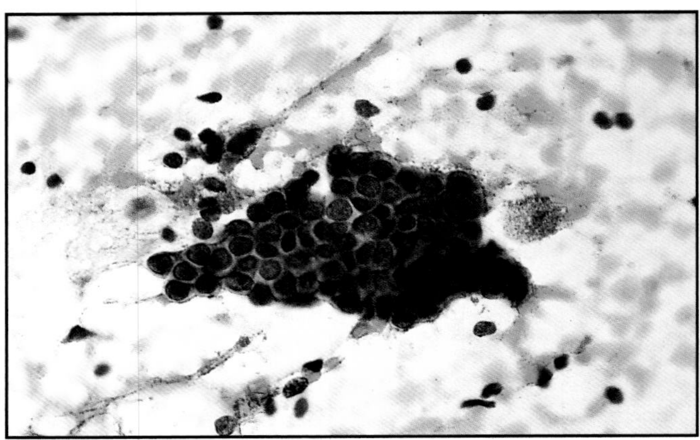

▮21.1

Normal ductal cells. Note small, regular nuclei, and honeycombed appearance (Papanicolaou, x100).

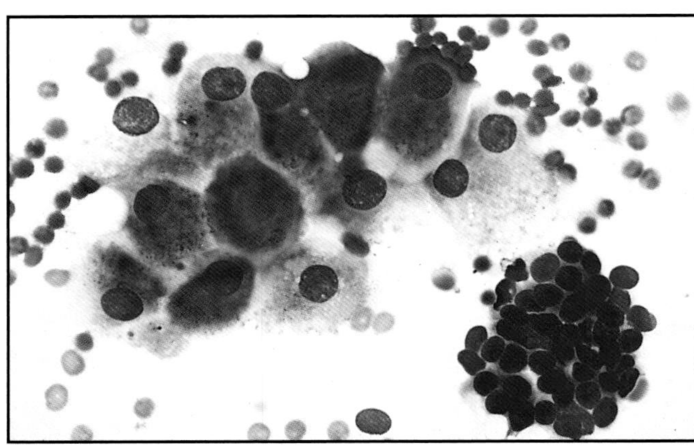

▮21.2

Fibrocystic changes. Cluster of normal ductal cells with small nuclei and scanty cytoplasm contrast with apocrine metaplastic cells (Diff-Quik, x100).

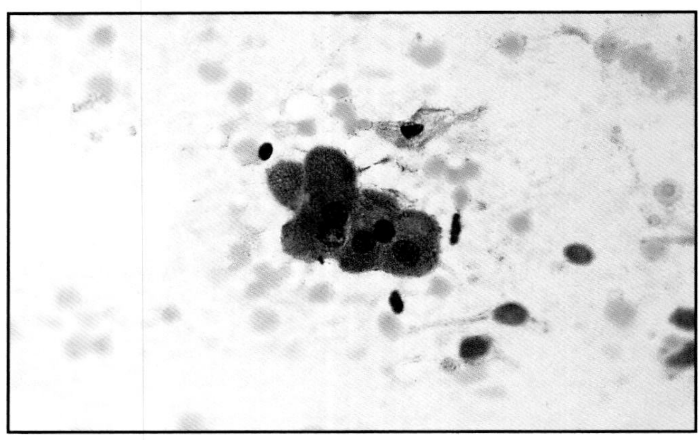

▮21.3

Apocrine metaplastic cells. Note scalloped borders, grayish-pink granular cytoplasm, and visible nucleoli (Papanicolaou, x100).

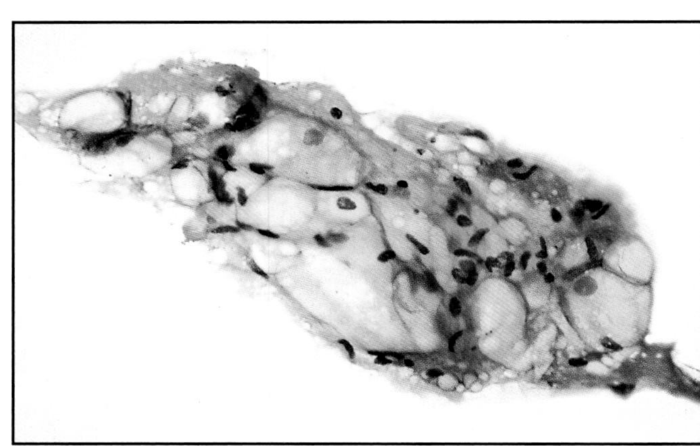

▮21.4

Adipose tissue fragment (Papanicolaou, x50).

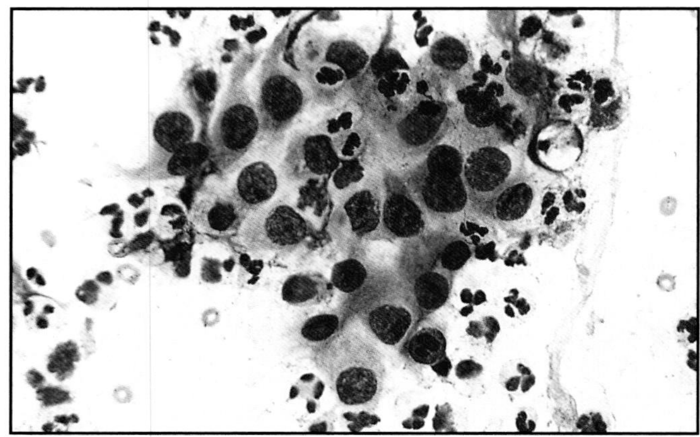

▮21.5

Mastitis and/or fat necrosis. Atypical epithelial cells in an inflammatory background may be a source of false-positive diagnosis (Diff-Quik, x100).

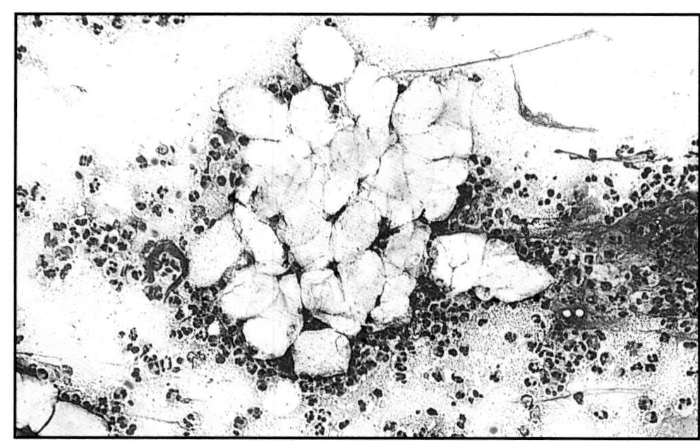

▮21.6

Subareolar abscess. Cluster of anucleated squamous cells with angular cell borders and many polymorphonuclear leukocytes in the background (Diff-Quik, x50).

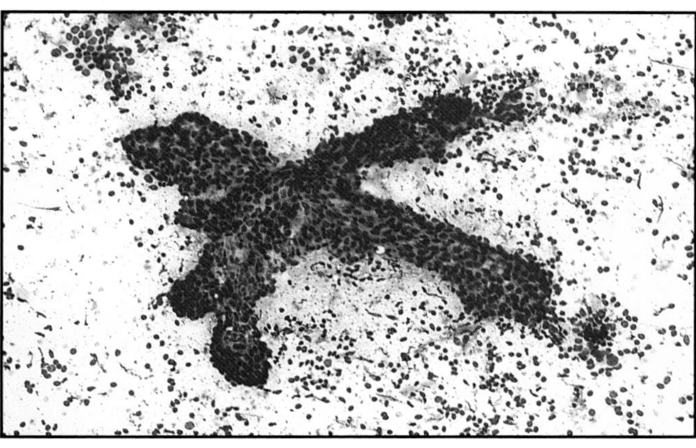

▮21.7

Fibroadenoma. Irregular tight cluster of epithelial cells with "blunt branching" and stripped bipolar nuclei in the background (Diff-Quik, x25).

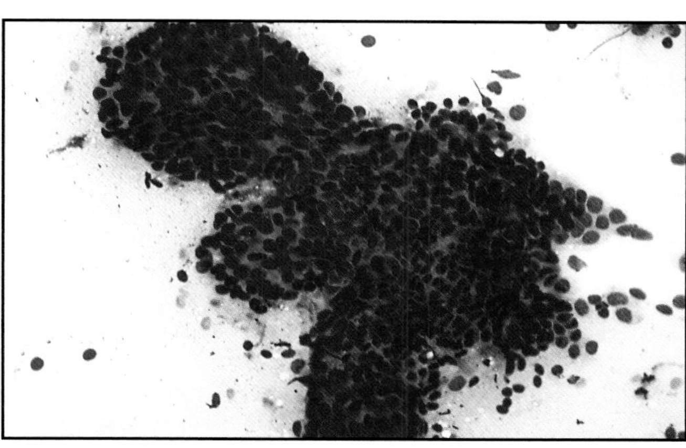

▮21.8

Fibroadenoma. Tightly cohesive epithelial cells with "blunt branching" (Diff-Quik, x50).

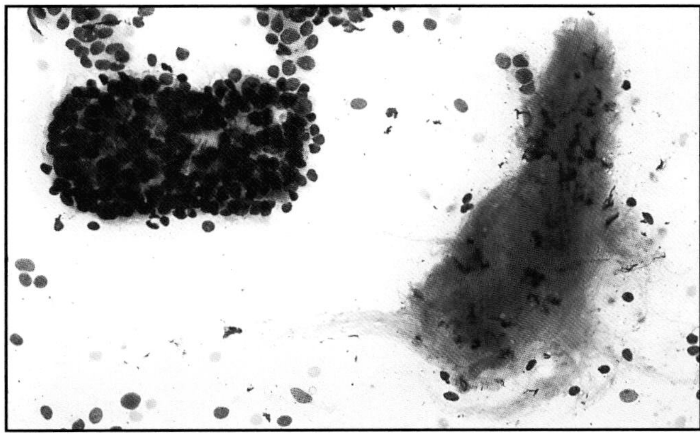

▮21.9

Fibroadenoma. Fibrocollagenous tissue fragment and tight cluster of ductal epithelial cells (Diff-Quik, x50).

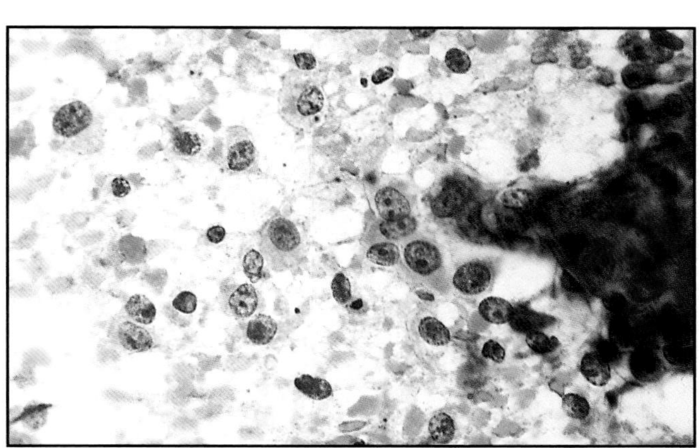

▮21.10

Ductal adenocarcinoma. Atypical epithelial cells arranged singly and in a large cluster (Papanicolaou, x100).

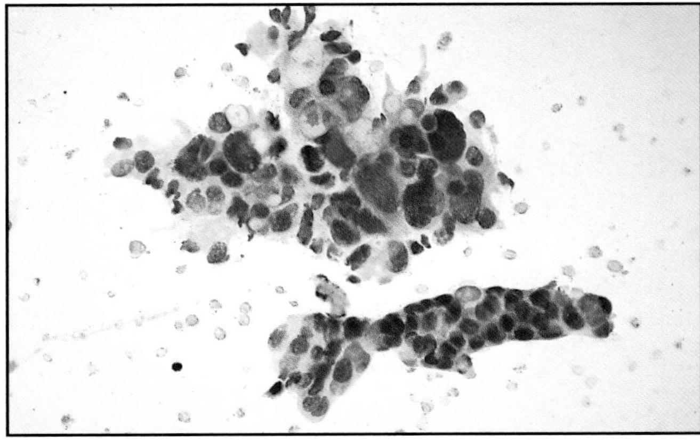

▮21.11

Ductal adenocarcinoma. Clusters of atypical ductal epithelial cells (Papanicolaou, x100). Compare with I21.1 (benign ductal cells).

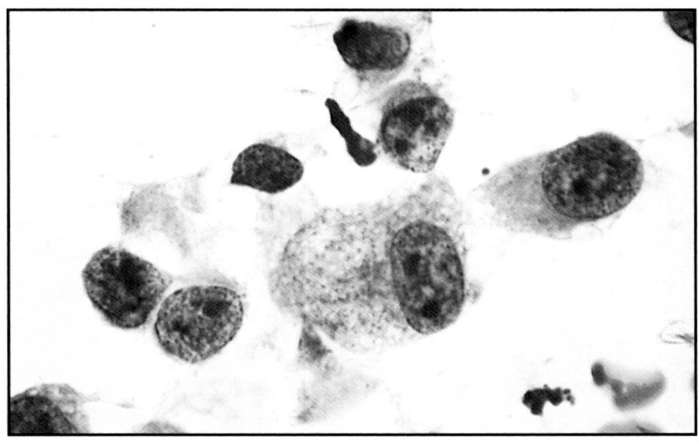

▮21.12

Ductal adenocarcinoma. Atypical cells with delicate cytoplasm, variable nuclear size and shape, and multiple nucleoli (Papanicolaou, x400).

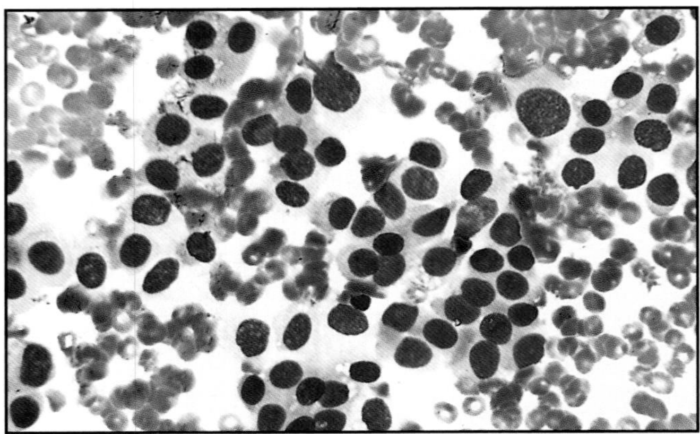

▌21.13

Ductal adenocarcinoma. Loosely cohesive atypical epithelial cells and erythrocytes in the background (Diff-Quik, x100).

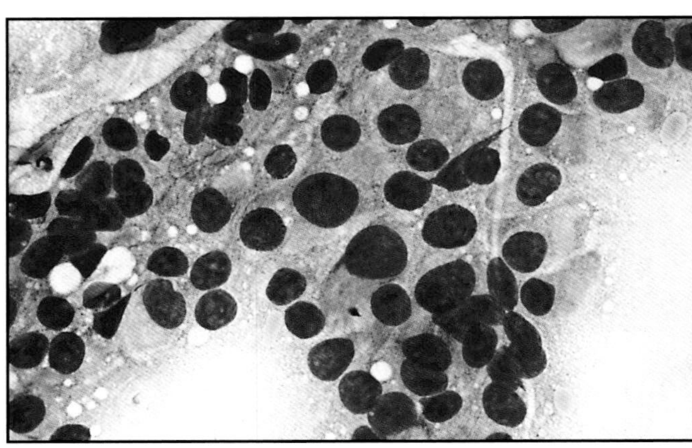

▌21.14

Ductal adenocarcinoma. Sheet of atypical epithelial cells with variable nuclear sizes and visible nucleoli (Diff-Quik, x100).

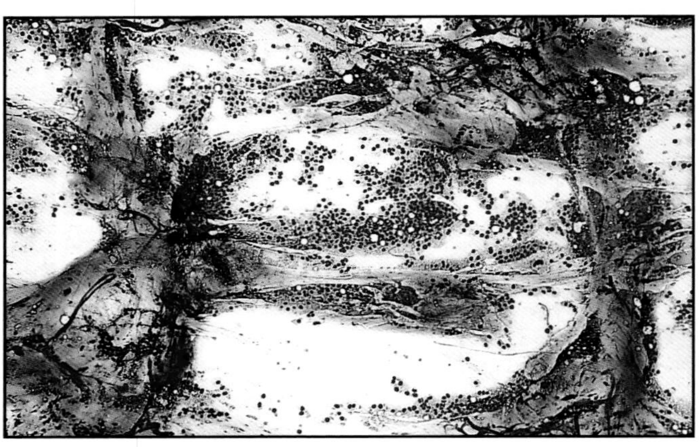

▌21.15

Colloid carcinoma. Note mucous pools and many neoplastic cells ("tumor cellularity") (Diff-Quik, x25).

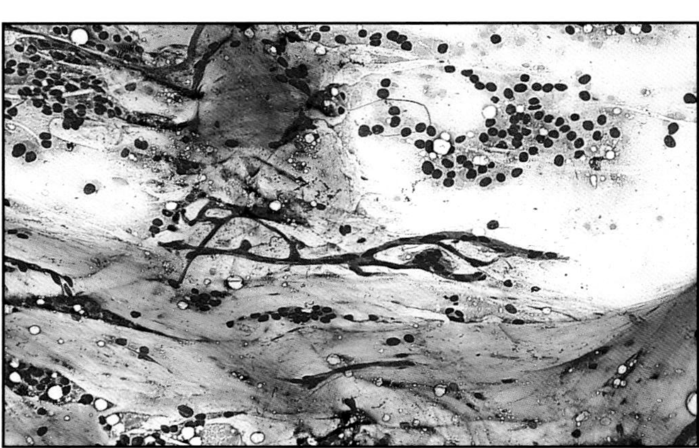

▌21.16

Colloid carcinoma. Mucous pools, branching capillary (center of the field), and neoplastic cells (Diff-Quik, x50).

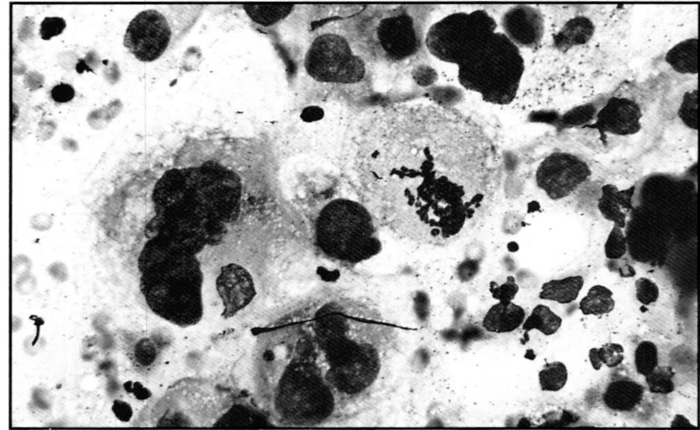

▌21.17

Atypical medullary carcinoma. Bizarre epithelial cells and atypical mitosis (Diff-Quik, x100).

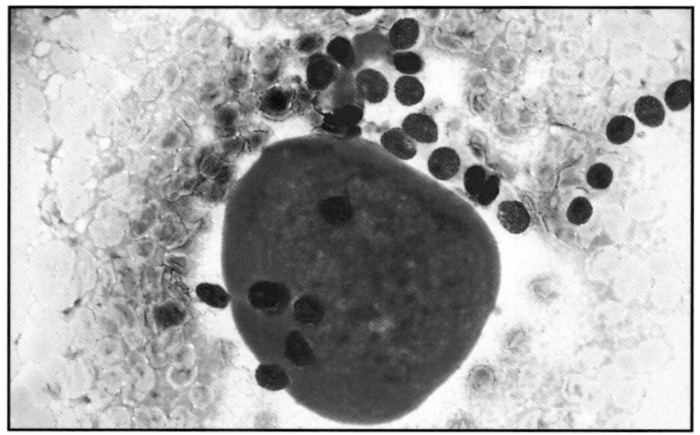

▌21.18

Adenoid cystic carcinoma. Pink, dense, homogeneous globule and small neoplastic cells with scanty cytoplasm (Diff-Quik, x100).

REVIEW EXERCISES

1. How valuable is the cytologic examination of a nipple discharge?
2. Is the cytologic examination of fluid aspirated from mammary cysts worthwhile?
3. Is the presence of some atypical cells in an inflammatory background pathognomonic of inflammatory carcinoma?
4. What are the cytologic diagnostic criteria of subareolar abscess?
5. A young woman presents with a movable nodule in the breast. Multiple aspirates reveal lymphoid tissue. What is the diagnosis?
6. What are the cytologic diagnostic criteria of fibroadenoma?
7. What are the cytologic diagnostic criteria of ductal adenocarcinoma?
8. How would you diagnose cellular smears with mucous pools traversed by capillaries?
9. Cellular smears have enlarged naked nuclei (with prominent nucleoli) and some clusters of atypical epithelial cells. What is the diagnosis?
10. Which mammary carcinoma is the most likely to cause a false-negative diagnosis?

SELECTED READINGS

Boring CC, Squires TS, Tong T. Cancer statistics, 1991. *CA.* 1991;41:19-36.

Ciatto S, Cariaggi P, Bulgaresi P. The value of routine cytologic examination of breast cyst fluids. *Acta Cytol.* 1987;31:301-304.

Feldman PS, Covell JL. *Fine Needle Aspiration Cytology and Its Clinical Applications: Breast and Lung.* Chicago, Ill: ASCP Press; 1985:25-118.

Frable WJ; Bennington JL, ed. *Thin-Needle Aspiration Biopsy.* Philadelphia, Pa: WB Saunders Co; 1983;14:20-73.

Galblum LI, Oertel YC. Subareolar abscess of the breast: diagnosis by fine-needle aspiration. *Am J Clin Pathol.* 1983;80:496-499.

Kline TS. *Handbook of Fine Needle Aspiration Biopsy Cytology.* 2nd ed. New York, NY: Churchill Livingstone Inc; 1988:199-252.

Kline TS, Kline IK. *Guides to Clinical Aspiration Biopsy: Breast.* New York, NY: Igaku-Shoin Medical Publishers Inc; 1989.

Koss LG, Woyke S, Olszewski W. *Aspiration Biopsy: Cytologic Interpretation and Histologic Bases.* New York, NY: Igaku-Shoin Medical Publishers Inc; 1984:53-104.

Leach C, Howell LP. Cytodiagnosis of classic lobular carcinoma and its variants. *Acta Cytol.* 1992;36:199-202.

Linsk JA, Franzen S. *Clinical Aspiration Cytology.* 2nd ed. Philadelphia, Pa: JB Lippincott Co; 1989:111-143.

Martin HE, Ellis EB. Biopsy by needle puncture and aspiration. *Ann Surg.* 1930;92:169-181.

Oertel YC. *Fine Needle Aspiration of the Breast.* Stoneham, Mass: Butterworth Publishers; 1987.

Orell SR, Sterrett GF, Walters MN-I, Whitaker D. *Manual and Atlas of Fine Needle Aspiration Cytology.* 2nd ed. New York, NY: Churchill Livingstone Inc; 1992:129-169.

Rama Rao C, Narasimhamurthy NK, Jaganathan K, et al. Cystosarcoma phyllodes: diagnosis by fine needle aspiration cytology. *Acta Cytol.* 1992;36:203-207.

Schöndorf H; Schneider V, trans. *Aspiration Cytology of the Breast.* Philadelphia, Pa: WB Saunders Co; 1978.

Söderström N. *Fine-Needle Aspiration Biopsy: Used as a Direct Adjunct in Clinical Diagnostic Work.* New York, NY: Grune & Stratton; 1966;14:109-115.

Zajicek J; Wied GL, ed. *Aspiration Biopsy Cytology, I: Cytology of Supradiaphragmatic Organs.* Switzerland: S Karger AG; 1974;4:136-194.

Zaloudek C, Oertel YC, Orenstein JM. Adenoid cystic carcinoma of the breast. *Am J Clin Pathol.* 1984;81:297-307.

CHAPTER 22

Thyroid

John R. Goellner, MD
Darwin A. Johnson, CT(ASCP), CMIAC

CONTENTS

Fine needle aspiration cytology is indicated when information is desired about the nature of a pathologic process in the thyroid: to confirm apparent malignancy, to rule out possible malignancy, to diagnose thyroiditis, etc.

PROCEDURE

The area to be aspirated is located by palpation. The skin is cleansed with antiseptic. Local anesthesia is not necessary. A 25-gauge needle on a 10-mL syringe is used to enter the thyroid while the gland is stabilized. The lesion is pierced and suction is applied while the needle is quickly jabbed in and out to dislodge cells. Suction is released, the needle is withdrawn, and the aspirated material is expelled as drops on slides. (The procedure is facilitated by use of a pistol-grip syringe holder.)

Depending on the amount of fluid obtained, different methods can be used for smearing. Small drops are simply smeared by using a second slide in a "bread-and-butter" fashion. Larger amounts need to be concentrated either by a two-step technique or by dabbing away excess fluid with a piece of gauze. After concentration, the residual semisolid cytologic material is smeared as above. The slide is then either immediately fixed in 95% ethanol or allowed to air-dry. Alcohol-fixed slides are stained by the Papanicolaou method and air-dried slides are stained by the May-Grünwald-Giemsa technique. Each of these staining techniques has some advantages and disadvantages. Nuclear detail and chromatin pattern are better visualized by Papanicolaou stain; some cell products and cytoplasmic features are easier to see in air-dried preparations. Comparison between Papanicolaou stain and hematoxylin-eosin stain on tissue sections is convenient because both preparations fix the cells, producing similar morphologic appearances.

Several punctures can be performed if desired, depending on the amount of material obtained. Cystic lesions may yield only fluid, which must be concentrated by either filtration or other methods. Some aspirates yield large amounts of bloody fluid, which can be added to a balanced salt solution or placed in a tube of anticoagulant. The material can then be filtered or centrifuged for cell block or smear preparations.

INTERPRETATION

Interpretation of aspirate cytology smears demands a different emphasis from that of traditional Papanicolaou smears of the cervix or sputum. Scanning and low-power viewing to appreciate cellularity, cell arrangements, and cell products (such as colloid and amyloid) are important; in contrast, individual cell detail is emphasized less (but may be crucial in some cases).

Benign Nodule

A negative or benign cytologic diagnosis may be made from an aspirate from a normal gland, a multinodular goiter, or a macrofollicular adenoma. The cytologic picture is characterized by small to moderate numbers of rather cohesive epithelial cells in sheets, clusters, or microbiopsy specimens. The cells contain small, round, and regular nuclei with "salt-and-pepper" chromatin and often show a "macrofollicular" architecture. Nucleoli are small or absent, mitoses are absent, and cytoplasm is scanty. Colloid is often visible and may be seen in follicles or as background material [▮*22.1*, ▮*22.2*]. Foam cells are often present and indicate degeneration.

Thyroiditis

Hashimoto's thyroiditis (chronic lymphocytic or autoimmune thyroiditis) is usually characterized by a hypercellular aspirate with a dispersed cell arrangement. Follicles, if they are present, are generally small, and colloid is scanty and often absent. There is a mixture of lymphoid elements and Hürthle cells. Hürthle cells are modified epithelial cells that show abundant finely granular cytoplasm and nuclei that are larger than normal with prominent nucleoli. These cells are often multinucleated and may show considerable "atypia." Ultrastructural examination reveals cytoplasm filled with mitochondria. Hürthle cells are a prominent part of Hashimoto's thyroiditis but can be seen in smaller numbers or show less complete development of Hürthle cell features in various other conditions. In addition, Hürthle cells are sometimes involved in neoplasia—another consideration for the cytomorphologist. The lymphoid cells should comprise a heterogeneous population (small and large lymphocytes, plasma cells, macrophages) indicative of a benign process. Attention should be given to any monotonous lymphoid population because of the possibility of malignant lymphoma. Streak or squish artifact ("lymphoid nesting") is often seen in Hashimoto's thyroiditis because of the fragility of the lymphoid cells [▮*22.3*, ▮*22.4*]. Multinucleated giant cells are not uncommon in Hashimoto's thyroiditis.

Subacute thyroiditis (de Quervain's thyroiditis, granulomatous thyroiditis) is diagnosed by the presence of a number of large multinucleated giant cells (often with 50 or more nuclei); a mixed inflammatory background, which often includes a fair number of neutrophils; and reactive epithelial cells (but not Hürthle cells) [▮*22.5*]. Fibrosing thyroiditis (Riedel's thyroiditis) may be expected to yield little material—mostly chronic inflammatory cells.

Neoplasms

Most neoplasms of the thyroid are primary and epithelial—benign (adenomas) or malignant (carcinomas). Aspiration cytology is useful in distinguishing a neoplasm from a non-neoplastic disease and in classifying the neoplasm in most cases. In some cases, the cytology is indicative of probable neoplasm or possible malignancy but definitive classification is impossible. Most benign tumors of the thyroid are variants of follicular adenomas, often subclassified on the basis of their resemblance to the normal follicular architecture of the thyroid and the presence or absence of a Hürthle cell component.

Carcinomas of the thyroid are divided into four major types: papillary, follicular, medullary, and anaplastic. Papillary carcinoma is the most common (85%-90%), tends to occur in young adults, and has a female predominance. It is an indolent, slow-growing malignancy, tends to metastasize to regional lymph nodes, and is locally invasive into structures of the neck. The primary management of papillary carcinoma is surgical, and most patients with this tumor enjoy a normal life expectancy.

Follicular carcinoma is less frequent (5%-10%), tends to occur in middle-aged to older adults, and has a female predominance. The disease is of low to intermediate aggressiveness, depending on the stage of disease at the time of presentation and the degree of invasiveness. Both papillary and follicular carcinomas are considered to be differentiated tumors of thyroid follicular epithelium, tend to take up radioactive iodine, and usually give positive results with immunostains for thyroglobulin.

Medullary carcinoma, in contrast, is a tumor of the "C cells" of the thyroid. C cells are neuroendocrine cells and produce calcitonin rather than thyroglobulin. Eighty percent of medullary carcinomas are sporadic and 20% are associated with familial syndromes (particularly multiple endocrine neoplasia [MEN] IIA and IIB). This tumor is moderately aggressive and prognosis depends on the stage of disease at presentation. Tumor cells give positive results with immunostains for calcitonin and are negative for thyroglobulin.

Anaplastic carcinoma is a rare but very aggressive, highly lethal tumor. This tumor occurs in older adults and presents as a rapidly growing, large neck mass, with symptoms referable to invasion of neck organs. Patients usually die within 1 year and the disease is refractory to therapy, including surgery, radiation, and chemotherapy. By immunostaining, anaplastic carcinomas may show epithelial differentiation (keratin and epithelial membrane antigen positivity) but may assume a morphologic appearance and immunostain pattern similar to sarcoma rather than carcinoma. Only a minority (20%) of anaplastic carcinomas are positive for thyroglobulin by immunostains. Areas of differentiated thyroid carcinoma are frequently seen in association with anaplastic carcinoma.

Metastatic carcinoma to the thyroid is also occasionally seen. The most common primary sites are kidney, lung, and breast.

Papillary carcinoma is characterized cytologically by cells arranged in papillary groups, monolayer sheets, or single cells (some papillary carcinomas show considerable follicular growth pattern and their arrangement in aspiration cytology may resemble that seen in follicular neoplasms). Papillary groups (elongated, finger-like cell aggregates with a central fibrovascular stromal core) strongly suggest papillary carcinoma but are not pathognomonic. Parenchymatous hyperplasia (Graves' disease) may show some papillary architecture, as do rare follicular adenomas. The nuclei in papillary carcinoma are generally enlarged and show irregular nuclear outlines with molding, flattening, and angulation of the nuclear membrane. The chromatin is usually pale, diffuse, and nongranular ("washed out"). There is often a prominent groove in the nuclear membrane (coffee bean grooving), which may appear as a notch in the nuclear outline if it is observed at the proper angle [▮*22.6*, ▮*22.7*]. Grooving is not exclusive to papillary carcinoma and may be seen in other conditions, particularly Hashimoto's thyroiditis. Intranuclear inclusions or holes (actually cytoplasmic invaginations and not true inclusions) are often, but not invariably, seen. These too are not unique to papillary carcinoma; intranuclear inclusions are present in medullary carcinoma and also, rarely, in benign conditions such as hyalinizing trabecular adenoma. Colloid may be unusually viscous and stringy. Multinucleated giant cells may also be present (these are nonspecific and are seen in degeneration, Hashimoto's thyroiditis, and, particularly, subacute thyroiditis, as noted above). Psammoma bodies may also be seen but are only present in approximately 20% of aspirates from papillary carcinoma. Importantly, psammoma bodies are not pathognomonic but only strongly suggestive of papillary carcinoma; they are rarely seen in benign conditions. Papillary carcinomas frequently undergo cystic degeneration (25%-30%). This should be kept in mind when examining cyst fluid.

Cellular follicular neoplasms (both benign and malignant) produce hypercellular aspirates that contain scanty colloid and in which the cells are arranged in a dispersed microfollicular pattern. Cohesive cell aggregates may also be present, but at least in areas the microfollicles are dispersed randomly across the slide [▮*22.8*, ▮*22.9*]. Nuclear details are relatively unimportant given this low-power cell pattern, although significant atypia increases the concern of malignancy. Necrosis (as opposed to foam cell degenerative features) suggests malignancy. Hürthle cell neoplasms are a variation of follicular neoplasms that show a relatively pure Hürthle cell epithelial population and generally a hypercellular aspirate [▮*22.10*]. A cytologic distinction of the benign or malignant nature of follicular neoplasms/Hürthle cell neoplasms is impossible because the diagnosis of malignancy rests on the histologic identification of capsular or vascular invasion and not on cytomorphologic features. In our experience, approximately 15% of these cases prove to be malignant at operation (90%-95% are neoplasms; most are benign adenomas).

Efforts have been made to further subclassify these lesions by techniques such as image analysis or ploidy studies in an attempt to distinguish preoperatively between follicular adenomas and follicular carcinomas. Computer-assisted image analysis (planimetry) of follicular neoplasms was initially thought to be promising in the preoperative distinction between follicular adenoma and follicular carcinoma. Subsequent studies, however, have failed to confirm diagnostic usefulness for image analysis because the diagnosis of benign and malignant lesions could not be reliably predicted. "Marker features" (nuclear morphology, nuclear chromatin texture, and nuclear staining density) have shown promise. DNA analysis (ploidy) has been studied as a predictor of adenoma vs carcinoma and has shown too much overlap between benign and malignant groups for diagnostic usefulness. Approximately 25% of follicular adenomas have aneuploid DNA patterns, and a significant fraction (30%-50%) of follicular carcinomas show a diploid DNA content. (Despite limitations in the use of ploidy analysis for diagnosis, the quantitation of DNA does appear to be useful as a prognostic indicator in the patient with established thyroid malignancy, particularly in papillary and medullary carcinoma.)

Medullary carcinoma is a histologically variable tumor and its cytology reflects this variability. The aspirates are generally hypercellular and have poor cell cohesion. The cells are oval to spindle shaped, as are the nuclei. Well-fixed material may show the typical granular chromatin pattern often seen in other neuroendocrine neoplasms such as carcinoid tumor. Some medullary carcinomas mimic lymphoid neoplasms in their cytologic pattern; eccentric nuclei may suggest plasma cells. Amorphous material staining for amyloid is often present in aspirates of medullary carcinoma [▮*22.11*]. Papanicolaou-stained slides can be restained with Congo red for amyloid in questionable cases. The results appear to be reliable, although amyloid is not invariably present in medullary carcinoma. Immunostains for thyrocalcitonin can also be used to confirm a suspected diagnosis in problem cases; however, false-negative results for thyrocalcitonin may be misleading.

Anaplastic carcinoma shows malignant cells by the classic cytologic criteria of cell pleomorphism, nuclear hyperchromatism, prominent nucleoli, mitotic activity, and evidence of necrosis. The background is often extensively necrotic and shows purulent inflammation secondary to the necrosis [▮*22.12*]. Classically, anaplastic carcinoma is divided into giant cell, sarcomatoid or spindle cell, and small cell types. Differentiation of small cell anaplastic carcinoma from malignant lymphoma is important and immunostains (keratin vs leukocyte common antigen) may be extremely helpful. Anaplastic carcinoma cells are highly malignant and, as mentioned above, may yield negative results on immunostains for epithelial markers (keratin and epithelial membrane antigen) and for thyroglobulin.

Lymphomas are occasionally encountered in thyroid aspiration cytology. Their identification may be difficult, and a conscious effort to consider lymphoma should be made when any significant lymphoid infiltrate is present. Clinical findings are helpful in establishing the diagnoses. Immunostaining of cytologic specimens has been reported to be helpful in confirming cases of lymphoma, or surgical biopsy may be needed for confirmation and typing.

Metastatic carcinoma also may be encountered on occasion. Usually there will be a history of a previous malignancy, although this information may not be communicated to the laboratory. Metastatic disease should be considered when malignant cells are present and they do not fit easily into one of the four major categories of primary thyroid carcinoma discussed above. Negative immunostaining for thyroglobulin and thyrocalcitonin may help establish that the lesion is metastatic. Clinical evaluation may be necessary to accurately diagnose metastatic disease, and open biopsy may be required for definitive diagnosis.

Other Findings

In addition to thyroid lesions discussed above, the microscopist may encounter nonthyroidal cells. These are most frequently benign contaminants from adjacent tissues such as skin, fat, or muscle. Less frequently, respiratory epithelium or hematopoietic cells are observed when the aspiration encounters tracheal or laryngeal tissues. In addition, pathologic conditions of nonthyroidal tissues may be found at aspiration. Hodgkin's disease or non-Hodgkin's lymphoma of adjacent lymph nodes, tumors originating from the nerves of the neck, or tumors related to the soft tissues of the adjacent structures all may be encountered.

STATISTICAL COMMENTS

Thyroid cytologic results may be placed into one of four broad categories: positive for malignancy, suspicious for malignancy, negative for malignancy, and nondiagnostic. Within these categories further descriptive comments are generally made (eg, Hashimoto's thyroiditis, follicular neoplasm). Our experience with more than 10,000 aspirations has found approximately 64% of aspirates negative for malignancy, 11% suspicious for malignancy, 4% positive for malignancy, and 20% nondiagnostic.

Unless a tissue diagnosis is obtained in every case, it is difficult to ascertain the accuracy rates of aspiration cytology. In our practice the false-positive rate is less than 1%. Our sensitivity rate is approximately 98% (ie, 98% of known malignancies had either a suspicious or positive cytologic result—discounting nondiagnostic specimens). Suspicious cytologic findings include several different situations: cases with cellular atypia not otherwise specified, cases suggestive but not conclusive for malignancy, and cases of follicular or Hürthle cell neoplasm. Ordinarily, surgical exploration is recommended when the cytologic results suggest malignancy, but this is tempered by the clinician's judgment as to the risk of malignancy in view of the patient's age, general health status, and expected operative risk. In our experience, approximately 29% of cases operated on because of suspicious cytologic results do prove to be malignant. The nondiagnostic or unsatisfactory category is used for aspirations that have too little cellular material to render a cytologic diagnosis. Approximately half these cases are cystic lesions that produce only cyst fluid and degenerative foam cells. A second aspiration yields diagnostic material in approximately 50% of cases that were initially nondiagnostic.

A rule of thumb for "diagnostic adequacy" is six or more groups of benign-appearing thyroid epithelial cells per case. These may be on one or more slides. A group is approximately 15 to 20 thyroid epithelial cells in a sheet or cluster. The presence of colloid is reassuring but not in itself adequate for a negative diagnosis. Large benign-appearing cell groups may be extrapolated to the appropriate numbers of minimum groups for the purpose of assessment of adequacy. Obviously, air-drying, inadequate fixation, or blood or inflammation obscuring the cell morphology may lead to a less than optimal or inadequate specimen.

RISKS

There is practically no risk to the patient from the fine needle aspiration technique. Several studies have shown that dissemination of tumor cells from the needle tract does not affect long-term prognosis and practically never causes implantation of tumor in the needle tract. Life-threatening, massive hemorrhage is not a problem—local pressure and normal clotting mechanisms usually control any defect in major vessels. Rarely, bleeding will not cease normally and a hematoma may develop. Our experience has confirmed the negligible morbidity reported in the literature.

SUMMARY

Cytologic examination of specimens obtained by fine needle aspiration of the thyroid is a safe, expedient, and useful diagnostic modality for studying thyroid abnormalities. Even in experienced hands there will be a fair number of nondiagnostic aspirates because of the nature of the underlying pathologic condition. Additionally, the clinicians and cytopathologists involved need to have experience and good communication to optimize the application of the technique.

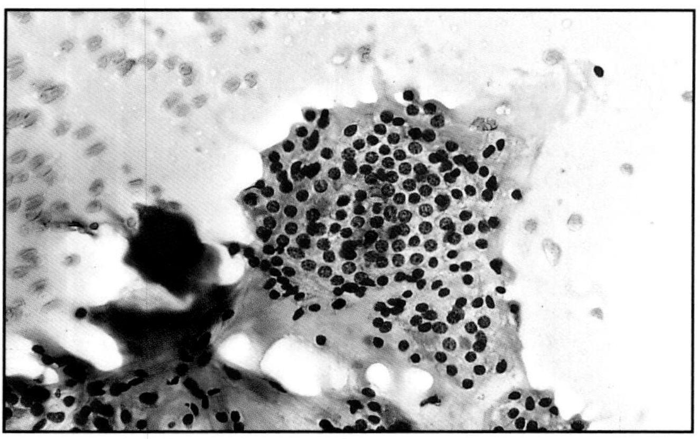

▮22.1

Benign thyroid nodule (colloid nodule) showing a sheet of regular cells with accompanying colloid, some of it in radial strands attached to the epithelial cells (Papanicolaou, x250).

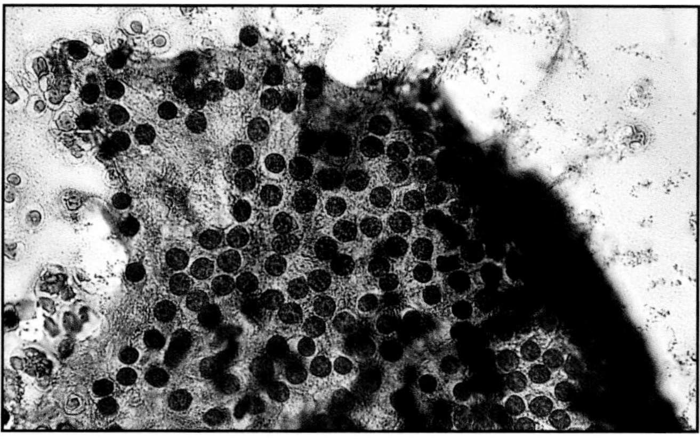

▮22.2

High-power view of benign thyroid epithelial cells illustrating the regular round nuclei, which are approximately twice the diameter of a red blood cell. Note the finely granular chromatin pattern (Papanicolaou, x400).

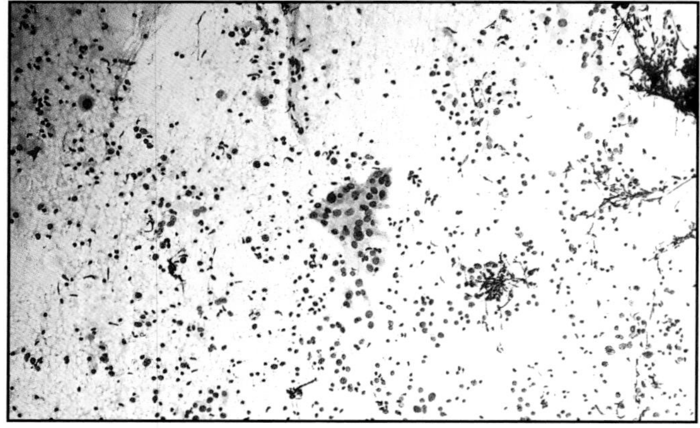

▮22.3

Scanning-power view of Hashimoto's thyroiditis showing dispersed hypercellularity. There is a suggestion of two cell populations (Papanicolaou, x100).

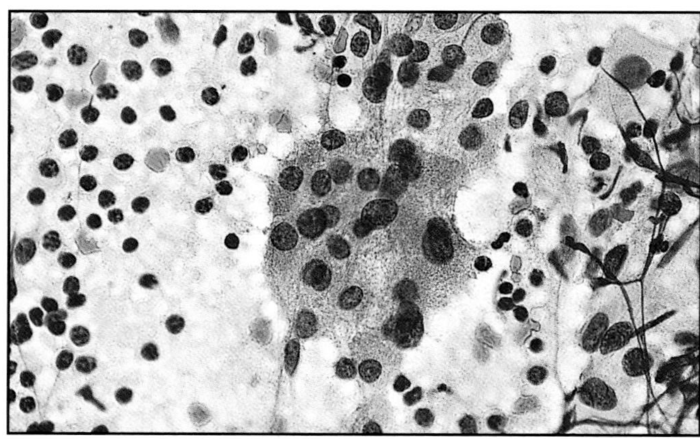

▮22.4

Hashimoto's thyroiditis showing Hürthle cells centrally with adjacent noncohesive lymphoid elements. Note the abundant finely granular cytoplasm and nuclear atypia of the Hürthle cells. Streaking artifact is present in the lymphoid cells (Papanicolaou, x400).

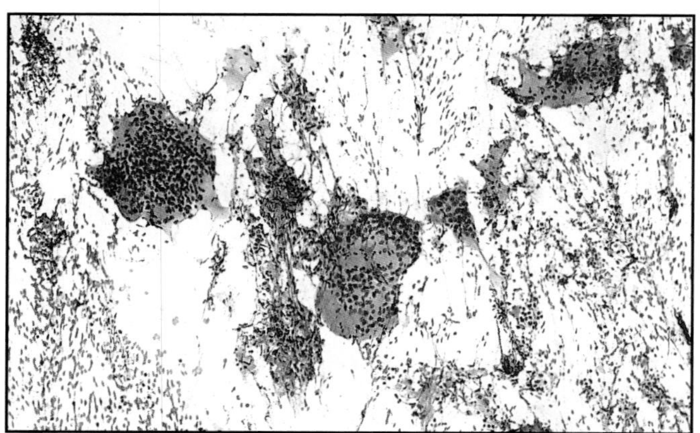

▮22.5

Subacute thyroiditis with several huge multinucleated histiocytic giant cells (Papanicolaou, x64).

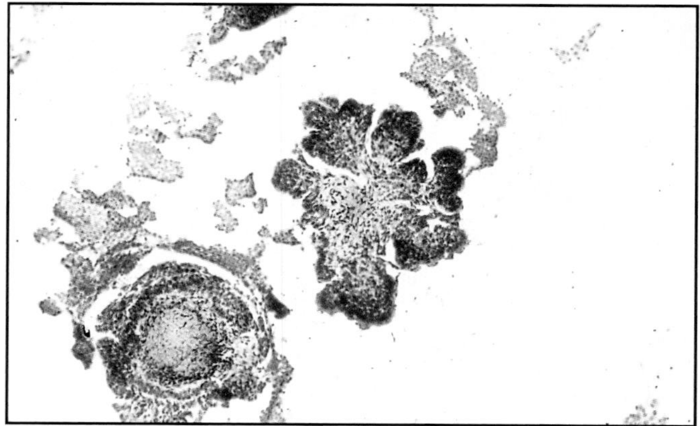

▮22.6

Low-power view of papillary cell groups aspirated from papillary carcinoma. Such groups often show distal clubbing, and a fibrovascular core can usually be seen with careful focusing (Papanicolaou, x64).

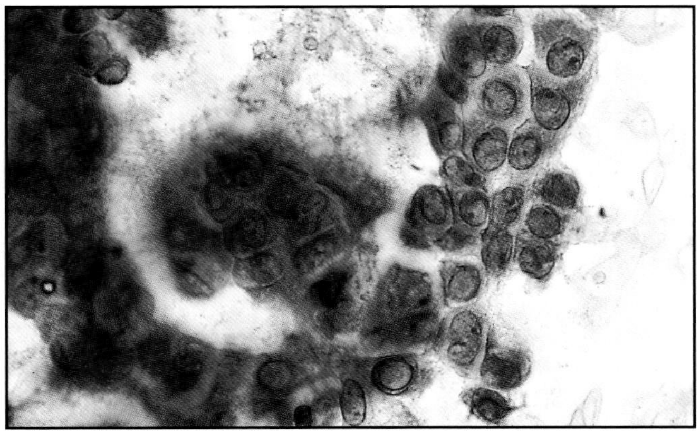

▮22.7

High-power view of papillary carcinoma cells. Nuclei are enlarged and show irregular nuclear outline. Nuclear grooving and notching are present; an intranuclear hole is also identified. Chromatin is pale and diffuse (Papanicolaou, x540).

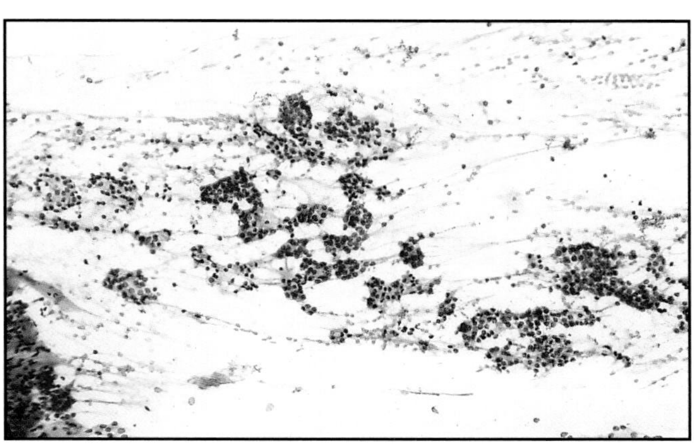

▮22.8

Low-power scanning view of follicular neoplasm showing hypercellularity in a dispersed microfollicular pattern with scanty colloid. This lesion subsequently proved to be a microfollicular adenoma (Papanicolaou, x100).

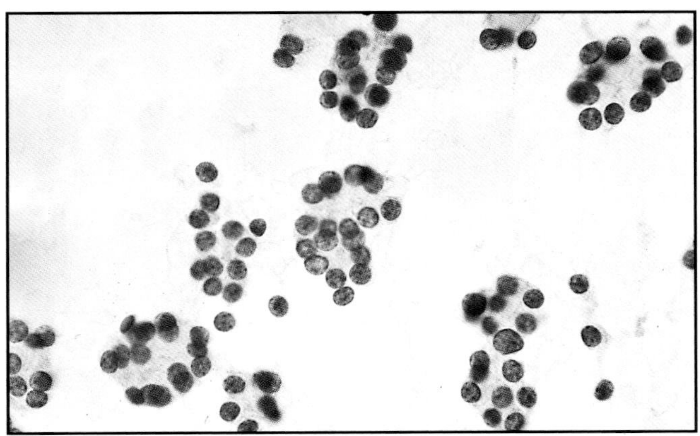

▮22.9

High-power view of follicular neoplasm showing dispersed microfollicles that do not contain colloid. Nuclear atypia is minimal. This lesion subsequently proved to be a follicular carcinoma (Papanicolaou, x400).

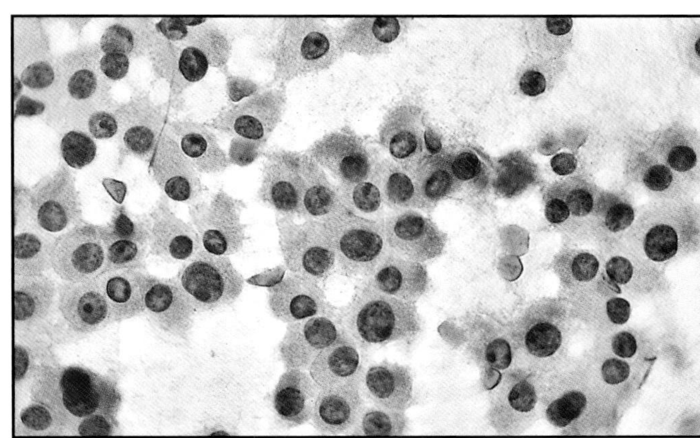

▮22.10

Hürthle cell neoplasm showing a hypercellular population composed almost entirely of Hürthle cells. There is mild nuclear pleomorphism; note the abundant cytoplasm. Hürthle cell adenoma was subsequently diagnosed at surgery (Papanicolaou, x540).

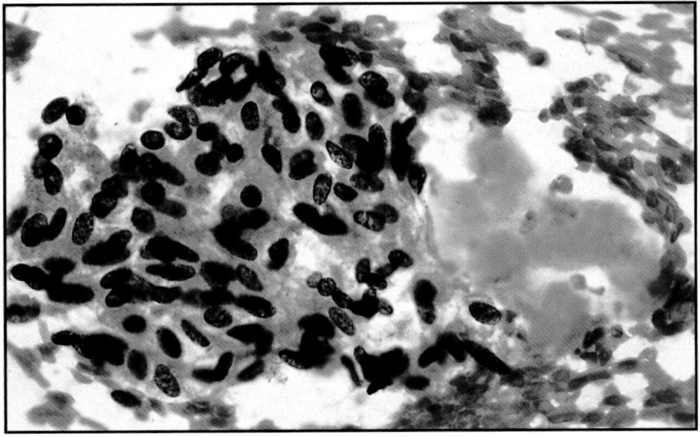

▮22.11

Cytologic smear from medullary carcinoma showing atypical spindle-shaped tumor cells with nuclear hyperchromasia. Amyloid is present on the right side (Papanicolaou, x400).

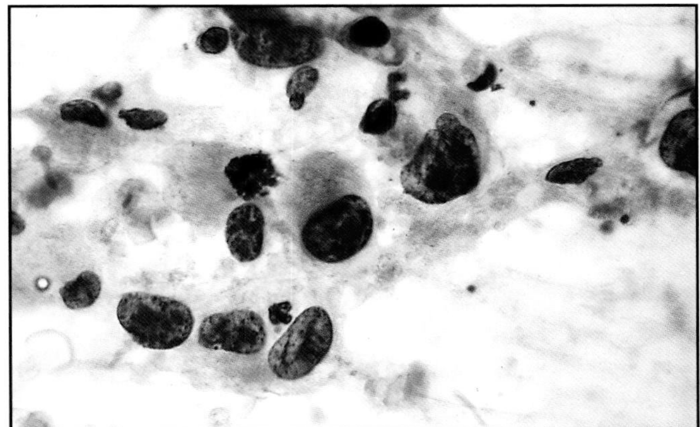

▮22.12

Aspiration cytology of anaplastic carcinoma showing large, extremely malignant-appearing cells accompanied by necrotic debris (Papanicolaou, x540).

REVIEW EXERCISES

1. Intranuclear holes are frequently seen in which of the following conditions?
   a) Hashimoto's thyroiditis
   b) Papillary carcinoma and medullary carcinoma
   c) Follicular carcinoma and follicular adenoma
   d) Subacute thyroiditis
   e) None of the above

2. Cytologic criteria important in the diagnosis of thyroid aspirates include which of the following?
   a) Overall cellularity
   b) Cell arrangement
   c) Nuclear size and shape
   d) Chromatin pattern
   e) All of the above

3. The differential diagnosis when histiocytic giant cells are present includes
   a) degeneration.
   b) papillary carcinoma.
   c) subacute thyroiditis.
   d) Hashimoto's thyroiditis.
   e) all of the above.

4. The differential diagnosis of a hypercellular smear containing prominent Hürthle cells includes
   a) Hürthle cell neoplasm.
   b) Hashimoto's thyroiditis.
   c) subacute thyroiditis.
   d) a) and b).
   e) a) and c).

5. Which of the following statements about the most common primary malignancy of the thyroid is false?
   a) It is generally a slow-growing, indolent tumor.
   b) Primary management is surgical.
   c) Immunostain is positive for calcitonin.
   d) It tends to occur in young adults.
   e) It most commonly spreads to regional lymph nodes.

SELECTED READINGS

Abele JS, Miller TR, King EB, et al. Smearing techniques for the concentration of particles from fine needle aspiration biopsy. *Diagn Cytopathol.* 1985;1:59-65.

Boon ME, Löwhagen T, Willems J-S. Planimetric studies on fine needle aspirates from follicular adenoma and follicular carcinoma of the thyroid. *Acta Cytol.* 1980;24:145-148.

Galera-Davidson H, Bibbo M, Bartels PH, et al. Differential diagnosis between follicular adenoma and follicular carcinoma of the thyroid by marker features. *Anal Quant Cytol Histol.* 1986;8:195-200.

Gharib H, Goellner JR. Fine-needle aspiration biopsy of the thyroid: an appraisal. *Ann Intern Med.* 1993;118:282-289

Gharib H, Goellner JR, Zinsmeister AR, et al. Fine-needle aspiration biopsy of the thyroid: the problem of suspicious cytologic findings. *Ann Intern Med.* 1984;101:25-28.

Goellner JR, Gharib H, Grant CS, et al. Fine needle aspiration cytology of the thyroid, 1980 to 1986. *Acta Cytol.* 1987;31:587-590.

Grant CS, Hay ID, Gough IR, et al. Long-term follow-up of patients with benign thyroid fine-needle aspiration cytologic diagnoses. *Surgery.* 1989;106:980-986.

Grohs HK. Fine needle aspiration of medullary thyroid carcinoma. *Cytology Check Sample*, C88-5 (C-179). Chicago, Ill: American Society of Clinical Pathologists; 1988.

Hamberger B, Gharib H, Melton LJ III, et al. Fine-needle aspiration biopsy of thyroid nodules: impact on thyroid practice and cost of care. *Am J Med.* 1982;73:381-384.

Hostetter AL, Hrafnkelsson J, Wingren SOW, et al. A comparative study of DNA cytometry methods for benign and malignant thyroid tissue. *Am J Clin Pathol.* 1988;89:760-763.

Kini SR, Miller JM, Hamburger JI, et al. Cytopathology of papillary carcinoma of the thyroid by fine needle aspiration. *Acta Cytol.* 1980;24:511-521.

Kini SR, Miller JM, Hamburger JI, et al. Cytopathology of follicular lesions of the thyroid gland. *Diagn Cytopathol.* 1985;1:123-132.

Koss LG, Zajicek J. The aspiration biopsy smear. In: Koss LG, ed. *Diagnostic Cytology and Its Histopathologic Bases.* 4th ed. Philadelphia, Pa: JB Lippincott Co; 1992;2:1268-1279.

Löwhagen T, Willems J-S. Aspiration biopsy cytology in diseases of the thyroid. In: Koss LG, Coleman DV, eds. *Advances in Clinical Cytology.* London, England: Butterworths; 1981:201-231.

Luck JB, Mumaw VR, Frable WJ. Fine needle aspiration of the thyroid: differential diagnosis by videoplan image analysis. *Acta Cytol.* 1982;26:793-796.

Nunez C, Mendelsohn G. Fine needle aspiration and needle biopsy of the thyroid gland. *Pathol Annu.* 1989;24:166-168.

Sprenger E, Löwhagen T, Vogt-Schaden M. Differential diagnosis between follicular adenoma and follicular carcinoma of the thyroid by nuclear DNA determination. *Acta Cytol.* 1977;21:528-530.

CHAPTER

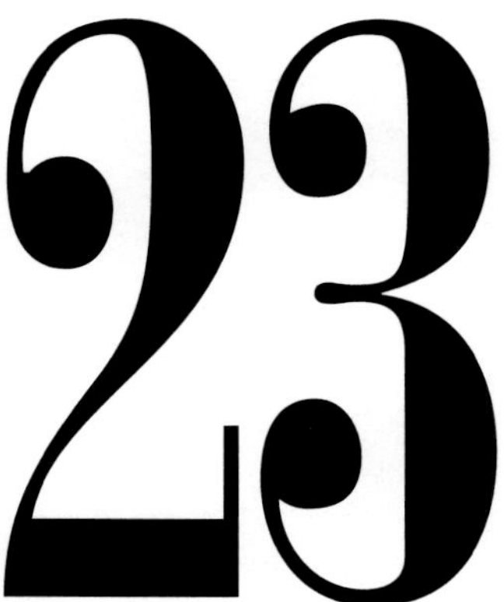

Lymph Nodes

MICHAEL D. GLANT, MD

DOUGLAS E. KING, MS, CT(ASCP), CMIAC

CONTENTS

The use of the needle aspiration biopsy technique to evaluate enlarged lymph nodes has been a subject of great debate ever since it was first introduced in the early 1900s. Equally controversial has been the ability of fine needle aspiration (FNA) to correctly make the diagnoses of lymphoma and Hodgkin's disease, and to distinguish them from some types of reactive lymphoid hyperplasia. It was initially used to diagnose trypanosomiasis in swollen nodes. Most of the early literature dealt with the cytomorphologic patterns associated with metastatic and primary lymphoid neoplasia in lymph nodes. Recently, cytologic criteria have been developed for the diagnosis of most primary adenopathy, especially those associated with reactive processes.

UTILIZATION

FNA offers numerous advantages over other methods in the assessment of lymphadenopathy. Traditionally, clinical observation (with or without antibiotic therapy) and surgical excision were the only accepted options to evaluate enlarged lymph nodes. Aspiration biopsy offers a method of cellular analysis to guide clinical observation or treatment and to prompt excision only when necessary.

As an extension of the clinical examination and patient history, FNA can provide a reliable diagnosis in over 90% of cases. In experienced hands a predictive value greater than 95% can be attained, which is comparable to surgical biopsy. Despite a definitive diagnosis for malignancy in primary disease, exact subtyping is less often conclusive. This includes both Hodgkin's disease and non-Hodgkin's lymphomas and is often due to the "nodular" or "diffuse" histologic growth patterns that are not visualized in aspirate samples of non-Hodgkin's lymphomas. In aspirates of metastatic neoplasms the predictive value is very high and the primary site can usually be suggested in most instances. In some cases of reactive lymphadenopathy, presumptive cause and the rate of clinical resolution can be predicted, which greatly assists the clinician in planning patient follow-up and treatment.

In body sites where surgery is risky or cosmetically unacceptable, FNA offers the possibility of immediate evaluation without significant trauma or risk. In the patient with very low risk of neoplasia, FNA can efficiently exclude the unlikely, allay the fears of the patient (or family), and avoid delay in treatment.

Complications, including needle track spread, are virtually nonexistent when the smallest gauge (23-25) needles are used. Minor hematoma is infrequent, and the procedure is rapid and only minimally uncomfortable.

TECHNICAL CONSIDERATIONS

When evaluating FNA specimens it is essential to obtain as much data as possible before rendering a diagnostic interpretation. While some authors utilize exclu sively air-dried Romanowsky or wet-fixed Papanicolao stained aspirate preparations, making paired slides for bo types of stains maximizes the morphologic data availab for evaluation. This is especially true when dealing wit aspirates of lymph nodes, since cytoplasmic characteristi of lymphoid cells are best visualized on air-dried prepar tions. Lymphoglandular bodies, which are markers fo lymphoid cells, are only seen reliably with Romanowsk stains. In addition, because air-drying causes cells to flatte and spread in the plane of the slide, their diamete increase two to three times when compared with wet-fixe lymphocytes. This makes the spectrum of lymphoid ce size much more pronounced and facilitates evaluation o the mixture of lymphocytes in the cellular populatio Ethanol-fixed, Papanicolaou-stained slides produce cel with crisp nuclear detail, which helps distinguish lymphoi cell types as they differentiate. The Papanicolaou stain als helps identify various epithelial cell types in metastat disease and other nonlymphoid cells such as epithelioi cells and connective tissue elements.

LYMPH NODE STRUCTURE AND FUNCTION

Like other body systems that are studied by the cyto logic method, an understanding of the basic anatomic an histologic structure of lymph nodes is necessary to accu rately evaluate specimens from this site. In addition, sinc lymph nodes are a major component of the body's periph eral immune system a brief review of basic immunology warranted. There is a direct relationship between the cyto logic patterns in lymph node aspirates and the immuno cyte population that develops after antigenic stimulatio Keep in mind the following three points when evaluatin aspirates of lymph nodes: (1) lymph node structure, (2 lymph node function and its role in the immune proces and (3) the morphogenesis and differentiation of stimu lated lymphocytes.

Lymph nodes are involved with the body's respons that generates "specific" products to a given antigenic stim ulus. As such, they are part of the body's peripheral immun system where lymphocytes can interact with antigen, an subsequently differentiate and ultimately assist in the elim nation of the antigenic (foreign) substance. A lymph node function, then, is to filter lymph fluid to sequester foreig antigens, to amplify the number of immunocompeten lymphocytes, and to recirculate lymphocytes.

These functions are accomplished through a series o sinuses that run from the connective tissue capsule of lymph node through the cortex, into the medullary sinu and eventually into the efferent lymphatics [**F**23.1]. Th sinuses are lined by phagocytic cells that recognize an engulf foreign substances. These cells present the antige to lymphocytes with specific receptors and stimulate th

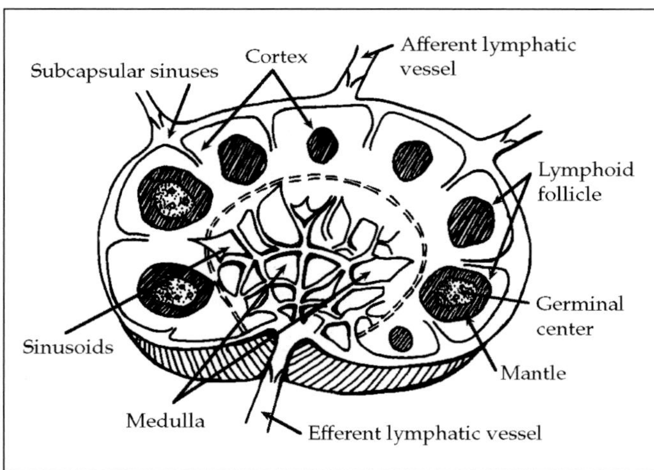

F23.1
Cross section of normal lymph node.

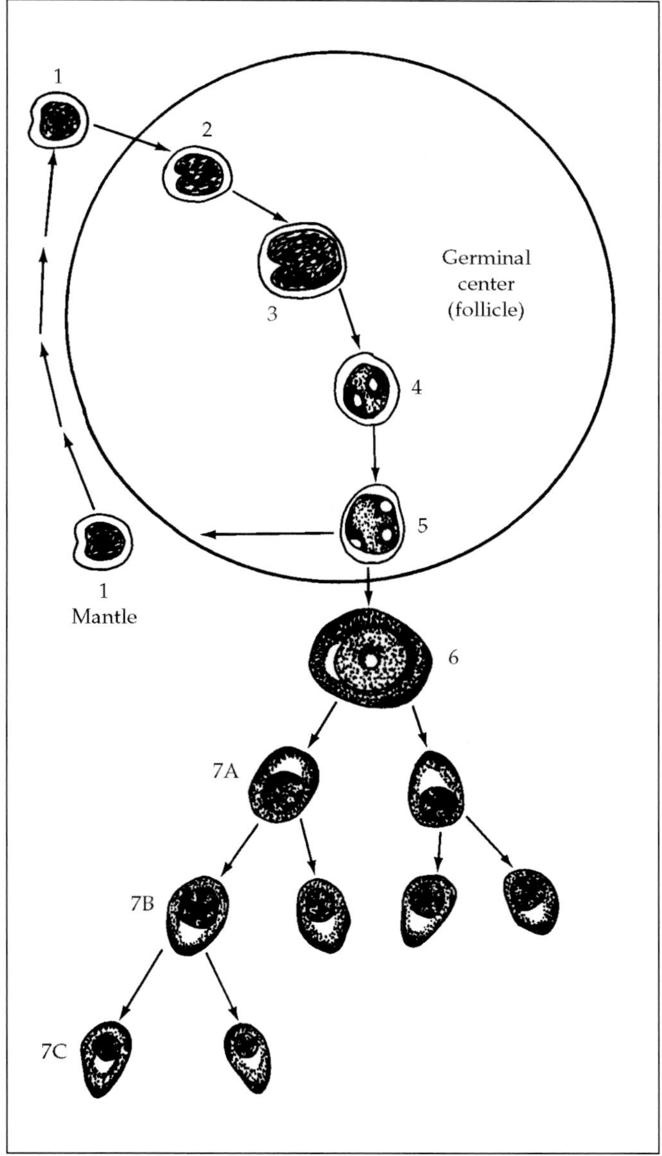

F23.2
Differentiation of stimulated lymphocytes. 1, small round lymphocyte; 2, small cleaved lymphocyte; 3, large cleaved lymphocyte; 4, small noncleaved lymphocyte; 5, large noncleaved lymphocyte; 6, immunoblast; 7A, plasmablasts; 7B, plasmacytes; 7C, plasma cells.

lymphocytes to undergo a series of morphologic and functional changes. This prepares them for one of a variety of interactions with antigen, resulting in antigen destruction.

There are two classes of lymphocytes that are involved in the immunologic response. B cells are lymphocytes that differentiate into plasma cells capable of manufacturing immunoglobulins (antibodies) specifically directed toward a given antigen. This is the humoral response to antigen. T cells are lymphocytes that do not produce antibodies but instead affect antigen destruction through cell-cell interaction (cell-mediated immune response). Different classes of antigen elicit a different type of immune response, either humoral or cell mediated, but many times the two systems work in concert with one another in a variety of ways.

In lymph nodes, B and T cells reside and differentiate in different sites. B cells and B cell reactions are located primarily in and around lymphoid follicles, in the cortex of the node. When B cell reactions occur these follicles increase in number, size, and shape and develop germinal centers. Germinal centers are the sites where the bulk of B cell differentiation from mature, small round lymphocytes to plasmacytoid cells takes place. Deep to the cortex (the paracortex or interfollicular zone) is the site of T cell activity and differentiation.

Lymphocyte Differentiation

T and B lymphocytes are morphologically indistinguishable when viewed by standard light microscopy. For this reason, only B cell stimulation and differentiation are described. Keep in mind that B cells generate antibody-producing plasma cells and T cells do not.

T lymphocytes make subsets of T cells with variable functions and constitute the majority of long-lived circulating blood lymphocytes. Mature lymphocytes or small round lymphocytes [**F**23.2; **T**23.1, **T**23.2] are found in primary lymphoid follicles or surrounding germinal centers in the so-called "mantle zone." Small round lymphocytes are about 4 to 6 µm in diameter on wet-fixed preparations [**I**23.1]. They have round nuclei with coarse or dense chromatin and no nucleoli. Cytoplasm is scanty [**I**23.2].

After stimulation by a random encounter with antigen, small round lymphocytes differentiate into small cleaved lymphocytes. Small cleaved lymphocytes are the first transformed cell type to be identified in germinal centers and are somewhat larger than small round lymphocytes [**I**23.1, **I**23.3]. Their nuclei may or may not be indented, and

Cell Type	Volume	Quality
Small round lymphocyte	Scant	Pale blue
Small cleaved lymphocyte	Scant	Pale blue
Large cleaved lymphocyte	Scant	Pale blue
Small noncleaved lymphocyte	Scant	Blue, vacuolated
Large noncleaved lymphocyte	Intermediate	Blue
Immunoblast	Abundant	Deep blue, vacuolated
Plasma cell	Moderately abundant	Deep blue

T *23.1*

Comparative Morphology of Differentiating Lymphocytes: Cytoplasmic Features (Air-Dried)

while the chromatin is usually coarse it may be "open," with fine granularity and parachromatin clearing on Papanicolaou stain.

Small cleaved lymphocytes transform into large cleaved lymphocytes [▮*23.4*, ▮*23.5*] with nuclei equal to or larger than histiocyte nuclei in wet-fixed preparations. Large cleaved lymphocytes, too, have coarse chromatin with rare nucleoli and differentiate into small noncleaved lymphocytes, which have nuclei the size of histiocyte nuclei and have fine, open chromatin and one to three small nucleoli. Small noncleaved lymphocytes are very mitotically active and are rarely seen in aspirate specimens. Large noncleaved lymphocytes are derived from small noncleaved lymphocytes and are about twice the size of small round lymphocytes. They have a finely granular chromatin and one to three large, usually membrane-bound nucleoli [▮*23.5*]. Large noncleaved lymphocytes differentiate into immunoblasts or may [▮*23.4*, ▮*23.5*] undergo morphologic and functional changes to small round lymphocytes (memory B cells), which usually occur outside of the germinal center.

Immunoblasts [▮*23.1*] are approximately three to four times the size of small round lymphocytes and have large nuclei with fine, open chromatin and one to two central or eccentric macronucleoli. They have moderately abundant cytoplasm, which on Romanowsky stain appears deep blue and vacuolated with a paranuclear clear zone (cytoplasmic hof). This hof contains the Golgi complex and is the primary site of immunoglobulin (antibody) production and modification. Immunoblasts differentiate into progressively smaller plasmacytoid lymphocytes and finally into plasma cells [▮*23.1*]. This final stage of B cell differentiation usually occurs in the medullary sinus of nodes. Plasma cells have small, round eccentric nuclei with coarse (often "clock face") chromatin and are devoid of nucleoli. The cytoplasm in plasma cells is deep blue on Romanowsky-stained smears and also has a cytoplasmic hof.

REACTIVE LYMPH NODE HYPERPLASIA

The reactive process in nodes is extremely heterogeneous from a histologic standpoint and involves a variety of lymphoid and nonlymphoid cells. Patterns of reactive lymph node hyperplasia (RLNH) may overlap one another and in some instances may overlap the morphologic picture seen in lymphoid neoplasia. For this reason lymph node aspirates should always be evaluated with complete knowledge of patient history and physical findings (prior illness, vaccinations, surgery, or malignancy, and the physical character of the lymph node). In the majority of cases, RLNH can be distinguished from lymphoma with a great deal of precision. The most useful and consistent cytologic criterion in RLNH is the finding of a polymorphic population of lymphoid cells with the full spectrum of morphologic forms present. It should be

Cell Type	Size/Shape	Chromatin	Nucleoli
Small round lymphocyte	Small/Round	Coarse/Dense	None
Small cleaved lymphocyte	Small/Grooves	Coarse/Moderately open	Rare/Small
Large cleaved lymphocyte	Large/Grooves	Coarse/Moderately open	Rare/Small
Small noncleaved lymphocyte	Intermediate/Round	Fine/Open	1-3 Small
Large noncleaved lymphocyte	Large/Grooves	Fine/Open	1-3 Large/Membrane bound
Immunoblast	Large/Round	Fine/Open	1-2 Large/Central
Plasma cell	Small/Round	Coarse/Dense "clock face"	None

T *23.2*

Comparative Morphology of Differentiating Lymphocytes: Nuclear Features (Ethanol Fixation)

remembered that the entire spectrum of cells, from small round lymphocytes to plasmacytoid cells, is usually seen. However, depending on the time frame of reaction in which a particular lymph node is sampled, the lymphoid hyperplasia may show different relative proportions of lymphoid cells [F23.3]. The relationship between these cell types can best be visualized on the Romanowsky-stained slides, using low power (x10). In nearly all RLNH the following relationship holds true:

small round lymphocytes + small cleaved lymphocytes >
large cleaved lymphocytes + large noncleaved lymphocytes >
immunoblasts + plasma cells

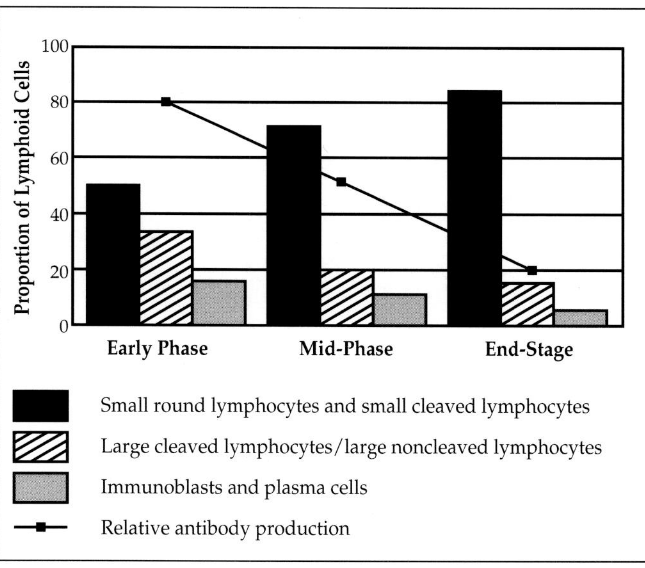

F23.3

Histogram showing relative proportion of lymphoid cells in reactive lymph node hyperplasia (RLNH).

Early-Phase Lymph Node Reaction

Once an antigenic substance has been recognized as foreign the initial response is to produce large amounts of antibody (usually IgM) directed specifically against the antigen. As such, in the earliest recognizable stages of RLNH (in B cell activation) numerous large cells (large cleaved and noncleaved lymphocytes, immunoblasts) are seen along with many plasmacytoid lymphocytes [I23.4, I23.5], indicating active antibody production. This pattern is infrequently seen in lymph node aspirates because the node is only first palpable at this stage. Clinically, antibiotics or observation are usually prescribed for 1 to 2 weeks before any biopsies are considered. The relative number of small round lymphocytes and small cleaved lymphocytes is still greater than the number of large cells and plasma cells and is consistent with a reactive pattern. The observation of numerous large lymphoid cells with their "ominous" cytologic features are at first quite alarming. Determining that the relative proportion of these cells is smaller than that for small round lymphocytes and small cleaved lymphocytes reassures that the process is benign.

Midphase Lymph Node Reaction

As the need for antibody to a specific antigen diminishes, the relative percentage of memory B cells and T cells (small round lymphocytes) increases and the number of large cells and plasma cells decreases. This is a midphase reactive process and signifies subsiding reactive hyperplasia and diminishing antibody production. Numerous small round lymphocytes are seen [I23.1, I23.3], many of which are probably memory B and T lymphocytes located in the mantle zone around the germinal center. A smaller population of large cells, including some large noncleaved lymphocytes, immunoblasts, and occasional plasmacytoid cells, are also identified in midphase node aspirates. Clinically, this is the most common period (second to fourth week after stimulation) when biopsy is sought.

End-Stage Lymph Node Reaction

End-stage (resolution-phase) patterns are observed as antibody production drops even further. This phase is characterized by a marked predominance of small round lymphocytes and small cleaved lymphocytes, and only rarely are large cells or plasmacytoid lymphocytes seen [I23.2, I23.6]. In some cases foci of dense connective tissue are seen and represent areas of fibrosis secondary to prior vascular hyperplasia from intense reactions. Clinically, this is often the lymph node that decreases in size but does not disappear over a period of 5 to 6 weeks or more.

Recurrent Lymph Node Stimulation

If a patient has had multiple, sequential antigenic stimulation over time, lymph node aspirates may show a variety of patterns. The easiest to recognize is the end-stage pattern with recurrent antigenic stimulation. An aspirate specimen from this node would be composed of an abundance of small round lymphocytes and an increased number of large cells (especially immunoblasts and large noncleaved lymphocytes) and plasmacytoid cells [I23.7]. The need for clinical information cannot be overemphasized in these cases. Knowing the onset of any infectious process, the duration of the palpable node, and any history of antibiotic therapy is essential. Clinically, these are usually persistent nodes that fluctuate somewhat over many months. Patients may have recurrent viral disease or other symptoms. Adenopathy in patients with chronic diseases such as systemic lupus erythematosus may have this pattern.

Other Morphologic Features of Lymph Node Aspirates

In addition to the polymorphous lymphoid population there are other morphologic features that are helpful in recognizing RLNH. Lymphohistiocytic aggregates [▮*23.8*] are usually indicative of RLNH and are composed of reticular cells, follicular center/germinal center cells, and tingible body macrophages. They are useful markers of B cell hyperplasias (follicular hyperplasia), since they contain elements found in follicles. Reticular cells are difficult to visualize in cytologic and histologic preparations without special techniques, including enzyme histochemistry. They are part of the connective tissue system that holds lymph nodes together, are stellate in shape with delicate cytoplasm, and contain oval, plump nuclei with small nucleoli. They provide the "matrix" to which the germinal center cells (small round, small cleaved, large noncleaved lymphocytes) and tingible body macrophages combine to form the "syncytia-like" lymphohistiocytic aggregates. Tingible body macrophages are phagocytic macrophages responsible for phagocytizing cell debris and other detritus, which usually fills their cytoplasm [▮*23.9*]. Tingible body macrophages can also be seen as isolated cells separate from lymphohistiocytic aggregates and are often but not always associated with RLNH. Occasionally, since increased vascularity is a histologic feature of RLNH, branching capillaries may be observed in node aspirates [▮*23.10*] and are often associated with lymphohistiocytic aggregates.

Lymphoglandular bodies were first described by Soderstrom in 1968 as 6- to 8-μm "flakes or spherules" in Romanowsky-stained lymph node aspirates. They are fragments of lymphocytic cytoplasm that stain gray-blue with Romanowsky [▮*23.7*] and are not reliably seen with the Papanicolaou stain. They are extremely useful indicators of lymphoid differentiation, especially when distinguishing nonlymphoid metastases (especially poorly differentiated carcinomas) in nodes. As such, they are not seen in lymph nodes that are entirely replaced by epithelial metastases. Their presence is not helpful in determining whether a node aspirate contains reactive or neoplastic lymphoid cells.

The lymph node response depends on the antigenic agent (fungus, bacterium, parasite, virus, chemical, etc). A granulomatous process is a variant of host response and may be seen in a variety of clinical scenarios. Granulomatous reactions are composed of clusters of histiocytes [▮*23.11*]. These are epithelioid cells with delicate, spindle cytoplasm, oval, grooved nuclei, and rare micronucleoli. These epithelioid cells differ from tingible body macrophages in that they are not phagocytic. They contain fibroblast-activating factors that help to stabilize granulomas and promote healing.

Multinucleate giant cells [▮*23.11*] are also a common feature of granulomata, and when seen in combination with epithelioid cells with or without caseous necrosis, are suggestive of tuberculosis, histoplasmosis, or sarcoidosis, in the appropriate clinical setting. Epithelioid cells without giant cells in a background of numerous polymorphonuclear leukocytes is characteristic of a suppurative granuloma. This pattern of microabscess formation is most often associated with cat scratch disease [▮*23.12*] but may be seen with tularemia, *Yersinia*, or brucellosis, etc. Toxoplasmosis is another granuloma-producing infectious process characterized by scattered clusters of epithelioid cells with neither giant cells nor evidence of suppuration [**T***23.3*].

Clinical history is needed to suggest possible causative agents in any of these cellular patterns. Serum studies may be helpful in confirming these agents. If abundant purulent material is obtained in any node aspirate, it should be submitted for routine culture and special cultures and stains for acid-fast bacillus, fungus, etc. Bacterial infection, the later stages of cat scratch disease, or mycobacterial infections may result in extensive suppuration without specific features.

MALIGNANT LYMPHOMAS

Hodgkin's disease and non-Hodgkin's lymphoma are well known malignancies involving lymphoid tissue. The diagnosis of Hodgkin's disease rests on the finding of unequivocal Reed-Sternberg cells and is discussed below. Because non-Hodgkin's lymphoma has a long history of controversial, contradictory, and often confusing classification systems, a broader set of morphologic criteria for light microscopic diagnosis is required. It is critical to remember that some physicians do not consider FNA an acceptable method for initial diagnosis of lymphoma. In well-trained, experienced hands, using appropriate procurement and processing techniques and utilizing immunocytochemical and/or flow cytometric methods (when necessary), malignant lymphoma can be accurately diagnosed in 85% to 90% of cases. Excisional biopsy may be required for precise subclassification and staging, especially if marker studies are not available.

The histologic classification of non-Hodgkin's lymphoma is strongly based on a predominant lymphoid cell population that is usually monomorphic or bimorphic in histologic sections. Lymph node architecture is variably altered, usually with effacement of cortical and medullary structure and outpouring of the neoplastic cells through the lymph node capsule. A nodular (follicular) pattern at low-power magnification may mimic reactive germinal centers and is usually a good prognostic sign for many subtypes of non-Hodgkin's lymphoma. Increased mitotic activity indicates a relatively poorer prognosis. This histologic picture is the result of a block in the differentiation process described earlier for B lymphocytes. This block apparently interferes with the progression of differentiation from one lymphoid

	Epithelioid Histiocytes	Giant Cells	Necrosis	Microabscess
Toxoplasmosis	+	−	−	−
Cat scratch disease	+	±	SUP	+
Lymphogranuloma venereum	+	±	SUP	+
Sarcoidosis	+	+	−	−
Tuberculosis	+	+	CAS	−

SUP, suppurative granuloma formation; CAS, caseous necrosis.
Note: Brucellosis, *Yersinia*, and tularemia also produce suppurative granulomas.

T*23.3*
Morphologic Features of Granulomatous Processes in Aspirate Specimens

cell type to the next, which results in a lymph node tissue section characterized by a disproportionate number of one or two proliferating cell types.

This monomorphic or bimorphic lymphoid tissue pattern for non-Hodgkin's lymphoma is in sharp contrast to the polymorphic pattern described above in aspirates from RLNH. This criterion, when observed in the context of clinical data, is the single most important characteristic that distinguishes most non-Hodgkin's lymphomas from RLNH. Usually, non-Hodgkin's lymphoma in aspirate specimens of lymph nodes is composed of a nearly "pure" population of a single cell type: the normal differentiation scheme of lymphocytes is disrupted. There is a disproportionate number of one proliferating cell type relative to the other cells in the differentiation process. For example, there may be a background of small round lymphocytes, an overabundance of small cleaved lymphocytes, and virtually no large cells [▮*23.13*]. With this number of small cleaved lymphocytes you would expect to see many more large cells. This "shift" in the relative numbers of a single lymphoid cell type is strong evidence for non-Hodgkin's lymphoma in the appropriate clinical setting.

In addition, except in the few instances in which a lymph node is only partially replaced by lymphoma or when a lymphoma induces a "granulomatous response," lymphohistiocytic aggregates are not usually seen. Lymphoglandular bodies are nearly always observed in non-Hodgkin's lymphoma and play an extremely important role in helping to distinguish poorly differentiated epithelial malignancy from lymphoma. Once again, clinical data, including peripheral blood and serum studies, physical examination, radiologic studies, and patient history, are required to make a confident diagnosis of non-Hodgkin's lymphoma in lymph node aspirates.

Cell Patterns in Non-Hodgkin's Lymphoma

For the purposes of this discussion, non-Hodgkin's lymphomas are broken down into typical cytologic patterns instead of histologic classification. This facilitates the understanding of the cytomorphologic features of the more commonly observed non-Hodgkin's lymphomas in node aspirates and enables us to separate them on a morphologic basis.

Small Round Cell Pattern

A monotonous population of small round cells (>80% small round lymphocytes) in a lymph node aspirate is suggestive of a small round cell lymphoma (well-differentiated lymphocytic lymphoma) [▮*23.14*], especially in older patients. This pattern is morphologically similar to the population of small round lymphocytes seen in end-stage RLNH. The best way (short of excisional biopsy) to distinguish these two processes in patients older than 45 years is through the use of immunocytochemistry or flow cytometry.

This small round cell lymphoma expresses a monoclonal light chain but may be very weakly expressed. Fortunately, the vast majority of neoplasms with small round cell pattern are B cell neoplasms and show a characteristic dual marking with pan–B cell antigen and a T cell antigen (Leu1/CD5). Histologically, this lymphoma always has a diffuse growth pattern. Cytologically, this pattern is essentially identical to chronic lymphocytic leukemia with node involvement, is a male-dominant lymphoma, and is rarely observed in patients under the age of 40 years.

Small Cleaved Cell Pattern

Another small cell lymphoma (poorly differentiated lymphocytic lymphoma) is composed of greater than 80% small cleaved cells in a background of scattered small round lymphocytes and few large cells [▮*23.13*]. Small cleaved cells are slightly larger than small round lymphocytes with scant cytoplasm, nuclear clefts or grooves, and a coarse or open chromatin pattern with occasional small nucleoli. This small cleaved lymphoma may appear in a follicular or diffuse pattern in histologic sections and is more mitotically active in the latter. While the relative number of mitotic figures can help distinguish follicular lymphoma from lymphoid hyperplasia in tissue sections (greater numbers of mitoses in reactive processes), it is generally not a useful feature in lymph node aspirates.

Tingible body macrophages and lymphohistiocytic aggregates are rarely seen in aspirates from this type of lymphoma. Morphologically, this neoplasm is nearly identical to small round cell lymphoma in air-dried preparations. Wet-fixed smears are more helpful in distinguishing these two types of lymphomas because of their distinctive chromatin patterns and nuclear shapes. Even so, it must be remembered that small cleaved lymphomas present with a spectrum of cell sizes that can cause diagnostic difficulty. Flow cytometry can be very helpful since small cleaved lymphomas are usually monoclonal B cell neoplasms that often express "common acute lymphocytic leukemia antigen" (CALLA/CD10) and do not coexpress T cell and B cell surface antigens. The median age for detection of small cleaved lymphoma is 54 years.

Mixed Small Cleaved, Large Cell Pattern

In contrast to the polymorphous lymphoid population observed in reactive lymphoid hyperplasia, in which the number of small round lymphocytes and small cleaved lymphocytes is greater than the number of large lymphoid cells, the mixed lymphoma has a bimorphic pattern in lymph node aspirates. Generally, 80% or more of the lymphoid cells are small cleaved lymphocytes and large cells (either large noncleaved or large cleaved lymphocytes) [▮*23.15*]. Tingible body macrophages and lymphohistiocytic aggregates are rarely seen. Of all the different types of lymphomas, the mixed type is most apt to be mistaken for a reactive process. It looks like a midphase reactive pattern. The key to correct interpretation is the virtual lack of small round lymphocytes and immunoblasts despite numerous small cleaved lymphocytes and large cells. Rarely, histiocytes may be abundant, which further complicates the pattern since this may mimic the polymorphous pattern seen in RLNH. Histologically, this neoplasm may present in either a follicular or diffuse pattern in tissue sections, with more mitoses seen in the diffuse type. Using immunocytochemical or flow cytometric techniques, mixed lymphomas are monoclonal for light chains in contrast to the polyclonal pattern in reactive hyperplasia.

Large Cell Pattern

Large cell lymphomas are composed of greater than 80% large cells (either large noncleaved or large cleaved lymphocytes) and in earlier literature were erroneously referred to as a "histiocytic" lymphoma. Fewer than 20% of the cells in the aspirate are small round lymphocytes or small cleaved lymphocytes, and immunoblasts are rarely seen [▮*23.16*]. This disproportionate number of large cells relative to small cells is a hallmark for this lymphoma. Rarely, an immunoblastic lymphoma is encountered in which 50% to 80% of the large cells are immunoblast forms [▮*23.17*, ▮*23.18*]. In this type, smaller plasmacytoid cells may be seen and an early-phase reactive pattern must be excluded. The rarity or lack of small round lymphocytes, small cleaved lymphocytes, large cleaved lymphocytes, and large noncleaved lymphocytes is helpful in making this differential diagnosis. Follicular or diffuse patterns may be observed in histologic sections of the large noncleaved lymphocytic type. Many clinicians believe however, that the large noncleaved lymphocytic and immunoblastic variants are equally aggressive and are treated similarly. The median age at detection for large cell lymphomas is approximately 56 years, and these neoplasms usually mark as monoclonal B cell populations.

Intermediate Cell Pattern

Some lymphomas are composed of cells with nuclei about the same size as a histiocyte nucleus. Two types are representative of this intermediate pattern: undifferentiated B cell lymphoma (Burkitt's and non-Burkitt's lymphoma) and lymphoblastic lymphoma. The undifferentiated type is composed of cells similar to small noncleaved lymphocytes [▮*23.19*], which are rarely observed in reactive processes because they are highly mitotically active. The African Burkitt's lymphoma of the jaw and the non-Burkitt's lymphoma that commonly occurs in the abdomen are also characterized by small noncleaved lymphocytes. These cells are intermediate in size with deep blue, finely vacuolated, lipid-positive cytoplasm. Mitotic figures may be frequent in aspirates of this neoplasm and account for its aggressive behavior. Flow cytometry usually demonstrates a monoclonal B cell neoplasm with IgM kappa surface markers.

Lymphoblastic lymphoma is a T cell lymphoma usually arising in the thymus of young adult males or teenagers. As a result, most patients present with a mediastinal mass. In the "nonconvoluted" variant of lymphoblastic lymphoma the cells are generally monotonously round with a dusty chromatin pattern and a single, medium-sized nucleolus. The cytoplasm is usually scant and pale blue. Mitoses are frequent [▮*23.20*]. Cells from the "convoluted" type are more variable in size and have a coarse chromatin; they may resemble the small cleaved cell lymphoma and frequently have leukemic involvement at the time of diagnosis. Aspirates or histologic sections from both the undifferentiated and Burkitt's lymphomas may contain tingible body macrophages, creating the so-called "starry sky" pattern. This histiocytic infiltrate reflects the high cell proliferation and cell death of these aggressive lymphomas. They always grow in a diffuse pattern histologically.

Hodgkin's Disease

In contrast to non-Hodgkin's lymphoma, Hodgkin's disease has been organized according to subtypes in a useful classification system (the Rye classification), which corresponds to the prognosis and often the clinical setting of the disease. The initial diagnosis of Hodgkin's disease, whether in tissue or aspirate specimens, relies solely on the finding of the classic Reed-Sternberg cell in a background of benign, reactive lymphocytes and/or leukocytes (host response). In recurrent or extranodal disease the finding of one of the Reed-Sternberg cell variants in the appropriate inflammatory background is considered sufficient evidence for the diagnosis of Hodgkin's disease. The exact histogenesis of the Reed-Sternberg cell is uncertain and remains controversial.

Nearly 50% of Hodgkin's disease occurs in patients between the ages of 20 and 40 years and is rarely seen before the age of 10 years or after the age of 60 years. It is somewhat male dominant. Many patients present with "B symptoms," which typically include fever, night sweats, or weight loss. Other presenting symptoms include pruritis, rashes, malaise, and alcohol-induced pain.

The Reed-Sternberg Cell and Its Variants

As stated above, for initial diagnosis of classic Hodgkin's disease, the finding of unequivocal Reed-Sternberg cells in the appropriate background is essential. The classic Reed-Sternberg cell [▮*23.21*] in cytologic material is best visualized in air-dried, Romanowsky-stained preparations because of the cellular flattening that occurs during air-drying. They are usually 40 to 70 µm in diameter and have abundant, pale blue or gray, delicate cytoplasm. A paranuclear cytoplasmic zone or hof is not seen. The nucleus in classic Reed-Sternberg cells is bilobed (often mirror image), with extremely large, irregular nucleoli often exceeding one third the diameter of the nucleus. They may appear in aspirates as bare or stripped nuclei. Reed-Sternberg cell variants include the mononuclear form (so-called Hodgkin's cell); the lacunar cell (seen predominantly in the nodular sclerosing type of Hodgkin's disease); the bizarre, polylobed "popcorn cell" often seen in the lymphocyte-predominant type of Hodgkin's disease; and the "mummified" Reed-Sternberg cell variant, a degenerated form with a smudged, pyknotic nucleus.

The Rye classification acknowledges four histologic subtypes of Hodgkin's disease: (1) lymphocyte predominant, (2) nodular sclerosing, (3) mixed cellularity, and (4) lymphocyte depleted. Each subtype has an inversely proportional population of Reed-Sternberg cells and host response: few Reed-Sternberg cells and abundant lymphocytes in the lymphocyte predominant subtype and many aberrant Reed-Sternberg cells and little evidence of host response in the lymphocyte depleted type. Epithelioid cells as part of a host granulomatous process may be abundant in the lymphocyte predominant subtype. Nodular sclerosing type, as its name suggests contains dense bands of fibrous connective tissue in a background of inflammatory cells and scattered Reed-Sternberg cells. Here, the mononuclear lacunar cell variant of the Reed-Sternberg cell may be observed. The cellularity of the aspirate sample from nodular sclerosing type is generally lower than the other subtypes. The mixed cellularity subtype usually contains numerous Reed-Sternberg cells or variants thereof, and a truly mixed inflammatory background composed of eosinophils, plasma cells, and neutrophils.

The Subtypes of Hodgkin's Disease

Cytologic features are not usually helpful in determining the subtypes of Hodgkin's disease in aspirate specimens. When they are evaluated in conjunction with clinical information, however, FNA may be useful in predicting these histologic variants. For example, Hodgkin's disease, lymphocyte predominant subtype, is often observed in young children who present with a single, large cervical lymph node. The background of the aspirate is filled with a monotonous population of small round lymphocytes that can mimic a well-differentiated lymphocytic lymphoma (a lymphoma usually seen in the elderly). Typical Reed-Sternberg cells or the polylobed Reed-Sternberg variant [▮*23.22*] may be readily identified in this subtype of Hodgkin's disease.

Nodular sclerosing Hodgkin's disease is seen in young adults (classically in females with a mediastinal mass) who present with firm, rubbery nodes. Aspirate samples from the larger, rubbery or hard nodes are scantly cellular, but samples from adjacent smaller, soft nodes will often yield a cellular population. Mononuclear Reed-Sternberg cell variants (the "Hodgkin's cell") often outnumber classic Reed-Sternberg cells in nodular sclerosing Hodgkin's disease and are seen in a reactive lymphoid background with or without eosinophils or plasma cells [▮*23.23*].

Mixed cellularity Hodgkin's disease is usually richly cellular in Reed-Sternberg cells in a mixed leukocytic background with many eosinophils [▮*23.23*]. Lymphocyte depleted Hodgkin's disease may be composed of many bizarre, polylobed Reed-Sternberg cells with almost no reactive background population. They are often observed in patients with recurrent Hodgkin's disease.

SOME PITFALLS IN THE ASPIRATION OF LYMPH NODES

Non-Hodgkin's lymphoma and Hodgkin's disease present with a wide spectrum of morphologic features. Since individual neoplastic lymphoid cells (with the exception of Reed-Sternberg cells) have most of the cellular characteristics of differentiating lymphoid cells, it is essential to make these diagnoses by evaluating the pattern of cells in lymph node aspirates. It may be difficult to make definitive diagnoses in some instances because reactive lymphoid cells may populate neoplastic lymph nodes or lymphoid neoplasms may only partially replace a reactive lymph node. As such, there are five patterns that should raise the possibility of a neoplasm even though most features suggest a reactive process: (1) when there are fewer than 10% small round lymphocytes in the lymphoid population, (2) when there are greater than 25% large cells without immunoblasts, (3) when there is a mixed population of large and small cells with pleomorphic nuclear shapes, (4) when there are numerous histiocytes without tingible body macrophages, and (5) when there are numerous eosinophils in the aspirate sample.

One of the hallmarks of reactive lymphoid hyperplasia is the predominance of small round lymphocytes in the aspirate sample. When small round lymphocytes and immunoblasts are absent, a mixed lymphoma should be considered. This is true especially when there are greater than 25% large cells and very few immunoblasts in the population. Pleomorphic nuclei, which are deeply indented with unusual finger-like projections, are observed in mixed lymphomas [▮*23.15*] and are rarely seen in reactive patterns. Eosinophils are rare findings in reactive lymphoid hyperplasias. The rare polymorphous T cell lymphoma, early reactions to or involvement with Hodgkin's disease, and the probable "premalignant" immunoblastic lymphadenopathies typically contain eosinophils. Despite a benign flow cytometric analysis with these processes, a surgical biopsy is recommended.

SELECTED METASTATIC TUMORS

The use of FNA to evaluate metastatic disease in patients with known or suspected malignancy is widespread and well accepted by the medical community. In general, metastatic disease is easily diagnosed in lymph node aspirates and primary site can be determined in the majority of cases. Since the morphologic features of the more common epithelial primary tumors are discussed in other chapters, only two areas are discussed here: (1) metastatic lesions or patterns that mimic a primary neoplasm and (2) metastatic neoplasms that are rarely sampled by FNA in their primary sites.

Several nonlymphoid malignancies can mimic lymphoma in lymph node aspirates. Metastatic seminoma consists of poorly cohesive large malignant cells with many features similar to a large cell lymphoma. Usually, a large testicular mass or a history of germ cell neoplasm is helpful in making the correct diagnosis. The most helpful cytologic finding in this case is the background on air-dried smears. Rather than finding lymphoglandular bodies characteristic of a lymphoma, an irregular, wavy pattern called "tigroid" background is seen.

On rare occasions a small cell neuroendocrine carcinoma (intermediate type small cell carcinoma) will present predominantly as isolated cells. On air-dried, Romanowsky-stained smears lymphoglandular bodies are absent and the chromatin pattern is not typical for lymphoma.

Finding true nuclear molding with angular compression is also helpful in excluding lymphoma. Rhabdomyosarcoma, embryonal type, can metastasize to lymph nodes and may be composed of many isolated, intermediate size cells. Finally, some leukemias (in addition to chronic lymphocytic leukemia) can involve lymph nodes. Generally, clinical data are usually known that can help avoid an erroneous interpretation of lymphoma.

There are several neoplasms that metastasize to lymph nodes and may be sampled by FNA before they are sampled in their primary site. These include nasopharyngeal carcinoma (lymphoepithelioma), melanoma, and urothelial carcinoma. Of these, melanoma is the only one seen with any frequency and has characteristic features: binucleation, macronucleoli, eccentric nuclei, and intranuclear cytoplasmic invaginations (holes), with scant or absent melanin.

Undifferentiated nasopharyngeal carcinoma in FNA specimens is composed of reactive lymphoid cells admixed with variable numbers of isolated and loosely cohesive aggregates of oval cells with whispy cytoplasm. These cellular aggregates may be infrequent and the diagnosis may be difficult to establish.

Urothelial carcinoma rarely metastasizes to lymph nodes outside of the pelvis. However, subcutaneous or even distant metastases can be observed. In aspirates from this neoplasm, two patterns can be seen. Most often a dimorphic population is seen, composed of large, binucleate or trinucleate cells (umbrella-like) and numerous small bipolar or columnar cells. Cohesive groups of cells that show palisading and papillary configurations are common. A poorly differentiated adenosquamous carcinoma is in the differential diagnosis. Less commonly, only the small columnar cells are observed without the larger cells.

A panel of immunocytochemical stains can help determine the primary site of metastatic neoplasms to lymph nodes. Cell blocks prepared from centrifuged aspirate material can be used for this purpose.

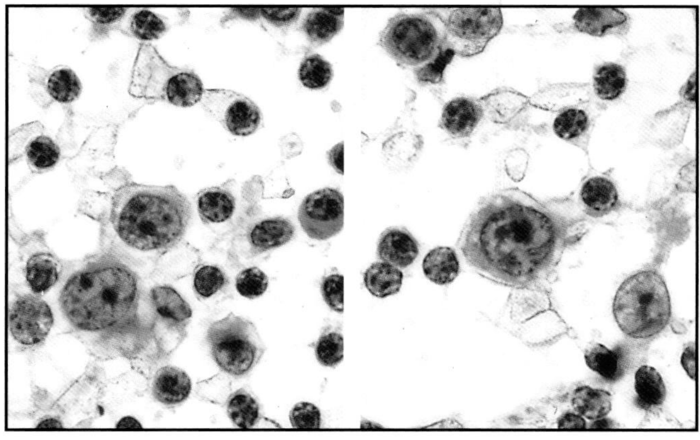

▌23.1

Reactive lymph node, midphase. Small round lymphocytes, small cleaved lymphocytes, large noncleaved lymphocytes, immunoblasts, plasma cells, and histiocytes are shown (Papanicolaou, x330).

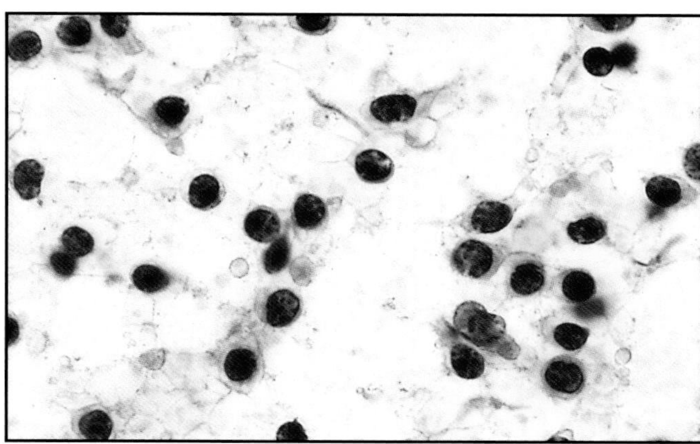

▌23.2

Reactive lymph node, end stage (Papanicolaou, x330).

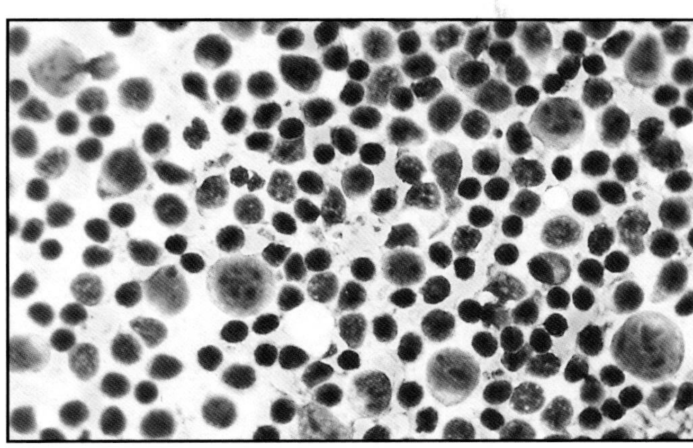

▌23.3

Reactive lymph node, midphase. Polymorphic population of lymphoid cells (small round lymphocytes, small cleaved lymphocytes, large noncleaved lymphocytes, immunoblasts, and plasma cells) are shown (Romanowsky, x330).

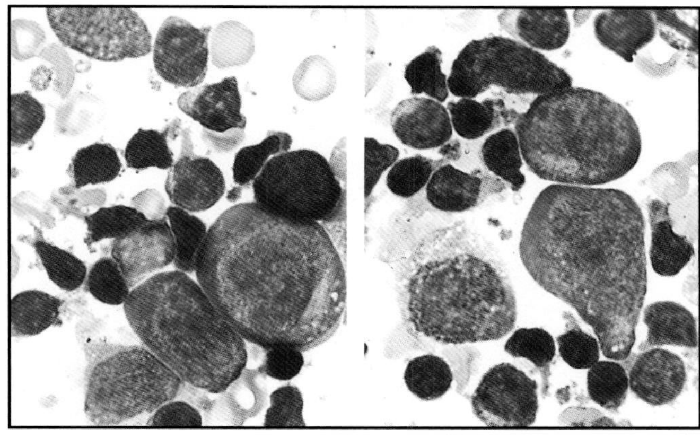

▌23.4

Reactive lymph node, early phase. There are prominent immunoblasts and large noncleaved lymphocytes, as well as small round lymphocytes. Note hofs and lymphoglandular bodies (Romanowsky, x330).

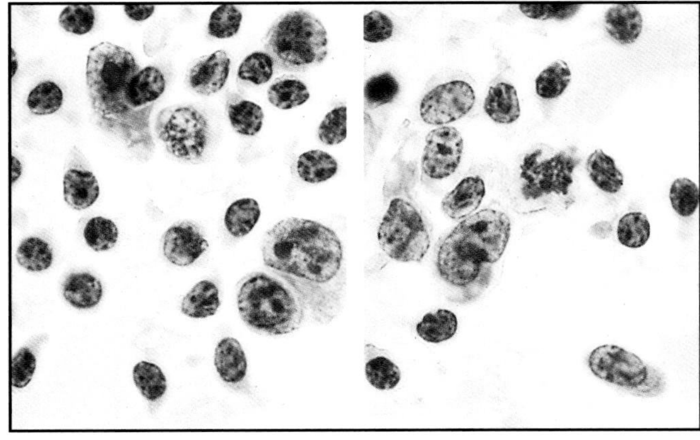

▌23.5

Reactive lymph node, early phase. There are several immunoblasts and large noncleaved lymphocytes in a background of small round lymphocytes (Papanicolaou, x330).

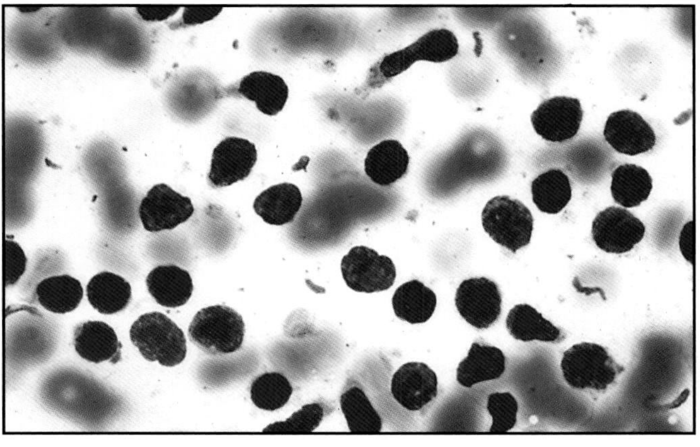

▌23.6

Reactive lymph node, end stage. Small round cells are predominantly seen (Romanowsky, x330).

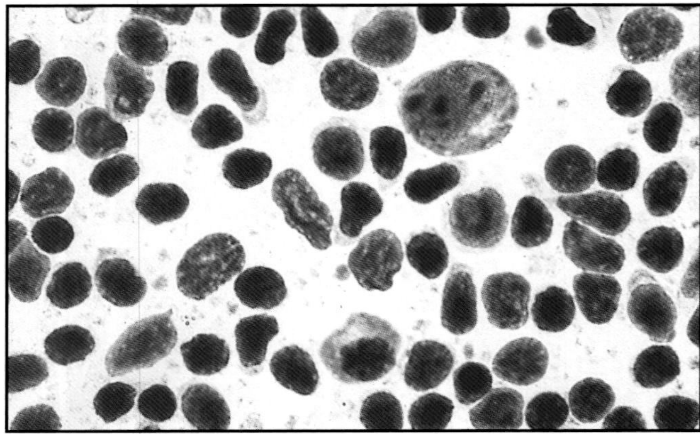

23.7

Reactive lymph node, recurrent stimulation. Numerous small round lymphocytes and small cleaved lymphocytes with rare immunoblasts and plasma cells are present. Note the lymphoglandular bodies (Romanowsky, x330).

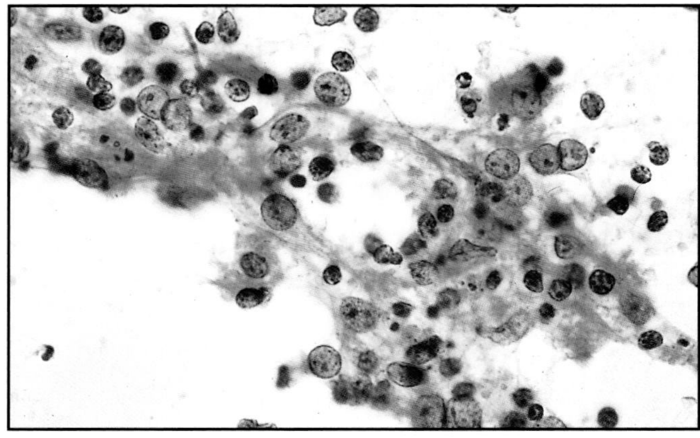

23.8

Reactive lymph node. A lymphohistiocytic aggregate is composed of reticular cells, tingible body macrophages, and follicular center cells (Papanicolaou, x198).

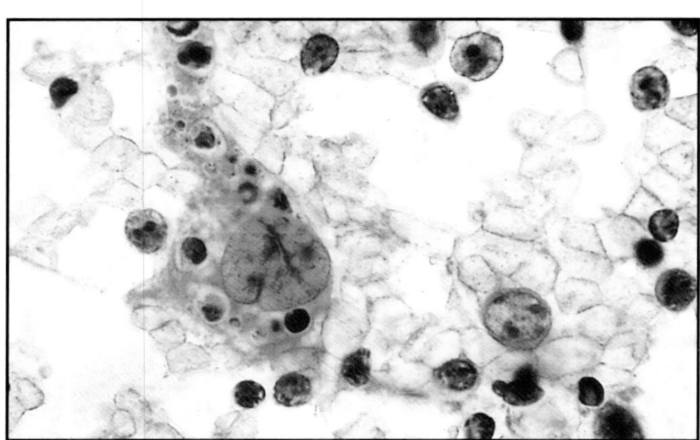

23.9

Reactive lymph node. Tingible body macrophage with phagocytized cell debris in cytoplasm is shown (Papanicolaou, x330).

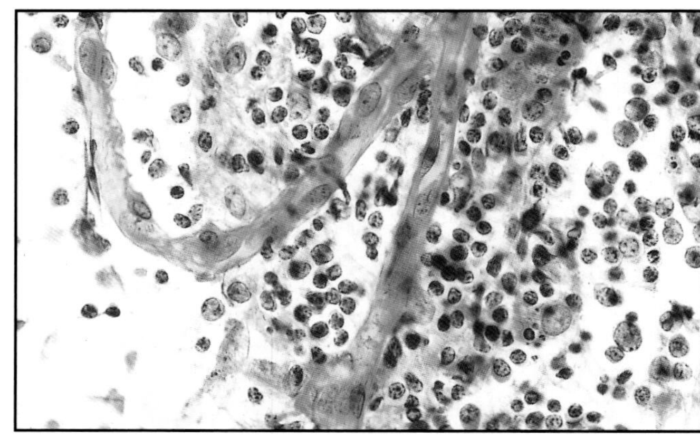

23.10

Reactive lymph node. Branching capillary in a mixed lymphoid population is depicted (Papanicolaou, x150).

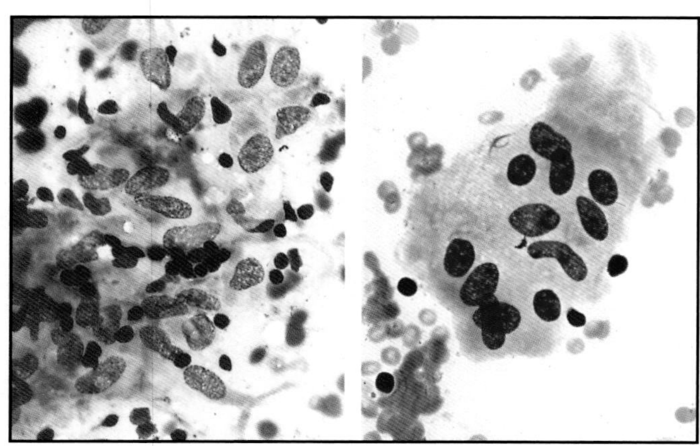

23.11

Reactive lymph node, granulomatous process. Left, histiocyte cluster (epithelioid cells); right, a multinucleate giant cell (Romanowsky, x132).

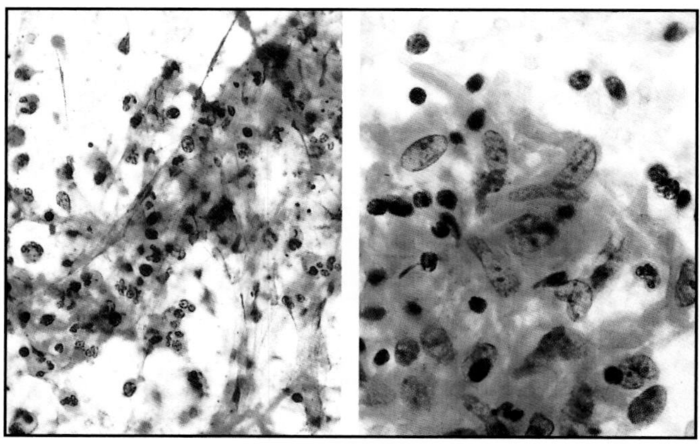

23.12

Reactive lymph node, granulomatous process. Epithelioid cells and aggregates of neutrophils (microabscess) suggestive of cat scratch disease are depicted (Papanicolaou, x198, x132).

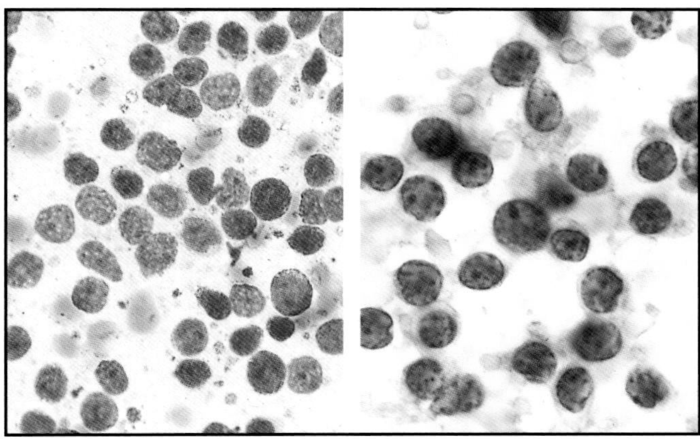

▌23.13
Small cleaved cell lymphoma (poorly differentiated lymphocytic lymphoma) is composed of more than 80% small cleaved lymphocytes with few small round lymphocytes or large cells. Note nuclear cleaves and coarse chromatin (Romanowsky/Papanicolaou, x330).

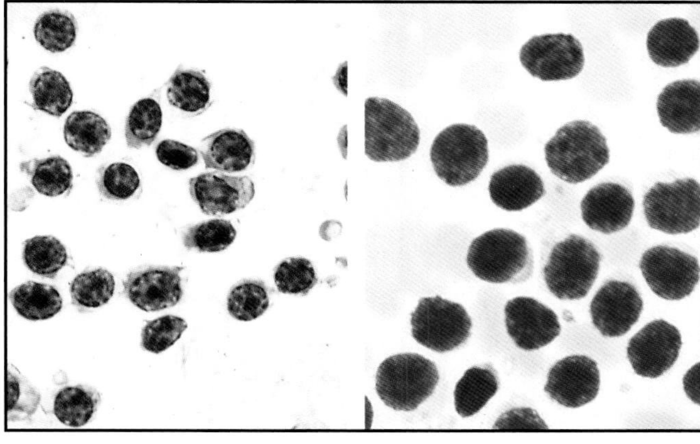

▌23.14
Small round cell lymphoma (well-differentiated lymphocytic lymphoma). A monomorphic pattern of small round lymphocytes is depicted (Romanowsky/Papanicolaou, x330).

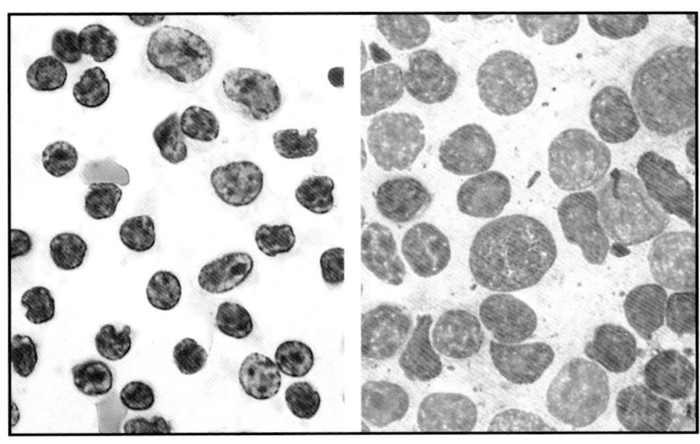

▌23.15
Mixed lymphoma composed of greater than 80% small cleaved and large noncleaved and cleaved cells. In some lymphomas a small number of normal small round lymphocytes and immunoblasts may be seen (Romanowsky/ Papanicolaou, x330).

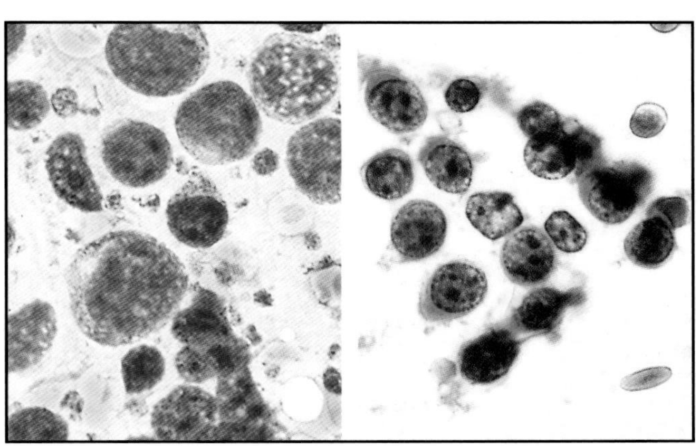

▌23.16
A large cell lymphoma is composed of greater than 80% large noncleaved or large cleaved cells. Note lymphoglandular bodies. As in other lymphomas, a small number of normal lymphoid cells may be seen (Romanowsky/Papanicolaou, x330).

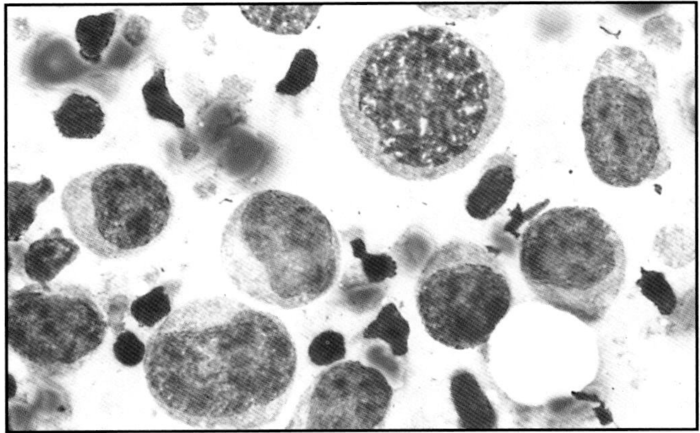

▌23.17
A large cell lymphoma, immunoblastic type, is composed of many atypical immunoblasts and occasional plasmacytoid cells (Romanowsky, x330).

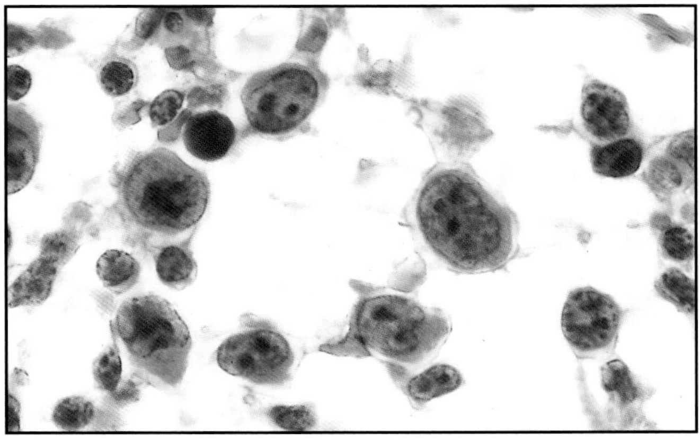

▌23.18
A large cell lymphoma, immunoblastic type, is composed predominantly of immunoblasts and plasmacytoid cells (Papanicolaou, x330).

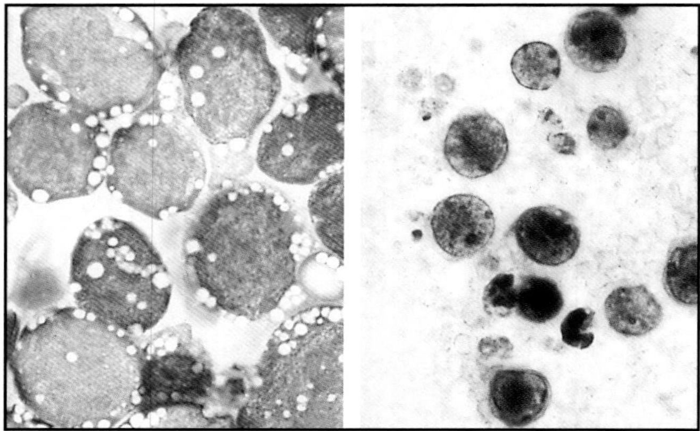

23.19

Undifferentiated lymphoma, Burkitt's type. A monomorphic population of small noncleaved lymphocytes is depicted. Note lipid vacuoles in cytoplasm (Romanowsky/Papanicolaou, x330).

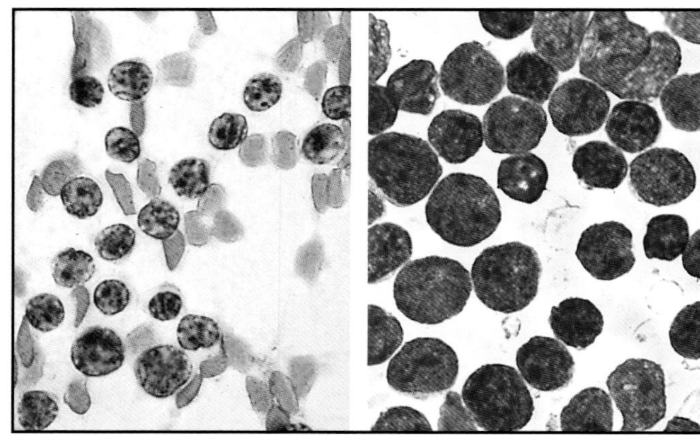

23.20

Lymphoblastic lymphoma, convoluted type. A monomorphous population of abnormal lymphoblasts is depicted (Romanowsky/ Papanicolaou, x330).

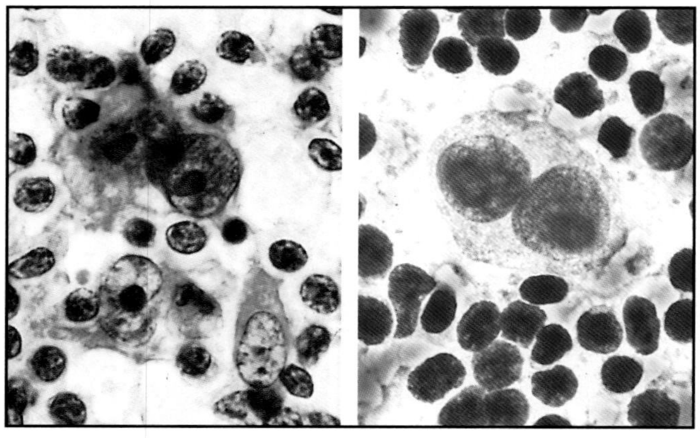

23.21

Hodgkin's disease. A classic Reed-Sternberg cell is shown: a bilobed nucleus with huge nucleoli and absence of "hof" (Romanowsky/ Papanicolaou, x330).

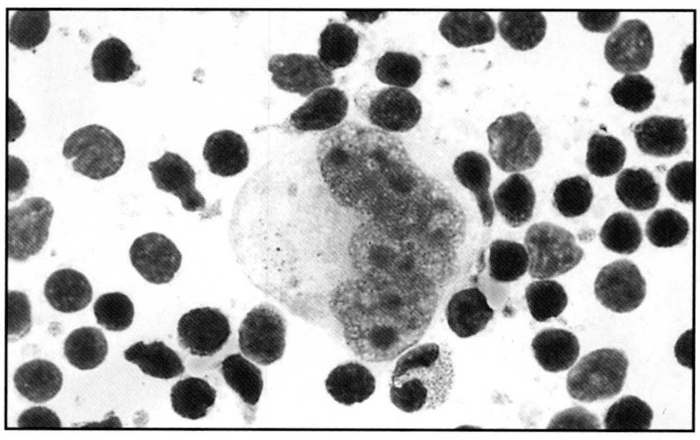

23.22

Hodgkin's disease. A "polylobed" Reed-Sternberg cell is shown. Note the adjacent eosinophil (Romanowsky, x330).

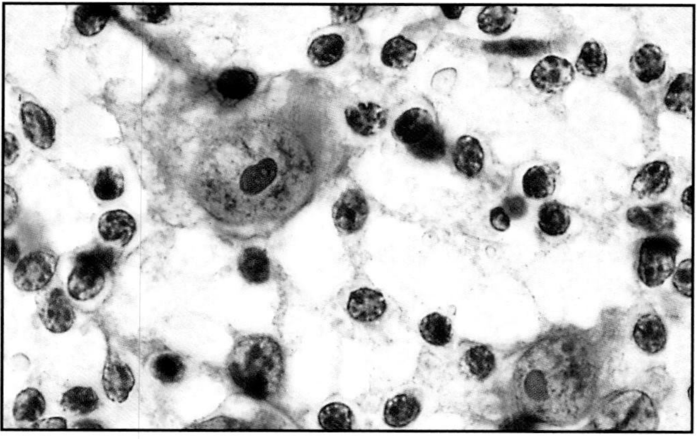

23.23

Hodgkin's disease. A mononuclear Reed-Sternberg cell variant is depicted (Papanicolaou, x330).

REVIEW EXERCISES

1. The most useful characteristic of reactive lymph node hyperplasia in lymph node aspirates that distinguishes it from most malignant lymphomas is
   a) the presence of many lymphohistiocytic aggregates.
   b) an absence of mitotic figures.
   c) a polymorphous lymphoid population.
   d) the presence of epithelioid histiocytes.

2. In most reactive lymphoid hyperplasias in lymph node aspirates, there is a greater relative proportion of
   a) small round lymphocytes.
   b) large cleaved lymphocytes.
   c) plasma cells.
   d) immunoblasts.
   e) large noncleaved lymphocytes.

3. Tingible body macrophages in lymph node aspirates are most often associated with
   a) malignant lymphoma.
   b) cat scratch disease.
   c) reactive lymph node hyperplasia.
   d) metastatic disease.

4. A lymph node aspirate specimen that is composed of many immunoblasts and plasma cells is most consistent with
   a) an early-phase lymphoid hyperplasia.
   b) a midphase lymphoid hyperplasia.
   c) an end-stage lymphoid hyperplasia.
   d) a granulomatous process.

5. A lymph node aspirate specimen from a 40-year-old man contained many large cells with bilobed nuclei and macronucleoli in an inflammatory background of eosinophils, neutrophils, and plasma cells. This cellular pattern is most consistent with
   a) large cell lymphoma.
   b) midphase reactive lymphoid hyperplasia.
   c) Hodgkin's disease.
   d) granulomatous lymphadenitis.

6. A lymph node aspirate specimen from a 59-year-old man was composed dominantly of lymphoid cells with nuclei in the size range of histiocyte nuclei. These nuclei were round and contained a fine chromatin pattern and several large nucleoli that were "membrane bound." The most consistent diagnosis for this population of lymphoid cells is
   a) Hodgkin's disease.
   b) small noncleaved lymphoma.
   c) cat scratch disease.
   d) large cell lymphoma.
   e) midphase reactive lymphoid hyperplasia.

SELECTED READINGS

Bellanti JA. *Immunology III.* 2nd ed. Philadelphia, Pa: WB Saunders Co; 1985.

Bizkak-Schwarzbartl M. Cytomorphologic characteristics of non-Hodgkin's lymphoma. *Acta Cytol.* 1988;32:216-220.

Cardozo PL. The cytologic diagnosis of lymphnode punctures. *Acta Cytol.* 1964;8:194-205.

Das DK, Gupta SK, Datta BN, Sharma SC. Fine needle aspiration cytodiagnosis of Hodgkin's disease and its subtypes, I: scope and limitations. *Acta Cytol.* 1990;34:329-336.

Das DK, Gupta SK, Datta BN, Sharma SC. FNA cytodiagnosis of non-Hodgkin's lymphoma and its subtyping under working formulation of 175 cases. *Diagn Cytopathol.* 1991;5:487-498.

Feldman P, Covell J, Kardos T. *Fine Needle Aspiration Cytology: Lymph Node, Thyroid and Salivary Gland.* Chicago, Ill: ASCP Press; 1989:13-94.

Glant MD, King DE. Aspiration biopsy of lymph nodes: reactive and primary neoplasia. In: *Atlas of Diagnostic Cytopathology.* Philadelphia, Pa: WB Saunders Co; 1992:485-529.

Glant MD, King DE. Fine needle aspiration cytology of reactive lymph node hyperplasia. *Cytotechnology Tech Sample No. CY-1.* Chicago, Ill: American Society of Clinical Pathologists; 1992.

Jaffe ES. *Surgical Pathology of the Lymph Nodes and Related Organs.* Philadelphia, Pa: WB Saunders Co; 1985.

Kardos TF, Vinson JH, Behm FG, Frable WJ, O'Dowd J. Hodgkin's disease: diagnosis by fine needle aspiration biopsy. *Am J Clin Pathol.* 1986;86:286-291.

O'Dowd GJ, Frable WJ, Behm FG. Fine needle aspiration cytology of benign lymph node hyperplasias. *Acta Cytol.* 1985;29:554-558.

Orell SR, Skinner JM. The typing of non-Hodgkin's lymphomas using fine needle aspiration cytology. *Pathology.* 1982;14:389-394.

Pontifex AH, Haley L. Fine needle aspiration cytology of lymphomas and related disorders. *Diagn Cytopathology.* 1989;5: 432-435.

Qizilbash AH, Young JEM. *Guides to Clinical Aspiration Cytology: Head and Neck.* New York, NY: Igaku-Shoin Medical Publishers Inc; 1988.

Silverman JF. Fine needle aspiration cytology of cat scratch disease. *Acta Cytol.* 1985;29:542-547.

Sneige N. Diagnosis of lymphoma and reactive hyperplasia by immunocytochemical analysis of fine needle aspiration biopsy. *Diagn Cytopathol.* 1990;6:39-43.

Soderstrom N. The free cytoplasmic fragments of lymphoglandular tissue (lymphoglandular bodies). *Scand J Haematol.* 1968;5:138-152.

Stani J. Cytologic diagnosis of reactive lymphadenopathy in fine needle aspiration biopsy specimens. *Acta Cytol.* 1987;31:8-13.

Stanley MW, Steeper TA, Horwitz CA, Burton LG, Strickler JG, Borken S. FNA of lymph nodes in patients with acute infectious mononucleosis *Diagn Cytopathol.* 1990;6:323-329.

CHAPTER 24

Salivary Glands

LESTER J. LAYFIELD, MD

CONTENTS

The salivary glands can be the site of a wide variety of pathologic changes, including inflammatory, degenerative, autoimmune, and neoplastic processes. Classically, therapeutic decisions have been based on physical findings alone. Fine needle aspiration cytology has become an increasingly popular technique for the preoperative diagnosis of salivary gland nodules. Numerous studies have documented the diagnostic accuracy of the method. Qizilbash and Young have shown that one third of all patients undergoing fine needle aspiration biopsy for diagnosis of salivary gland enlargement can be spared subsequent operative intervention. In addition, preoperative cytologic diagnosis of salivary gland neoplasms can aid in the selection of the type and extent of surgery performed.

ANATOMY

The salivary glands are represented by the three major glands (parotid, submandibular, and sublingual) as well as numerous minor glands distributed throughout the oral cavity. The secretion product varies and serves to classify the glands into three types: (1) mucous cells elaborating a viscid secretion composed primarily of mucin, (2) serous cells secreting a watery liquid containing salts and protein, and (3) mixed glands with both serous and mucous cells. The parotid gland is composed of serous cells, while the submandibular and sublingual glands are of mixed type. The microanatomy of all salivary glands [▮*24.1*, left] is similar, with serous or mucous acini draining into the intercalated ducts. Myoepithelial cells surround the acini and intercalated ducts, where they perform the functions of contraction and formation of basement membrane. The acinar cells contain well-developed rough endoplasmic reticulum, Golgi bodies, and secretory granules. The intercalated ducts drain into the striated ducts, which themselves empty into the excretory ducts. The striated ducts play a role in electrolyte and water transportation. The excretory ducts are lined proximally by columnar and goblet cells and distally by squamous cells. Understanding the microstructure of the salivary glands is important, since many neoplasms appear to arise from or differentiate toward specific portions of the salivary gland.

Cytologic material obtained from normal salivary gland tissue is composed of grape-like clusters of acini and connecting ducts [▮*24.1*, right]. The acini are composed of large uniform cells with abundant, finely granular cytoplasm and small dark peripheral nuclei. The segments of ducts appear as "honeycomb" sheets or short tubular segments composed of oval to columnar cells with small dark nuclei surrounded by modest amounts of cytoplasm. The background often contains many small dark nuclei devoid of cytoplasm.

INFLAMMATORY LESIONS

Acute suppurative sialadenitis is characterized by the rapid onset of swelling of the gland and surrounding soft tissues. The area is firm, tender, and warm to the touch. If the parotid is involved, a purulent discharge may drain from Stensen's duct. While seldom a diagnostic problem, needle aspirates may be obtained from such glands for culture of the causative organisms. Bacteria most often obtained include *Staphylococcus aureus*, *Streptococcus viridans*, and pneumococcus.

In immunocompromised individuals, the parotid gland may play host to a variety of uncommon organisms, including cytomegalovirus and fungal organisms. Cytomegalovirus involvement of the parotid is characterized by large nuclear inclusion bodies within ductal and acinar cells [▮*24.2*].

Needle aspiration specimens obtained from chronic recurrent sialadenitis are generally nonspecific but often show a prominent population of mature lymphocytes scattered among clusters of ductal cells. The ductal cells may show mild nuclear hyperchromasia and crowding. Acinar cells are rarely seen. Careful clinical correlation is important since chronic sialadenitis may be seen in the area of a small tumor obstructing a duct.

Autoimmune Sialadenitis

Historically, Mikulicz's disease has been associated with bilateral swelling of the lacrimal and salivary glands secondary to a variety of causes but is pathologically ill defined. The benign lymphoepithelial lesion and Sjögren's syndrome are more specifically defined entities and have nearly identical histopathologic and cytologic findings. In these two processes, a reactive lymphoid infiltrate is associated with acinar atrophy and ductal changes culminating in the characteristic "epimyoepithelial island." Patients affected are usually women in the fifth and sixth decades; many present with bilateral or unilateral disease. While the swelling is usually diffuse, some cases may present as a unilateral discrete nodule, making distinction from a neoplasm difficult.

Aspirates obtained from these glands show a mixed population of small and large lymphocytes, plasma cells, and histiocytes. Lymphohistiocytic aggregates may be seen [▮*24.3*]. Small clusters of ductal epithelium forming short tubular segments are rarely seen; acinar epithelium is generally absent.

Cystic Benign Lymphoepithelial Lesion

Cystic benign lymphoepithelial lesions of the parotid have recently been described in patients at risk for or suffering from the acquired immune deficiency syndrome. Histologically, these lesions are characterized by a marked lymphoid hyperplasia surrounding squamous lined cysts. Material obtained by fine needle aspiration biopsy contains a heterogeneous population of small and large lymphocytes, foamy or debris-laden macrophages, and scattered benign squamous cells [▮24.4]. The latter cells may be anucleate, parakeratotic, superficial, or intermediate. On occasion, no epithelial component is found, or the epithelial component will have a "mucoepidermoid," columnar, or cuboidal appearance.

BENIGN NEOPLASMS

Benign mixed tumors make up about 65% of all tumors of the parotid gland. They occur most often in women, with the majority of patients in the fifth decade, but no age group is immune. This tumor presents as a painless slow-growing mass that may have been present for years. On palpation, the tumor appears firm, smooth, and mobile. These neoplasms are characterized by their morphologic diversity but are composed of varying proportions of both epithelial and mesenchymal elements. The component epithelial and myoepithelial cells form tubules, islands, and sheets within a myxoid, chondroid, or fibrous background. Peripherally, the tumor margin is bosselated.

Cytologically, aspirated material may be mixed or dominated by the epithelial-myoepithelial or stromal elements. Generally, the smears have a mixture of epithelial and myxoid-chondroid elements [▮24.5]. The epithelial cells are uniformly small and cuboidal and form cohesive clusters, tubules, and sheets. The epithelial cells are well seen on Papanicolaou staining but are smudged and poorly seen in preparations stained by the May-Grünwald-Giemsa technique [▮24.5]. The nuclei of the epithelial cells (Papanicolaou staining) are small and oval to round, and have fine chromatin and a small nucleolus. Occasionally, aspirates contain prominent numbers of squamous, columnar, or oncocytic cells. The stromal component is best seen on May-Grünwald-Giemsa where it stains an intense magenta. Fine fibers can generally be appreciated within the stromal matrix. Trapped within the myxoid matrix are bland spindle cells. Occasionally, tyrosine crystals are found within aspirated material.

Monomorphic Adenomas

The monomorphic adenomas (basal cell adenoma, trabecular adenoma, dermal anlage tumor) have similar cytologic appearances, varying predominantly in the amount of stroma present. Their distinction from adenoid cystic carcinomas can be difficult. Aspirates from both trabecular adenomas and dermal anlage tumors contain stromal cylinders [▮24.6], resembling those seen in adenoid cystic carcinomas. Distinction of these adenomas from adenoid cystic carcinoma is achieved by recognizing the slightly greater nuclear atypia of the carcinoma (best seen with Papanicolaou stain) and the more abundant stroma of the monomorphic adenomas. In addition, the stroma associated with the adenomas often has a tubular or branching pattern and a finely fibrillar consistency.

Basal cell adenomas, like solid adenoid cystic carcinomas, are composed of tight clusters or tubules of small cells with a high nuclear/cytoplasmic ratio and small dark nuclei. Cytologic distinction may be impossible but the carcinomas usually have slightly larger nuclei and more prominent nucleoli. In many cases, distinction between monomorphic adenomas and adenoid cystic carcinomas can only be made after careful clinical correlation. Some authors will only definitively diagnose an adenoid cystic carcinoma when neural symptoms are present.

Oncocytoma (Oxyphilic Adenoma)

Oncocytomas are rare neoplasms, accounting for less than 1% of salivary gland tumors. These neoplasms occur most frequently in elderly women who present with a discrete slowly growing nodule. Rarely, bilateral tumors have been reported. Cytologically, these neoplasms are characterized by numerous clusters of large polygonal cells with abundant finely granular cytoplasm lying in a clean background free of lymphocytes [▮24.7]. The nuclei are round with frequently prominent nucleoli. The nuclei may be central or eccentrically located. Rarely, clear forms are seen that must be differentiated from metastatic renal cell carcinomas. This distinction is achieved by recognizing the greater nuclear atypia present in renal cell carcinoma. Distinction of oncocytoma from oncocytosis depends on clinical features (solitary nodule vs diffuse involvement) and the intimate admixture of oncocytic epithelium and normal acinar epithelium seen in the same smear obtained from cases of diffuse oncocytosis.

Warthin's Tumor

Warthin's tumors (papillary cystadenoma lymphomatosum, adenolymphoma) arise almost exclusively within the parotid, where they represent between 6% and 10% of tumors. Approximately 10% of cases are bilateral, and multifocal involvement of a gland has been frequently reported. This neoplasm is more common in men and is thought to arise from salivary gland inclusions within intraparotid lymph nodes. Patients present with a soft "doughy" mass that may be partially cystic. Smears are often watery, with rare to many clusters of large polygonal cells lying in a "dirty" proteinaceous background rich in mature lymphocytes with occasional mast cells. The individual epithelial cells have abundant granular cytoplasm with central or eccentric nuclei. Nucleoli are often prominent. In rare cases, metaplastic squamous epithelium is present and may show reactive nuclear atypia. This metaplastic change can be secondary to spontaneous infarction or prior needle aspiration.

Lipomas

Lipomas may occasionally arise within the parotid gland and represent a problem in differential diagnosis. Aspirated material grossly appears yellow and oily. Cytologic examination discloses fragments of mature adipose tissue indistinguishable from normal subcutaneous fat. Clinical and radiographic correlation are necessary to firmly establish this diagnosis.

Juvenile Hemangioma (Benign Hemangioendothelioma)

Vascular tumors are the most common neoplasms occurring in the parotid glands of infants and children. Despite their rapid growth and high cellularity, these lesions behave in a benign fashion and often regress with age. While most cases are recognized clinically, occasional patients need to undergo needle aspiration. Aspirates are bloody but contain occasional individual and small clusters of bland spindle cells. These cells have modest amounts of wispy cytoplasm extending from both ends of bland oval or bacillary nuclei. The nuclei are slender and the cytoplasmic margins are indistinct.

MALIGNANT NEOPLASMS

Adenoid Cystic Carcinoma

Adenoid cystic carcinoma is a slow-growing neuroinvasive carcinoma accounting for approximately 4% of all parotid gland neoplasms and 15% to 30% of submandibular and sublingual gland tumors. Patients with these neoplasms frequently present with pain and, despite the neoplasm's slow growth, have a poor long-term prognosis.

Smears are cellular, with numerous ring-like clusters of epithelial cells surrounding central cores of homogeneous hyaline material [▮*24.8*]. These clusters may form overlapping three-dimensional masses. The individual cells are bland with round to oval nuclei. On Papanicolaou staining, small but distinct nucleoli are seen. In more poorly differentiated examples, nuclear atypia is greater and less acellular material is seen. Adenoid cystic carcinomas must be distinguished from cellular pleomorphic adenomas and some monomorphic adenomas. Clinical findings including pain are most helpful in this separation.

Mucoepidermoid Carcinoma

Mucoepidermoid carcinoma comprises 5% to 10% of all tumors arising in the major salivary glands and is the most frequent primary salivary gland malignancy in children. These neoplasms are histologically subdivided into low-, intermediate-, and high-grade lesions. Low-grade lesions are predominantly cystic and slow-growing, while high-grade lesions are solid and infiltrative with a tendency to recur and metastasize.

Aspirates from low-grade carcinomas usually yield a small amount of cyst fluid, microscopic examination of which discloses a mucoid background in which are scattered a small number of mucus-secreting goblet or columnar cells [▮*24.9*]. These epithelial cells have small bland nuclei associated with pale mucus-rich cytoplasm. Bland squamous cells can also be found. A small population of polygonal intermediate cells with scant cytoplasm is seen in association with the mucous cells. In some cases only mucus is obtained.

Smears of high-grade mucoepidermoid carcinomas are highly cellular, with scattered intermediate cells and lesser numbers of mucin-containing cells. Neoplastic squamous cells are numerous. These cells have abundant cytoplasm with distinct cell borders. Their nuclei are enlarged, hyperchromatic, and may contain prominent nucleoli [▮*24.10*]. Keratinization is seen, but the presence of squamous whorls should suggest a pure squamous cell carcinoma rather than a high-grade mucoepidermoid carcinoma.

Intermediate-grade mucoepidermoid carcinomas have a prominent number of intermediate cells with lesser numbers of metaplastic squamous cells and scattered mucin-producing cells. True keratinization is uncommon.

Acinic Cell Carcinoma

Acinic cell neoplasms are low-grade tumors accounting for less than 3% of all salivary gland tumors. They are found almost exclusively in the parotid and may be bilateral. Acinic cell neoplasms are slow-growing lesions, and cytologic features are poorly predictive of behavior. Aspirates from these neoplasms are frequently cellular and composed of clusters and sheets of finely vacuolated to clear cells with distinct cytoplasmic margins [▮*24.11*]. The nuclei are uniform in size and generally bland in appearance. In some cases, prominent nucleoli may be seen. On May-Grünwald-Giemsa staining, bright red or magenta intracytoplasmic granules may be demonstrated.

Polymorphous Low-Grade Adenocarcinomas

These neoplasms arise almost exclusively in the minor salivary glands of the oral cavity and account for up to 11% of minor salivary gland tumors. Aspirates are characterized by a mixed population of relatively bland epithelial cells.

These cells may lie in tight clusters, tubules, or broad sheets. The nuclei are small and uniform, and nucleoli are tiny or absent. Some cells have a cuboidal appearance, while others are columnar. Most cells have fine granular cytoplasm but others appear vacuolated or mucin-containing. Few cases have been described in the literature.

Epithelial-Myoepithelial Cell Carcinoma

These rare carcinomas must be distinguished from other clear cell neoplasms, including metastatic renal cell carcinoma. Epithelial-myoepithelial cell carcinomas are characterized on aspiration by cellular smears composed of clusters of large polygonal cells often associated with background necrosis. The individual cells have moderate to abundant amounts of clear cytoplasm surrounding large hyperchromatic nuclei. The nuclei are uniformly large and may contain prominent nucleoli [▮*24.12*]. A second population of smaller cells with lesser amounts of cytoplasm and bland nuclei may be seen.

Lymphoma

Rarely, lymphomas may arise within the parotid gland and may be associated with a history of Sjögren's syndrome. Aspiration smears obtained from such patients show a monomorphous population of large or small atypical lymphocytes. Since the vast majority of parotid lymphomas are of a B cell type, immunohistochemical demonstration of light chain clonality is diagnostically useful.

Metastatic Carcinoma

The intraparotid lymph nodes play host to a wide variety of metastatic lesions. Aspiration biopsy of such masses may raise difficult diagnostic problems. Most commonly such metastases represent squamous cell carcinomas or melanoma, but occasional deposits of renal cell, gastric, and breast carcinoma may be seen. Careful clinical history and immunohistochemical studies may be helpful in making the diagnosis.

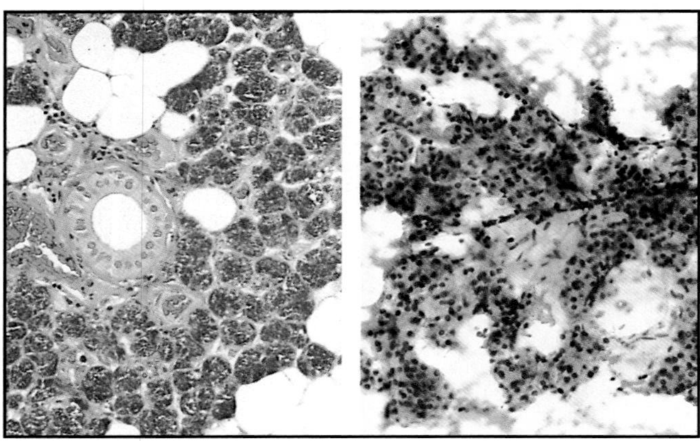

24.1

Left, Histologic section of normal parotid gland showing serous acini and duct (hematoxylin-eosin, x40). Right, Cytologic specimen of normal salivary gland acini and intercalated ducts (hematoxylin-eosin, x40).

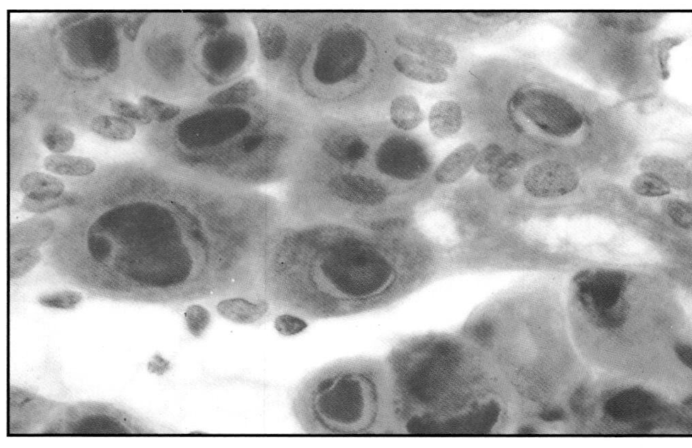

24.2

Salivary gland acinar cells infected by cytomegalovirus (Papanicolaou, x400).

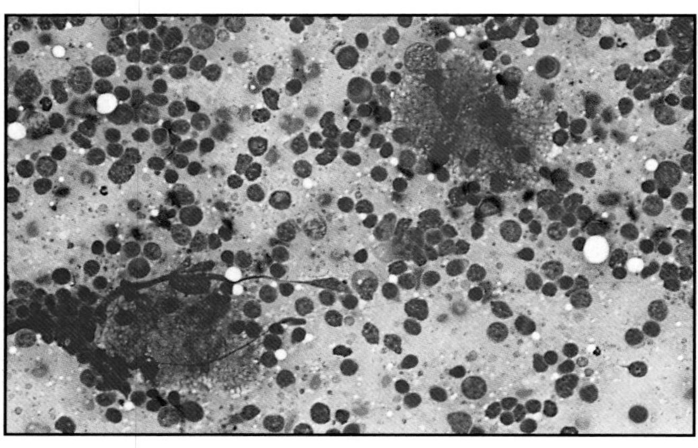

24.3

Mixed lymphoid infiltrate with scattered histiocytes characteristic of Sjögren's syndrome (May-Grünwald-Giemsa, x100).

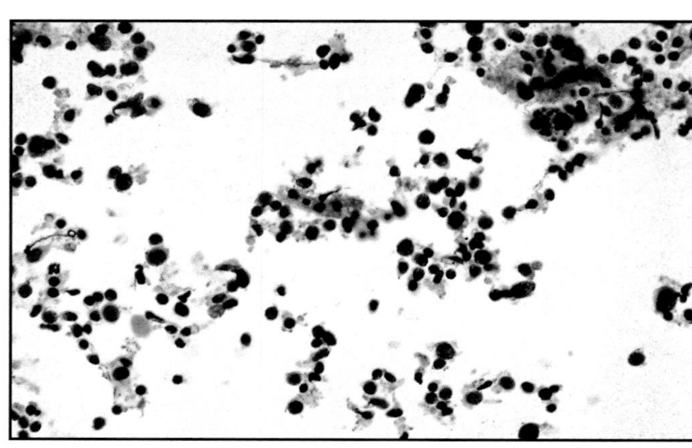

24.4

Benign cystic lymphoepithelial lesion of the parotid. Note keratinized squamous cell (Papanicolaou, x100).

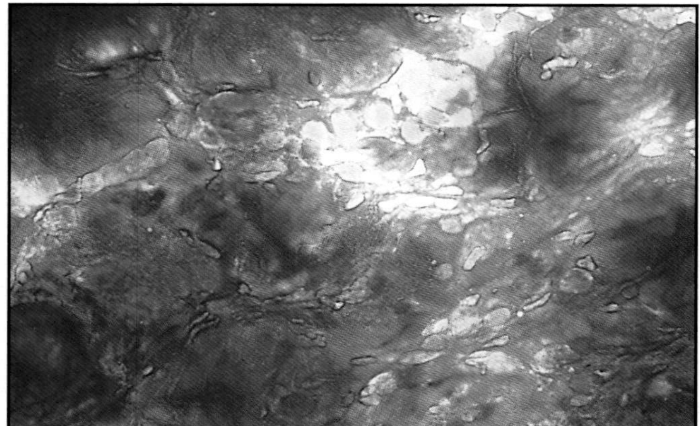

24.5

Pleomorphic adenoma (May-Grünwald-Giemsa, x200).

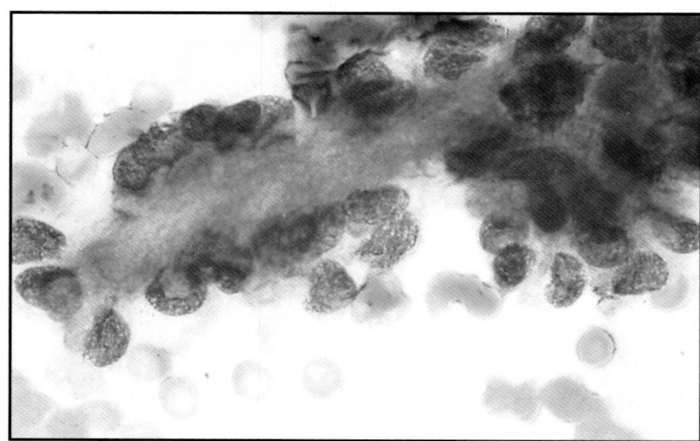

24.6

Monomorphic adenoma (May-Grünwald-Giemsa, x400).

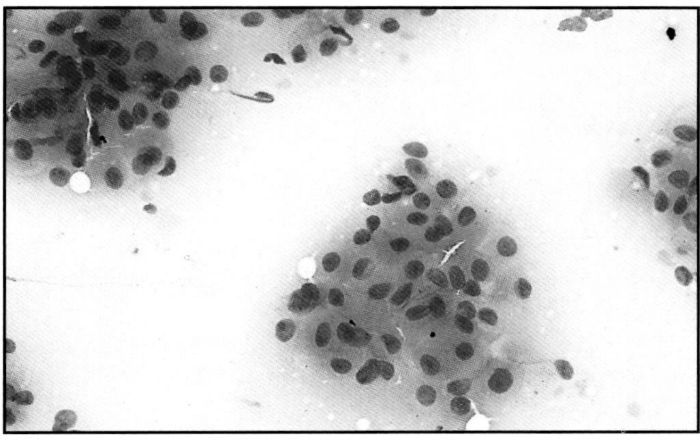

24.7
Oncocytoma (May-Grünwald-Giemsa, x100).

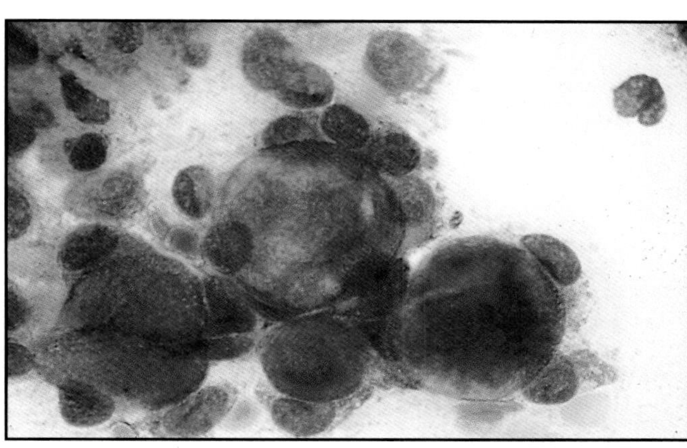

24.8
Adenoid cystic carcinoma (May-Grünwald-Giemsa, x400).

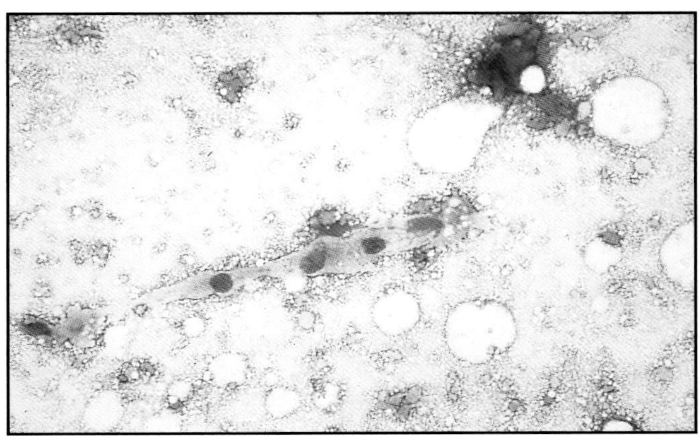

24.9
Low-grade mucoepidermoid carcinoma (May-Grünwald-Giemsa, x100).

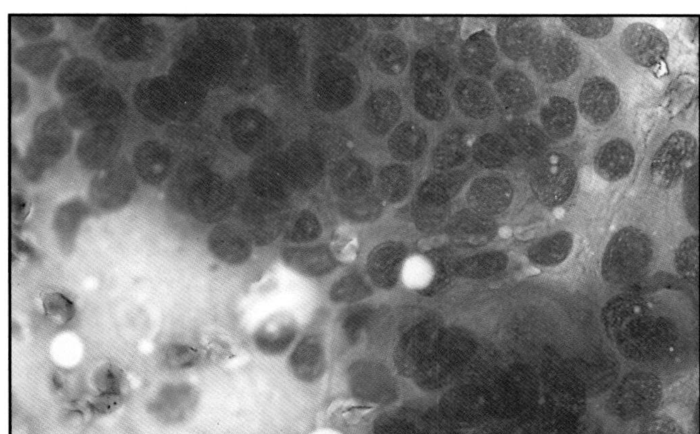

24.10
High-grade mucoepidermoid carcinoma (May-Grünwald-Giemsa, x400).

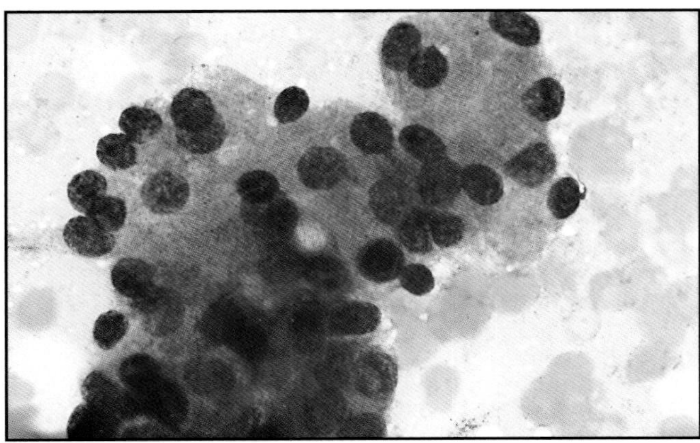

24.11
Acinic cell carcinoma with granular and foamy cytoplasm (May-Grünwald-Giemsa, x400).

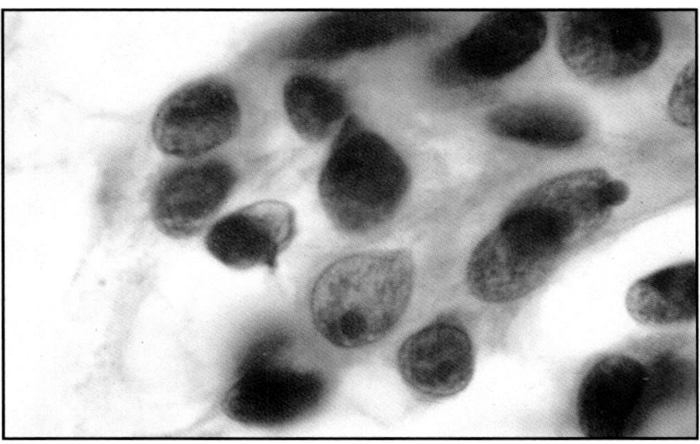

24.12
Clear cell form of epithelial-myoepithelial cell carcinoma (Papanicolaou, x640).

REVIEW EXERCISES

1. Small red or magenta intracytoplasmic granules are characteristic of
   a) pleomorphic adenoma.
   b) adenoid cystic carcinoma.
   c) mucoepidermoid carcinoma.
   d) acinic cell carcinoma.

2. Separation of Warthin's tumor from oncocytoma is best achieved by recognition of
   a) prominent nucleoli in oncocytomas.
   b) high mitotic activity in oncocytomas.
   c) background lymphocytes in Warthin's tumors.
   d) granular cytoplasm of epithelial cells in Warthin's tumors.

3. Reported metastatic lesions to the parotid gland include all the following except which one?
   a) Melanoma
   b) Renal cell carcinoma
   c) Leiomyosarcoma
   d) Squamous cell carcinoma

4. Bloody aspirates with rare spindle cells obtained from a parotid gland nodule in an infant should suggest which one the following diagnoses?
   a) Pleomorphic adenoma
   b) Mucoepidermoid carcinoma
   c) Hemangioma
   d) Insufficient specimen

5. The presence of abundant myxoid-chondroid matrix on a smear from a parotid mass should suggest the diagnosis of
   a) Warthin's tumor.
   b) adenoid cystic carcinoma.
   c) pleomorphic adenoma.
   d) mucoepidermoid carcinoma.

SELECTED READINGS

Batsakis JG. *Tumors of the Head and Neck: Clinical and Pathological Considerations.* 2nd ed. Baltimore, Md: Williams & Wilkins; 1979:4,105-112.

Bibbo M, ed. *Comprehensive Cytopathology.* Philadelphia, Pa: WB Saunders Co; 1991:632-634.

Bottles K, Ferrell LD, Miller TR. Tyrosine crystals in fine needle aspirates of a pleomorphic adenoma of the parotid gland. *Acta Cytol.* 1984;28:490-492.

Bottles K, Lowhagen T, Miller TR. Mast cells in the aspiration cytology differential diagnosis of adenolymphoma. *Acta Cytol.* 1985;24: 513-515.

Enroth CM, Franzen S, Zajicek J. Cytologic diagnosis on aspirates from 1,000 salivary gland tumors. *Acta Otolaryngol.* 1967;224(suppl):168-172.

Enroth CM, Zajicek J. Aspiration biopsy of salivary gland tumours, IV: morphologic studies on smears and histologic sections from 45 cases of adenoid cystic carcinomas. *Acta Cytol.* 1969;13:59-63.

Feldman PS, Covell JL, Kardos TF, eds. *Fine Needle Aspiration Cytology: Lymph Node, Thyroid and Salivary Gland.* Chicago, Ill; ASCP Press; 1989:178.

Finfer MD, Galle L, Perchick A, et al. Fine needle aspiration biopsy of cystic benign lymphoepithelial lesions of the parotid gland in patients at risk for the acquired immune deficiency syndrome. *Acta Cytol.* 1990;34:821-826.

Layfield LJ, Tan P, Glasgow BJ. Fine needle aspiration of salivary gland lesions. *Arch Pathol Lab Med.* 1987;111:346-353.

Palma O, Torri AM, deCristofaro JA, et al. Fine needle aspiration cytology in two cases of well differentiated acinic cell carcinoma of the parotid glands: discussion of diagnostic criteria. *Acta Cytol.* 1985;29:516-521.

Qizilbash AH, Young JEM. *Guides to Clinical Aspiration. Biopsy: Head and Neck.* New York, NY: Igaku-Shoin Medical Publishers Inc; 1988:15-16,64-70.

Webb AJ. Cytologic diagnosis of salivary gland lesions in adult and pediatric surgical patients. *Acta Cytol.* 1973;17:51-58.

Zajicek J, Enroth CM, Jakobssen P. Aspiration biopsy of salivary gland tumors, VI: morphologic studies on smears and histologic sections from mucoepidermoid carcinoma. *Acta Cytol.* 1976;20:35-41.

CHAPTER 25

Liver and Pancreas

Denise Frias-Hidvegi, MD, FIAC
Carol Isoe, SCT(ASCP)IAC
Ricardo Cajulis, MD, MIAC

CONTENTS

LIVER

With the development of new imaging techniques, detection of benign liver growths as well as primary and metastatic liver neoplasms can be diagnosed by samples obtained by fine needle aspiration (FNA) of the liver. There are several advantages of FNA biopsy over core biopsy. The main advantage is easy accessibility of lesions in the left lobe of the liver and the porta hepatis, which is difficult using large-bore needles. The ability to obtain multiple samples and visualize the needle inside the tumor prior to obtaining the aspirate makes this an important technique in the care of patients with liver neoplasms.

Several works published in the last decade discuss the cytomorphology of benign and malignant primary neoplasms of the liver, and equate the diagnostic cytologic results with the diagnoses obtained from histologic biopsy samples. The correlation depends on the adequacy of the specimen and the cytopathologist's ability to interpret the aspirate.

Histology and Cytology

The liver is composed of lobules formed by radiating rows of trabeculae containing single-file cords of hepatocytes. In the center of each lobule is the central efferent vein. In the periphery of the lobules lie the portal triads, which contain branches of the bile ducts, hepatic artery, portal vein, lymphatics, and nerves. The liver cords are separated by sinusoidal spaces, which are lined by alternating endothelial cells and Kupffer cells [**F**25.1].

Cytologically, hepatocytes are polygonal cells usually arranged in monolayers. Their cytoplasm is granular due to abundant organelles. The cell borders are well defined. Nuclei are round or slightly oval with a symmetric outline. Large single or double nucleoli are present against a background of granular chromatin [**I**25.1, right]. Approximately 40% of the hepatocytes are binucleate, and in some of these cells the cytoplasm is slightly enlarged. Intranuclear inclusions are observed in some nuclei [**I**25.1, right]. A low nuclear/cytoplasmic ratio is maintained. The bile duct cells are columnar nonciliated cells. In liver aspirates these cells can be seen in a honeycomb arrangement or in palisade formation. The nuclei are round or oval with symmetric outlines, and the chromatin is granular with inconspicuous nucleoli [**I**25.1, left].

Monolayers of mesothelial cells from Glisson's capsule are a frequent finding in liver aspirates. When liver necrosis is present, mesothelial cells may become markedly reactive, especially in Giemsa-stained smears [**I**25.2].

According to some authors, the endothelial cells deriving from the sinusoidal spaces are morphologically identical to mesothelial cells. In contrast, endothelial cells from the large blood vessels are elongated and easily recognized as to their site of origin.

Cytoplasmic Organelles and Pigments

Normally, several pigments can be found in hepatocytes. In well-fixed smears stained by the Papanicolaou technique, small red granules representing cytoplasmic organelles are seen. The most frequent cytoplasmic pigment encountered in hepatocytes is lipofuscin (lipochrome). It is usually found in livers of elderly patients. It is golden-brown in Papanicolaou-stained smears [**I**25.3, left] and green in Giemsa-prepared samples [**I**25.3, right]. This material represents the undigested residue of autophagic vacuoles formed during cell aging.

Other pigments found in the liver are bile and iron. The latter is found in hemosiderosis, a disease caused by an overload of iron pigment in several organs. Iron particles are brown-black in smears stained by the Papanicolaou method [**I**25.4, left], and blue-green in Giemsa-stained aspirates [**I**25.4, right]. Bile is seen in Papanicolaou-stained smears as homogeneous green globules of varying sizes [**I**25.5, left], located in the cytoplasm or in the bile canaliculi between hepatocytes. In Giemsa-stained smears this pigment is seen as greenish-black homogeneous deposits [**I**25.5, right] in the same locations as described above.

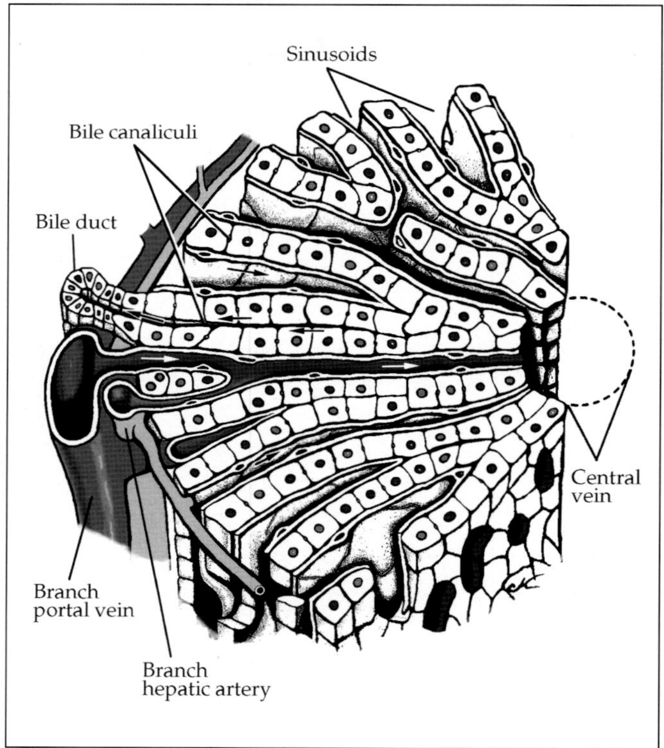

F25.1

Liver lobule depicting single cords of hepatocytes, central vein, and portal spaces with normal structures found in those areas. (Adapted from Fawcett D. Bloom & Fawcett: A Textbook of Histology. *11th ed. Philadelphia, Pa: WB Saunders Co; 1986:683.)*

Nuclear and Cytoplasmic Findings Common to Benign and Malignant Hepatocytes

Intranuclear cytoplasmic inclusions are found in benign, reactive, and malignant hepatocytes. Other tumors from a variety of body sites may show the same type of inclusions, and some of those neoplasms may cause liver metastasis [▮*25.1*, right].

Intracytoplasmic inclusions are encountered in benign and malignant liver disease such as alpha-1-antitrypsin deficiency, and in some hepatocellular carcinomas [▮*25.6*]. Additionally, livers severely damaged by cirrhosis may depict hepatocytes with similar cytoplasmic inclusions.

Benign Epithelial and Mesenchymal Processes

There are several neoplastic and hamartomatous benign processes that can occur in the liver. They can be subclassified as epithelial and mesenchymal [**T***25.1*]. In practically all of these epithelial processes, liver aspirates show benign hepatocytes and bile duct cells. Aspirations of mesenchymal liver neoplasms yield endothelial and/or fibrous tissue, mature adipose tissue, or a mixture of several of those elements, depending on the nature of the process sampled.

Adenomas

Adenomas have been reported as a possible source of error in diagnosis, since the cells may mimic well-differentiated hepatocellular carcinoma. However, several reports indicate that the nuclei of hepatocytes aspirated from liver cell adenomas are normal and the cytoplasm is abundant and clear due to increased amounts of fat and glycogen.

Other Benign Disorders

Fatty Metamorphosis

Fatty metamorphosis occurs when there is accumulation of triglycerides in the hepatocytes. There are numerous causes of fatty metamorphosis—for example, excessive alcohol intake, diabetes mellitus, obesity, and malnutrition. There are two major morphologic features seen in hepatocytes with fatty metamorphosis. A large single vacuole may displace normal nuclei to the cell periphery or numerous small vacuoles of variable sizes may surround a centrally located nuclei. It is important to establish the normal appearance of the nuclei, since clear cell hepatocellular carcinoma may have similar cytoplasmic features, with its nuclei having highly abnormal nucleoli.

Cirrhosis

Cirrhosis refers to the regeneration of liver tissue after destruction of the hepatic parenchyma. The tissue response is similar despite various causes of injury (eg, alcoholism, viral hepatitis, hemochromatosis), except for the size of the regenerative nodules. Regenerative nodules are present throughout the damaged area and the normal architecture of central veins and portal triads is lost. Regenerative nodules are formed by normal-appearing cords of hepatocytes that maintain some degree of organization [▮*25.7*]. In the active process, bile ductular proliferation and an inflammatory infiltrate occur in the fibrotic tissue that surrounds the regenerative nodules [▮*25.7*, left]. As the process is inactivated, the inflammatory infiltrate, proliferating bile ductules, and liver cell necrosis subside. In spite of some reports of pitfalls involving aspirates obtained from cirrhotic livers, other studies found that the aspirates yield normal-appearing hepatocytes [▮*25.7*, right]. Fragments of fibroconnective tissue and normal bile ducts may also be present, which correlates with the histologic appearance of active cirrhosis. Occasionally, foci of atypical hepatocytes may be seen among the normal cells; this finding is called liver cell dysplasia.

Epithelial
- Hepatocellular adenoma
- Focal nodular hyperplasia
- Bile duct hamartoma (von Meyenburg's complex)
- Bile duct adenoma
- Cystic processes
- Biliary papillomatosis

Mesenchymal
- Cavernous hemangioma
- Tumors of adipose tissue
- Fibrous mesothelioma
- Benign mesenchymoma
- Inflammatory pseudotumor

T*25.1*

Neoplastic and Hamartomatous Benign Processes

Liver Cell Dysplasia and Well-Differentiated Hepatocellular Carcinoma

Liver cell dysplasia refers to the presence in diseased livers of foci of atypical hepatocytes, depicting enlarged nuclei and nucleoli, hyperchromasia, multinucleation, and pleomorphism. This entity can be found frequently in patients with viral hepatitis. Authors have reported that some of these atypical cells may remain dormant, and some dysplastic cells have the potential to develop into hepatocellular carcinoma. In fact, the most frequent mistake in interpreting liver aspirates is to confuse cells from liver cell dysplasia with those from well-differentiated hepatocellular carcinoma.

Liver cell dysplasia is also associated with a variety of processes and entities, such as viral hepatitis, regenerative nodules from cirrhotic livers, cell changes due to some chemotherapeutic agents, and cells found in the vicinity of metastatic tumors to the liver.

If some general rules are followed, the differentiation between liver cell dysplasia and hepatocellular carcinoma is quite simple. In liver cell dysplasia, the cell distribution frequently occurs in a monolayer, with the atypical hepatocytes distributed randomly [▮*25.8*]. The nuclear, nucleolar, and cytoplasmic features of dysplastic hepatocytes are identical to those of normal-appearing hepatocytes, except for their large size but with their nuclear/cytoplasmic ratio maintained. The nuclear outlines are symmetrical; when irregularity does occur, it is infrequent and minimal.

In solid, nontrabecular hepatocellular carcinomas, atypical hepatocytes are numerous, not random like those found in liver cell dysplasias. The nuclei may maintain symmetrical outlines and a low nuclear/cytoplasmic ratio is present. Distinguishing features are the frequent irregular distribution of chromatin and the appearance of several malignant hepatocytes with enlarged ("stop sign") nucleoli. In comparison with normal liver structure, trabecular well-differentiated hepatocellular carcinomas show liver cords forming numerous confluent rows of abnormal hepatocytes with high nuclear/cytoplasmic ratios [▮*25.9*]. Nuclear atypia is frequently absent and the size of the nucleoli is usually smaller than that of normal hepatocytes. Attached to the periphery of these structurally abnormal agglomerates of hepatocytes are endothelial cells [▮*25.9*, ▮*25.10*]. This architectural abnormality is seen better at low power [▮*25.10*]. Occasionally, especially in air-dried, Giemsa-stained smears, a whole capillary is seen surrounding the malignant group of hepatocytes, or it is seen as a vascular core with neoplastic cells attached.

Metastatic Disease

Metastatic disease to the liver is the most frequent reason for obtaining an FNA of deep organs. Usually, the primary site is known. Frequently, the tissue section of the original biopsy is available. The cells present in the liver aspirate should be compared with the cells from the original tissue biopsy sample for a site-specific diagnosis to be established. Occasionally, the primary tumor is not known and the burden of identification of the cell of origin is placed on the cytopathologist. Frequently, the therapeutic approach is based on the tumor type. In some instances, this assessment is not difficult; however, there are circumstances in which it is impossible on morphologic grounds alone to predict the origin of a metastatic tumor.

Poorly Differentiated Squamous Carcinoma and Adenocarcinoma

Depending on the degree of differentiation, squamous carcinomas and adenocarcinomas may be easy or difficult to classify. Well-differentiated squamous carcinomas are characterized by cells with dense, well-defined cell borders, coarse chromatin, and nucleoli of variable size. Opaque nuclei are a frequent finding. Cytoplasmic keratinization lines can occasionally be found [▮*25.11*]. Keratinization is variable and aspirations containing numerous keratinized cells are infrequent. Well-differentiated adenocarcinomas frequently show delicate cyanophilic cytoplasm and enlarged nucleoli against the background of a fine nuclear chromatin pattern. When epithelial tumors are poorly differentiated, a problem may arise as to how to differentiate them from each other. In instances where the cytoplasm is not differentiated, it is good practice to evaluate the quality of the chromatin, search for occasional acinar formations, or evaluate the cells on the periphery of the cell clusters for cytoplasmic definition. Also, adenocarcinomas of very large size frequently have compromised vascularization with areas of necrosis. Through a process of schematic necrosis, the glandular cells may assume a squamoid appearance; however, the cells are very small and mimic atypical parakeratosis of the uterine cervix.

Colonic Carcinoma

The cellular pattern of metastatic adenocarcinoma is very easy to identify. The cells are seen arranged in palisade formation or in a honeycomb arrangement. In the former arrangement, one can appreciate the elongated shape of the nuclei, which is characteristic of this neoplasm [▮*25.12*]. The chromatin is granular and single or multiple nucleoli are present, their size depending on the degree of differentiation of the tumor. In addition, there is frequently an abundance of necrotic debris associated with the tumor cells.

Breast Carcinoma

The easiest type of breast carcinoma to identify in liver aspirates from patients with metastatic disease is lobular carcinoma containing intracytoplasmic lumina [▮*25.13*]. These structures are not exclusive to lobular carcinoma but are most frequently seen in this type of neoplasm. Normally, lumina are formed between glandular cells by apposition of their cell borders. In malignancy the morphologic and functional characteristics of the cells are disturbed, and the lumina may be formed within the cytoplasm of the neoplastic cells. Intracytoplasmic lumina should be assessed in well-preserved and stained smears to avoid pitfalls in diagnosis secondary to spaces formed in the cytoplasm by degeneration or an air-drying artifact. The space has to have well-defined borders, and usually a globule of secretion is present in the luminal space.

Small Cell Undifferentiated Carcinoma of Lung

The easiest tumor to diagnose in an FNA of the liver is a small cell undifferentiated carcinoma from the lung. Occasionally, when the tumor is not necrotic, the cells may be dispersed, and while molding is not a prominent feature, it can always be found in the aspirate [▮*25.14*, right]. The chromatin is granular and pleomorphism is frequently present. When cytoplasm is present, it is delicate, transparent, and cyanophilic. The differential diagnosis is of a lymphoma, usually of a high-grade type ▮*25.14*, left].

Lymphoma

In lymphoma, a dispersed pattern is the rule. High-grade lymphoma cells, when devoid of cytoplasm, have a tendency to mold, which may mimic a small cell undifferentiated carcinoma. The diagnosis should be based only on well-preserved cells. The chromatin of aggressive lymphomas is granular but open. The nucleoli are frequently larger than in small cell undifferentiated carcinoma. This is especially true in immunoblastic lymphomas. The cytoplasm of cells from malignant lymphoma has a dense, blue color, which is quite characteristic of this neoplasm.

Renal Cell Adenocarcinoma

Characteristically, renal cell adenocarcinoma of the clear cell variety has distinctive cytoplasmic features. The cytoplasm is usually abundant with a clear appearance due to the fat particles dissolved during processing [▮*25.15*, right]. Nuclei are round. The texture of the chromatin and the size of nucleoli are variable depending on the degree of differentiation of the tumor. In Giemsa-stained slides, prior to application of the mounting media and coverslip, a quick look under the microscope shows the fat droplets quite clearly. The granular variety of renal cell adenocarcinoma is more difficult to evaluate. Fortunately, the characteristics of nuclei and nucleoli are identical to those of the clear cell variety. Very frequently these two varieties are found together [▮*25.15*, left]. Malignancies of primary sites from practically all over the body can be expected to metastasize to the liver. Enumeration of the most likely sites can narrow the search to a few organs.

Neuroendocrine Tumors

Numerous cytologic features are recognized in the diagnosis of neuroendocrine tumors metastatic to the liver. A specific diagnosis can be reached provided all morphologic types are known. This knowledge is of utmost importance, since the chemotherapeutic approach to these tumors is based on an accurate diagnosis. Patients with neuroendocrine tumors may have a long survival with adequate therapy even when large metastases to the liver are encountered. Single or multiple hormones, such as insulin, glucagon, and corticotropin, can be produced on initial analysis. When producing active substances, the detection of hormones in the serum supports, and may even predict, the FNA diagnosis of the tumor. The ability of the cell to produce hormones is unrelated to cell morphology.

Round or Oval Cell Type

The most frequent cell type seen and described in the literature is the small round or oval cell type with a "salt-and-pepper" chromatin pattern. The smears are usually cellular and the differential diagnosis is lymphoma [▮*25.16*]. However, there are small cell aggregates arranged in rosette-like fashion. The presence of eccentric nuclei and a small comet-like cytoplasmic tail may indicate the neuroendocrine nature of the cells.

Polygonal Type

In the polygonal cell type, the cytoplasm can either be homogeneous or granular. The cytoplasm is abundant, thus a low nuclear/cytoplasmic ratio is evident. Nuclei are round or oval and the chromatin is granular. The size of the nucleoli is variable according to the degree of differentiation [▮*25.17*].

Fusiform Type

In the fusiform type, the nuclei are elongate with variable degrees of chromatinic granularity. The cytoplasm can either be delicate or granular following the contours of the nuclear shape [▮*25.18*]. This cell type is frequently aspirated from tumors that histologically show trabecular features. Viewed by light microscopy, the cells can be seen singly or in rows mimicking the trabecular arrangement.

Clear Cell Type

The clear cell type is rare. Cases described in the literature have been benign insulinomas. The aspirates of clear cell neuroendocrine tumors are hypocellular. The cells are distributed mainly in small groups. Occasionally, isolated cells are noted. The cellular characteristics are similar to those of the clear cell variant of adenocarcinoma of renal origin. However, the cells of clear cell neuroendocrine tumors are quite small and the nuclear atypia is less marked when compared with the neoplasms of renal origin.

PANCREAS

The pancreas is located in the retroperitoneum, at the level of the second and the third lumbar vertebrae. On the right, the pancreatic head adheres to the midportion of the duodenum. At this site, the ductal system excretes the secretions of the acinar cells through the papilla of Vater into the duodenum. The body of the pancreas transverses the posterior aspect of the abdomen, and its tail is close to the spleen. Because of its location and surrounding viscera, the pancreas is difficult to evaluate radiologically and occasionally even during laparotomy.

Wedge biopsy during surgical exploration may fail to sample the lesion in up to 54% of patients harboring carcinoma of the pancreas. This sampling technique has serious complications; eg, hemorrhage, fistulas, pseudocyst formation, and onset of pancreatitis may occur. Occasionally, there is a fatal outcome; the morbidity rate during and after wedge biopsies ranges from 3% to 20%.

In the last decade FNA has become an excellent diagnostic tool for the management of pancreatic malignant neoplasms. There has been tremendous development of FNA techniques to assess pancreatic disease. Additionally, cytologic diagnosis has generally become acceptable as a means by which to care for patients with pancreatic disease.

Normal Histology and Cytology

The pancreas is composed of several compartments that serve different functions.

Acinar Cells

Acinar cells produce digestive enzymes that are excreted by the ductal system. Acinar cells have abundant granular cytoplasm, round nuclei with granular chromatin, and symmetrical nuclear outlines. The nucleoli are prominent. Acinar cells can be seen in small groups [▮*25.19*] or in large clusters.

Ductal Cells

Ductal cells line the excretory ducts of the pancreas. Cytologically, they usually occur in monolayered groups either in a honeycomb arrangement or in a palisade formation [▮*25.20*, ▮*25.21*]. Isolated cells are less frequently present in aspirates and have a tall nonciliated columnar shape resembling endocervical cells. The basally located nuclei are round or oval with fine and evenly distributed chromatin. There is no nuclear pleomorphism or macronucleolus.

Intercalated and Centroacinar Cells

Intercalated and centroacinar cells are located between the acinar and ductal cells and are considered less mature than acinar cells.

Islets of Langerhans

The endocrine compartment is formed by the islets of Langerhans, which are dispersed throughout the pancreatic parenchyma but are more concentrated in the pancreatic body and tail.

The cells of the islets of Langerhans are small and monomorphic [▮*25.21*]. The cells have different functions but similar morphology. The alpha cells produce glucagon; the beta cells, insulin; the delta cells, somatostatin; the pancreatic polypeptide cells, pancreatic polypeptide; and the enterochromatin cells, 5-hydroxytryptamine. Another endocrine cell type named P cell has not yet been assigned a specific function.

The three main hormones secreted by the cells of the Langerhans islets—namely, insulin, glucagon, and somatostatin—are involved in the control of the blood glucose levels. When glucose is below normal levels, the alpha cells secrete glucagon, which raises the glucose levels. The opposite occurs when the beta cells release more insulin to lower the glucose in the blood. The role of somatostatin is not yet well established. This substance is known to suppress insulin and glucagon, thus modulating the functional activity of the alpha and beta cells.

Electron microscopy studies show that insulin, glucagon, and somatostatin have different types of cytoplasmic neurosecretory granules, depending on the cell function. Immunohistochemistry studies demonstrate the presence of specific hormones or polypeptides.

Benign Processes

The most frequent benign morphologic alteration involving the pancreas is pancreatitis, which can be seen in various stages and intensity from acute to chronic subsiding forms. Frequent sequelae are fistulous processes and pseudocyst formation. At the early stages, during the acute onset, there is damage of the acinar cells with the release of digestive enzymes, resulting in destruction of the pancreatic parenchyma and surrounding tissues. Necrosis and infiltration of the tissue by polymorphonuclear leukocytes, as well as areas of fat necrosis and calcification, are encountered. The clinical findings of acute abdominal pain, coupled with high levels of blood amylase, usually indicate the presence of pancreatitis.

When aspiration is done at this stage of the disease, necrotic epithelial cells are seen intermixed with neutrophils. Enzymes escaping from the destroyed acinar cells induce necrosis of the mature adipose tissue within the pancreatic substance or elsewhere, which is known as fat necrosis [▮*25.22*].

The reparative process takes place in the form of granulation tissue. There is an exuberant proliferation of capillaries surrounded by lymphocytes, plasma cells, and histiocytes. There is a proliferation of myofibroblasts whose function is to lay collagen to form scar tissue. Aspirates of granulation tissue yield endothelial cells, myofibroblasts, and arborization of capillaries [▮*25.23*].

Cysts

There are a variety of cystic structures that can occur in the pancreas. Some are sequelae of inflammatory processes, others are of congenital or neoplastic nature, and (rarely in the United States) parasitic cysts can be seen. The most frequent pancreatic cysts are the result of inflammation and necrosis, eg, pseudocysts and retention cysts. Pseudocysts are associated with resolving stages of acute pancreatitis, surgical trauma, and reflux of bile into the pancreatic duct, as a consequence of gallbladder and ductal abnormal processes.

The histogenesis of pseudocysts is the result of destruction of the acinar cells with the release of enzymes, which in turn causes further damage of the other cellular elements of the pancreatic parenchyma. Pseudocysts are of variable size, and when they enlarge they may spread into the lesser peritoneal cavity. They are formed by a wall of fibroconnective tissue and characteristically lack a luminal epithelial lining. Mononuclear and multinucleated histiocytes are frequently attached to the luminal surface or are embedded in the fibrous wall.

Aspiration of pseudocysts yields debris, histiocytes, and variable numbers of white blood cells.

Retention cysts result from blockage of large ducts due to inflammation, necrosis, or tumor. The dilated cyst may assume large proportions and the epithelial lining may be present or dislodged due to various causes, such as fluid distention and necrosis. When the obstruction is due to neoplasia, aspiration may disclose malignant cells.

Benign Neoplasms

Benign neoplasms of the pancreas are microcystic adenomas, mucinous cystadenomas, and papillary cystic neoplasms.

Microcystic Adenomas

Microcystic adenomas, also known as glycogen-rich neoplasms, are invariably benign serous tumors. They can attain very large sizes, are frequently seen in elderly patients, and are located mainly in the head of the pancreas. Histologically, the microcystic adenomas are composed of numerous small cysts, lined by low cuboidal epithelium. The aspirates are hypocellular, and small groups of cells containing clear cytoplasm and round nuclei with benign features are found. The cytoplasm is periodic acid–Schiff positive and digestible by diastase, indicating the glycogen content. Mucin stains are negative.

Mucinous Cystadenomas

Mucinous tumors are multiloculated cystic lesions lined by tall columnar mucoproducing cells. Frequently seen in middle-aged patients, these neoplasms can become sizable and are considered potentially malignant, since careful sampling usually discloses areas of malignant transformation. Because their biologic behavior is uncertain, the term *mucinous cystic tumor* is preferred to *mucinous cystadenoma*.

It is important to remember that when mucinous tumors are sampled by FNA the areas of malignant transformation may be missed. For this reason, surgical resection is the treatment of choice for mucinous cystic tumors.

Aspirates show small clusters of mucus-producing cells with a low nuclear/cytoplasmic ratio [▮*25.24*]. Single cells with eccentric nuclei resembling histiocytes are degenerated epithelial cells aspirated with mucus from the luminal aspect of the glands. Fragments of cellular stroma, resembling ovarian stroma, can also be encountered in the aspirates.

Solid and Papillary Epithelial Neoplasms

Other terms for solid and papillary epithelial neoplasms include *papillary solid neoplasms* and *papillary cystic epithelial neoplasms of the pancreas*. These rare, low-grade neoplasms are seen in young women; age at diagnosis ranges from 12 to 33 years, with a median age of 24 years. They are found most frequently in the tail of the pancreas. Patients complain of abdominal discomfort and pain; the tumors are sometimes an incidental finding during clinical and radiologic examination.

The histologic pattern consists of solid areas of papillary fronds with fibrovascular stalks and/or cores of mucous substances. Aspirates contain slender papillary fronds composed of fibrovascular tissue surrounded by metachromatic material and rows of monomorphic cells attached to its surface. The rounded, light-blue globules seen in specimens stained by the Papanicolaou technique that are metachromatic when stained by the Giemsa method are visible among the epithelial cells. The cells are small and round or oval. Indentation of the nuclear envelope is not observed or is reported infrequently. The chromatin is fine, granular, and evenly distributed, and one or two small nucleoli are seen.

Adenocarcinoma

A large majority of pancreatic malignant tumors are adenocarcinomas that arise in the ductal system. They have various degrees of differentiation, ranging from very well-differentiated tumors to anaplastic neoplasms. The dedifferentiated tumors may be difficult to differentiate from sarcomas. Fortunately, the most frequent ductal neoplasm falls into the category of moderately differentiated adenocarcinoma, which is easily diagnosed. Well-differentiated mucoproducing adenocarcinomas are formed by tall columnar cells with eccentric nuclei. The cells are arranged in monolayers and the cytoplasm is distended by mucus, where the neoplastic cells are seen in an exaggerated honeycomb formation. The nuclei are hypochromatic, and the chromatin is fine. Single or multiple minute nucleoli may be present.

The main features useful in diagnosing well-differentiated mucoproducing adenocarcinomas [▮*25.25*, ▮*25.26*] are the pronounced infolding of the nuclear envelope and the high nuclear/cytoplasmic ratio present in all cells.

Nonmucoproducing well-differentiated tumors are infrequent and are characterized on aspirates by monolayers of cells similar to normal ductal cells. At close scrutiny, slight pleomorphism is noticeable and mitotic figures are frequent [▮*25.27*, ▮*25.28*].

Moderately differentiated adenocarcinomas can be seen as monolayer, three-dimensional, and isolated [▮*25.29*]. Frequently, there are severe atypical features, including marked pleomorphism, irregularities of the nuclear envelope, and single or multiple macronucleoli. The cytoplasm is variable; there may be pronounced mucus production or more cytoplasmic density.

Pleomorphic Adenocarcinoma

This neoplasm is classified as a giant cell tumor and has poor biologic behavior. Such neoplasms usually come to clinical attention after distant metastases have developed.

Pleomorphic adenocarcinoma has a predilection for the body and tail of the organ and an unusually high incidence of hematogenous spread. Because of its unusual morphologic features, this tumor can be easily confused with sarcoma, hepatocellular carcinoma, and poorly differentiated carcinoma [▮*25.30*].

Histologic examination shows mononuclear giant cells that have a large number of mitotic figures in a loose sarcomatoid pattern. Pleomorphic, multinucleated giant cells that have markedly atypical nuclei may also be encountered in association with poorly or well-differentiated adenocarcinoma, squamous carcinoma, or spindle components.

Aspirates contain numerous cells because of the small amount of tumor stroma. Mainly solitary cells are seen, unless a second cell population composed of classical-appearing glandular cells is present, in which case the tumor cells are in clusters. The mononuclear cells are large, and most of them are oval. The cytoplasm is finely granular and cyanophilic and has well-defined borders.

The round or oval nuclei contain coarsely granular chromatin and sometimes have irregular outlines. There are one or more large nucleoli. A large number of mitotic figures can be seen. Multinucleated malignant cells are occasionally encountered, but mononuclear cells predominate, outnumbering the multinucleated giant cells. The cytoplasm of the multinucleated cells has the same qualities as that of the mononuclear cells. The large nuclei contain coarse chromatin, frequently distributed unevenly, and often have irregular outlines. There are one or more large nucleoli.

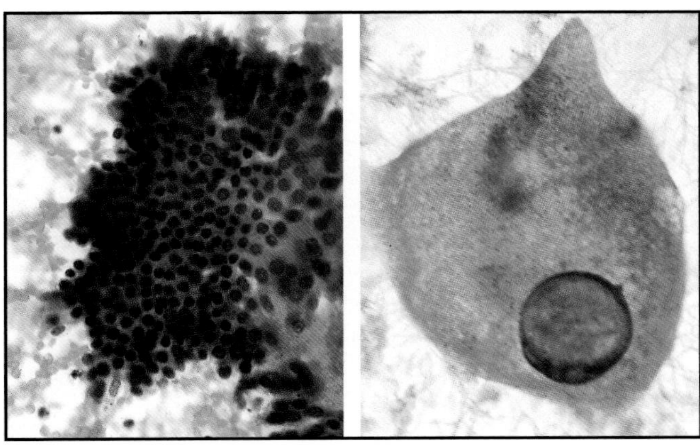

▮25.1

Benign hepatocyte showing abundant, well-defined dense cytoplasm. Left, A monolayer of benign bile duct cells (Papanicolaou). Right, The nucleus is symmetrical and a large intranuclear cytoplasmic inclusion occupies most of the nuclear area (Papanicolaou).

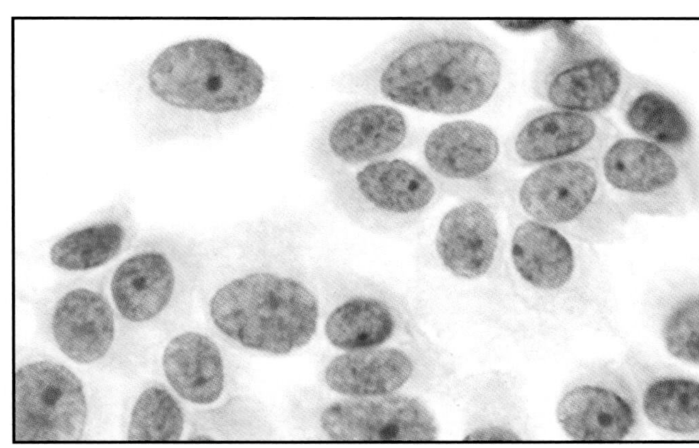

▮25.2

Group of pleomorphic mesothelial cells (Papanicolaou).

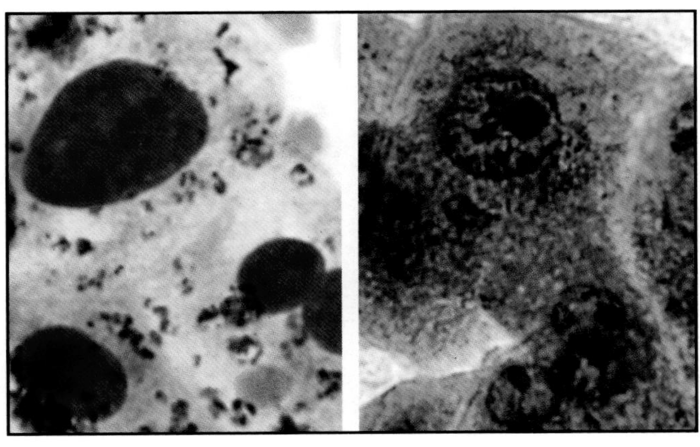

▮25.3

Hepatocytes depicting cytoplasmic lipochrome pigment (left, Papanicolaou; right, Giemsa).

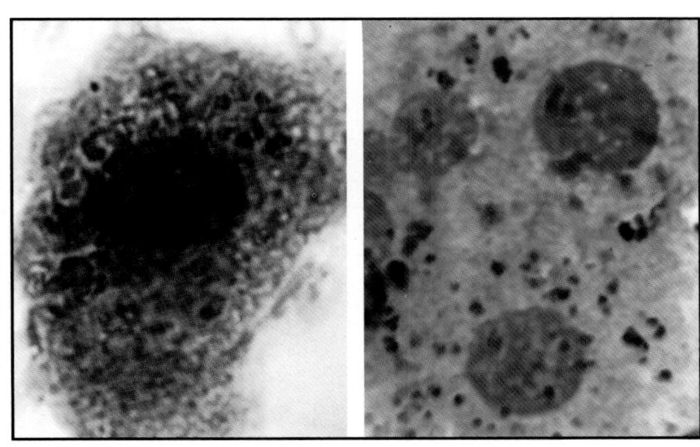

▮25.4

Benign hepatocytes showing iron pigment in their cytoplasm (left, Papanicolaou; right, Giemsa).

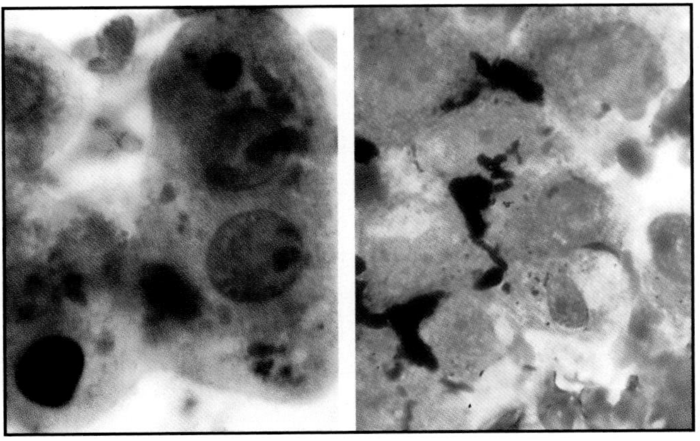

▮25.5

Benign hepatocytes showing bile pigment in their cytoplasm and in the bile canaliculi (left, Papanicolaou; right, Giemsa).

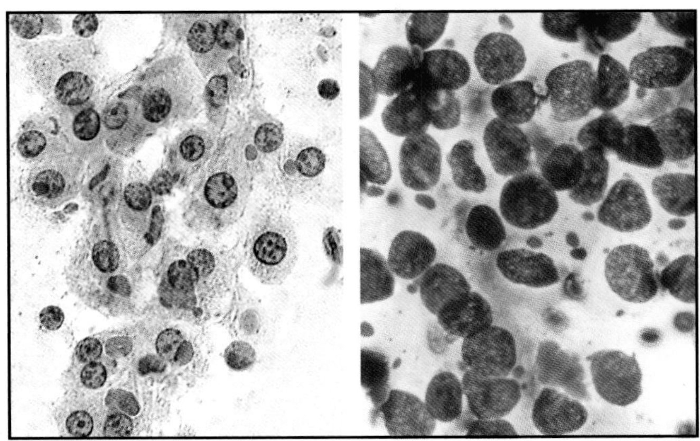

▮25.6

Aspirate of a well-differentiated hepatocellular carcinoma showing cytoplasmic inclusions (left, Papanicolaou; right, Giemsa).

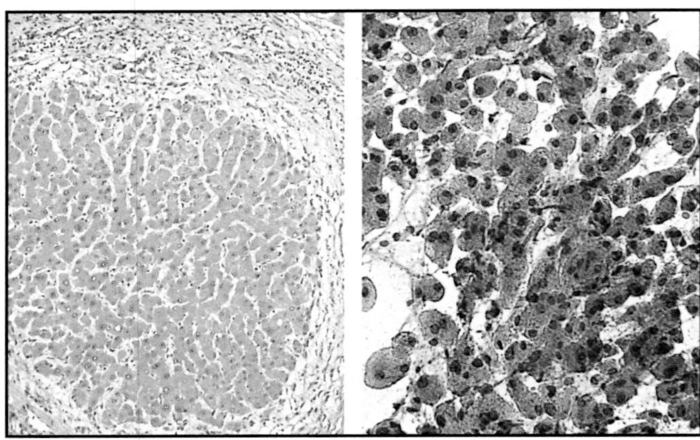

▌25.7

Left, Histologic section of cirrhotic liver showing regenerative nodule surrounded by fibrosis (hematoxylin-eosin). Right, Aspirate of a cirrhotic nodule showing benign hepatocytes arranged in rows (Papanicolaou).

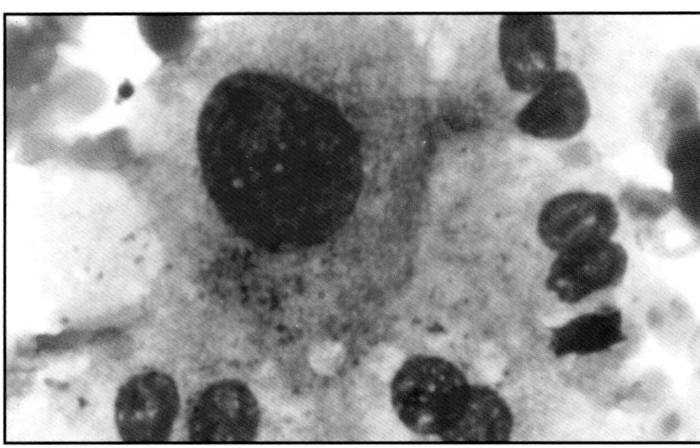

▌25.8

Liver aspirate showing dysplastic hepatocyte surrounded by normal binucleated cells (Giemsa).

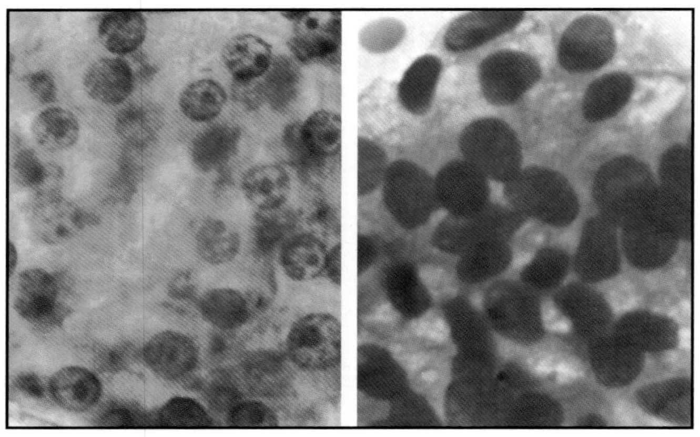

▌25.9

Aspirate of a well-differentiated hepatocellular carcinoma. Thick trabeculae of malignant hepatocytes with high nuclear/cytoplasmic ratio are surrounded by endothelial cells (left, Papanicolaou; right, Giemsa).

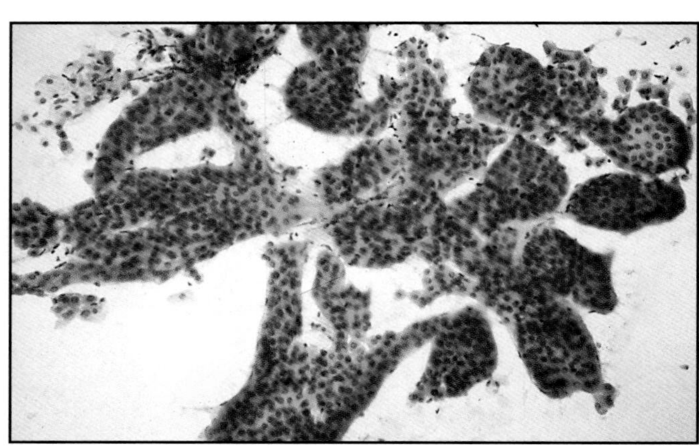

▌25.10

Low-power view of an aspirate of a well-differentiated trabecular hepatocellular carcinoma. Thick cords of small hepatocytes are surrounded by endothelial cells (Papanicolaou).

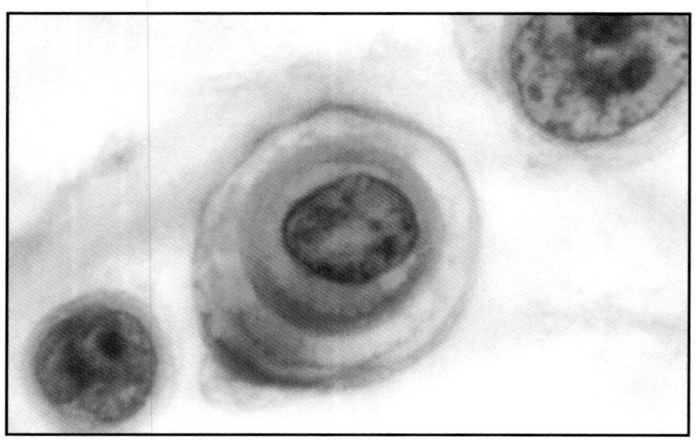

▌25.11

Individual neoplastic squamous cells showing keratinizing lines (Papanicolaou).

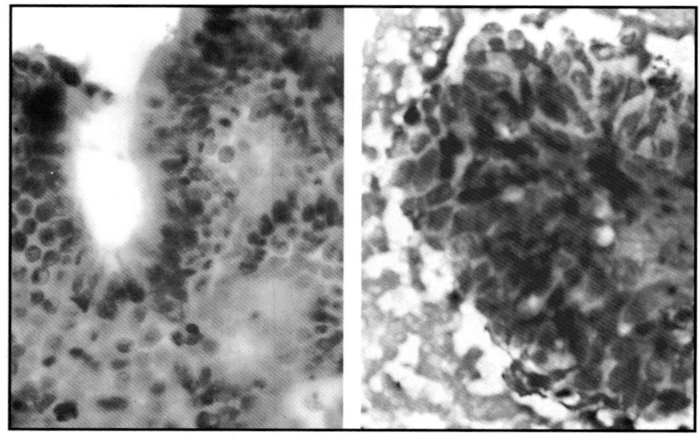

▌25.12

Colonic carcinoma is seen in aspirates as columnar cells in palisade formation (left, Papanicolaou; right, Giemsa).

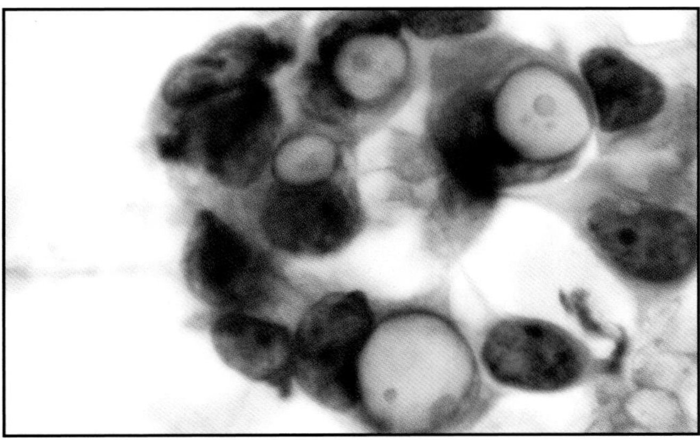

▮25.13

Adenocarcinoma of breast depicting intracytoplasmic lumina (Papanicolaou).

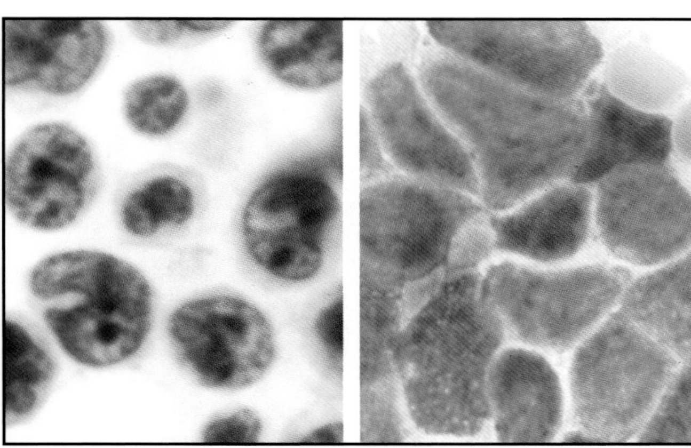

▮25.14

Left, Malignant lymphoma seen in a dispersed pattern (Papanicolaou). Right, Small cell undifferentiated carcinoma depicting nuclear molding (Giemsa).

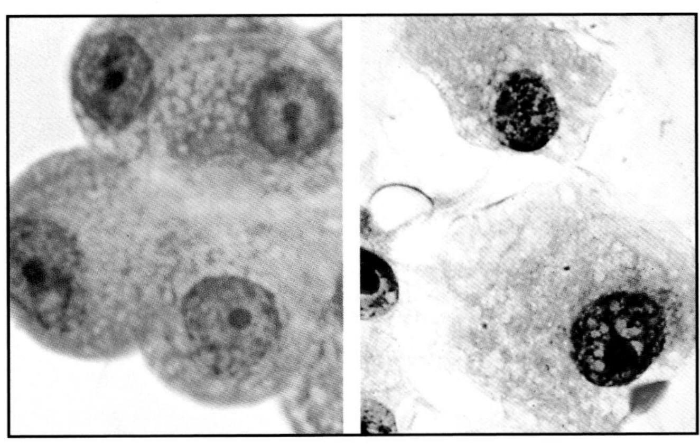

▮25.15

Granular (left) and clear cell (right) renal cell adenocarcinoma (Papanicolaou).

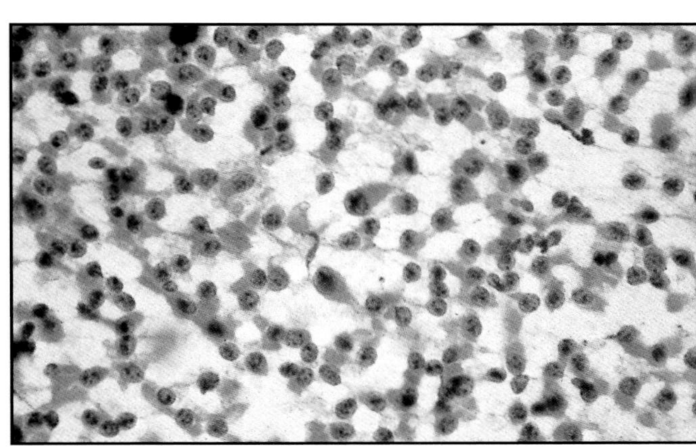

▮25.16

Aspirate of a metastatic neuroendocrine tumor to the liver showing the increased cellularity of the smear (Papanicolaou).

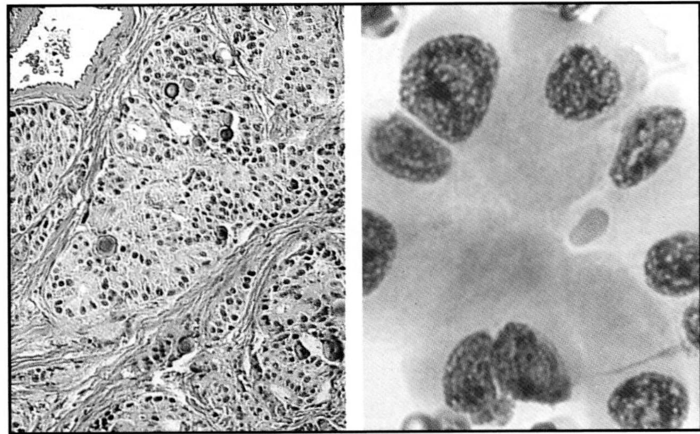

▮25.17

Polygonal type of neuroendocrine tumor (right, Giemsa) and histologic section (left, hematoxylin-eosin).

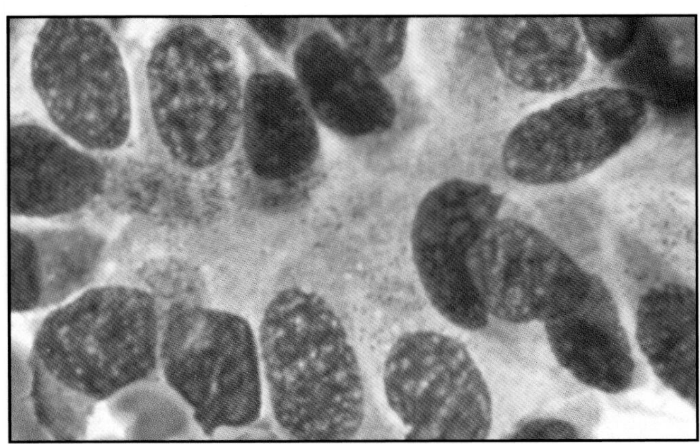

▮25.18

Fusiform pattern of neuroendocrine tumor showing elongated cells and granular cytoplasm (Giemsa).

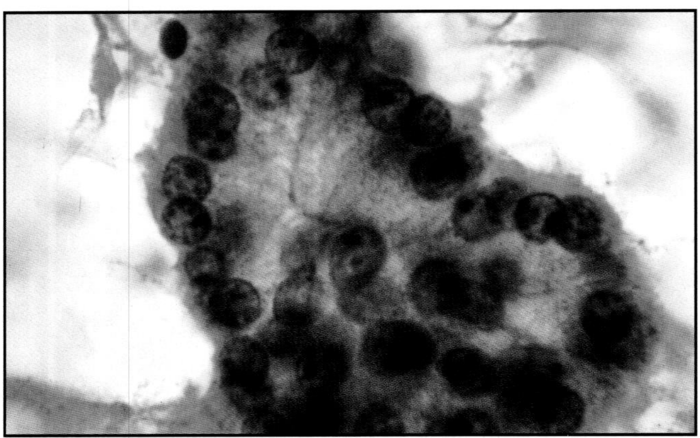

25.19

Benign acinar cells. Acinus is formed by cells containing round nuclei with enlarged nucleoli. The cytoplasm is abundant and granular (x1300).

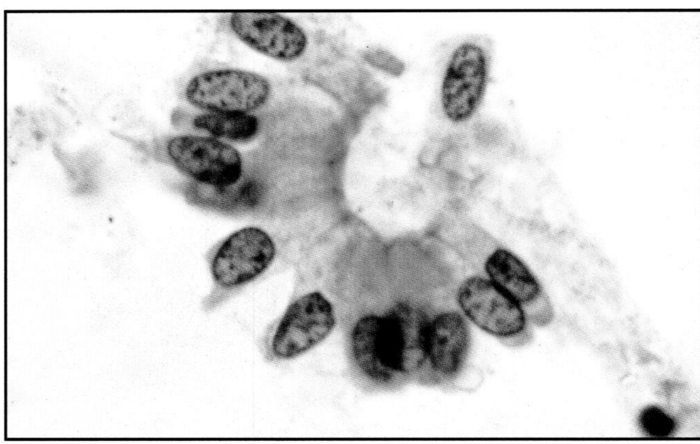

25.20

Benign ductal cells. Cluster of ductal cells on palisade formation showing monomorphic nuclei and elongated cyanophilic cytoplasm (x450).

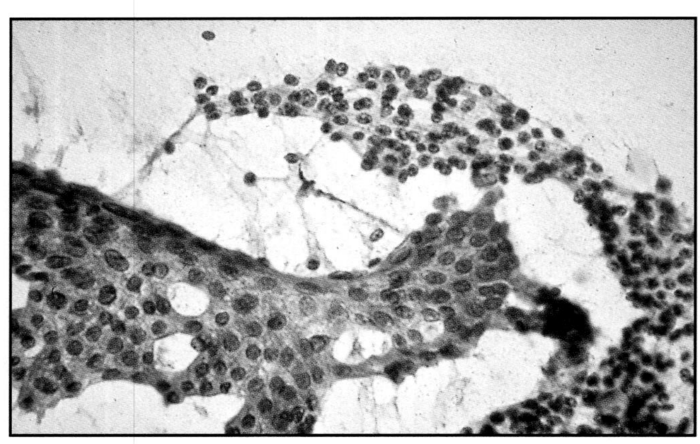

25.21

Benign ductal and islet cells. Monolayer of ductal cells seen in honeycomb arrangement with well-defined cell borders. At right a group of islet cells shows single or multiple enlarged nucleoli and ill-defined cellular borders (x940).

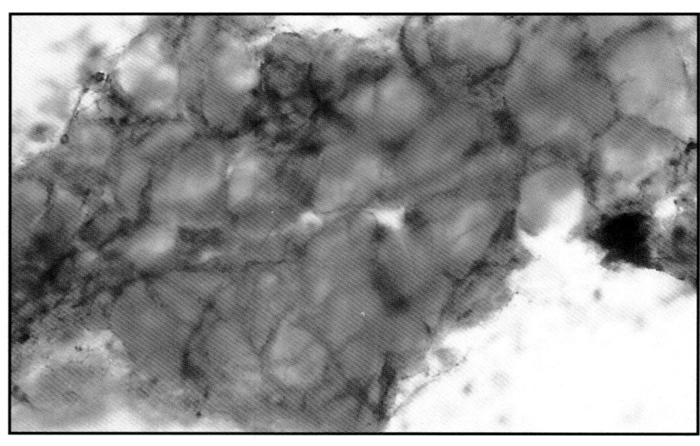

25.22

Aspiration of fatty necrosis. Ghosts of adipose tissue cells with a background of calcium deposits are shown (x450).

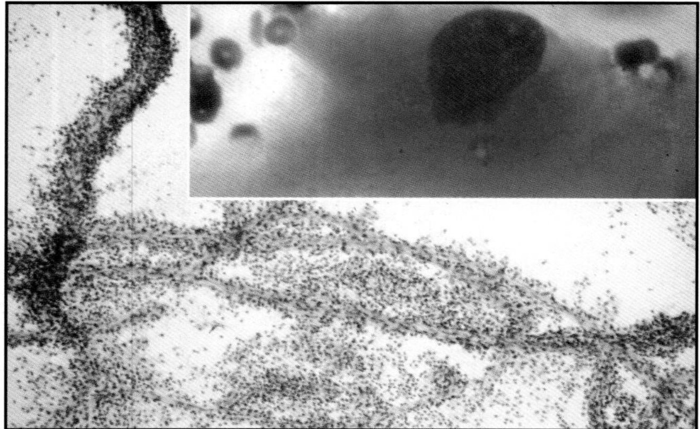

25.23

Granulation tissue. Capillaries are surrounded by histiocytes and round inflammatory cells (Papanicolaou, x250). Inset, Myofibroblasts. Mesenchymal cells have ill-defined cytoplasmic borders, rounded nuclei, and enlarged nucleoli (Giemsa, x960).

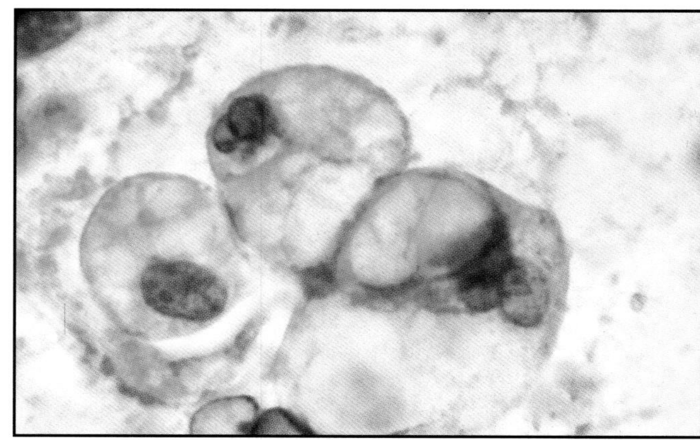

25.24

Mucinous tumor. Aspirate shows cells with abundant clear cytoplasm distended by mucus. The nuclei are small, maintaining a low nuclear/cytoplasmic ratio (Papanicolaou, x960).

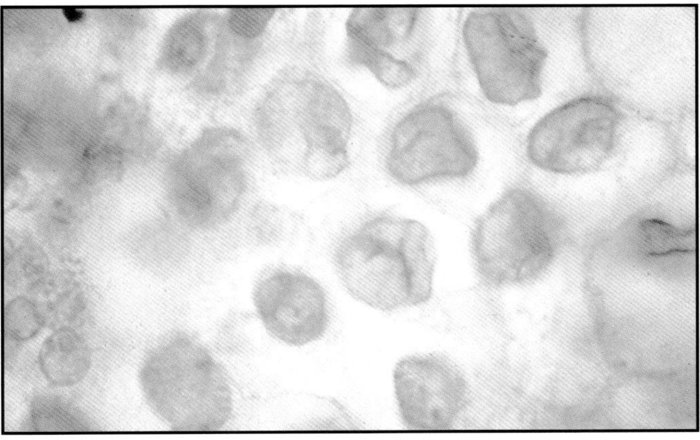

▌25.25

Well-differentiated mucoproducing adenocarcinoma. Clusters of cells have a small amount of clear cytoplasm distended by mucus, emphasizing the honeycomb pattern. The nuclei are infolded and the nuclear/cytoplasmic ratio is very high (Papanicolaou, x940).

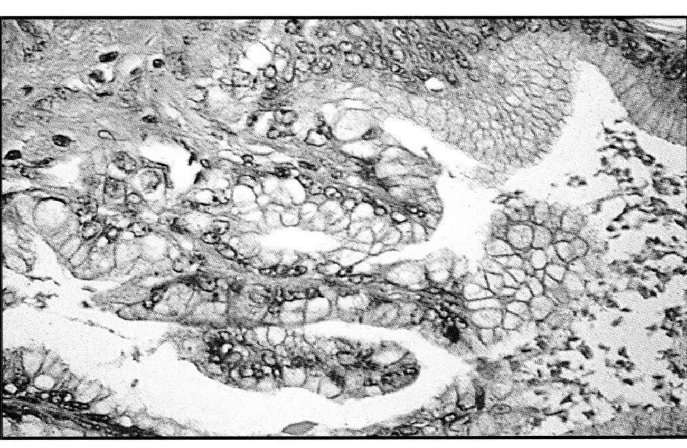

▌25.26

Well-differentiated mucoproducing adenocarcinoma. Fronds of tall columnar cells project into the luminal space (hematoxylin-eosin, x450).

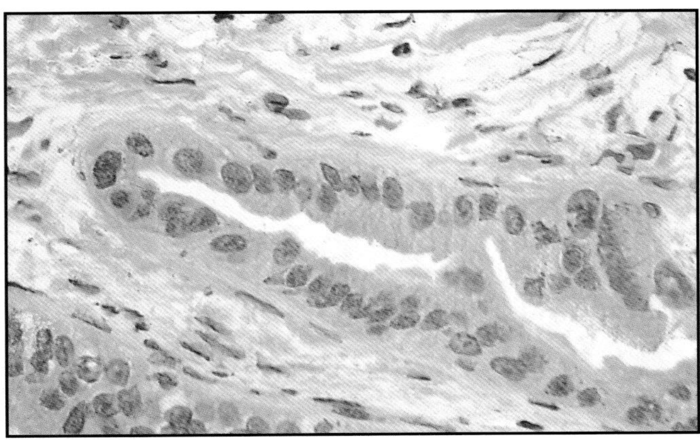

▌25.27

Well-differentiated nonmucoproducing adenocarcinoma. Histologic section shows glands composed of cuboidal cells with dense cytoplasm (hematoxylin-eosin, x450).

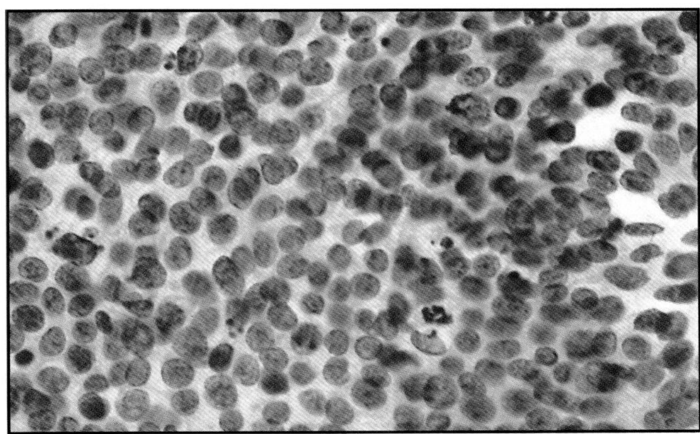

▌25.28

Well-differentiated nonmucoproducing adenocarcinoma. Aspirate shows monolayer of cells with slight pleomorphism and numerous mitoses (Papanicolaou, x450).

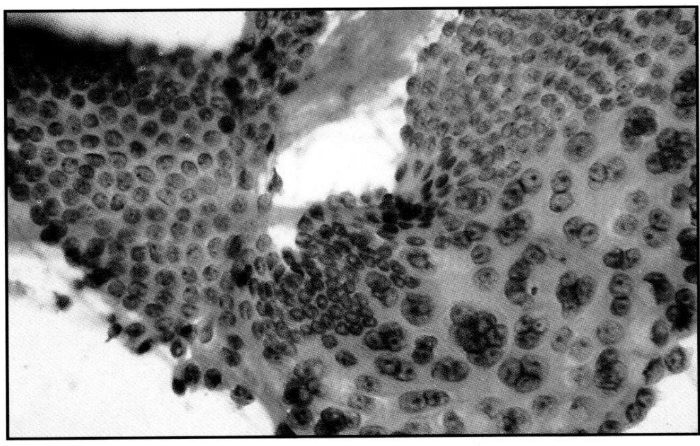

▌25.29

Moderately well-differentiated adenocarcinoma. A cluster of highly pleomorphic cells has macronucleoli alongside morphologically benign-appearing cells (Papanicolaou, x450).

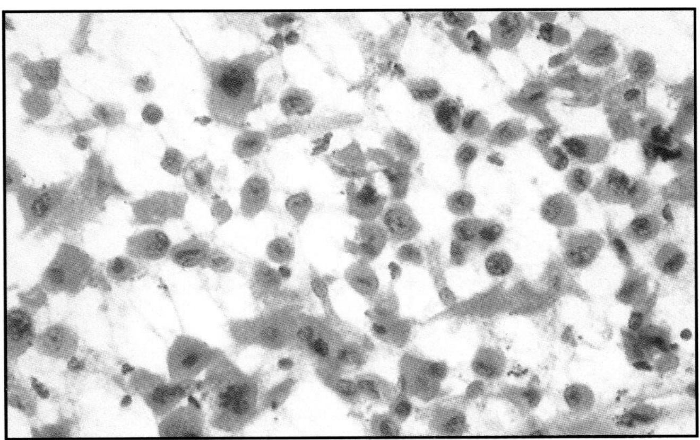

▌25.30

Anaplastic carcinoma. An aspirate shows highly pleomorphic cells arranged in a dispersed pattern (Papanicolaou, x450).

SELECTED READINGS (LIVER)

Anthony PP, Vogel CL, Barker LF. Liver cell dysplasia: a premalignant condition. *J Clin Pathol.* 1973;26:217-223.

Anthony PP, Vogel CL, Nayak NC, et al. The morphology of cirrhosis. *J Clin Pathol.* 1978;31:395-414.

Berman JJ, McNeill RE. Cirrhosis with atypia: a potential pitfall in the interpretation of liver aspirates. *Acta Cytol.* 1988; 32:11-14.

Bognel C, Rougier P, Leclere J, et al. Fine needle aspiration of the liver and pancreas with ultrasound guidance. *Acta Cytol.* 1988;32:22-26.

Brechot C, Hadchouel M, Scotto J. Evidence that hepatitis B virus has a role in liver-cell carcinoma in alcoholic liver disease. *N Engl J Med.* 1982;306:1384-1387.

Chandrasoma P. Fine needle aspiration of the liver. In: Astarita RW, ed. *Practical Cytopathology.* New York, NY: Churchill Livingstone Inc; 1990:chap 9.

Cohen C. Intracytoplasmic hyaline globules in hepatocellular carcinoma. *Cancer.* 1976;37:1754-1758.

Craig JR, Peters RL, Edmondson HA, et al. Fibrolamellar carcinoma of the liver: a tumor of adolescents and young adults with distinctive clinicopathologic features. *Cancer.* 1980;46:372-379.

Ekelund P, Wasastjerna C. Cytological identification of primary hepatic carcinoma cells. *Acta Med Scand.* 1971;189:373-375.

Gupta SK, Das DK, Rajwanslin A, et al. Cytology of hepatocellular carcinoma. *Diagn Cytopathol.* 1986;2:291-294.

Hidvegi-Frias D. Liver and pancreas. In: Kline TS, ed. *Guides to Clinical Aspiration Biopsy.* New York, NY: Igaku-Shoin Medical Publishers Inc; 1988.

Ho CS, McLoughlin MJ, Tao LC, et al. Guided percutaneous fine-needle aspiration biopsy of the liver. *Cancer.* 1981;47:1781-1785.

Jaffe BM. Factors influencing survival in patients with untreated hepatic metastases. *Surg Gynecol Obstet.* 1968;127:1-6.

Kline TS. Liver. In: Kline TS, ed. *Handbook of Fine Needle Aspiration Biopsy.* 2nd ed. New York, NY: Churchill Livingstone Inc; 1988:chap 11.

Koss GL, Woyke S, Olszewski W. The liver. In: *Aspiration Biopsy Cytologic Interpretation and Histological Bases.* New York, NY: Igaku-Shoin Medical Publishers Inc; 1984:350-374.

Linsk JA, Franzen S. Abdominal aspiration. In: *Clinical Aspiration Cytology.* Philadelphia, Pa: JB Lippincott Co; 1983:182-195.

Marion PL, Salazar FH, Alexander JJ, et al. State of hepatitis B viral DNA in a human hepatoma cell line. *J Virol.* 1980;33:795-806.

Parker SH, Hopper KD, Yakes WF, et al. Image-directed percutaneous biopsies with a biopsy gun. *Radiology.* 1989; 171:663-669.

Perry MD, Johnston WW. Needle biopsy of the liver for the diagnosis of non-neoplastic liver diseases. *Acta Cytol.* 1985; 29:385-390.

Pilotti S, Rilke F, Claren R, et al. Conclusive diagnosis of hepatic and pancreatic malignancies by fine needle aspiration. *Acta Cytol.* 1988;32:27-38.

Pinto MM, Avila NA, Heller CI, et al. Fine-needle aspiration of the liver. *Acta Cytol.* 1988;32:15-21.

Prince AM. Hepatitis B virus and hepatocellular carcinoma: molecular biology provides further evidence for an etiologic association. *Hepatology.* 1981;1:73-75.

Rosenblatt R, Kutcher R, Moussouris HF, et al. Sonographically guided fine-needle aspiration of liver lesions. *JAMA.* 1982;248:1639-1641.

Saul SH. Neoplasms of liver. In: Sternberg SS, ed. *Diagnostic Surgical Pathology.* New York, NY: Raven Press; 1989.

Schwartz MR. Gastrointestinal tract. In: Ramzy T, ed. *Clinical Cytopathology and Aspiration Biopsy.* East Norwalk, Conn: Appleton & Lange; 1990.

Schwerk WB, Schmitz-Moormann P. Ultrasonically guided fine-needle biopsies in neoplastic liver disease. *Cancer.* 1981;48:1469-1477.

Soderstrom N. *Fine Needle Aspiration Biopsy.* Stockholm, Sweden: Almqvist & Wiksell; 1966.

Suen KC. Diagnosis of primary hepatic neoplasms by fine-needle aspiration cytology. *Diagn Cytopathol.* 1986;2:99-109.

Suen KC, Magee JF, Halparin LS, et al. Fine needle aspiration cytology of fibrolamellar hepatocellular carcinoma. *Acta Cytol.* 1985;29:867-872.

Tao LC. Liver and pancreas. In: Bibbo M, ed. *Comprehensive Cytopathology.* Philadelphia, Pa: WB Saunders Co; 1991.

Tao LC, Donat EE, Ho CS, et al. Percutaneous fine-needle aspiration of the liver: cytodiagnosis of hepatic cancer. *Acta Cytol.* 1979;23:287-291.

Tao LC, Ho CS, McLoughlin MJ, et al. Cytologic diagnosis of hepatocellular carcinoma by fine-needle aspiration biopsy. *Cancer.* 1984;53:547-552.

Tao LC, Kline TS. Liver. In: Kline TS, ed. *Handbook of Fine Needle Aspiration Biopsy Cytology.* 2nd ed. New York, NY: Churchill Livingstone Inc; 1988:chap 11.

Tatsuta M, Yamamoto R, Kasugai H. Cytohistologic diagnosis of neoplasms of the liver by ultrasonically guided fine-needle aspiration biopsy. *Cancer.* 1984;54:1682-1686.

Wasastjerna C. Liver. In: Zajicek J, ed. *Aspiration Biopsy Cytology, II: Cytology of Infradiaphragmatic Organs.* Basel, Switzerland: S Karger; 1979:167-193. Monographs in Clinical Cytology.

Whitlach S, Nunez C, Pitlik DA. Fine needle aspiration biopsy of the liver: a study of 102 consecutive cases. *Acta Cytol.* 1984;28:719-725.

SELECTED READINGS (PANCREAS)

American Cancer Society. *Cancer Facts and Figures—1990.* Atlanta, Ga: American Cancer Society; 1990.

Arnesjo B, Stormby N, Akerman M. Cytodiagnosis of pancreatic lesions by means of fine-needle biopsy during operation. *Acta Chir Scand.* 1972;138:363-369.

Ascoli V, Newman GA, Kline TS. Grimelus stain for cytodiagnosis of carcinoid tumor. *Diagn Cytopathol.* 1986;2:157-159.

Banner GF, Myrent KL, Menioli BA, et al. Neuroendocrine carcinoma of the pancreas diagnosed by aspiration cytology: a case report. *Acta Cytol.* 1985;29:442-448.

Bognel C, Rougier P, Leclere J, et al. Fine needle aspiration of pancreas with ultrasound guidance. *Acta Cytol.* 1988;32:27-38.

Bondeson L, Bondeson A, Genell S, et al. Aspiration cytology of a rare solid and papillary epithelial neoplasm of the pancreas: light and electron microscopic study of a case. *Acta Cytol.* 1984;28:605-609.

Bouredeau C, Sylvestre J, Levesque HP, et al. Computerized axial tomography and fine needle biopsy in surgery of the pancreas. *Can J Surg.* 1979;22:29-33.

Bowden L. The fallibility of pancreatic biopsy. *Ann Surg.* 1954; 139:403-408.

Campagno J, Oertel JE. Mucinous cystic neoplasm of the pancreas with overt and latent malignancy (cystadenocarcinoma and cystadenoma): a clinicopathologic study of 41 cases. *Am J Clin Pathol.* 1978;69:573-580.

Combs S, Hidvegi DF, Ma Y, et al. Evaluation of a pleomorphic adenocarcinoma of the pancreas with the monoclonal antibody 44-3A6. *Diagn Cytopathol.* 1988;4:316-322.

Evander A, Ihse I, Lunderquist A, et al. Percutaneous cytodiagnosis of carcinoma of the pancreas and bile duct. *Ann Surg.* 1978;188:90-92.

Fawcitt RA, Forbes W St C, Isherwood I, et al. Computed tomography in pancreatic disease. *Br J Radiol.* 1978;51:1-4.

Foote A, Simpson JS, Stewart RJ, et al. Diagnosis of the rare solid and papillary epithelial neoplasm of the pancreas by fine needle aspiration cytology: light and electron microscopic study of a case. *Acta Cytol.* 1986;30:519-527.

Forsgren L, Orell S. Aspiration cytology in carcinoma of the pancreas. *Surgery.* 1973;73:38-42.

Frederiksen P, Thommesen P, Skjolborg H. Fine needle aspiration biopsy of the pancreas. *Scand J Gastroenterol.* 1976;11:785-791.

Geng JZ, Qin PR, Hui LD, et al. Ct guided fine needle aspiration biopsy of biliopancreatic lesions: report of 30 cases. *Jpn J Surg.* 1987;17:461-464.

Goldstein HM, Zornoza J. Percutaneous transperitoneal aspiration biopsy of pancreatic masses. *Dig Dis.* 1978;23:840-843.

Gudjonsson B, Livstone EM, Spiro HM. Cancer of the pancreas: diagnostic accuracy and survival statistics. *Cancer.* 1976;42:2492-2506.

Hall-Craggs MA, Lees WR. Fine needle aspiration biopsy: pancreatic and biliary tumors. *AJR.* 1986;147:399-403.

Hancke S, Holm HH, Kock F. Ultrasonically guided percutaneous fine needle biopsy of the pancreas. *Surg Gynecol Obstet.* 1975;140:361-364.

Harter LP, Moss AA, Goldberg HI, et al. CT guided fine needle aspirations for diagnosis of benign and malignant disease. *AJR.* 1983;140:363-367.

Hidvegi DF. *Guides to Clinical Aspiration Biopsy of Liver and Pancreas.* New York, NY: Igaku-Shoin Medical Publishers Inc; 1988.

Hidvegi D, Nieman HL, Demay RM, et al. Percutaneous transperitoneal aspiration of pancreas guided by ultrasound: morphologic and cytochemical appearance of normal and malignant cells. *Acta Cytol.* 1979;23:181-184.

Hsiu JG, D'Amato NA, Sperling MH, et al. Malignant islet cell tumor of the pancreas diagnosed by fine needle aspiration biopsy: a case report. *Acta Cytol.* 1985;29:576-579.

Karoda C, Yoshioka H, Tokunaga K, et al. Fine needle aspiration biopsy via percutaneous transhepatic catheterization technique and clinical results. *Gastrointest Radiol.* 1986;11:81-84.

Kini SR. Aspiration biopsy cytology of unusual lesions of the pancreas. *ASCP Cytopathology Check Sample, No. C84-4.* Chicago, Ill: American Society of Clinical Pathologists; 1984.

Kline TS. *Handbook of Fine Needle Aspiration Biopsy Cytology.* 2nd ed. New York, NY: Churchill Livingstone Inc; 1988.

Kline TS, Neal HS. Needle aspiration: a critical appraisal. *JAMA.* 1978;239:36-39.

Kline TS, Neal HS. Needle aspiration biopsy: a pilot study. *JAMA.* 1973;224:1143-1146.

Kocjan G, Rode J, Lees WR. Percutaneous fine needle aspiration cytology of the pancreas: advantages and pitfalls. *J Clin Pathol.* 1989;42:341-347.

Kozowski W, Hadju SI, Melamed MR. Cytomorphology of carcinoid tumors. *Acta Cytol.* 1979;23:36-365.

Kreel L. Computerized tomography of the pancreas. *Comput Axial Tomogr.* 1977;1:287-297.

Kuo T-T, Su I-J, Chien C-H. Solid and papillary neoplasm of the pancreas: report of three cases from Taiwan. *Cancer.* 1984; 54:1469-1474.

Lee Y-N. Tissue diagnosis for carcinoma of the pancreas and periampullary structures. *Cancer.* 1982;49:1035-1039.

Lightwood R, Reber HA, Way LW. The risk and accuracy of pancreatic biopsy. *Am J Surg.* 1976;132:189-194.

McLoughlin MJ, Ho CS, Langer B, et al. Fine needle aspiration biopsy of malignant lesions in and around the pancreas. *Cancer.* 1978;41:2413-2419.

Mitchell ML, Bittner CA, Wills JS, et al. Fine needle aspiration cytology of the pancreas: a retrospective study of 73 cases. *Acta Cytol.* 1988;32:4447-4451.

Mitty HA, Efremidis SC, Yeh H-C. Impact of fine needle biopsy on management of patients with carcinoma of the pancreas. *AJR.* 1981;137:1119-1121.

Neff CC, Simeone JF, Wittenberg J, et al. Inflammatory pancreatic masses: problems in differentiating focal pancreatitis from carcinoma. *Radiology.* 1984;15:35-38.

Oland J, Rosen A, Reif R, et al. Fine needle aspiration cytology of the pancreas. *J Surg Oncol.* 1988;38:14-15.

Parsons L Jr, Palmer CH. How accurate is fine needle biopsy in malignant neoplasia of the pancreas? *Arch Surg.* 1989;124:681-683.

Schultz NJ, Sanders RJ. Evaluation of pancreatic biopsy. *Am J Surg.* 1963;158:1057-1058.

Schwerk WB, Durr HK, Schmitz-Moormann P. Ultrasound guided fine needle aspiration in pancreatic and hepatic neoplasms. *Gastrointest Radiol.* 1983;8:219-225.

Simms MH, Tindall N, Allan RN. Pancreatic fistula following operative needle aspiration. *Br J Surg.* 1982;69:548.

Sneige N, Ordonez NG, Veanatt U, et al. Fine needle aspiration cytology in pancreatic endocrine tumors. *Diagn Cytopathol.* 1987;3:35-40.

Tao L-C, Ho C-S, McLoughlin JJ, et al. Percutaneous fine needle aspiration biopsy of pancreas. *Acta Cytol.* 1978;22:215-220.

Tylen U, Arnersjo B, Lindberg LG, et al. Percutaneous biopsy of carcinoma of the pancreas guided by angiography. *Surg Gynecol Obstet.* 1976;142:737-739.

Wilander E, Norheim I, Oberg K. Application of silver stains to cytologic specimens of neuroendocrine tumors metastatic to the liver. *Acta Cytol.* 1985;29:1053-1057.

Wittenberg J, Simeone JF, Ferrucci JT, et al. Non-focal enlargement in pancreatic carcinoma. *Radiology.* 1982;144:131-135.

Zornoza J. *Percutaneous Needle Biopsy.* Baltimore, Md: Williams & Wilkins; 1981.

CHAPTER 26

Bone and Soft-Tissue Tumors

STANLEY J. RADIO, MD
KAREN D. BOHL, CT(ASCP)
JAMES LINDER, MD

CONTENTS

Bone and soft-tissue tumors comprise a group of greater than 200 reactive, benign, and malignant lesions with a wide array of morphologic patterns. The reason for this heterogeneity is multifactorial. These tumors are derived from mesoderm, which is the progenitor to such diverse normal cells as muscle, fat, connective tissue, and bone. Mesodermal tumors can sometimes contain different and varying proportions of these cell types. Also, the appearance of tumor cells is modified by the local tissue and other host factors. Thus, the cell morphology and pattern of any single tumor might fulfill criteria for a number of bone or soft-tissue lesions.

Fine needle aspiration is a reliable method to diagnose bone and soft-tissue tumors, with a sensitivity and specificity similar to histologic diagnoses from open biopsy. Needle aspiration has several potential advantages over incisional biopsy when limb-sparing surgical approaches are contemplated: there is (1) minimal disruption of the tumor, reducing the potential for tumor seeding and dissemination; (2) less wound contamination; (3) shorter healing time; (4) simplicity; (5) relative lack of discomfort to the patient; (6) immediate assessment of specimen adequacy; and (7) enhancement of nuclear detail otherwise lost in decalcification of core biopsy specimens. Also, tissue procured by fine needle aspiration can be used for ultrastructural, cytometric, molecular diagnostic, or cytogenetic analysis.

A widely accepted tenet of fine needle aspiration diagnosis is that the final diagnosis must include consideration of the patient's age, sex, predisposing risk factors, and radiologic findings as well as findings at presentation and clinical course. This premise is perhaps even more imperative in the interpretation of bone and soft-tissue tumors. The overlap between reactive, benign, and malignant morphology on both cytologic and histologic specimens demands that the cytotechnologist and cytopathologist consider clinical features before a diagnosis is rendered.

In particular, the radiologic appearance of the tumor assumes a priority otherwise reserved for gross tissue characteristics in other specimens. The bone radiologist is a treasured ally of the cytopathology laboratory. One should never render a cytomorphologic interpretation of a bone tumor without knowledge of the radiographic appearance of the lesion. This includes both the location within the bone (eg, shaft vs metaphysis vs epiphysis) and what bone is affected. Different bone tumors have predilections for different locations. For example, intraskeletal osteosarcoma almost exclusively arises in long bones adjacent to the knee, whereas osteoblastoma commonly arises in the vertebral column. Information provided by the radiograph is invaluable in narrowing the differential diagnosis of bone lesions.

Bone and soft-tissue tumors are uncommon in most practice settings. A prudent approach, when previous experience with these tumors is limited, may be the provision of a differential diagnosis and exclusion of diseases not meriting further consideration. It is important to remember that reactive or benign bone or soft-tissue neoplasms outnumber malignant neoplasms nearly 100 to 1.

A description of common representative tumors from each group of bone and soft-tissue tumors is presented. A modified World Health Organization classification of bone tumors is also presented [**T** *26.1*]. Readers should remember that metastatic carcinoma is the most common malignant tumor involving bone. Tumors of the breast, lung, prostate, or other sites should be considered based on the patient's sex, age, and clinical setting.

SAMPLING TECHNIQUES

Aspiration of soft-tissue masses is usually performed with 22-gauge needles. Bone, because of its density, may require larger and rigid 18- or 20-gauge needles. Radiographic guidance of the biopsy may be required for deep retroperitoneal or axial skeleton lesions. Immediately after obtaining the specimen, air-dried Romanowsky-stained slides can be prepared to assess specimen adequacy. This stain is beneficial in demonstrating osteoid or chondroid tumor matrix. Additional smears are immediately fixed in 95% alcohol for subsequent staining by the Papanicolaou technique. Multiple aspirations allow for fresh tissue samples to be further triaged for possible special procedures such as flow or imaging cytometry, electron microscopy, and cytogenetics.

NORMAL BONE

Normal bone generally consists of a dense outer cortex surrounding a soft central medulla. The bone cortex is formed by the mineralization of a cartilaginous matrix by osteoblasts and osteocytes. During bone formation, and after bone injury, there is active remodeling of bone by osteoclasts.

Osteoblasts are found in many reactive and reparative lesions of bone as well as in primary bone tumors. Aspiration of bone often separates strips of osteoblasts from the osteoid seams, thus in smears they may appear as loose aggregates or in loosely cohesive linear strips. Osteoblasts tend to have single hyperchromatic eccentric nuclei and abundant cytoplasm with an eccentric zone of clearing that corresponds to a well-developed Golgi complex [**I** *26.1*]. Osteoblasts mature to osteocytes, which are relatively small cells with round nuclei that reside within small lacunae in bone.

Osteoclasts are large cells with ample basophilic cytoplasm. Multinucleation is the most conspicuous feature of osteoclasts. Typically, 10 to 20 or more oval nuclei are

I. Bone-Forming Tumors
- A. Benign
  1. Osteoma
  2. Osteoid osteoma
  3. Osteoblastoma
- B. Malignant
  1. Osteogenic sarcoma (osteosarcoma)
     - a. Osteoblastic, chondroblastic, fibroblastic
     - b. Low-grade intramedullary
     - c. Telangiectatic
     - d. Small cell type
  2. Parosteal osteogenic sarcoma (juxtacortical osteosarcoma)
  3. Periosteal osteosarcoma

II. Cartilage-Forming Tumors
- A. Benign
  1. Chondroma (enchondroma)
  2. Osteochondroma (osteocartilaginous exostosis)
  3. Periosteal chondroma
  4. Chondroblastoma
  5. Chondromyxoid fibroma
- B. Malignant
  1. Chondrosarcoma
  2. Clear cell chondrosarcoma
  3. Mesenchymal chondrosarcoma
  4. Dedifferentiated chondrosarcoma

III. Giant Cell Tumor (Osteoclastoma)

IV. Marrow Tumors
  1. Malignant lymphoma
  2. Myeloma
  3. Ewing's sarcoma

V. Vascular Tumors
- A. Benign
  1. Hemangioma
  2. Lymphangioma
  3. Glomus tumor (glomangioma)
  4. Hemangiopericytoma
- B. Malignant
  1. Angiosarcoma
  2. Malignant hemangiopericytoma

VI. Other Connective Tissue Tumors
- A. Benign
  1. Fibrous histiocytoma (nonossifying fibroma)
  2. Desmoplastic fibroma
  3. Lipoma
- B. Atypical fibrous histiocytoma
- C. Malignant
  1. Fibrosarcoma
  2. Malignant fibrous histiocytoma
  3. Leiomyosarcoma
  4. Liposarcoma
  5. Neurofibrosarcoma
  6. Malignant mesenchymoma
  7. Undifferentiated sarcoma

VII. Other Tumors
  1. Chordoma
  2. "Adamantinoma" originating in long bones
  3. Neurilemoma (schwannoma)
  4. Neurofibroma

VIII. Unclassified Tumors

IX. Tumor-like Changes
  1. Solitary bone cyst
  2. Aneurysmal bone cyst
  3. Intraosseous ganglion (juxta-articular bone cyst)
  4. Fibrous defect in metaphysis
  5. Eosinophilic granuloma
  6. Fibrous dysplasia
  7. Other fibro-osseous lesions
  8. Myositis ossificans
  9. Brown tumor in patients with hyperparathyroidism (osteitis fibrosa)
  10. Reparative giant cell granuloma

X. Metastatic Malignant Neoplasms

* Adapted from Spjut HJ, Ayala AG. Neoplasms and tumor-like lesions of bone. In: Silverberg S, ed. *Principles and Practice of Surgical Pathology.* New York, NY: Churchill Livingstone Inc; 1990.

T26.1
*Modified World Health Organization Classification of Tumors**

present with finely granular chromatin and small prominent nucleoli [**I**26.2]. Osteoid is used to describe matrix material that has undergone calcification but is not yet mature bone. It is a sharply defined material that may contain entrapped cells. Osteoid appears metachromatic in Romanowsky-stained smears, and usually orangeophilic with the Papanicolaou stain. Cartilage (or chondroid matrix material) may be recovered by bone aspiration. In contrast to osteoid, masses of cartilage are basophilic and less well defined. Chondrocytes are usually present within chondroid material, as described below.

Bone marrow within the medulla is an important and plentiful element of normal bone. Marrow contains immature hematopoietic cells and megakaryocytes. These cells can complicate the interpretation of fine needle aspirates of bone. Myeloid blast cells may resemble non-Hodgkin's lymphoma or metastatic breast carcinoma. The large, hyperchromatic nuclei of megakaryocytes can be particularly troublesome and easily confused with metastatic carcinoma [▮*26.3*]. It is important to be familiar with the appearance of these normal components of bone before attempting to interpret bone tumor aspirates.

BONE-FORMING TUMORS

Callus

Callus describes the reparative process that occurs at fracture sites. The microscopic appearance of callus differs according to the age of the injury, so that it may mimic several different benign or malignant osseous tumors. Within the first 2 weeks of injury, mononucleate and multinucleate histiocytes and slender fibroblasts in a myxoid and necrotic stroma predominate. Osteoblasts, uniform cells with round, somewhat hyperchromatic nuclei and abundant granular cytoplasm, then deposit osteoid to form woven or immature bone. Lamellar bone appears at approximately 6 weeks as calcium is deposited onto the osteoid. At this stage osteoblasts are transforming to polygonal osteocytes. Bizarre-appearing osteoblasts may be seen at any time during the healing process and may extend into surrounding soft tissues.

Osteoid Osteoma

Osteoid osteoma is a painful, solitary neoplasm most commonly seen in the second decade of life, usually in the long bones of males. Because of its small size (less than 1 cm) and benign radiologic appearance, biopsy is not commonly performed on these lesions before resection. Microscopically, it consists of a central nidus of myxoid connective tissue surrounded by a zone of sclerosis and osteoid with variable mineralization. If aspirated, a variable number of osteoclast-type giant cells and slender fibroblasts may be recovered from the nidus. Thus, the cytology may closely resemble an osteoblastoma.

Osteoblastoma

Osteoblastoma is an uncommon tumor that often arises in the vertebral column, usually in the second or third decade of life. It is composed of uniform cells with round, somewhat hyperchromatic nuclei and abundant granular cytoplasm (osteoblasts) and interlacing bone trabeculae and islands of osteoid. Multinucleated giant cells, each containing 10 to 20 or more nuclei, are also present along with slender spindle cells within a vascular and myxoid background that makes up the intertrabecular matrix.

Osteosarcoma

Osteosarcoma is the most common nonhematopoietic primary malignancy of bone. Osteosarcoma is predominantly a tumor of young males that demonstrates a strong predilection for sites of rapidly growing long bones. The metaphyseal ends of the distal femur, proximal tibia, proximal humerus, and proximal femur are the most common sites. Osteosarcoma can also arise in soft tissues away from bone. These extraskeletal tumors are most common in the sixth decade of life.

A variety of cells and matrix patterns occur in osteosarcoma. The unifying diagnostic features are malignant spindle shape sarcomatous cells [▮*26.4*] and malignant osteoid [▮*26.5*]. The names ascribed to morphologic variants of osteosarcoma describe the predominate cell type or material, such as (1) osteoblastic osteosarcoma, with round epithelioid osteoblasts with granular cytoplasm; (2) chondroblastic osteosarcoma, with islands of neoplastic cartilage and sheets of neoplastic fibroblasts; (3) fibroblastic osteosarcoma, consisting of sheets and fascicles of plump spindle cells and malignant osteoblasts; (4) telangiectatic osteosarcoma, characterized by a loose vascular mesh containing malignant osteoblasts with irregular trabeculae of osteoid; (5) pleomorphic osteosarcoma, characterized by cells ranging from mononucleated spindle cells to multinucleated epithelioid cells; and (6) sclerosing osteosarcoma, containing anastomosing trabeculae of calcified osteoid with scant intertrabecular matrix and a limited number of widely dispersed malignant osteoblasts.

CARTILAGE-PRODUCING TUMORS

Chondroblastoma

Chondroblastoma is a benign lesion of bone commonly occurring in the epiphysis of long bones, typically in the region of the knee. The tumor is composed of round to polygonal chondroblasts and chondrocytes [▮*26.6*, ▮*26.7*]. These cells have dense, glassy, well-defined cytoplasm, and a single round or oval nucleus often with a distinct longitudinal groove or indentation. Some chondroblasts have eccentrically placed indented or reniform nuclei, whereas others have deeply lobulated nuclei. Scattered binucleated chondroblasts are common. Osteoclast-type multinucleate giant cells are a prominent feature of chondroblastoma. Cartilaginous matrix material is often present and stains bright magenta with Romanowsky stain.

Chondroma

Chondroma (enchondroma if the tumor is within bone) is usually a well-defined solitary lesion. Aspiration of a chondroma yields amorphous basophilic chondroid matrix material. This benign tumor has low cellularity, with chondrocytes appearing to reside within vacuoles in the matrix material. These cells have indistinct cell borders, abundant clear vacuolated cytoplasm, and small round pyknotic nuclei [▮*26.8*].

Osteochondroma

Osteochondroma is the most common benign cartilage-producing neoplasm. It is usually seen in children during the second decade and has a distinct radiographic picture. Microscopically, it is composed of well-differentiated chondrocytes with a distinct, trabecular endochondro-ossification. Chondrocytes are seen in cohesive nests or rows with a hyalinized matrix.

Chondrosarcoma

Chondrosarcoma, a malignant cartilaginous tumor, may arise primarily in either soft tissue or bone. Most chondrosarcomas occur in the flat bones of the pelvis or the proximal ends of the femur and humerus. Extraskeletal chondrosarcomas are usually seen in the deeper regions of the extremities. Chondrosarcomas usually present in the fifth to seventh decades of life. The four major histologic variants of chondrosarcoma include well-differentiated, myxoid, chondroblastic, and pleomorphic types. Well-differentiated chondrosarcomas are composed largely of immature chondrocytes with clear cytoplasm and prominent plump oval or round nuclei and invariably a few small round epithelioid cells and chondroblasts in an abundant myxoid matrix [▮*26.9*-▮*26.11*]. Binucleated chondrocytes are a common finding. Myxoid chondrosarcomas are defined by a pale, low cellularity matrix. The chondroid cells have indistinct cell borders in short cords or small coalescent lobules. The nuclei are round, oval, or slightly elongated or crescent shaped. Chondroblastic chondrosarcoma is composed almost exclusively of round or oval chondroblasts with granular cytoplasm. In pleomorphic or dedifferentiated chondrosarcoma, the dominant elements may show no resemblance to chondrocytes and chondroblasts. Pleomorphic fibrous histiocytic forms and spindle cells resembling neoplastic fibroblasts are usually admixed with vaguely outlined pleomorphic neoplastic chondrocytes and chondroblasts.

OTHER BONE TUMORS

Giant Cell Tumor

Giant cell tumor of bone most often involves the epiphysis or metaphysis of long bones, usually in patients between 20 and 40 years of age. Aspirates contain numerous multinucleated giant cells of the osteoclastic type, and numerous small, round, oval, or spindly stromal cells [▮*26.12*]. The dispersed to loosely clustered giant cells have abundant cytoplasm and 10, 20, or more central nuclei. The nuclei are oval with finely granular chromatin and small, conspicuous nucleoli. The stromal cells have oval nuclei with finely granular chromatin and delicate, scanty cytoplasm. The cytologic diagnosis of giant cell tumor of bone relies on clinical and radiologic findings since similar appearing giant cells can be seen in several benign and malignant tumors as well as non-neoplastic lesions such as fracture callus and reparative granuloma.

Ewing's Sarcoma

Ewing's sarcoma is an undifferentiated malignancy that may affect any bone but typically presents in young males in the second decade of life as painful swelling associated with underlying lytic destruction of the long bones of the lower extremities, vertebrae, or ribs. Ewing's sarcoma consists of solidly packed small round cells with well-defined sparse granular cytoplasm. Cytologic smears usually contain numerous poorly cohesive tumor cells, approximately twice the size of mature lymphocytes [▮*26.13*]. Cells may be arranged in small clusters or form rosettes. The tumor cells have round nuclei with coarsely granular chromatin and inconspicuous nucleoli [▮*26.14*]. Tumor necrosis is commonly widespread. Intracytoplasmic glycogen aids in differentiating this tumor from other small cell neoplasms, namely, neuroblastoma, small cell carcinoma, rhabdomyosarcoma, lymphoma, or small cell osteosarcoma.

Malignant Lymphoma

Malignant lymphoma of bone or soft tissues is usually a manifestation of disease arising in the lymph nodes or other sites. Primary bone lymphoma is usually seen in adults in the fifth to sixth decades, and sites include deep soft tissues, femur, pelvic bones, and ribs. The morphology of primary or secondary lymphoma is similar and consists of a monotonous population of single, noncohesive cells with lymphocytic to lymphoblastic features. Aspirates from well-differentiated or small lymphocytic lymphoma present the most difficult differentiation from inflammatory conditions. Fortunately, non-Hodgkin's lymphoma, especially when it involves the soft tissues, tends to be of the cell types with grooved, cleaved, or large vesicular nuclei and thus is readily identified as malignant. Histochemical and immunohistochemical stains can be quite useful in narrowing the differential diagnosis of small round cell tumors in this setting, depending on the patient's age and sex. Small cell carcinoma can be excluded with negative keratin and carcinoembryonic antigen stains; Ewing's sarcoma is less likely when glycogen is absent on periodic acid–Schiff stain or electron microscopy; rhabdomyosarcoma can be excluded with negative desmin and muscle-specific actin immunohistochemical stains; and neuroblastoma would express neuron-specific enolase or other neuroendocrine markers. Positive leukocyte common antigen staining and B or T cell markers would confirm the diagnosis of lymphoma.

Reactive lymphocytes, such as occur in chronic osteomyelitis, can possibly cause confusion with non-Hodgkin's lymphoma. Reactive lymphocytes usually lack the monomorphic appearance of lymphoma. If osteomyelitis is suspected, bacterial, fungal, and acid-fast stains should be performed. Also, as previously mentioned, immature myeloid and lymphoid cells from normal bone marrow can simulate lymphoma.

Metastatic Carcinoma

Metastatic carcinoma often presents as multifocal lesions most frequently located in the bodies of the thoracic and lumbar vertebrae, the bony pelvis, the ribs, the calvarium, and the proximal part of the femur and humerus. The typical radiologic picture of an osteolytic or, less commonly, osteoblastic lesion usually confirms the clinical suspicion of a metastasis. When morphologic confirmation is necessary, the aspirate is usually similar in appearance to the primary tumor. Abundant tumor cells are usually present in small groups and clusters, or occasionally in large, irregular sheets [▮*26.15*, ▮*26.16*]. The cytologic features of specific tumors are the same as described for their primary sites, although the aspirates often also contain osteoclasts, fibroblasts, endothelial cells, fat, and sometimes marrow elements.

TUMOR-LIKE CONDITIONS OF BONE

Aneurysmal Bone Cysts

Aneurysmal bone cysts are a common cause of lytic lesions within bone. If aspirated, blood, giant cells, and stromal cells may be recovered. The major differential diagnostic consideration is giant cell tumor.

Eosinophilic Granuloma

Eosinophilic granuloma is a process that may involve any bone but most commonly involves the skull, mandible, ribs, vertebrae, femur, and humerus. The lesion contains a large number of eosinophils, mononucleated histiocytes, occasional foam cells, and pigmented multinucleated cells. Charcot-Leyden crystals, which are proteinaceous crystals formed during eosinophil degeneration, may be seen. Birbeck granules, which are cytoplasmic inclusions seen by electron microscopy, are considered pathognomonic.

Osteomyelitis

Osteomyelitis usually presents as a systemic febrile illness affecting the ends of long bones in children and the midportion in adults. Aspirates performed during the acute phase yield innumerable polymorphonuclear neutrophils and scattered lymphocytes along with marrow elements. The cytologic picture from patients with chronic osteomyelitis may include a variable number and mix of plasma cells, lymphocytes, fibroblasts, histiocytes, and varying amounts of necrotic debris and bone fragments, and thus is difficult to differentiate from such tumors as malignant lymphoma or Ewing's sarcoma.

SOFT-TISSUE TUMORS

Benign Fibrous Histiocytoma

Benign fibrous histiocytoma has three subtypes, the most common of which is the fibroblastic type that is usually a solitary, cutaneous lesion of the extremities that is rarely found in deep soft tissues or bone. The tumor is composed of short fibroblasts arranged in a storiform pattern. Along with fibroblasts, histiocytes are arranged around numerous thin-walled capillary vessels. The histiocytic form is less common, occurs in middle-aged patients, and is characterized by abundant osteoclast-type multinucleated giant cells and round to elongate mononuclear stromal cells. Both types of cells possess granular cytoplasm. Hemosiderin-laden or lipid-rich foam cells may also be present. These features are nonspecific and can also be seen in varying patterns in solitary or aneurysmal bone cysts, granulomas, malignant fibrous histiocytomas, and nodular tendosynovitis.

Hemangiomas

Hemangiomas are commonly found on the trunk, extremities, and the head and neck region, and may occur at any age. The typical clinical presentation and highly vascular nature with great propensity for hemorrhage greatly limits any benefit of fine needle aspiration of these tumors. Microscopically, they consist of capillary vessels lined by flattened endothelial cells surrounded by pericytes and reticulum fibers in the capillary type and dilated, distended anastomosing vascular channels in the cavernous type.

Malignant Fibrous Histiocytoma

Malignant fibrous histiocytoma is the most common sarcoma in adults. It can occur at any body site, but shows preference for the extremities, head and neck region, and retroperitoneum. Several variants are seen with varying combinations of the following cell types: mononuclear histiocytic round cells, multinucleated Touton giant cells, slender or plump fibroblastic cells, bizarre polymorphic tumor giant cells, and stromal components. The inflammatory variant is characterized by numerous chronic inflammatory cells, including lymphocytes. The differential diagnosis includes entities with giant pleomorphic cells, such as pleomorphic liposarcoma, osteosarcoma, pleomorphic fibrosarcoma, melanoma, large cell carcinomas, and such benign lesions as proliferative myositis and myositis ossificans [▮*26.17*].

Liposarcoma

Liposarcoma, the second most common sarcoma of adult life, presents in the extremities or retroperitoneum with a peak incidence between 40 and 60 years of age. Liposarcomas are known for their frequent large size and variable histologic picture. Subtypes include myxoid, round cell, pleomorphic, and well-differentiated. Aspirates of myxoid liposarcoma yield round and slender neoplastic adipocytes with eccentrically placed round or oval nuclei and occasional monovacuolated or granular lipoblasts. The tumor cells are held together by a trabecular network of fine capillary vessels. Pleomorphic liposarcoma tends to be a large, deep-seated tumor comprised of cells of varying size and shape, including small round lipoblasts and slender fibroblastic forms to monovacuolated distended adipocytes and multinucleated, granular cytoplasmic tumor giant cells. The tumor cells are arranged in loosely formed clusters and ill-formed, irregular sheets. Aspirates from well-differentiated liposarcoma are comprised of distended monovacuolated adipocytes similar to those seen in benign lipomas, and thus the distinction between these is best made on evaluation of histologic pattern.

Angiosarcomas

Angiosarcomas often present as cutaneous tumors but can also be seen rarely in the liver, spleen, breast, or bone. Histologically, the tumor is composed of closely packed nests of epithelioid cells and a complex network of anastomosing blood vessels lined by pleomorphic endothelial cells. Cytologic preparations contain numerous clusters of pleomorphic endothelial cells, some of which may appear frankly malignant; however, definitive diagnosis and grading is best accomplished by histologic evaluation.

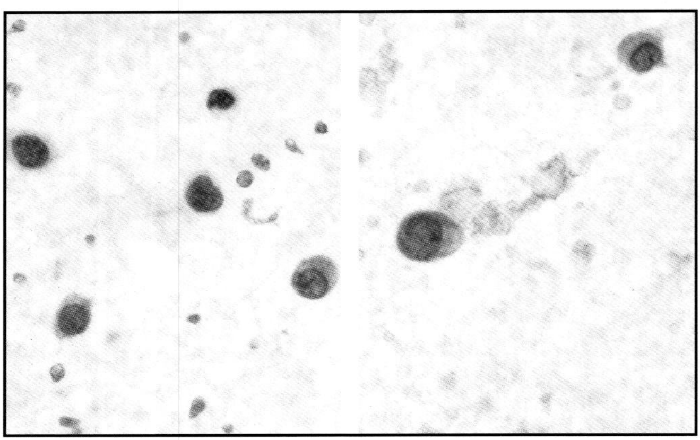

26.1
Osteoblasts with single eccentric hyperchromatic nuclei and abundant cytoplasm with slight cytoplasmic clearing (Papanicolaou, left, x200; right, x400).

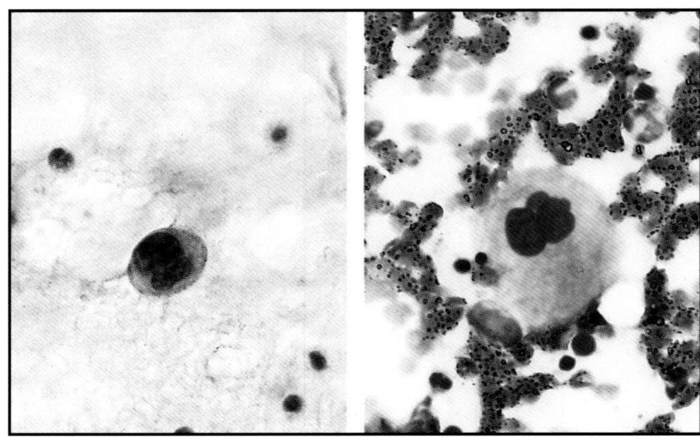

26.2
Osteoclast with multiple central nuclei with finely granular chromatin and conspicuous small nucleoli and dense cytoplasm (left, Papanicolaou, x400; right, Romanowsky, x400).

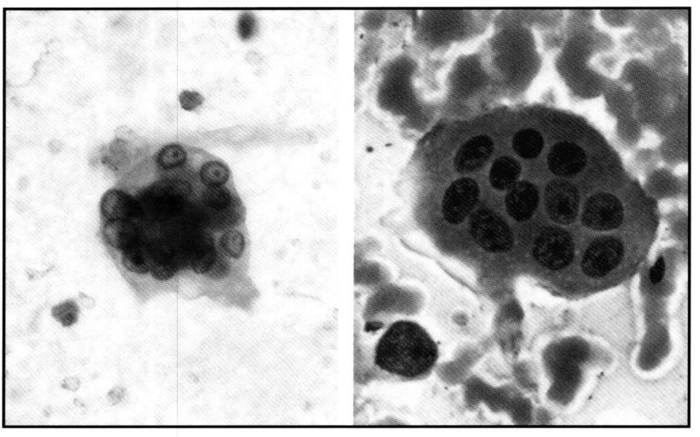

26.3
Large megakaryocyte with hyperchromatic, multilobated nuclei and well-defined cytoplasm (left, Papanicolaou, x400; right, Romanowsky, x500).

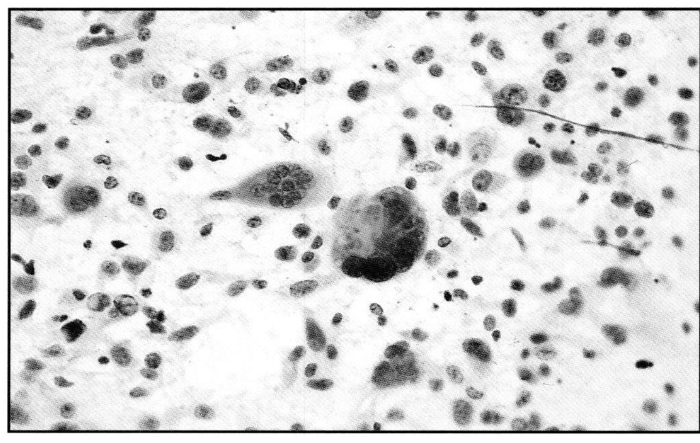

26.4
Aspirate from osteosarcoma with tumor cells of varying sizes and hyperchromatic nuclei, some with sharply defined cytoplasm that portrays an epithelioid appearance. Numerous large bizarre-appearing giant tumor cells are present (Papanicolaou, x200).

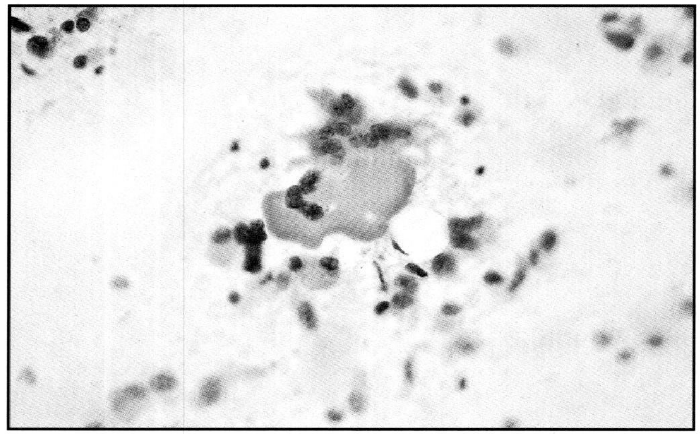

26.5
Malignant cells in aspirate from osteosarcoma with many pleomorphic forms, some of which are embedded in a discrete aggregate of osteoid (Papanicolaou, x400).

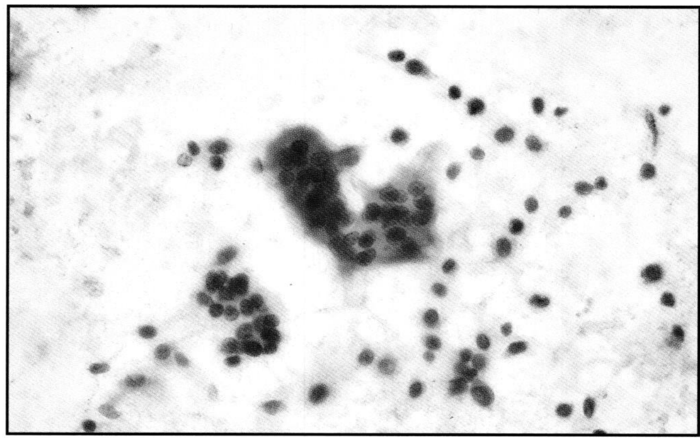

26.6
Numerous round to polygonal chondrocytes and chondroblasts with well-defined granular to glassy cytoplasm and small round to oval nuclei, along with osteoclast-type multinucleated giant cell in aspirate from chondroblastoma (Papanicolaou, x400).

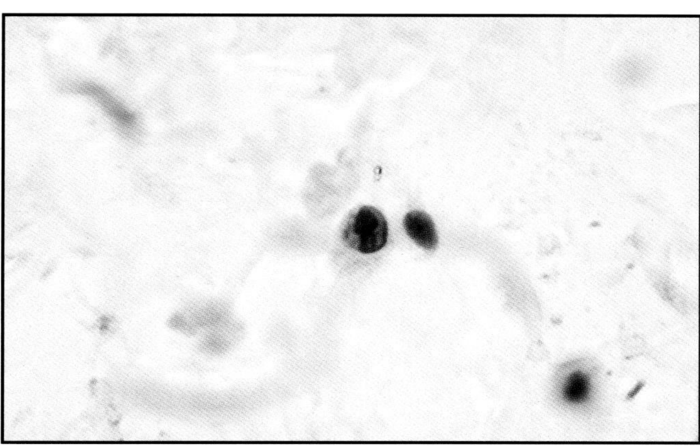

▮26.7
Chondroblasts from chondroblastoma with slight nuclear groove or indentation (Papanicolaou, x500).

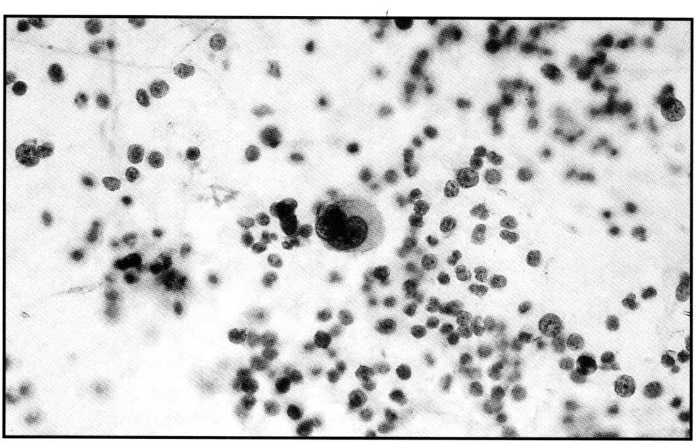

▮26.8
Cellular aspirate from enchondroma containing chondrocytes with indistinct cell borders, abundant clear vacuolated cytoplasm, and small round pyknotic nuclei. A large megakaryocyte is also present with multilobated nuclei (Papanicolaou, x400).

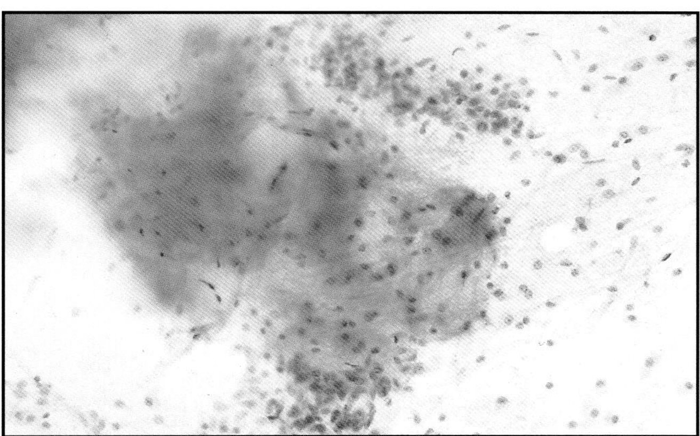

▮26.9
Fine needle aspirate of well-differentiated chondrosarcoma containing immature chondrocytes with prominent plump oval to round nuclei and atypical chondroblasts in an abundant myxoid matrix (Papanicolaou, x100).

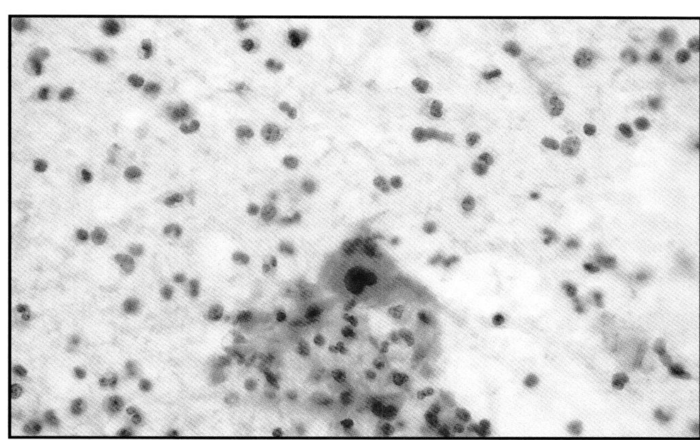

▮26.10
Malignant chondroblast with hyperchromatic and irregular nuclei (Papanicolaou, x400).

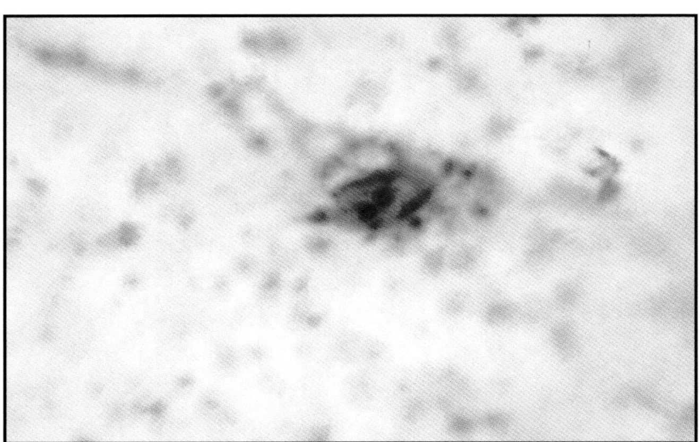

▮26.11
Binucleated atypical chondrocyte within lacuna (Papanicolaou, x400).

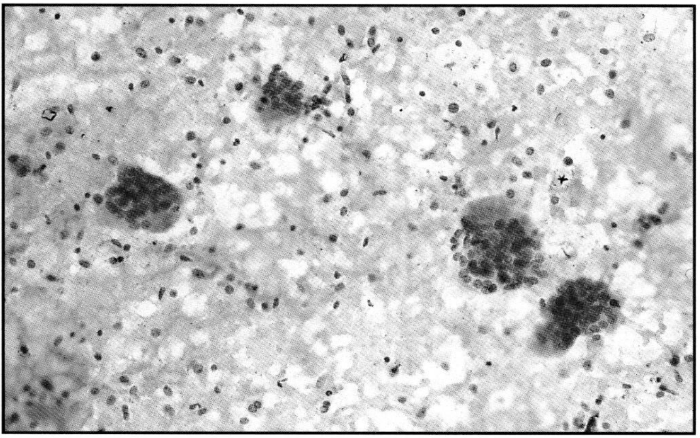

▮26.12
Fine needle aspirate of giant cell tumor of bone with numerous loosely clustered multinucleated giant cells of the osteoclastic type, and numerous small, round, oval, or spindly stromal cells (Papanicolaou, x400).

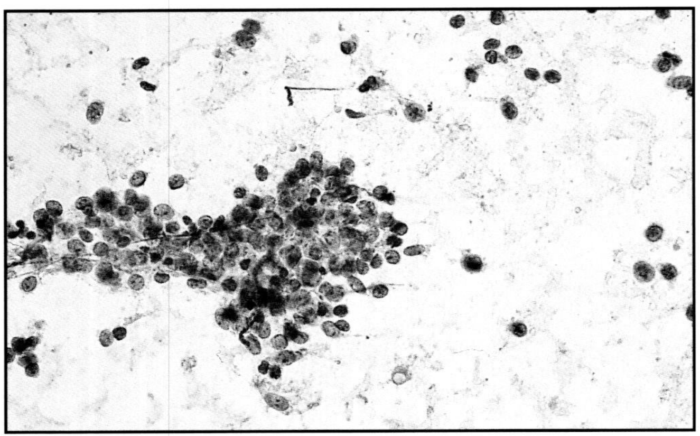

26.13

Loosely cohesive group of small tumor cells with sparse granular cytoplasm from lytic bone lesion in patient with Ewing's sarcoma (Papanicolaou, x200).

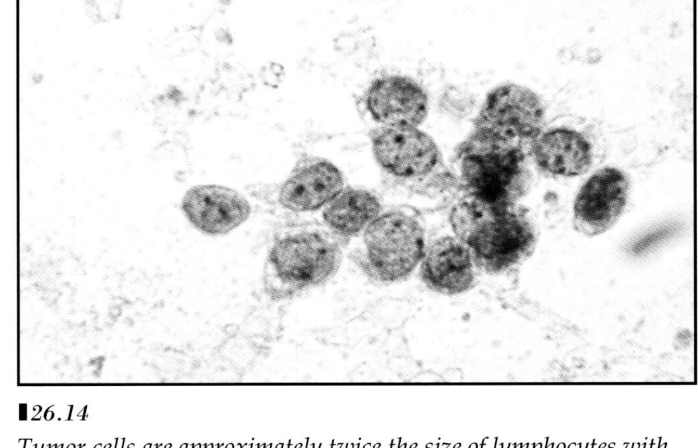

26.14

Tumor cells are approximately twice the size of lymphocytes with round nuclei with coarsely granular chromatin and inconspicuous nucleoli (Papanicolaou, x400).

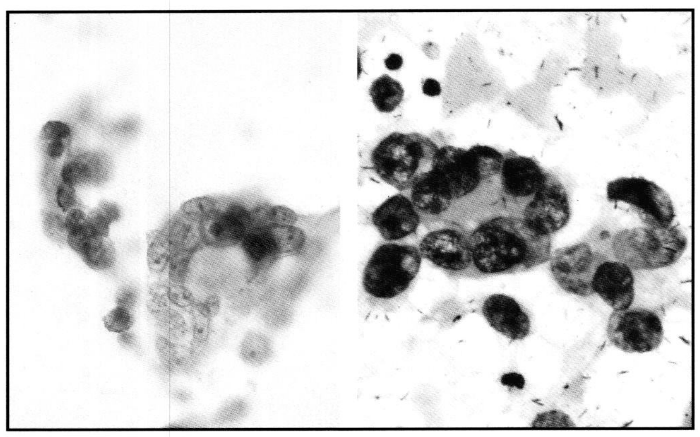

26.15

Cluster of tumor cells forming gland-like structure in aspirate of moderately well-differentiated colon adenocarcinoma metastatic to bone (left, Papanicolaou, x400; right, Romanowsky, x400).

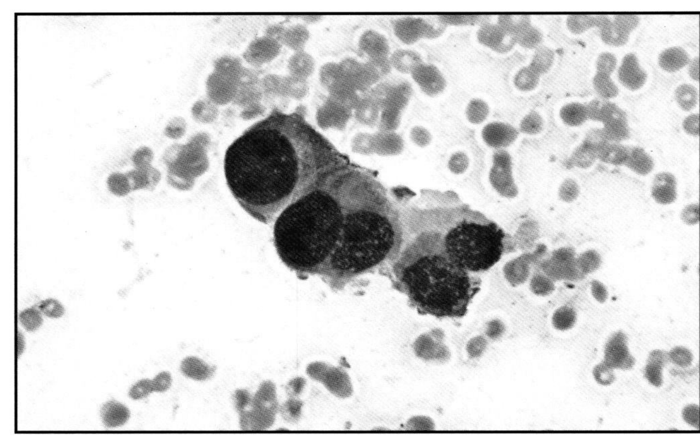

26.16

Metastatic carcinoma in fine needle aspiration from bone lesion with tumor cells arranged in linear array characteristic of breast carcinoma (Romanowsky, x400).

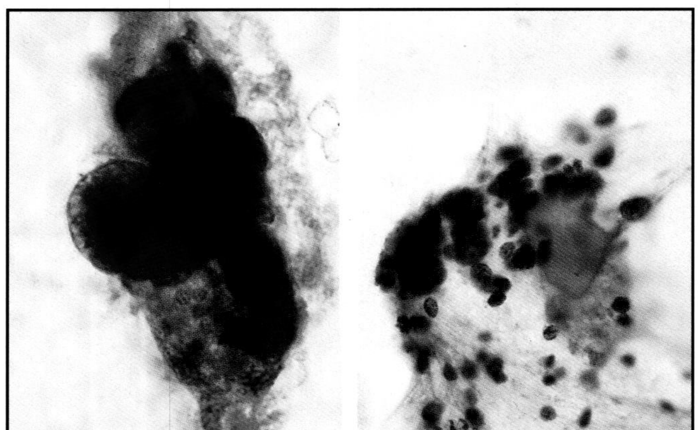

26.17

Bizarre giant tumor cell with hyperchromatic nuclei in aspirate of pleomorphic malignant fibrous histiocytoma (Papanicolaou, left, x400; right, x500).

SELECTED READINGS

Agarwal PK, Wahal KM. Cytopathologic study of primary tumors of bones and joints. *Acta Cytol.* 1983;27:23-27.

Akerman M, Berg NO, Persson VM. Fine needle aspiration biopsy in the evaluation of tumor-like lesions of bone. *Acta Orthop Scand.* 1976;47:129-136.

Akhtar M, Alii MA, Sabba HR. Aspiration cytology of Ewing's sarcoma: light and electron microscopic correlations. *Cancer.* 1985;56:2051-2060.

Bondeson L, Andreasson L. Aspiration cytology of adult rhabdomyoma. *Acta Cytol.* 1986;30:679-682.

Dahl I, Ackerman M. Nodular fasciitis: correlative, cytologic and histologic study of thirteen cases. *Acta Cytol.* 1981;25:215-222.

Enzinger FM, Weiss SW. *Soft Tissue Tumors.* 2nd ed. St Louis, Mo: CV Mosby Co; 1988.

Fanning CV, Sneige NS, Carrasco CH, et al. Fine needle aspiration cytology of chondroblastoma of bone. *Cancer.* 1990;65:1847-1863.

Hajdu SI, Ehya H, Frable WJ, Gissenger KR, et al. The value and limitations of aspiration cytology in the diagnosis of primary tumors. *Acta Cytol.* 1989;33:741-790.

Hajdu SI, Hajdu EO. Cytopathology of soft tissue in bone tumors. New York, NY: S Karger; 1989.

Hajdu SI, Melamed MR. Needle biopsy of primary malignant bone tumors. *Surg Gynecol Obstet.* 1971;133:829-832.

Hales M, Bottles K, Miller T, et al. Diagnosis of Kaposi's sarcoma by fine needle aspiration. *Cancer.* 1987;88:20-25.

Hales MS, Ferrell LD. Fine-needle aspiration of tibial adamantinoma: a case report. *Diagn Cytopathol.* 1988;4:67-70.

Hood IC, Qizilbash AH, Young JEM, et al. Fine needle cytology of a benign and malignant schwannoma. *Acta Cytol.* 1984;28:157-164.

Kannan V, von Ruden D. Malignant fibrous histiocytoma of bone: initial diagnosis by aspiration biopsy cytology. *Diagn Cytopathol.* 1988;4:262-264.

Katz RI, Sylva EG, de Santos LA, et al. Diagnosis of eosinophilic granuloma of bone biopsy by cytology, histology, and electron microscopy of transcutaneous bone aspiration biopsy. *J Bone Joint Surg.* 1980;62:1284-1290.

Koss LG, Woyke S, Olszewski W. *Aspiration Biopsy: Cytologic Interpretation and Histologic Bases.* New York, NY: Igaku-Shoin Medical Publishers Inc; 1984.

Layfield LJ, Glasgow BJ, Du Puis MH, et al. Aspiration cytology of primary bone lesions. *Acta Cytol.* 1987;31:177-184.

Lefer LG, Roseer PR. Cytology of chordoma. *Acta Cytol.* 1978;22:51-53.

Nickels J, Koivuniema A. Cytology of malignant hemangiopericytoma. *Acta Cytol.* 1979;23:119-125.

O'Dowd G, Schumann GB. Aspiration cytology and cytochemistry of coccygeal chordoma: a case report and review of the literature. *Acta Cytol.* 1983;27:178-183.

Olszewski W, Woyke S, Musiatowicz B. Fine needle aspiration biopsy and cytology of chondrosarcoma. *Acta Cytol.* 1983;27:345-349.

Popok SM, Naib ZM. Fine needle aspiration cytology of myositis ossificans. *Diagn Cytopathol.* 1985;1:236-240.

Sneige N, Ayala AG, Carrasco CH, et al. Giant cell tumor of bone: a cytologic study of 24 cases. *Diagn Cytopathol.* 1985;1:111-117.

Thommesen P, Frederiksen P. Fine needle aspiration biopsy of bone lesions: clinical value. *Acta Orthop Scand.* 1976;47:137-143.

CHAPTER 27

Inflammatory Diseases

JAN F. SILVERMAN, MD

CONTENTS

Although fine needle aspiration (FNA) has been used primarily for the diagnosis of neoplasia, it has become increasingly apparent that many inflammatory mass lesions can be sampled by this procedure. Until recently, the main emphasis in the literature and practice has been on the FNA diagnosis of benign and malignant neoplasms, even though the technique was originally used to obtain material for the diagnosis of infectious diseases. Leyden was the first to report transthoracic aspiration biopsy for the diagnosis of pneumonia in 1882. Around the turn of the century, Grieg and Gray described aspiration biopsy for the diagnosis of infectious diseases in a series of biopsy samples of lymph nodes from patients with sleeping sickness. In the early 1900s, other investigators utilized lymph node aspiration as a valuable means of documenting the presence of filariasis, bubonic plague, spirochetes, and secondary syphilis, tuberculosis, and bacterial infections. It was only starting in 1925 that physicians began to use FNA primarily for the diagnosis of neoplastic conditions. Beginning in the 1940s, European physicians, many of whom were clinician-cytopathologists, described their experience with aspiration biopsy of numerous benign and malignant lesions.

In the last 10 years, FNA has undergone a phenomenal revival in the United States. Although aspiration biopsy has been employed primarily to diagnose neoplastic conditions, a number of reports have described its use for the diagnosis of infectious and inflammatory diseases. Recently there has been renewed interest in non-neoplastic/inflammatory aspiration biopsy, perhaps due to the increasing need for rapid diagnosis of opportunistic infections in immunocompromised patients, eg, those who have undergone organ transplantation, received aggressive treatment of malignant diseases, or contracted the acquired immune deficiency syndrome. It is anticipated that wider application of FNA for the evaluation of superficial and deep masses will lead to more non-neoplastic, inflammatory diagnoses.

This chapter details the procedures and techniques utilized in the workup of inflammatory aspirates, describes the cytomorphologic patterns of inflammatory aspirates, and discusses the cytologic criteria used to avoid potential false-negative or false-positive diagnoses of malignancy. In those inflammatory cases of infectious etiology, cytologic features of specific infectious agents are described that allow prompt appropriate treatment and avoid unnecessary surgery.

WORKUP

General procedures of FNA are discussed in Chapter 20. For superficial and deep lesions, we recommend a 22-gauge needle attached to a disposable 20-mL syringe fitted into a commercially available holder, allowing one-handed aspiration. For superficial lesions, at least two aspirations ("passes") are performed on almost all cases. The aspirated material is expressed onto slides and smeared with another slide, similar to the preparation of a bone marrow aspirate (Chapter 26). Approximately half the smears are wet-fixed with 95% ethanol for Papanicolaou staining. The remaining smears are air-dried and stained by a modified rapid Wright stain (Diff-Quik, Dade Diagnostics Inc, Aquada, Puerto Rico). Usually two air-dried smears from each pass are chosen for rapid Diff-Quik staining, which can be performed within 30 seconds and thereby lends itself to a quick interpretation of the material. The critical step in the workup of the FNA is the rapid examination of the Diff-Quik–stained smears. The immediate interpretation can answer a number of questions, such as: (1) Is the specimen adequate or representative? (2) Is the lesion inflammatory or neoplastic? (3) Are additional ancillary studies needed?

The workup of potential inflammatory lesions begins when the immediate interpretation of the Diff-Quik–stained smears is negative for malignant cells or shows cytomorphologic features consistent with an infectious or inflammatory process. When this occurs, needle rinses for culture are performed [▮*27.1*]. It is recommended that once an infectious lesion is suspected, a separate aspiration or "pass" should be done for microbiologic examination. If the quantity of the aspirate is limited, the cytopathologist, clinician, or clinical microbiologist should determine the priority for special stains and for inoculation of media for different groups of microbes, since the volume of the sample will be the limiting factor in determining the number of cultures that can be obtained. With limited specimens, transportation in a holding medium will be necessary, although it may be less than optimal for all potential microorganisms. If *Legionella* is suspected in a lung aspirate, transportation in water rather than saline is required because salt solutions may inhibit the growth of some members of that genus.

In our laboratory we utilize previously prepared, sterile 2-mL tubes of balanced saline solution for most needle rinses. The needle itself should not be sent to the laboratory, since it exposes the collectors and others to a risk of needle-stick injury. In addition, organisms may dehydrate in the needle during transportation of the aspirated material to the microbiology laboratory, resulting in loss of viability or in misleading culture results secondary to survival and overgrowth of a more hardy microorganism present in low numbers in the tissue.

The microbiology workup for pulmonary cases includes Gram stain, routine culture, fungus culture and smear, acid-fast bacillus culture and smear, and legionella culture and smear. For nonpulmonary cases, legionella culture and smear are not performed. If the clinical or cytologic findings suggest a viral process, then aspirated material should be submitted to the virology laboratory. The microbiology workup can be tailored when specific organisms or granulomatous processes are identified in the immediate Diff-Quik–stained smears. If a cell block is available, hematoxylin-eosin and special stains for organisms can be performed on the histologic portion of the specimen. Special stains for organisms can also be performed on the direct smears.

Romanowsky-type stains such as Diff-Quik stain have some advantages in the workup of inflammatory lesions. The Diff-Quik stain can be performed rapidly since immediate fixation is not required for staining of the air-dried smears. In general, less cell loss occurs than with the Papanicolaou stain. Cytologic advantages of the Diff-Quik stain include larger size of cells because shrinkage from immediate fixation does not occur. Hematologic processes can be better evaluated with Diff-Quik staining than Papanicolaou staining since cytoplasmic cell fragments called lymphoglandular bodies, a feature of lymphoid lesions, are more readily appreciated. In infectious cases, bacteria are better appreciated in Diff-Quik–stained smears due to the larger size and tinctorial quality of the organisms. In general, fungi and intranuclear inclusions of viruses are better identified in Papanicolaou-stained material. While the Papanicolaou stain details the honeycomb cast of *Pneumocystis carinii*, the Diff-Quik stain better identifies the intracystic trophozoites of the organism. Although we use both Diff-Quik and the Papanicolaou staining in our FNA cytology cases, we believe that the Diff-Quik stain has special value in the evaluation of infectious and inflammatory cases. However, cytotechnologists and cytopathologists should use the stain that most readily allows them to make a correct diagnosis.

IDENTIFICATION

Many different types of organisms have been seen in FNA specimens. Identification of the organisms is based on their morphologic features in the routine Papanicolaou and Romanowsky-type stained smears, along with those features seen by special stains. Some cases may require culture for precise identification. In immunocompromised patients, more than one type of organism may be present in the specimen. General classification of organisms that can be encountered include bacteria such as mycobacteria, legionella, actinomyces, nocardia, and numerous species of gram-negative and gram-positive bacilli and cocci [▮*27.2*]. Fungi such as aspergillus [▮*27.3*], candida, zygomyces [▮*27.4*], dematiaceous fungi, blastomyces [▮*27.5*], cryptococcus [▮*27.6*], histoplasma, and coccidioides may be encountered. Parasites such as pneumocystis, leishmania, and amoeba have been described, while tissue helminths such as filaria, trichinella, echinococcus, and cysticercosis have rarely been reported. Viruses to consider include cytomegalovirus and herpes simplex virus, along with the papovavirus seen in progressive multifocal leukoencephalopathy of the brain.

It is important not to confuse nonmicrobial foreign material with true infectious organisms, whether found in the body tissues with a secondary host response such as in aspiration pneumonia and talc granulomatosis, or if it presents in the form of a foreign body reaction to suture material or as a contaminant introduced into the FNA specimen during handling and processing. Morphologic features that suggest nonmicrobial elements include the recognition of angulated structures with thick refractile cell walls containing numerous basophilic round bodies in the cytoplasm as plant material [▮*27.7*] or polarizable talc or suture material in a granulomatous process. Microscopic fibers can simulate fungal hyphae but have a more haphazard size, lack an internal structure, and are polarizable in contrast to fungi. Starch granules from glove powder are refractile and have a characteristic "Maltese cross" configuration under polarized light. Some pollen granules may simulate coccidioides. Red blood cells coated with petroleum-based material may arrange themselves into saccular structures, causing the lesion referred to as myospherulosis, which may be confused with fungi such as *Coccidioides immitis*.

CYTOLOGIC PATTERNS

Inflammatory processes may be a more common target of FNA biopsies than neoplasms. An infectious or inflammatory process should be suspected when the smears contain a background of inflammatory cells and/or necrosis. However, there are a number of neoplasms that have a prominent inflammatory component that could be a pitfall for a false-negative diagnosis if the diagnostic neoplastic cells are obscured by the inflammatory cells or are few in number in the smears. Conversely, epithelial and mesenchymal repair and inflammatory atypia can be potential pitfalls for a false-positive diagnosis of malignancy in non-neoplastic aspirates. The basic inflammatory patterns include acute inflammation, chronic inflammation, granulomatous inflammation, and necrosis.

Acute Inflammation

Acute inflammation can be due to a number of different factors, such as microbes, chemicals, immunologic reactions, and physical causes that include burns, irradiation, and trauma. Acute inflammation is clinically characterized by its short duration. Cytologically, numerous neutrophils and other inflammatory cells are present; necrosis is a common finding in the inflammatory process.

Epithelial and mesenchymal repair and inflammatory atypia are often much more pronounced in acute inflammation than in other inflammatory processes. Therefore, one should be more conservative in diagnosing malignancy in the setting of severe acute inflammation. Conversely, some malignancies can have a prominent associated acute inflammatory response. Metastatic and primary keratinizing squamous cell carcinomas are notorious for having increased numbers of associated neutrophils with or without the presence of foreign body histiocytes [▮*27.8*]. In some pulmonary aspirates, the malignant squamous cells may be obscured by the extensive acute inflammatory process, leading to a false-negative diagnosis of a lung abscess. Subtle cytologic clues that suggest the correct diagnosis of squamous cell carcinoma include the presence of keratinous fragments or ghost cells along with rare dysplastic or malignant cells. However, diagnosis should be conservative, since acute inflammation can lead to degeneration and inflammatory atypia of epithelial cells, which may potentially cause a false-positive diagnosis of malignancy. A diagnosis of malignancy should not be made if only degenerating or poorly preserved atypical cells are present. Primary and metastatic colon cancer are also associated with acute inflammation.

Chronic Inflammation

Chronic inflammation may be the sequelae of acute inflammation caused by the persistence of the inciting stimulus, interference with the healing process, repeated bouts of acute inflammation, or a low-grade smoldering inflammatory process. Chronic inflammation is cytologically characterized by varying numbers of mononuclear cells, including lymphocytes, plasma cells, and macrophages [▮*27.9*]. In chronic inflammatory processes, proliferation of fibroblasts and small blood vessels may be present along with fibrosis and tissue destruction. Misinterpretation of granulation tissue in an aspiration can be a potential source for a false-positive diagnosis of malignancy, especially in Diff-Quik–stained material where the nuclear enlargement and atypia of endothelial cells and histiocytes may be accentuated. Fortunately, the epithelial and mesenchymal repair and atypia are less pronounced in chronic inflammation. Generally, these cells and tissue fragments in the Papanicolaou-stained smears have a much less ominous appearance and therefore can serve as a conservative check to avoid a false-positive diagnosis of malignancy. Inflammatory atypia of epithelial cells, fibroblasts, and histiocytes has been reported as a potential cause for false-positive diagnosis of malignancy in a number of chronic inflammatory processes such as tuberculosis, aspergillosis, and actinomycosis. An unequivocal diagnosis of malignancy should not be rendered when there are a limited number of atypical epithelial cells and the cellular material is not well preserved.

Metaplastic cells can be mistaken for malignant squamous cells, especially in aspirates of cavitary lesions of the lung. Atypical squamous metaplasia in Warthin's tumor has also been misinterpreted as representing squamous cell carcinoma in some salivary gland aspirates. Helpful diagnostic clues include the presence of groups of oncocytic cells along with the atypical metaplastic cells. Inflammatory pseudotumors of the lung can clinically, radiologically, and cytologically mimic a neoplastic process. Cytologic findings include the presence of uniform spindle-shaped fibroblasts arranged in small clusters and large groups, along with uniform sheets of pneumocytes. A potential for false-positive diagnosis of malignancy exists when the atypical histiocytic-type cells and fibroblasts are misinterpreted as malignant.

Nonlymphoid neoplasms associated with increased numbers of lymphocytes include Warthin's tumor, lymphoepithelioma, seminoma, thymoma, and medullary carcinoma of the breast [▮*27.10*]. A potential for a false-negative diagnosis of malignancy exists if the nonlymphoid elements are obscured by a prominent lymphoid population or are few in number. The differentiation of reactive lymphadenopathy from lymphoma is based on appreciating the nonuniform appearance of the lymphocytes, which may vary according to the type and degree of stimulus and the duration of the process. Findings in favor of chronic lymphadenitis include a range of lymphoid cells with small lymphocytes almost always predominating, a progressive transition in size of the lymphoid cells, a cell population of plasmacytoid lymphocytes, and the presence of tingible-body macrophages, either isolated or as part of reactive follicular center fragments [▮*27.11*]. Lymphomas, in contrast, are characterized cytologically as monotonous in appearance, although there are exceptions to this guideline. Monotonous populations of small lymphocytes may be seen in aspirates from mildly reactive or indolent lymph nodes, while mixed cell lymphomas may present with a heterogeneous population of lymphoid cells that can vary in size and sometimes in type. Hodgkin's disease may also be quite polymorphous. Features in favor of lymphoma include the presence of bizarre cells, marked nuclear irregularity, and individual cell necrosis.

Granulomatous Inflammation

Granulomatous inflammation is cytologically characterized by the presence of epithelioid histiocytes arranged individually or in clusters with or without the presence of multinucleated histiocytes (giant cells) [▮*27.12*]. The epithelioid histiocytes are round, oval, or elongated and have nuclei that can be oval, elongated, or bent resembling boomerangs or snowshoes. With the Diff-Quik stain, the cytoplasm is pale grayish-blue and the nuclear chromatin is granular and evenly distributed with small blue nucleoli. With the Papanicolaou stain, the cytoplasm is pale greenish-blue with an evenly distributed granular chromatin and inconspicuous small nucleoli. When the cells are present in aggregate, the cytoplasm may be arranged in a syncytial pattern. Granulomatous inflammation is one of the leading causes of a false-positive diagnosis of malignancy in FNA because epithelioid histiocytes tend to aggregate and therefore be confused with a clump of tumor, especially if the smears are overstained [▮*27.13*]. In addition, a false-positive diagnosis of malignancy can occur when there is associated inflammatory atypia of the epithelial cells in granulomatous inflammation. Conversely, a number of neoplastic processes are associated with the presence of epithelioid histiocytes and granuloma formation.

The most common neoplasms having a granulomatous component include Hodgkin's and non-Hodgkin's lymphoma, seminoma, and thymoma. Occasional cases of carcinoma can be associated with nearby granulomas, and a granulomatous response may be seen in the draining lymph nodes. Products produced by the tumor such as keratin in squamous cell carcinoma or amyloid in medullary carcinoma may also elicit a granulomatous reaction. Hodgkin's disease, in contrast to benign granulomatous lymphadenitis, is characterized by having scattered bizarre cells (Reed-Sternberg cells and their variants) along with granulomatous inflammation. Non-Hodgkin's lymphoma with granulomas generally lacks the spectrum of lymphoid cells seen in reactive lymphadenitis, and bizarre cells or cells with marked nuclear irregularity may be present. Seminomas are characterized by the presence of large germ cells with a moderate amount of pale cytoplasm and central nuclei with prominent nucleoli along with variable numbers of mature lymphocytes and a peculiar stripped or "tigroid" background frequently seen in the Romanowsky preparations.

Whenever granulomatous inflammation is identified in the smears, a thorough search for underlying organisms should be undertaken. Special stains for fungi (Gomori methenamine silver, periodic acid–Schiff, etc) and tuberculosis (Ziehl-Neelsen, auramine-rhodamine, etc) should be performed on the smears and/or cell block and a separate specimen should be submitted for microbiologic examination. The smears should also be polarized to identify foreign material. Neoplasms associated with acute, chronic, and granulomatous inflammation are detailed [**T***27.1*].

Acute Inflammation
- Squamous cell carcinoma
- Colon carcinoma

Chronic Inflammation
- Warthin's tumor
- Lymphoepithelioma
- Seminoma
- Thymoma
- Medullary carcinoma of the breast

Granulomas
- Lymphoma
- Hodgkin's disease
- Seminoma
- Some carcinomas

T*27.1*
Neoplasms Associated With Inflammatory Cells

Necrosis

Varying types of necrosis can be appreciated in the aspirated material. Coagulative necrosis is defined when the cells have lost their nuclei with preservation of the basic shape of the cells. These ghost cells may suggest an ischemic process or necrosis. Coagulative necrosis is also seen in tumor necrosis. In contrast, caseous necrosis represents a combination of coagulative and liquefactive necrosis converting the cellular material into granular and amorphous debris. Cytologically, this material takes on a fluffy, granular appearance [**I***27.14*].

Necrosis can be seen in both benign or malignant processes. In some aspirates of malignancy, a prolonged search is sometimes required before preserved malignant cells are found. If the lesion is suspected to be neoplastic, reaspiration of the peripheral portion of the mass is recommended in an attempt to find more viable malignant cells. Necrosis may also be associated with granulomatous and acute inflammation. Any aspirate consisting predominantly of necrotic material, especially if it has the appearance of caseation, should be submitted for culture and special stains for organisms obtained.

Fat necrosis may be secondary to trauma (especially involving the breast or soft tissue) or due to acute pancreatitis, in which pancreatic enzymes destroy the adipose tissue. Collections of vacuolated histiocytes may be present, which potentially can be confused with a clear cell carcinoma. However, histiocytes have a lower nuclear/cytoplasmic ratio with eccentrically placed reniform-shaped nuclei in addition to the vacuolated cytoplasm. Occasional necrotic processes such as pulmonary or renal infarcts can lead to a false-positive diagnosis of malignancy. Epithelial repair of bronchioloalveolar cells or renal tubular cells can be misinterpreted for malignancy. Diagnosis should be quite conservative if only a limited number of atypical cells are present and the cells show features of a repair reaction.

ATYPICAL REACTION PATTERNS

The potential for a false-positive diagnosis of malignancy exists when aspiration of a repair reaction is obtained. In conventional exfoliative gynecologic and nongynecologic cytology, cells derived from epithelial repair and regeneration are quite common, since the cells are obtained from an epithelial mucosal surface. In contrast, in aspirated material, mesenchymal and/or epithelial repair secondary to inflammation and wound healing can be present. An epithelial and/or mesenchymal repair reaction may occur following a biopsy, surgical procedure, irradiation, chemotherapy, infection, ischemia, or foreign body reaction [**T***27.2*].

Criteria applicable to the recognition of epithelial repair in aspirated material are the same as those outlined

Postsurgical biopsy changes or surgical procedure
Ischemia or infarction
Chemotherapy and/or irradiation
Infections
Foreign body reaction

T27.2

Causes of Inflammatory Atypia and Epithelial and/or Mesenchymal Repair

in conventional exfoliative cytology. These criteria include recognition of groups of cells arranged in cohesive flat sheets with distinct cell borders and maintenance of cellular polarity [▮*27.15*]. Single cells when present should be quite few in number. The worrisome features of epithelial repair are based mainly on the atypical nuclear changes consisting of enlarged nuclei with prominent nucleoli and mitotic activity [▮*27.16*]. Cytologic features favoring the diagnosis of benign epithelial repair include uniform appearance of nuclei within the groups, oval to round nuclei with a smooth nuclear border, and an evenly distributed chromatin pattern that can vary from vesicular to hypochromatic. A diathesis is usually not present and the presence of mitotic figures is normal.

Atypical cells may also be present secondary to irradiation or chemotherapy. We have encountered them in aspirates from the lung and other sites in patients who have received chemotherapy or irradiation; these changes could be misinterpreted as malignant if the cytologic features of the treatment effect are not appreciated. Helpful cytomorphologic findings of irradiation/chemotherapy effect include the repair-like arrangement of the cells along with atypical cells demonstrating nuclear or cytoplasmic vacuolization and a degenerative quality to the nuclei [▮*27.17*]. Cells often show a loss of sharp cytoplasmic border with amphophilia and cytophagocytosis. The worrisome cytologic features include nuclear and cytoplasmic enlargement, but the overall nuclear/cytoplasmic ratio is within normal limits. Macronucleoli and anisonucleosis along with binucleation to multinucleation may be present.

Mesenchymal repair is another source for false-positive diagnosis of malignancy because of the variability and atypicality of the mesenchymal cells. In general, mesenchymal repair is characterized by sparse cellularity of spindled to stellate-shaped cells arranged singly or in loose clusters along with inflammatory cells in the background. The cytomorphologic features can vary, depending on whether the repair reaction consists of loose aggregates and individually scattered fibrous tissue, skeletal muscle, adipose tissue, or bone. Fibrous tissue repair consists of fibroblasts having centrally located nuclei that expand the midportion of the cell along with bipolar tapering cytoplasm [▮*27.18*]. The cytologic features can overlap with aspirates of nodular fasciitis and fibromatosis. Skeletal muscle repair can be more problematic due to the fact that there is greater

Atypical squamous metaplasia (especially in cavitary lesions of lungs and salivary gland lesions)
Atypical repair (epithelial or mesenchymal)
Inflammatory atypia
Fat necrosis with degenerating macrophages
Granulation tissue
Granulomatous inflammation
Some viral cytopathic changes
Atypical reserve cell hyperplasia, bronchioloalveolar cell hyperplasia, irritated bronchial cells ("Creola bodies") in respiratory FNAs

T27.3

Cytologic Pitfalls for False-Positive Diagnosis of Malignancy in FNA Biopsies

morphologic variation seen in muscle repair than in other types of mesenchymal regeneration and repair reactions. The skeletal muscle cells can vary from spindle to fusiform in shape and be mononuclear to multinucleated. Soft tissue neoplasms generally are much more cellular and show a greater degree of atypicality. The cytologic features of benign and malignant soft tissue neoplasms have been described in a few recent reports, including some articles stressing the helpful diagnostic role of ancillary studies performed on the aspirated material. A summary of epithelial and mesenchymal cytologic pitfalls for a false-positive diagnosis of malignancy is presented [**T***27.3*].

Finally, universal precautions apply to performing the FNA, handling the smears, and preparing the specimen, since all patients are potentially infectious with the human immunodeficiency virus (HIV) and other agents. It has been estimated that the risk of HIV transmission from a single percutaneous exposure to HIV-infected blood is 0.4%. General precautions include double gloving when performing the FNA, although there is generally no need to wear protective gowns, masks, or eye wear. Most needlestick injuries occur when drawing the blood and especially when one is resheathing the needle. There are devices that allow positioning of the needle and attached syringe into rigid holders and containers that provide a mechanism to decrease exposure of the hands to the needle when recapping. Following the aspiration, the needle must be handled with extreme care and promptly placed in a rigid puncture-proof container that contains a disinfecting solution. Fortunately, the usual pathology fixatives inactivate the HIV. It has been reported that ethanol used as a fixative for cytologic preparation inactivates HIV at a concentration as low as 20% and neutral-buffered formalin inactivates the virus at a concentration as low as 1%. After the FNA has been processed, the working preparatory area needs to be decontaminated using commercial and simple disinfectants such as 0.5% sodium hydrochloride (1:10 dilution of household bleach).

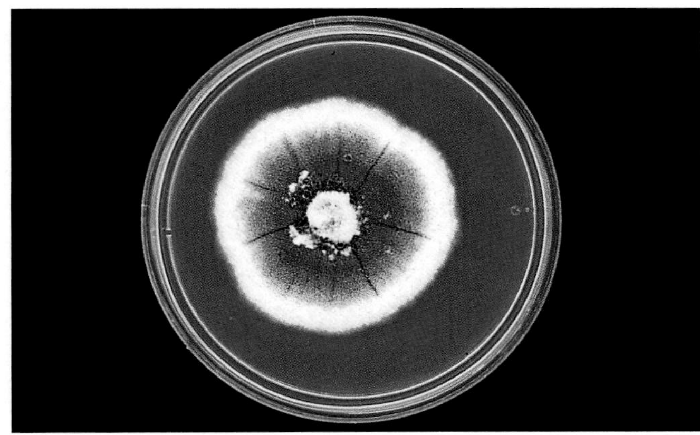

▮27.1

Culture plate demonstrating cottony growth of Aspergillus *from aspirate of lung.*

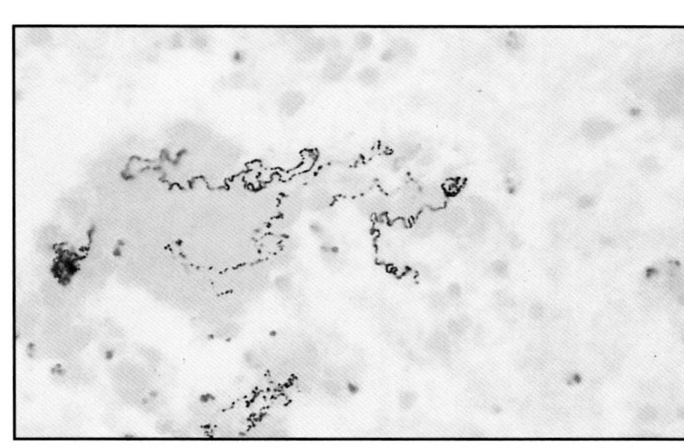

▮27.2

Gram stain performed on lung aspirate smear demonstrating chains of gram-positive organisms (x200).

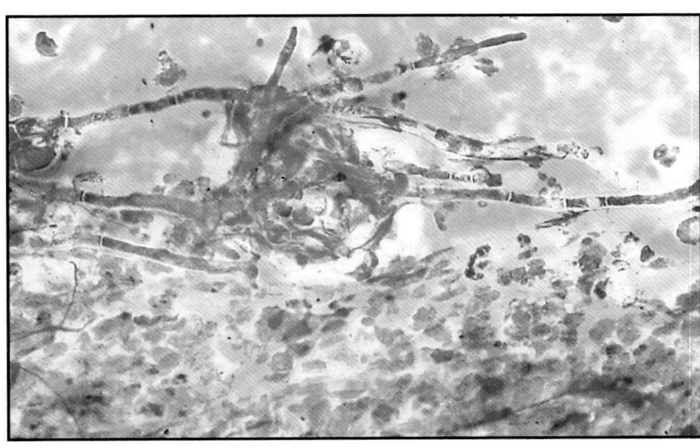

▮27.3

FNA of lung demonstrating presence of Aspergillus *characterized by septated hyphae with acute-angle branching (Diff-Quik, x200).*

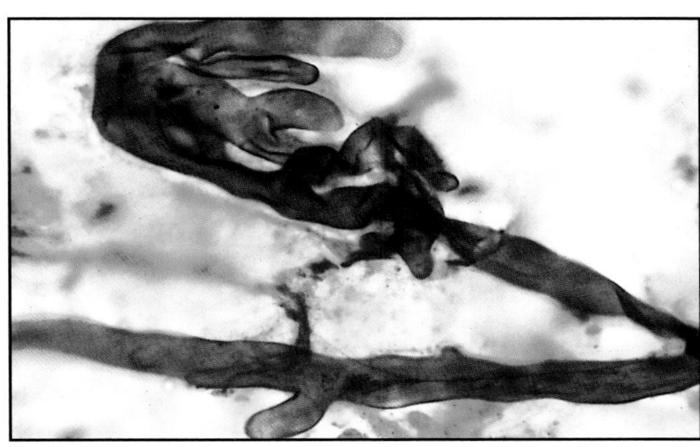

▮27.4

Lung aspirate containing mucormycosis (zygomycoses), characterized by thick ribbons of hyphae with 90°-angle branching (Papanicolaou, x400).

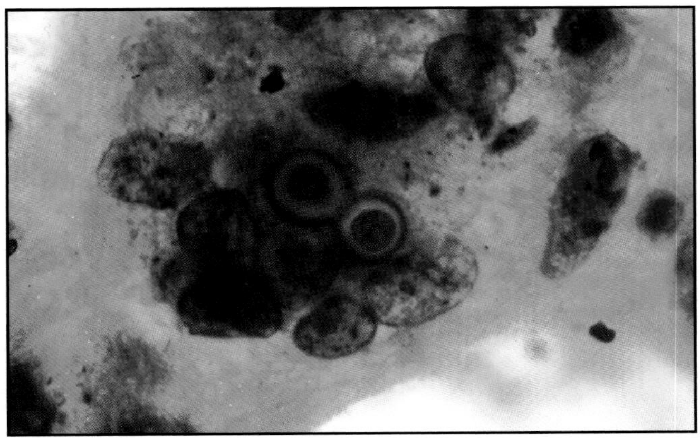

▮27.5

Aspirate of blastomycosis in which multinucleated giant cells contain intracytoplasmic broad-based budding yeasts having well-defined internal structure and outer cell wall (Papanicolaou, x400).

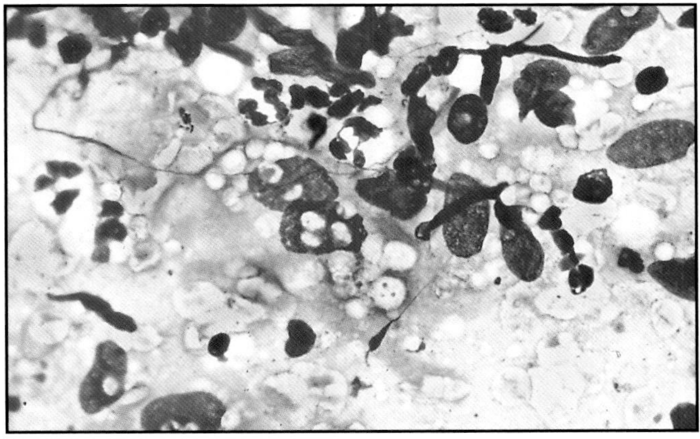

▮27.6

Aspirate of lung in which scattered histiocytes contain numerous small fungal yeast forms with well-defined capsule giving a vacuolated appearance to the cells (Diff-Quik, x200).

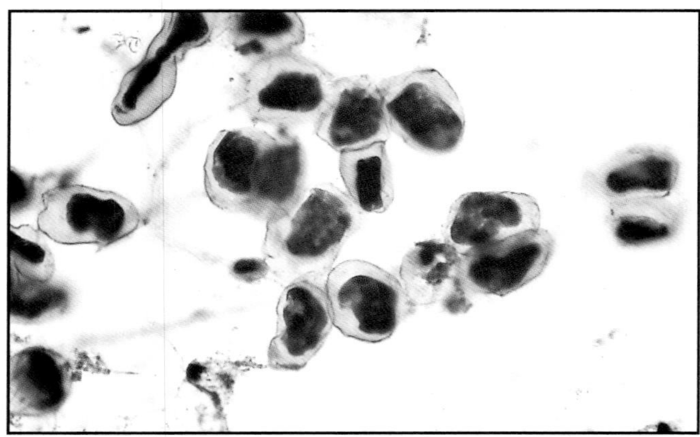

27.7

Aspirate of lung in patient with aspiration pneumonia in which food particles are present having hyperchromatic internal structures with well-defined cell walls that potentially could be misinterpreted as malignant cells (Papanicolaou, x400).

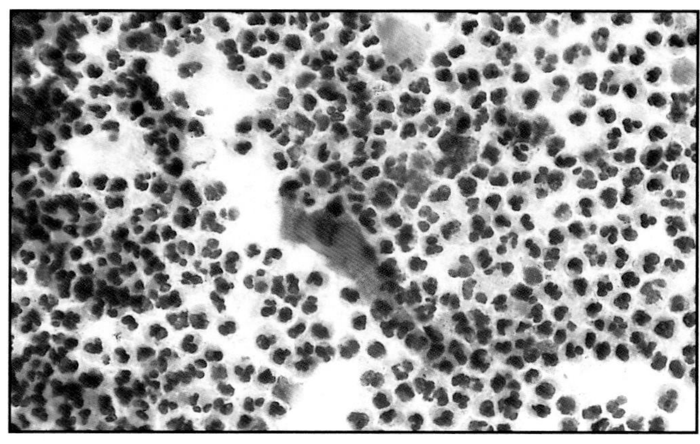

27.8

FNA of metastatic squamous cell carcinoma of the esophagus to cervical lymph node in which only rare malignant keratinized squamous cells are seen associated with sheets of neutrophils (Papanicolaou, x200).

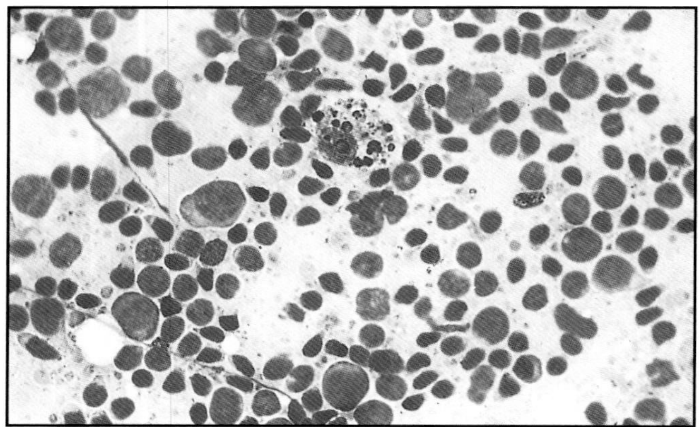

27.9

Aspirate of chronic lymphadenitis in which a polymorphic population of cells is present, including small lymphocytes, larger immunoblastic cells, and tingible body macrophage (Diff-Quik, x200).

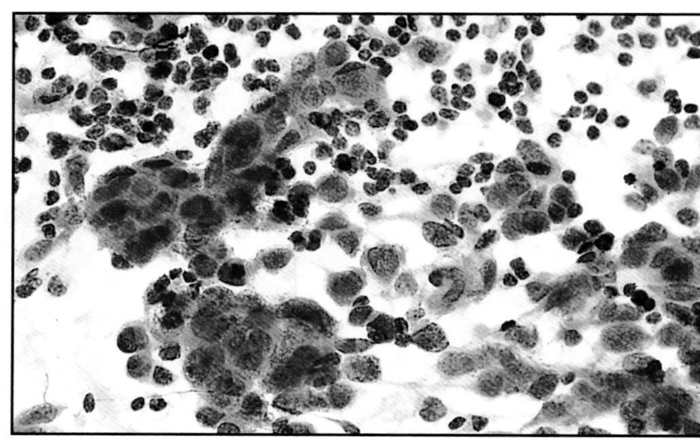

27.10

FNA of medullary carcinoma of the breast in which syncytial groups of malignant epithelial cells are present along with numerous chronic inflammatory cells in the background (Papanicolaou, x200).

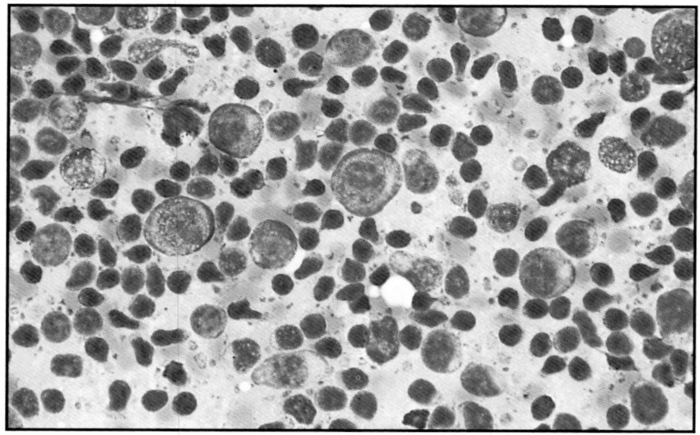

27.11

Aspirate of chronic lymphadenitis in which mature to reactive appearing immunoblastic lymphoid cells are present (Diff-Quik, x200).

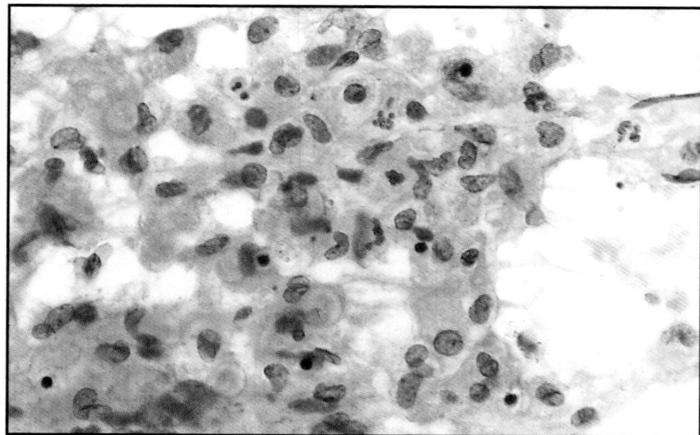

27.12

FNA of well-formed granulomas in case of sarcoid. Note the elongated to boomerang-shaped nuclei with surrounding amphophilic cytoplasm of the epithelioid histiocytes (Papanicolaou, x400).

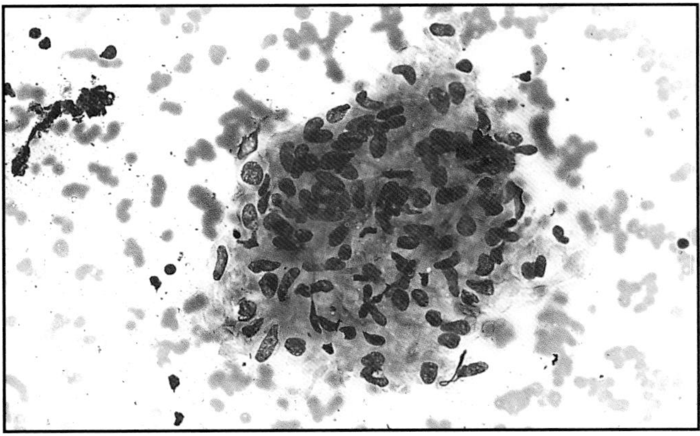

27.13

FNA of lymph node in patient with sarcoidosis. Tight cluster of epithelioid cells could potentially be mistaken for metastatic carcinoma, especially when the nuclei are overstained (Diff-Quik, x200).

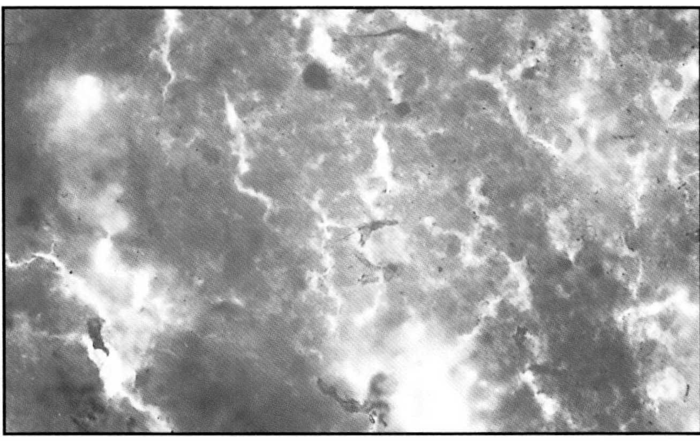

27.14

FNA of lung nodule in which extensive caseation necrosis is characterized by granular and amorphous debris. Special stains (Ziehl-Neelsen and auramine-rhodamine) demonstrated numerous mycobacteria, and culture of the aspirate was positive (Diff-Quik, x200).

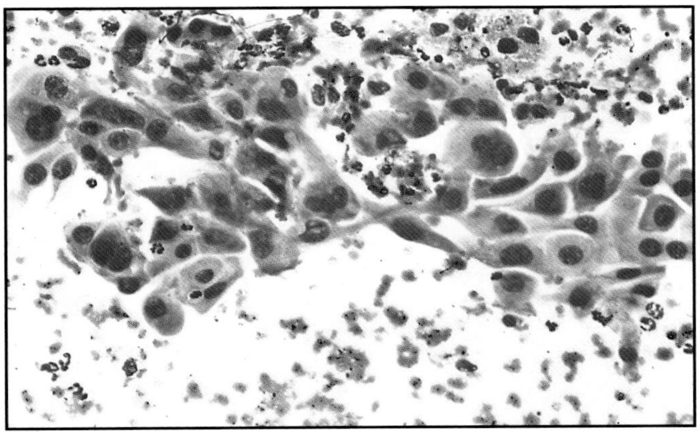

27.15

FNA of lung showing classic repair reaction characterized by loose sheet-like fragment of cells with well-defined cell borders (Diff-Quik, x200).

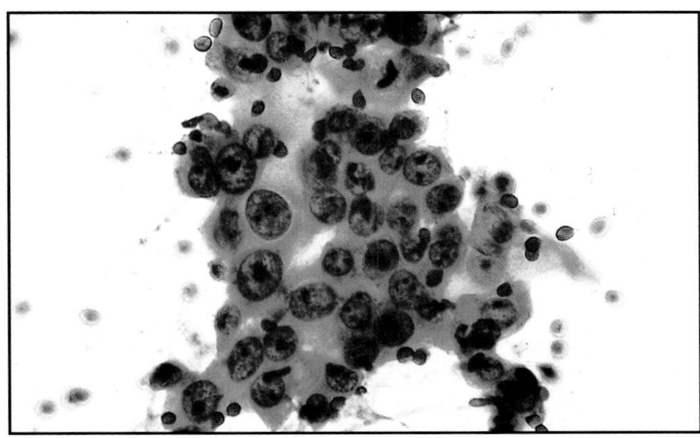

27.16

Aspirate of lung in which atypical repair is present characterized by sheet-like group of epithelial cells demonstrating a greater degree of hyperchromasia and more prominent nucleoli (Papanicolaou, x400).

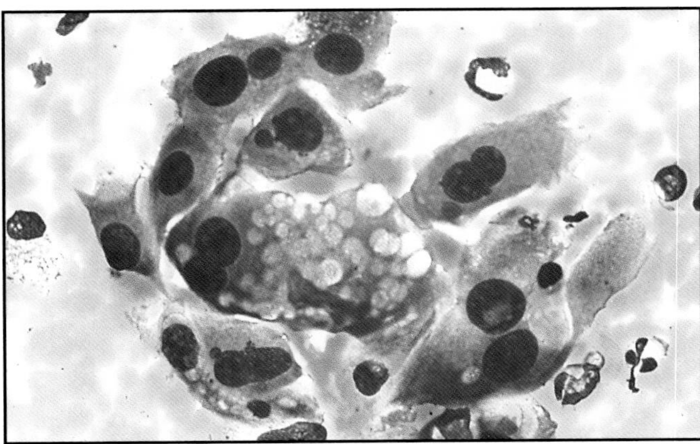

27.17

Aspirate of lung in patient treated with chemotherapy and irradiation. Note irradiation effect, including repair-like grouping of cells in which there is nuclear and cytoplasmic vacuolization, binucleation, and nuclear and cytoplasmic enlargement (Diff-Quik, x400).

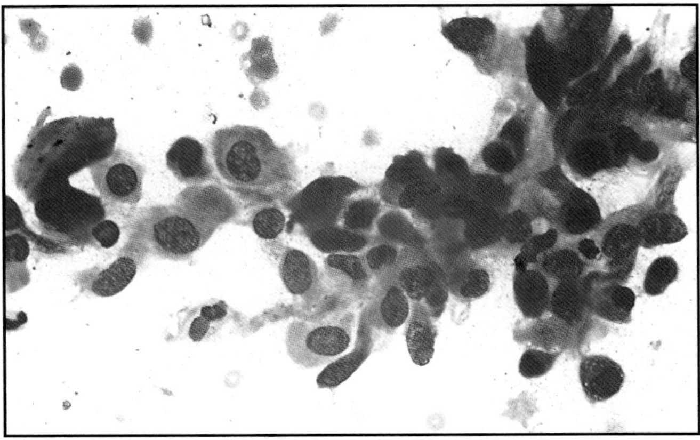

27.18

Aspirate of soft tissue in region of biopsy site from patient previously treated for primitive neuroectodermal tumor of chest wall. Loose cluster of spindle-shaped cells is characteristic of mesenchymal repair (Diff-Quik, x400).

REVIEW EXERCISES

1. Sterile saline holding media for culture of FNA inhibits the growth of which one of the following organisms?
   a) Mycobacteria
   b) *Aspergillus*
   c) *Pseudomonas*
   d) Streptococci
   e) Some species of *Legionella*

2. Which neoplasms can have an associated acute inflammatory cell response?
   a) Small cell carcinoma of the lung
   b) Squamous cell carcinoma of the lung
   c) Hepatoma
   d) Colon carcinoma
   e) Non-Hodgkin's lymphoma

3. Which neoplasms are often associated with chronic inflammation, including lymphocytes and plasma cells?
   a) Medullary carcinoma of the breast
   b) Thymoma
   c) Seminoma
   d) Warthin's tumor
   e) All of the above

4. Epithelial repair in FNA is characterized by all of the following except?
   a) Sheet-like groups
   b) Syncytial fragments
   c) Enlarged nuclei
   d) Prominent nucleoli
   e) Mitotic figures

5. Differential diagnosis of mesenchymal repair includes all of the following except?
   a) Nodular fasciitis
   b) Fibromatosis
   c) Some low-grade fibrous sarcomas
   d) Malignant fibrous histiocytoma
   e) Granulation tissue

6. Most needle-stick injuries occur when
   a) performing the biopsy.
   b) preparing the smears.
   c) transporting the needle to the laboratory.
   d) resheathing the needle.
   e) rinsing the needle.

SELECTED READINGS

Christie JD, Callihan DR. The role of the clinical microbiology laboratory. In: Silverman JF, ed. *Guides to Clinical Aspiration Biopsy: Infectious and Inflammatory Diseases and Other Nonneoplastic Disorders.* New York, NY: Igaku-Shoin Medical Publishers Inc; 1991:21-46.

Covell JL, Feldman PS. Identification of infectious microorganisms. In: Silverman JF, ed. *Guides to Clinical Aspiration Biopsy: Infectious and Inflammatory Diseases and Other Nonneoplastic Disorders.* New York, NY: Igaku-Shoin Medical Publishers Inc; 1991:47-83.

James LP. Cytopathology of mesenchymal repair. *Diagn Cytopathol.* 1985;1:91-104.

Silverman JF. Cytologic diagnosis in acquired immunodeficiency syndrome. In: Joshi VV, ed. *Pathology of AIDS and Other Manifestations of HIV Infection.* New York, NY: Igaku-Shoin Medical Publishers Inc; 1991:347-365.

Silverman JF. Thoracic and superficial and deep lesions of soft tissue, bone, and prostate. In: Silverman JF, ed. *Guides to Clinical Aspiration Biopsy: Infectious and Inflammatory Diseases and Other Nonneoplastic Disorders.* New York, NY: Igaku-Shoin Medical Publishers Inc; 1991:218-230,277-322.

Silverman JF, Finley JL, O'Brien KF, et al. Diagnostic accuracy and role of immediate interpretation of fine needle aspiration biopsy specimens from various sites. *Acta Cytol.* 1989;33:791-796.

Silverman JF, Frable WJ. The use of Diff-Quik stain in the immediate interpretation of fine-needle aspiration biopsies. *Diagn Cytopathol.* 1990;6:366-369.

Silverman JF, Kardos TF. Cytomorphologic patterns of inflammatory aspirates. In: Silverman JF, ed. *Guides to Clinical Aspiration Biopsy: Infectious and Inflammatory Diseases and Other Nonneoplastic Disorders.* New York, NY: Igaku-Shoin Medical Publishers Inc; 1991:85-104.

CHAPTER

28

Organization and Inspection

FLORENCE WOODWORTH PATTEN, MT(ASCP), CT(ASCP), CFIAC

CONTENTS

Development of a smoothly functioning cytopathology laboratory requires full knowledge and thoughtful evaluation of community needs, available professional and support staff, financial limitations, and physical facilities for service, preparatory, and record-keeping systems.

The "perfect laboratory" does not exist. However, guidelines for accreditation of cytopathology laboratories, both foreign and domestic, provide the necessary framework on which the laboratory can build and improve the quality of health care delivery.

LABORATORY ACCREDITATION

In the evaluation of laboratory performance, various terms become important and must be clearly defined before credentialing procedures are undertaken.

Certification is the process by which a nongovernmental agency or organization conveys recognition that an individual has demonstrated competence in certain tasks and has met certain predetermined qualifications specified by that body. In cytotechnology, generally those qualifications are (1) graduation from an accredited or approved school of cytotechnology, (2) completion of a given amount of work experience, and (3) acceptable performance on a qualifying examination or battery of related examinations.

Licensure is the mechanism by which an agency or governmental body awards permission to persons meeting predetermined qualifications to engage in a specific occupation and to assume a specific professional title, or awards permission to an institution to perform specific procedures.

Accreditation is the mechanism by which an agency or organization evaluates and verifies that a program of study or service meets specific predetermined qualifications and standards. Accreditation applies only to institutions and related programs of study and service, whereas certification applies only to individuals. Licensure may apply either to individuals or institutions but is generally related to governmental initiation and control, be it on the local, state, or federal level.

Two factors clearly differentiate licensure by governmental agencies from nongovernmental laboratory accreditation. In the process of licensure, evaluation is mandatory for continuing operation of the facility, and the evaluation process is funded by public monies. With nongovernmental laboratory accreditation, however, the accreditation procedure is essentially voluntary and is usually supported by private funds. The nongovernmental laboratory accreditation procedures designed by the American Society of Cytology (ASC) and the International Academy of Cytology (IAC) are limited to the practice of cytopathology, while those procedures offered by the Joint Commission on Accreditation of Healthcare Organizations (JCAHO) and the College of American Pathologists (CAP) include cytopathology service facilities as one part of the total laboratory facility.

In the past, governmental agencies involved in licensure included the Centers for Disease Control (CDC) and the Health Care Financing Administration (HCFA), which jointly monitored the qualifications and services of interstate laboratory practices, and also monitored Medicare/Medicaid (Social Security Administration) coverage reimbursable to laboratories for services when such laboratories processed in excess of 100 interstate specimens annually. More recently, an ever-increasing number of states (generally state departments of health) are designing and implementing state licensure procedures, some including challenge examinations involving all laboratory personnel and including on-site inspections based on predetermined performance standards.

In March 1990, the HCFA issued the Clinical Laboratory Improvement Amendments of 1988 (CLIA '88), which were designed to overhaul and recodify federal regulations as applied to clinical laboratories currently reimbursable by Medicare/Medicaid or licensed under the Clinical Laboratory Improvement Act of 1967 (CLIA '67). CLIA'88 attempted to simplify administration and unify health and safety requirements, providing a single set of regulations applicable to all appropriate laboratories.

Health care services today are publicly discussed and, therefore, monitored and "accountable." The processing of patient samples for which a fee is collected is a topic for careful scrutiny by the public and by the health care system. Of course, by far the more important factor is the occasional error in specimen processing or evaluation that compromises a patient's health.

By accepting the challenge of numerous agencies to permit on-site inspection of facilities, record-keeping and diagnostic practices, and personnel qualifications, a laboratory can state that it has performed at least at the level of competence designated as satisfactory by the agency conveying accreditation. One would anticipate fewer incidents of poor performance in laboratories that have recognized accreditation than in laboratories that elect not to seek voluntary or mandatory accreditation, or in laboratories that have an insufficient volume to permit individual accreditation.

With the initiation of CLIA '88, uniform, stringent regulations apply to most clinical laboratories, regardless of variations in governmental or private agency requirements that existed in the past. Private accrediting agencies may still inspect laboratories, but this accreditation will be recognized and honored by governmental bodies only if the regulations used by such nongovernmental inspections are equal to or more stringent than those contained in CLIA '88. Accreditation, like certification of individuals, merely acknowledges that certain criteria have been met and specific requirements have been addressed and answered.

Specific details concerning laboratory accreditation can be obtained directly from the following:

College of American Pathologists
325 Waukegan Road
Northfield, Illinois 60093

American Society of Cytology
1015 Chestnut Street, Suite 1518
Philadelphia, Pennsylvania 19107

Health Standards and Quality Board
Health Care Financing Administration
6325 Security Boulevard
Baltimore, Maryland 21207

How can one best prepare for what appears to be an inevitable and virtually endless series of evaluations, critiques, and on-site visits? Whether licensure or accreditation or both are to be achieved—and the likelihood of both being necessary is very great—careful attention should be paid to the laboratory components described in this chapter for the on-site laboratory inspection and performance evaluation.

The *Accreditation Manual for Hospitals* is the least specific in regard to cytology laboratory approval. This text states:

"A cytopathology service that is adequate to meet the needs of the hospital shall be available. The quality of this service shall be assured through the direct supervision of a pathologist or other physician qualified in cytology. This individual shall review all slides of extragenital origin and a random sample of negative reproductive tract slides. All abnormal smears shall be evaluated by a pathologist or other designated qualified physician. Abnormal smears shall be kept on file for as long as they are needed for patient care purposes and in accordance with federal and state regulations. Normal smears shall be kept on file in accordance with federal, state, and local requirements. Reports of abnormal or suspicious smears shall be authenticated by a physician who is qualified in pathology or cytology."

This single paragraph states the objectives of accreditation of hospital-based laboratory facilities but does not attempt to define the fine points of achieving those objectives. Nor does it address the question of nonhospital-based laboratories, although these facilities should be comparable in quality.

CLIA '88 contains numerous regulations already widely accepted by the laboratory community. Of note to the field of cytopathology are several new regulatory measures that impact significantly on the professional component of the discipline. Expanded proficiency testing requirements, methods applicable to rehabilitation of proficiency testing failures, and very specific daily screening volume limitations are prominent factors.

A brief discussion of the accreditation standards follows, with emphasis that all of these points, to one degree or another, are included in any on-site inspection after formal application for accreditation or renewal of existing accreditation.

PHYSICAL FACILITIES OF THE LABORATORY

Physical facilities provide the framework for all service functions. If they are well designed and convenient, capable professional and support personnel can perform their duties with ease. If hindered by ill-equipped or inconvenient laboratory and clerical facilities, service is invariably less than optimal.

Microscopic areas should be well lighted and ventilated, with disconcerting noise of nearby traffic or equipment minimized. Microscopes should be maintained in prime condition with regular cleaning. Technologists should have ample space to do microscopy and necessary record-keeping comfortably.

Proper ventilation and lighting of staining and specimen preparation areas are of utmost importance because of potential health hazards inherent in the use of volatile solutions and chemicals and in the processing of contaminated specimens. Installation of effective exhaust hoods over coverslipping areas and biohazard hoods for the cytopreparation areas are essential. Adequate counter space and sinks should be planned to provide for separation of staining procedures for gynecologic and nongynecologic specimens.

Clerical and record-keeping facilities should be located near screening and preparatory areas to permit rapid transmittal and retrieval of clinical and diagnostic data. Laboratories employing computerized record-keeping systems may find the availability of adjacent floor space inadequate for immediate needs. In this case, data retrieval terminals in the laboratory permit access to information stored elsewhere.

Health, fire, and safety regulations of state and local authorities, as well as those enforced by the Occupational Safety and Health Administration, must be observed for the personal safety of all laboratory personnel. Specific protocols include the following points for inspection of the physical facilities.

Laboratory Space

The laboratory has adequate floor, bench, and desk space; is clean, well lighted, and properly ventilated; and has adequate utilities available if appropriate (sinks, gas, suction, and electrical outlets). Work areas are adequate to allow proper specimen preparation, microscopy, record-keeping, and slide storage without interruption or health hazard. Microscopy facilities are conducive to high-quality performance, furniture is comfortable, and noise levels (interruptions) are minimal.

Laboratory Safety Procedures

See Chapter 31 on laboratory safety for a detailed discussion of appropriate safety precautions for laboratory performance. All accrediting agencies or organizations and delegated inspection teams pay particular attention to the application of strict safety precautions.

Laboratory Equipment

All equipment must be in good working condition. An active program of preventive maintenance is observed and log books recording such maintenance are up to date and available. Microscopes are cleaned at least annually and proper illumination is monitored.

LABORATORY OPERATION

Written Procedures

A laboratory procedure manual must be available in the laboratory outlining such procedures as collection, receipt, and preparation of specimens, with documented references where pertinent. This manual should be reviewed annually, updated, approved in writing, and dated by the laboratory director.

Written instructions on the proper collection of specimens from all body sites shall be made available to all physicians, paramedical personnel, and patient care units or clinics.

Personnel and Management Practices

Specimens are accepted by the laboratory only if collected by authorized personnel (persons authorized by law to collect such material and use medical information, ie, licensed physicians, dentists, medical house officers in an approved medical facility, or allied health personnel; or patients in an authorized health program).

Unsatisfactory specimens (ie, inadequate identification or inadequate preservation) should be noted immediately by the laboratory, which should then notify the originator so that repeated samples can be submitted.

Sound personnel practices are followed, including maintenance of current employee records complete with the individual's education, experience, certification, and health records (periodic physical examinations, illnesses, and accidents).

Work is assigned according to employee qualifications. Employee orientation and professional continuing education programs are conducted routinely for the staff, or there are provisions for participating in national and/or regional professional society meetings, workshops, and seminars.

Retention of Laboratory Records

In the past, the length of time the laboratory retained specimen reports varied with the different credentialing agencies, but with current regulations now in effect all final reports must be retained for a minimum of 10 years from the date of issuance. The laboratory copy should include the interpretation and signature or initials of the cytopathologist or cytotechnologist, or both, who examined the preparation and determined the final interpretation.

Prior to CLIA '88, retention of all slides and cell blocks by the laboratory was mandatory for various lengths of time. A minimum of 5 years was specified by both the ASC and the IAC, while the CAP indicated a minimum of 2 years for "all slides," with all "significantly abnormal" slides filed and retained indefinitely. With the enactment of CLIA '88, effective September 1, 1992, cytologic slides are kept no less than 5 years from the date of examination. In some cases, slides may be loaned to a proficiency testing program as long as they are retrievable on request. No distinction is made between gynecologic and nongynecologic specimens.

LABORATORY PERSONNEL QUALIFICATIONS

Individual personnel needs of the laboratory in terms of cytotechnologists depend on overall volume and diversification of specimens processed. However, several key positions must be identified and filled with highly competent professionals.

Laboratory Director

The laboratory director, as defined in CLIA '88, is a physician certified in anatomic and/or clinical pathology by the American Board of Pathology or the American Osteopathic Board of Pathology, or the equivalent. In certain instances, he or she may be a licensed physician or dentist who is certified to practice cytopathology, providing the laboratory performs such tests only on those anatomic sites for which that individual is certified.

The director is responsible for the proper preparation and reporting of all tests performed in the laboratory and for the employment of qualified staff members. In the absence of the director, these duties are performed by an associate physician or dentist designated by the director who has met the same requirements as the director or who is eligible for the examinations and certification indicated.

Technical Supervisor

In many facilities, laboratory activity may be monitored by one or more technical supervisors who are responsible for technical performance of all tests or procedures in each of the laboratory disciplines, general laboratory operation, and quality control. The laboratory director may serve in this capacity or someone who possesses qualifications equivalent to the laboratory director, or who is a physician or dentist certified by the ASC to practice cytopathology. This individual is responsible for confirming non-negative gynecologic samples and reports, and for reviewing all nongynecologic preparations regardless of diagnostic status.

General Supervisor

The general supervisor is responsible for the performance of all laboratory procedures in the absence of the laboratory director and technical supervisor. This position is filled by someone meeting one of the following educational requirements:

1. MD, DO, DDS, or PhD (with an academic major in one of the chemical, physical, or biologic sciences) with at least 2 years' experience in the laboratory specialty to be supervised
2. MS or MA degree with 4 years' experience, of which at least 2 years' experience is in the specialty to be supervised
3. BS or BA degree with at least 6 years' experience, of which at least 2 years' experience is in the specialty to be supervised
4. CT(ASCP) or equivalent with at least 4 years' full-time experience in cytology within the preceding 10 years; or, if qualified prior to July 1, 1971, has had at least 15 years of pertinent, full-time laboratory experience prior to January 1, 1968.

Cytotechnologist

The cytotechnologist classification is frequently divided into fairly arbitrary categories of responsibility. To aid in laboratory management and preparatory supervision, cytotechnologists with CT(ASC), CT(IAC), or equivalent certification and 5 years of full-time experience are often referred to as senior cytotechnologists, while individuals possessing similar certification but with less experience may be designated as staff cytotechnologists. The specific duties of these individuals may be the same or may vary, depending on the laboratory's service commitments.

Cytotechnologists employed in licensed or accredited laboratories must meet one of the following requirements in addition to possessing a current license issued by the state, if such state licensure exists:

1. 2 years in an accredited college with at least 12 semester hours in science, 8 of which are in biology, and
   a) 12 months of training in a school of cytotechnology accredited by an accrediting agency approved by the Department of Health and Human Services (HHS), or
   b) 6 months of formal training in a school of cytotechnology approved by HHS and 6 months of full-time experience in cytotechnology in a laboratory acceptable to the director of the formal training program, or
2. before January 1, 1969, had
   a) graduated from high school,
   b) completed 6 months of training in a laboratory directed by a pathologist or other physician recognized as a specialist in cytology, and
   c) completed 2 years of full-time supervised experience in cytotechnology, or
3. achieves a satisfactory grade in a proficiency examination approved by HHS and designed to qualify persons as cytotechnologists.

Laboratories outside the United States fall within the jurisdiction of regulations designed by the individual country or by the IAC.

The cytology laboratory shall employ enough qualified cytotechnologists to process all the tests performed by the laboratory.

Support Personnel

Cytopreparatory technicians lacking the qualifications for technologists may be employed in staining and specimen preparation of cell samples. They may perform highly skilled, repetitive procedures, but only under the supervision of a supervisor or technologist.

There should be enough support personnel to carry out effectively all other aspects of the laboratory operation. Clerical and secretarial functions in a large laboratory may be performed by specialized support personnel or, in small multipurpose laboratories, by technical personnel. Accurate clerical and filing needs are performed most competently by well-trained personnel who have sole responsibility for such duties, rather than by a technologist or preparatory technician whose technical responsibilities leave insufficient time for added duties. In laboratories with automated record-keeping systems, the support personnel vary according to the specific system used, and in many laboratories, cytotechnologists may be expected to be experienced in the use of data-entry and retrieval systems.

RECORD-KEEPING PRACTICES

The record-keeping system of the laboratory, whether manual or computerized, need not be complicated. However, it must be accurate and easily accessible to all laboratory personnel. Minimum needs include a specimen accession log that lists specimens in numerical order as they are received for processing, a patient cross-file for history and follow-up that is most frequently in alphabetical order, and copies of the original requisitions and final reports. The latter components are addressed in the following manner by CLIA '88:

1. Copies of all final reports shall be retained for 10 years.
2. Original requisitions are retained for 2 years. (Microfilm preservation is generally considered acceptable if accurate reproductions of the original document are possible.)
3. Biopsy and autopsy reports are to be included in the patient file as available.

When received in the laboratory, each specimen must be accompanied by an examination request form containing at least the following information:

1. Full name and identification of the patient from whom the specimen was taken
2. Name of the physician or other authorized person or clinic submitting the specimen
3. Collection date of the specimen
4. Type of examination requested (hormonal indices, sex chromatin studies, routine examination, etc)
5. Clinical history, including anatomic site, method of sampling (scrape, aspiration, etc), age of patient, previous therapy (endocrine, surgical, radiation, etc), gynecologic history on cervical/vaginal specimens, and other pertinent patient information

The following information must be added to the examination request form during laboratory processing:

1. Laboratory accession number
2. Date the specimen was received in the laboratory
3. Condition of the specimen when received, including fixation, quantity, and nature of cellular material when indicated
4. Result of the laboratory examination, date of final report, and identification of individual or individuals evaluating the sample

At the time of microscopic evaluation, knowledge of the patient's previous examinations is desirable and may be retrieved from the laboratory cross-files. For optimal usefulness, cross-files should contain documentation of all prior specimens, normal or abnormal, including examination dates, specimen source, cytologic interpretation, and any biopsy or therapeutic follow-up procedures as noted above.

Laboratories processing specimens from hospital inpatient and outpatient clinics exclusively often find that coordinating their cross-filing system with the hospital medical record system is extremely useful, especially when seeking follow-up data. In this case, cross-filing is generally done by patient unit number rather than alphabetically by patient name. When laboratory service extends to the private patient, other means of identification are necessary; filing by social security number is usually preferred.

Specimen reports issued from the laboratory should be as explicit as is cytologically feasible. Deficiencies observed in specimen adequacy, sampling procedures, cellular preservation, etc, should be included in the report. Recommendations for repeated studies or further diagnostic procedures should also be included in the final report when appropriate. The Bethesda System of reporting for gynecologic samples addresses this aspect in considerable detail. The results of follow-up procedures should be obtained and inserted in the patient's record along with correlations between cytologic and histologic findings. Cases in which histologic and cytologic interpretations do not correlate should be reviewed and the results of the review entered in the laboratory records.

Annual reports should be prepared by the laboratory to show total service load, the number of cases processed in each body site, and follow-up data as well as cytologic-histologic correlation. Additional figures usually requested by certifying and accreditation agencies include the number of malignant specimens and the number of unsatisfactory specimens processed per year. Therefore, an annual report of specimens processed, listed by diagnostic category as well as by body site, is virtually essential.

The laboratory director is responsible for the final laboratory report, but each report or laboratory copy should include the signature, initials, or other identification code of the cytotechnologist and/or cytopathologist who examined the preparation and made the final interpretation. Duplicate reports or a similar record should be readily accessible in the laboratory, whether in standard files or on miniaturized formats such as microfilm or microfiche when laboratory space is restricted. As noted earlier, final reports must be retained for at least 10 years, and from a practical standpoint, the use of microfilm methods provides easy access to previous records in a minimum of time and space.

Retention of Microscopic Slides and Report Forms

As noted previously, retention of microscopic slide preparations and cell blocks is essential for proper patient care and follow-up. Previous normal or abnormal specimens must be readily available for review when evaluating follow-up specimens and surgical or therapeutic reports.

Glass slides may be filed numerically in cabinets designed for this purpose. Cell blocks should be filed numerically in containers or cabinets located in a cool, well-ventilated room approved for such storage under local fire regulations.

Congestion in the laboratory due to accumulation of files can be reduced by separation of slides into two numerically filed systems. All non-negative specimens could be maintained permanently in one file within the service laboratory, allowing retrieval of slides for review or study at any time. In a second file system, negative specimens could be filed numerically with current specimens kept in the service laboratory for 6 to 12 months, then sent to long-term storage in ancillary support or separate storage facilities. Old material may be discarded after the required retention period has elapsed, or specimens may be kept for use in teaching collections or other study facilities.

With implementation of CLIA '88, cytologic slides are retained for no less than 5 years from the date of examination. Slides may be loaned to a proficiency testing program provided they are retrievable. No distinction has been made between gynecologic and nongynecologic specimens.

Computerization of Record-Keeping Systems

Adoption of a computerized record-keeping system in the cytopathology laboratory should be considered only with full knowledge of the ultimate capabilities and limitations of the particular system, the personnel required to maintain the system, and the expense involved. Laboratory computers must be expertly programmed, meticulously maintained, and precisely monitored.

Hardware (including computers, keyboards, display terminals) is produced by many firms, each with basic storage capacities and electronic variables. Software (including programs, core language, data storage and retrieval systems, data banks) may be purchased from commercial concerns or may be tailored to the specific needs of the laboratory by computer consultants.

Basic requirements for design of an effective computerized record-keeping system duplicate those for manual systems: storage of accurate and complete patient records, access to patient records by a variety of means, documentation of patient follow-up and histologic confirmation, and retrieval of annual statistical reports. Some laboratories also distribute computer-generated final diagnostic reports. Billing and book-keeping procedures adapt well to computers in many instances.

In the fully automated record-keeping system, all clinical data from the specimen requisition are stored in the computer, allowing rapid generation of "hard copy" (printed page) log records, often listed both numerically by accession number and alphabetically by patient name. Recall of prior patient records by hard copy search of the files or visual display by remote terminal is desirable for optimal evaluation when interpreting specimens.

Code	Description
001	No pathologic diagnosis
002	Acute cervicitis
003	Chronic cervicitis
004	Reserve cell hyperplasia
005	Squamous metaplasia
006	Immature squamous metaplasia
007	Mature squamous metaplasia
008	Condyloma acuminatum
009	Hyperkeratosis
010	Parakeratosis
011	Specimen unsatisfactory due to:
012	Limited cellular material
013	Marked drying artifact
014	Obscuring inflammatory exudate
161	Cellular changes consistent with:
162	*Trichomonas vaginalis*
163	Herpes simplex
164	Cytomegalovirus
165	Human papillomavirus cytopathic effect
166	*Candida albicans*
167	Unidentified mycotic organisms
168	Chronic lymphocytic cervicitis

T *28.1*
Cytopathology Registry Vocabulary

Inserting the final cytologic interpretation into each patient's record may be done in two basic ways. Frequently used diagnostic terms or entire phrases may be assigned simple number codes, permitting reduced time and effort required for data entry. Other system formats employ the word-processing method of "free text" data entry, affording somewhat greater flexibility in final report terminology. While more flexible, this latter method is often more time-consuming. When these two systems are used together, the blend may be both flexible and efficient. One factor must be addressed if free text is part of the final report. In the case of long-term computer report storage, free text should be preserved as well as numerical phrases for the duration of storage to allow factual reproduction of reports at a later time.

Laboratories issuing computer-generated final reports have developed "menus" of frequently used phrases, each numerically coded, which may be inserted individually or in combination with other phrases to produce the final interpretation. These lists of phrases may be simple or highly complex depending on the needs of the laboratory. Examples from such a vocabulary menu are shown [**T** *28.1*].

Retrieval of statistical data is especially suited to computerization. Often time-consuming when done manually, annual reports and statistical studies are readily available with a minimum of effort when the system is properly designed. In addition to overall laboratory statistics, individual cytotechnologist screening volumes, in cases per day, per week, or per year, or numbers of slides per day, per week, or per year, is rapidly available, a record now required for laboratory certification by the CLIA '88 regulations.

Several questions remain unanswered: Which laboratory should use a computerized record-keeping system? Which system is best? Who should design the system for laboratory use? There are no absolute answers to these questions, only guidelines for consideration.

Laboratories with large service volumes requiring expanded filing systems may adapt well to automation. Laboratories with access to automated systems used by other support or service complexes may find that adoption of compatible systems will be to their advantage. Individual assessment of the circumstances must form the basis for final decisions.

Like the "perfect laboratory," the "perfect system" does not exist. Good systems are to be found in many institutions, designed for the needs of that institution. Before final commitments are made, a thorough evaluation of laboratory needs, physical facilities, cost, personnel requirements, and system capabilities must be made. Observation of existing systems is advisable, with attention paid to strong points and weaknesses.

QUALITY CONTROL PRACTICES

One aspect of quality control involves reexamination of negative specimens and confirmation of non-negative specimen evaluations by supervisory personnel or the laboratory director. But quality control also includes precise monitoring of equipment, instruments, reagents, and stains with appropriate preventive maintenance and documented inspection; strict adherence to local health and safety codes; and adequate physical facilities in which to perform specimen preparation and evaluation. Once achieved, these conditions must be maintained at optimal levels. Additionally, performance evaluations must be kept for future reference.

Specimen Preparation

The laboratory must maintain optimal technical quality in preparation and staining of cytologic specimens and use the Papanicolaou staining method or its equivalent.

All stains and working solutions must be dated when prepared and initialed by the person making the solution or stain; for commercial solutions, the date they are received and opened must be recorded. All reagents must be labeled for identity, titer, strength or concentration, recommended storage, and expiration date. Staining quality must be checked at least daily, deficiencies corrected immediately, and checks recorded. All solutions must be filtered or replaced at least once each day. All staining solutions and mounting media must be covered when not in use and stored at the proper temperature.

Gynecologic specimens must be processed separately from nongynecologic specimens.

Volumetric measuring equipment and hydrometers must be of such quality and maintained in such condition as to assure accuracy and precision of results.

Microscopy

All optical equipment must be maintained in good operating order. All slides or specimens submitted to the laboratory must be processed, stained (if unstained at receipt), properly labeled, examined microscopically, and stored (or returned if consultation is required).

The cytotechnologist must evaluate each preparation to determine specimen adequacy and consistency with the patient source. For satisfactory samples, the cytotechnologist must render a cytologic interpretation using a reporting system (see "Record-Keeping Practices") that is as explicit as possible. This may constitute the final report for gynecologic material if normal.

The laboratory director or designee with equivalent qualifications must personally examine and report the diagnosis for all nongynecologic cases and all gynecologic cases with abnormal or questionable cytologic findings or with significant clinical abnormalities. If the sample is unsatisfactory or equivocal, an accompanying statement should indicate why, eg, there is limited cellular material or lack of history. In appropriate cases, some recommendation for follow-up of the patient should be issued with each report, eg, repeated cytologic studies at specific time intervals or further diagnostic studies.

Daily work load limitations for cytotechnologists have been debated for years, and in the case of voluntary accreditation criteria of the ASC have been set at "an average of 12,000 gynecologic cases, or 3000 nongynecologic cases per full-time cytotechnologist per year. Aspiration cytology specimens, cell block specimens and others not normally examined...are not included in this tabulation." These guidelines have been available since 1971, but as a voluntary measure have not resulted in realistic work load restrictions in laboratories not seeking such credentialing.

Several state departments of health have recently required adherence to specific work load limitations, most notably New York State in 1988. The experience of New York State may provide insight into events anticipated at the national level as a result of the work load limits implemented by CLIA '88. The limitations of CLIA '88 indicate that not more than 100 slides shall be examined in any 24-hour period and in no less than 6 hours. Work load limitations published in the February 28, 1992, *Federal Register* for active implementation on September 1, 1992, are as follows:

1. No more than 100 slides may be screened in any 24-hour period. This is to be done on the premises and may include either or both gynecologic or nongynecologic specimens. This slide evaluation must be completed in no less than 8 hours per 24-hour period.
2. Individual work load limitation for cytotechnologists working less than an 8-hour day or who have duties other than slide examination alone will have individual slide limits prorated for their schedules based on the 8-hour day compared with their specific work periods.
3. Within the 100-slide work load, the distribution of gynecologic to nongynecologic samples shall be determined for each cytotechnologist by the technical supervisor, who reviews this distribution at least every 6 months.

The laboratory must retain a record of the number of slides evaluated by each cytotechnologist during each 24-hour period, and the number of hours during that 24-hour period devoted to the evaluation of slides by that individual. Retention of these records, as well as evaluation and revision of work load distribution at monthly intervals where indicated, is required.

Specimen Sign-Out Procedures

As with all phases of laboratory organization, the mechanism for arriving at a final interpretation for each specimen varies with the laboratory. Ultimate responsibility for diagnostic accuracy rests with the laboratory director, but the initial responsibility for identification of abnormal conditions remains with the cytotechnologist.

The sign-out of specimens reviewed by the director or designee should be planned to include the cytotechnologist who originally evaluated the cell sample. The evaluation of unsatisfactory specimens may be performed by the director or designee, or by a supervisory or senior cytotechnologist at the direction of the laboratory director.

Cytologic, Histologic, and Clinical Correlations and Follow-up

The laboratory should establish a system for obtaining both tissue and clinical confirmation of cytologic findings on all abnormal cases and selected negative cases.

The laboratory should maintain records of false-negative and false-positive results for each category of specimens.

Proficiency Testing

Under CLIA '88 guidelines, proficiency testing is required of all participating cytopathology laboratories. As noted in CLIA '67, proficiency testing was specified as necessary in "exfoliative cytology, histopathology, and oral pathology," but was never enforced, most probably due to insufficient volumes of refereed test samples and the complex nature of test administration.

The February 28, 1992, printing of CLIA '88 states that each laboratory must enroll in an approved proficiency testing program for each of its specialty and subspecialty areas of test processing by January 1, 1994, and the laboratory must notify the Health Care Financing Administration (HCFA) of the program, authorizing that program to release to HCFA all data verifying compliance.

Each person examining cytologic preparations must be tested annually. Each test event is composed of 10 glass slides, to include slides representing some but not necessarily all of the following: unsatisfactory preparations, normal samples, infectious agents, benign reactive processes, premalignant processes, and malignant processes. All slides have been refereed in a scientifically defensible manner, and all premalignant and malignant slide preparations have been confirmed histologically.

If the laboratory fails to participate at all or fails to perform successfully in an HFCA-approved testing program for a given specialty or subspecialty, the laboratory's Medicare approval or licensure under CLIA, or both, will be terminated, revoked, suspended, or limited for that specialty or subspecialty. To be reinstated, the laboratory must then demonstrate sustained successful performances on consecutive proficiency testing events, after which HCFA will consider reinstatement.

An individual achieving less than 90% correct on a test set is considered to have failed that event. Failure will necessitate retesting, and repeated failure will require the laboratory to provide the individual with immediate remedial training and/or education. All such remedial work must be documented and all subsequent cytologic screening prohibited until the individual is retested and scores at least 90% on the next testing event. If the laboratory fails to take the necessary remedial actions, HHS will terminate Medicare approval for gynecologic cytology testing or revoke licensure under CLIA, or both.

These portions of CLIA '88 pertaining to compliance, like those concerning proficiency testing in general, have generated extensive discussion in view of fiscal implications of potentially large retraining requirements. At the same time, work load limitations are being imposed that will further reduce the number of cytotechnologists available to perform adequate evaluations of gynecologic samples now being processed annually in the United States. In February 1992, CLIA '88 was modified to include the statement that the entire proficiency testing program will be subject to reevaluation 2 years following implementation on January 1, 1994. Therefore, revision of testing frequency and other requirements may be considered in 1996.

Personnel Performance

The laboratory should maintain an active program of internal quality control, including individual evaluation of each cytotechnologist's performance and that of other technical support personnel.

Personnel performance should be evaluated by a standardized method to monitor quantity and quality of work, applying criteria to determine inappropriate or substandard performances. Procedures for taking corrective measures should be included in documentation of this quality control system.

The long debated "10% review" of negative gynecologic specimens remains a prominent requirement of CLIA '88. To be included in this 10% review are cases identified as "high risk" for developing cervical neoplasia, or so-called "focused" rather than "random" rescreening. Focused rescreening should include patients with abnormal histories, prior abnormal cellular studies, etc, rather than totally random rescreening practices. Previously reported negative cell studies performed within the past 5 years, if available, should be reviewed for each patient with a current premalignant or malignant cellular study. Cytologic/histologic correlation studies are recommended where appropriate, and careful records are to be kept of all such studies, including correlations and discrepancies.

As noted before, all non-negative slide preparations must be retained for a minimum of 5 years from the date of sampling. All final reports, or copies of final reports, must be kept for 10 years from the date of the examination, while all original requisitions, or copies, must be kept for at least 2 years from the date of the examination. Reports may be stored off the premises but must be retrievable within 2 hours of the initiation of a request for the document.

The laboratory director or supervisor may prefer to have all samples evaluated by the cytotechnologist available at the time of abnormal specimen sign-out. Focused selection of 10% of the negative gynecologic specimens may be done at this time for reexamination at a later time. Or, on the other hand, those cases selected may be reexamined immediately, documented on the report as quality control samples, and returned to the cytotechnologist for filing with the routine specimens. If time permits, this latter method affords "instant" quality control and reduces the need for revised reports at a later date should an error in initial evaluation be discovered. Discussion of an improperly evaluated specimen with the cytotechnologist is essential for elimination of future errors and improvement of general laboratory performance.

Another method is random or focused selection of gynecologic cases from the slide files. Reexamination is accomplished as before, and documentation of reexamination is recorded in the permanent logs and patient records. If any discrepancies in evaluation are considered significant to clinical management of the patient, they must be discussed with the initial cytotechnologist and a revised report issued.

Recirculating previously diagnosed and documented negative or non-negative cases as "unknowns" is an equally useful and perhaps more beneficial exercise for diagnostic skill determination. One or more cases may be directed to each cytotechnologist during a set period (weekly or monthly) as a "routine case" for routine evaluation. The cytotechnologist should be unaware of the nature of the case and the prior evaluation, thereby eliminating any bias in interpretation.

If cases are to be recirculated among the staff in a well-publicized manner, both negative and non-negative cases should be introduced into the screening system so that the idea that "if it's a test slide it must be abnormal" will prove to be an inappropriate and inaccurate diagnostic crutch. In obvious test situations, stress sometimes prompts an individual to overcall a negative case rather than provide the correct evaluation when logic and actual diagnostic knowledge confirm the negative nature. Because of this, selection of the former method of unannounced resubmission of "unknown" cases is preferred for unbiased evaluation of screening performance.

LABORATORY COMPLIANCE WITH GOVERNMENTAL REGULATIONS

The laboratory must comply with all applicable state, federal, and local laws and must hold valid licensure where licensing laws apply, or must be approved as meeting the standards established for licensure.

LABORATORY ETHICS

The laboratory director must adhere to the ethical practice of his or her profession and not solicit specimens in a manner that would be unethical for other physicians or dentists.

It should be noted here that cytotechnologists, as professionals on the health care team, must also adhere to the ethical practice of their profession. A discussion of ethics for cytotechnologists can be found in Chapter 1.

CONTINUING EDUCATION

Continuing education for cytotechnologists and cytopathologists is considered essential for high-quality professional performance. Certain states require documentation of participation by licensed physicians in acceptable continuing education programs for renewal of state licensure. Certain medical specialties outside the field of pathology also require such documented participation for continued credentialing.

Cytotechnologists certified by the Board of Registry of the American Society of Clinical Pathologists (ASCP), as CT(ASCP), are encouraged to participate in voluntary education programs such as the Professional Acknowledgment for Continuing Education Program (PACE) of the American Society for Medical Technology (ASMT), or the Continuing Education Certification for Cytotechnologists Program (CECC) of the ASC. Continuing education credits can also be obtained through participation in ASCP workshops, seminars, and self-study programs. However, annual reregistration by the ASCP is not dependent on acquisition of a predetermined number of credit hours of participation.

Cytotechnologists who successfully complete the IAC examination participate in a program of continuing education and submit documentation of this participation for renewal of certification. Failure to acquire the number of educational credits required results in withdrawal of CT(IAC) certification unless the individual elects to sit for the examination again.

Over and above the question of required vs recommended continuing education is the desirability for personal and professional enrichment and general upgrading of knowledge and skills. Internal programs for continuing education are addressed in accreditation standards for laboratories and considered an essential component within the general management of the laboratory. These programs may take many forms, eg, microscopic review sessions with histologic correlation of recent interesting cases, formal lecture sessions, and informal sessions reviewing 35-mm transparencies available from workshops, seminars, and atlases prepared by experts in the field. The important element is allocation of time expressly for the broadening and refining of the employee's level of expertise.

Concern is frequently expressed that continuing education programs are available only in large or academic centers, but this need not be true. Small facilities are equally able to mount such a program and maintain it for the benefit of both technologists and physicians. Cooperation among all members of the laboratory staff is essential in developing and sustaining a program regardless of the size of the facility.

Participation in workshops, seminars, tutorials, and scientific meetings is strongly recommended. Teleconferences provide on-site educational programs and are a convenient way for cytotechnologists to obtain continuing education without traveling. Local, regional, and national organizations frequently sponsor educational sessions; when feasible, cytotechnologists should be encouraged to attend.

When developing an internal program for continuing education, several factors should be taken into consideration. Identification of any areas of technical or diagnostic weakness would be useful in selecting general subject matter and format for a program. The time allotted to the program must be convenient and the location easily accessible for all who will be participating. Responsibility for the entire program and individual sessions may rest with the laboratory director, the laboratory supervisor, or several members of the staff. A rotational system of this responsibility may be employed to permit the active involvement of all staff.

Once a program format has been selected and topics noted, application should be made to the PACE program of ASMT, the CECC program of ASC, or the approval program of the ASCP, or all three, for acknowledgment of specific credits allowed for each individual session of the entire program. Attendance at each session should then be recorded, an evaluation of each session made, and the number of continuing education credits awarded for attendance entered in the employee's file. These credits, together with those obtained through participation in outside workshops, seminars, and scientific meetings, may be applied toward medical licensure renewal and CT(IAC) recertification as well as toward voluntary achievement programs.

When the decision has been made to implement a program of continuing education, the selected areas for emphasis must be suited to the participants. The interests of all participants and the needs of the laboratory, community, and surrounding area should be reflected in the final format. For any program of continuing education to survive and prove beneficial, the people for whom it is designed must participate actively and regularly. Therefore, the program must be interesting, easily accessible, reliably scheduled, and challenging. To prepare such a program can be a challenge in its own right, but the results of such a program should be rewarding to all who plan, prepare, and participate. It should also be kept in mind that professional enrichment ultimately results in superior health care delivery, which, after all, is the goal of this profession.

LABORATORY PREPARATION FOR ACCREDITATION OR LICENSURE

The following checklist may prove helpful when preparing a laboratory for inspections and accreditation or licensure. The answers to these questions should provide a basic outline of laboratory needs that could then be expanded for in-depth advance preparation for laboratory evaluations.

Physical Facilities	Yes	No	Pending
Is space adequate for specimen preparation?	❑	❑	❑
Is workbench space adequate?	❑	❑	❑
Is there adequate storage (shelves and cupboards)?	❑	❑	❑
Are utilities convenient (water, sink, etc)?	❑	❑	❑
Does each cytotechnologist have an adequate desk or microscopy bench area?	❑	❑	❑
Are chairs and benches comfortable?	❑	❑	❑
Are distractions and noises minimized?	❑	❑	❑
Are traffic patterns efficiently designed?	❑	❑	❑
Are slides and records stored conveniently?	❑	❑	❑
Is sufficient space available for clerical functions (reporting, filing)?	❑	❑	❑

Check One

Cytopreparatory Area: General Safety

	Yes	No	Pending
Are fire extinguishers within easy reach?	❑	❑	❑
Are fire extinguishers designed to combat fires from volatile and explosive substances?	❑	❑	❑
Is a fire blanket available?	❑	❑	❑
Are volatile substances stored in safety cans (small quantities), safety rooms, or fire cabinets (bulk storage)?	❑	❑	❑
Is disposal of xylene, etc, approved by the Environmental Protection Agency?	❑	❑	❑
Are procedures for disposal of contaminated material (sputum, cerebrospinal fluid, etc) written and approved by the Department of Health?	❑	❑	❑
Are fume and exhaust hoods available?	❑	❑	❑
Are these hoods used regularly?	❑	❑	❑
Are safety goggles or face shields available and in use?	❑	❑	❑
Are international safety precautions observed in all specimen preparation?	❑	❑	❑
Are appropriate disinfecting solutions applied to workbench space?	❑	❑	❑
Are preparatory implements sterilized or discarded after use?	❑	❑	❑

(*Note:* For additional suggestions, see Chapter 31, "Safety in the Laboratory.")

Equipment

	Yes	No	Pending
Is all equipment on a routine maintenance schedule?	❑	❑	❑
Are log books kept of maintenance checks?	❑	❑	❑
Are microscopes in good working order?	❑	❑	❑
Are there adequate numbers of microscopes?	❑	❑	❑
Are microscopes cleaned frequently?	❑	❑	❑
Is a log of microscope cleaning available?	❑	❑	❑
Is microscope illumination adequate?	❑	❑	❑

	Check One		
	Yes	No	Pending
Specimen Collection Procedures			
Is a preparatory procedure manual available, dated, and initialed by the laboratory director?	❑	❑	❑
Are instructions on gynecologic specimen collection techniques available for clinicians and staff?	❑	❑	❑
Are fixation and transportation instructions included?	❑	❑	❑
Are instructions available for collection and preparation of:			
Sputum?	❑	❑	❑
Bronchial washings?	❑	❑	❑
Bronchial brushings?	❑	❑	❑
Bronchoalveolar lavages?	❑	❑	❑
Gastric washings?	❑	❑	❑
Gastric brushings?	❑	❑	❑
Colonic washings?	❑	❑	❑
Colonic brushings?	❑	❑	❑
Urine samples?	❑	❑	❑
Body cavity fluids?	❑	❑	❑
Fine needle aspirations (where applicable)?	❑	❑	❑
Barr body studies?	❑	❑	❑
Amniocentesis (fetal dating)?	❑	❑	❑
Cerebrospinal fluids?	❑	❑	❑
Other miscellaneous samples?	❑	❑	❑
(*Note:* Not all laboratories will process all the specimens listed here; check only those that apply to your institution.)			
Are the preparations mentioned above included in the laboratory manual?	❑	❑	❑
If a procedure is discontinued, is the procedure protocol allowed to remain in the manual for 2 years before being deleted?	❑	❑	❑
Are the preparations mentioned included in ward or clinic manuals?	❑	❑	❑
Are all specimens properly identified with the patient's name?	❑	❑	❑
Are written policies for receipt and acceptance of specimens available?	❑	❑	❑
Are specimens listed in an accession log and given accession numbers?	❑	❑	❑
Is this log book available at all times?	❑	❑	❑
Are specimens accepted from authorized sources only?	❑	❑	❑
Are written policies including criteria for rejecting specimens available (eg, inadequate identification, quality of preservation)?	❑	❑	❑
Are specimens received from across state lines and so identified?	❑	❑	❑
Personnel			
Does the laboratory have a qualified director?	❑	❑	❑

	Check One		
	Yes	No	Pending
Does the laboratory have a qualified technical supervisor?	❑	❑	❑
Does the laboratory have a qualified general supervisor?	❑	❑	❑
Are the cytotechnologists certified or eligible for certification by a recognized agency?	❑	❑	❑
Are any cytologic samples evaluated by persons not qualified by a recognized agency?	❑	❑	❑
(*Note:* A "yes" to the preceding question will be an automatic deficiency!)			
Are properly trained cytopreparatory technicians employed?	❑	❑	❑
Is the laboratory director available daily?	❑	❑	❑

General Laboratory Procedures

Is the procedure manual for specimen collection procedures available at the workbench?	❑	❑	❑
Are all laboratory policies and procedures reviewed annually?	❑	❑	❑
Are all changes approved, initialed, and dated by the director or supervisor?	❑	❑	❑
Does the manual have a complete and up-to-date list of references?	❑	❑	❑
Are all reagents, working solutions, and stains properly labeled?	❑	❑	❑
Are all reagents, working solutions, and stains dated and initialed by the person preparing them?	❑	❑	❑
Are all storage requirements and expiration dates visible on each item?	❑	❑	❑
In the Papanicolaou procedure, are all solutions filtered or changed daily?	❑	❑	❑
Are the stains changed or filtered daily?	❑	❑	❑
Are gynecologic samples stained separately from nongynecologic specimens?	❑	❑	❑
Are all solutions covered when not in use?	❑	❑	❑
If an inspector selects a slide from the daily work load to check, note the following:			
Will the Papanicolaou stain (or a modified version) be in use?	❑	❑	❑
Will the nuclear detail be sufficient for detailed interpretation?	❑	❑	❑
Will the cytoplasmic stains be appropriate for the cell line?	❑	❑	❑
Will the smear be properly cleared?	❑	❑	❑
Will the coverslip be large enough to cover the cell spread?	❑	❑	❑
Will the coverslip be clean?	❑	❑	❑
Will enough mounting medium be used to prevent air bubbles?	❑	❑	❑
Will the slide be properly labeled?	❑	❑	❑

Reports and Records

Does the final cytologic report show			
Full name of the patient?	❑	❑	❑
Accession number of the specimen?	❑	❑	❑
Name of physician or clinic?	❑	❑	❑

	Check One		
	Yes	No	Pending
Adequate clinical data?	❑	❑	❑
Pertinent history?	❑	❑	❑
Date of specimen collection?	❑	❑	❑
Date sample received in laboratory?	❑	❑	❑
Condition of sample on receipt?	❑	❑	❑
Specific site (type) of sample?	❑	❑	❑
Type of test requested?	❑	❑	❑
Result of cytologic examination?	❑	❑	❑
Date report issued?	❑	❑	❑
Identification of individual(s) who evaluated the cell sample?	❑	❑	❑
Is space available for comments or recommendations by the pathologist?	❑	❑	❑
Is the reporting terminology explicit?	❑	❑	❑
Are equivocal reports explained?	❑	❑	❑
Are unsatisfactory reports explained?	❑	❑	❑
Are copies of all reports retained by the laboratory for 10 years?	❑	❑	❑
Are original requisitions (or approved copies) kept for 2 years?	❑	❑	❑
Is a patient history/report file available for rapid retrieval at the time of repeat studies?	❑	❑	❑
Are biopsy reports and/or autopsy reports entered or maintained with the patient file?	❑	❑	❑
Are abnormal reports followed up systematically?	❑	❑	❑
Are annual statistical reports prepared?	❑	❑	❑
Are cytotechnologist work load volumes recorded?	❑	❑	❑

Quality Control

Are all cytologic slides examined?	❑	❑	❑
Are all non-negative gynecologic smears reviewed by the pathologist?	❑	❑	❑
Are all nongynecologic samples reviewed by the pathologist?	❑	❑	❑
Is there a systematic surveillance of routine examination accuracy, for example:			
Random 10% negative gynecologic rescreening?	❑	❑	❑
"Focused" 10% negative rescreening?	❑	❑	❑
Circulation of "unknowns"?	❑	❑	❑
Other (explain)?	❑	❑	❑
Is clinical correlation available for both normal and abnormal cases?	❑	❑	❑
Are cytologic/histologic correlations determined?	❑	❑	❑
Are correlation studies reviewed periodically as personnel performance measurements?	❑	❑	❑
Are all slides retained for the recommended time?	❑	❑	❑

	Check One		
	Yes	No	Pending
If an inspector randomly selects a laboratory report nearly 2 years old, will he or she be able to go to the slide file and retrieve the slide?	❑	❑	❑
Are slides removed from the file for teaching, etc, identified, and a record kept of their location?	❑	❑	❑
Are prior slides pulled for review when repeat specimens are evaluated?	❑	❑	❑
Are slide files orderly?	❑	❑	❑
Are slide files easily accessible?	❑	❑	❑
Is the quality control defined and documented?	❑	❑	❑
Are written records of quality control slide review maintained?	❑	❑	❑
Are written records of intradepartmental and extradepartmental consultations maintained?	❑	❑	❑
Does the laboratory subscribe to a proficiency testing program?	❑	❑	❑
Does the laboratory maintain a program of continuing education?	❑	❑	❑

REVIEW QUESTIONS

1. What clinical data must accompany each sample on receipt in the laboratory; why is each item necessary for ultimate specimen evaluation?

2. What are the basic requirements, professional and educational, for a laboratory director? For a general supervisor? For a cytotechnologist?

3. What are the quality control requirements for reevaluation of gynecologic and nongynecologic specimens?

4. What major factors should be considered when designing a computerized record-keeping system?

5. How long must cytologic preparations, cell blocks, and reports be maintained in the laboratory before disposal?

SELECTED READINGS

Clinical Laboratory Improvement Act of 1967. *Federal Register.* October 15, 1967;33:15297-15303.

Clinical Laboratory Improvement Amendments of 1988 (CLIA '88, Public Law 100-578). *Federal Register.* March 14, 1990; Vol 55, No. 50.

Clinical Laboratory Improvement Amendments of 1988 (CLIA '88, Public Law 100-578). *Federal Register.* February 28, 1992; Vol 57, No. 40.

Commission on Laboratory Accreditation. *Inspection Manual: Laboratory Accreditation Program and Inspection Checklist.* Skokie, Ill: College of American Pathologists; 1989.

Laboratory Accreditation Committee. *Criteria for Cytopathology Laboratory Accreditation.* Philadelphia, Pa: American Society of Cytology; 1988.

Monitoring and evaluation: pathology and medical laboratory services. *Accreditation Manual for Hospitals.* Oakbrook Terrace, Ill: Joint Commission on Accreditation of Healthcare Organizations; 1988.

CHAPTER 29

The Cytotechnologist and the Workplace

Carol Carriere, SCT(ASCP), CMIAC

CONTENTS

Too often it is thought that the primary means to achieve ideal laboratory performance is to learn appropriate cytologic criteria, look through a microscope, and make an astute diagnosis. In truth, ideal laboratory performance involves a multiplicity of factors, many of which are frequently overlooked.

The ergonomics (physical setup) of the laboratory must be considered, standards for performance and work load limits must be addressed, and methods for monitoring the quality of the work have to be observed. Neglect of these factors will inevitably affect the quality of the work performed.

ERGONOMICS IN THE WORKPLACE

Before the cytotechnologist or cytopathologist begins the process of examining a cellular sample, the microscope and work area need to be properly prepared. Major medical problems have been documented for those who spend long hours at a microscope or workstation that is poorly designed. Carpal tunnel syndrome, which can be a severely disabling wrist injury, occurs as a result of repetitive wrist motions such as those used in manipulating the controls of the mechanical stage, in the constant twirling of the fine-focus knob, or in the repetitive wrist motion of manual nonstage screening. Permanent neck and back problems have been seen in those who must use poorly designed workplace chairs or utilize poor posture at the microscope. Some of these medical problems can be corrected surgically, but some may result in permanent disablement. The design of the microscope, the design of the desk or table on which the microscope sits, and the type of chair that the individual uses are now being addressed by the microscope and laboratory equipment vendors, in large part due to lawsuits and legislation that have come about with the use of computers in the workplace.

Chairs should have proper cushioning with complete seat and back angle adjustment and adjustable height. Contoured adjustable back support alleviates strain and fatigue, and back height adjustment will fit the user's lumbar area. Most new chairs come with pneumatic height adjustment and a five-legged base that is more stable than the old four-legged variety. Purchasers of laboratory equipment should be aware that chairs need to be tried out before purchasing to analyze their appropriateness not only to the general laboratory situation, but to each individual. What may work for one person may be totally uncomfortable for another, and a laboratory may need to purchase a variety of chairs to accommodate the various needs of the individuals working in the laboratory. Manufacturers are often willing to ship a chair to a laboratory on a trial basis, giving the laboratory a chance to test it out on-site. Short individuals may find that even with the built-in height adjustment it may be necessary to use a footstool so that their legs are supported and not dangling while they are sitting for long hours. Slanted moveable foot rests are available for those who need them and greatly relieve back strain.

More microscopes are designed with flexibility and human comfort in mind. Adjustable-tilt heads and tilted bases allow an individual to sit erect and have the microscope directly at eye level without having to stretch the neck upward or downward to accommodate the position of the scope. For older microscopes that lack a tilted base, a small pad of paper or something the thickness of a slide folder placed under the rear of the microscope will raise the position of the scope just enough to correctly bring the eye pieces to eye level and will alleviate strain and tension on the neck muscles. Newly developed rubber knobs on the focusing mechanisms allow a lighter or one-finger touch that lessens harmful strain on the wrists. Soft padded cushions on the microscope base can serve as arm rests, eliminating the need for foam pillows placed under the elbows. Microscope tables may be purchased that have curved front sections cut out allowing the individual to pull up close to the microscope, yet leaving desk space at the sides for arms or elbows to rest. The individual can sit erect and have the microscope close and at direct eye level without leaning forward. Strain on the neck or back is minimized. Electrical plugs have been build into some of these tables for added convenience. A few companies will design workstations and customize equipment to fit individual needs.

The microscope should be clean and properly illuminated. Each microscopist should know the principles of Koehler illumination and should check the adjustment of the microscope frequently. Daily cleaning of oculars should be performed using cotton-tip applicator sticks slightly moistened with commercial lens cleaner. Evidence of regular cleaning and maintenance is required by many of the laboratory accrediting agencies such as the College of American Pathologists (CAP). The work area should be located away from direct sunlight, and surrounding illumination should be diffuse and of moderate intensity. A nonreflecting table surface of a neutral color, eg, gray or green, helps to avoid eye fatigue.

EXAMINING THE SLIDE

Distractions need to be kept to a minimum so the individual can concentrate on evaluating the slide systematically and thoroughly. Modular furniture systems can create individual cubicles or workstations that reduce distractions and noise in the work area. Laboratory procedures that produce noxious or harmful fumes (xylene, formalin, alcohols) should be strictly separated from areas where microscopic work is performed. The environment should be comfortable and free of drafts.

The time required to examine a slide may take from a few minutes to a half hour or more, depending on the characteristics of the cell population and the experience of the cytologist. Abnormal cells may stand out and catch the eye, but in thick preparations and samples containing many leukocytes, a more tedious search must be made to detect their presence. The ability to differentiate cell forms quickly improves with practice.

Some cytotechnologists use a vertical [**F** *29.1*] while others use a horizontal [**F** *29.2*] movement of the slide. Most commonly a mechanical stage is used, but some individuals prefer manual nonstage movement of the slide. Whichever method is used, the entire cell sample must be systematically and thoroughly examined by the cytotechnologist.

Examination is usually performed with the low-power (x10) objective and either x10, x12, or x10 wide-field oculars. The high-power (x40) objective is utilized for close inspection of atypical cells or, occasionally, unusual microbiologic findings.

An initial overview of the cell sample is suggested. This can be achieved by moving the slide across the microscope stage once or twice prior to the systematic search for tumor cells. The cytologist may then assess the background and overall cellular content. As one gains experience, one will have a better indication of the possibilities contained within the cell sample, eg, a tumor diathesis, an inflammatory exudate, a scant cell sample.

Atypical cells are always marked for future reference. They may be marked with a pen, a split-tip applicator stick, a waterproof smearproof marking pencil, or an object marker that fits directly into the microscope's rotating head like an objective. The marker tip contains a circle that is inked and brought down to form a ring around the significant cells. Dots made with pen and ink can be placed to the side, top, or bottom of the significant cells, but within each laboratory the placement of the dots should be consistent so there is no confusion as to where to find the significant cells [**F** *29.3*].

After the atypical cells have been located and marked, the impression of the total cytologic assessment should be recorded by the examining cytologist. Quality as well as quantity is required, and regardless of the method used, alertness, thoroughness, and consistency are qualities needed to perform the daily cytologic evaluation.

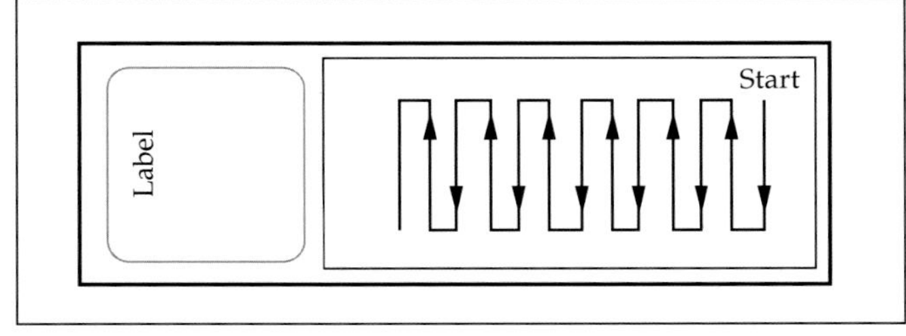

F *29.1*

Vertical screening pattern.

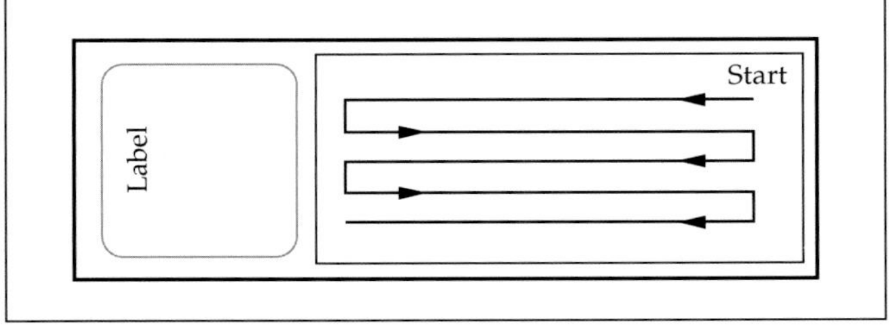

F *29.2*

Horizontal screening pattern.

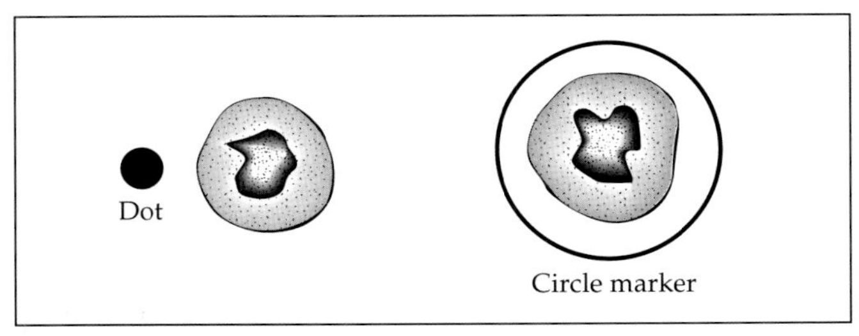

F *29.3*

Left, marking cells with pen and ink; right, marking cells with object marker.

QUALITY ASSURANCE/QUALITY CONTROL MEASURES AND PRACTICES

Regulations implementing CLIA '88 include specific quality assurance measures and quality control practices that must be observed for the laboratory to maintain proper licensure and/or accreditation (see Chapter 28). The full text of the regulations implementing CLIA '88 should be consulted for a complete discussion of quality assurance and quality control requirements.

Laboratory manuals need to be maintained that include specimen collection requirements and processing details; criteria for microscopic examination, including the adequacy of a specimen; cytopreparation procedures; quality control and quality assurance measures; known limitations in methodology; actions to be taken when quality control procedures indicate a problem; alternate test methods; how patient results are reported; and how long specimens are stored in the laboratory. Guidelines for the format of laboratory procedure manuals are regularly published by the National Committee for Clinical Laboratory Standards.

A number of training facilities and individual laboratories have established parameters by which they attempt to make specific measurements related to laboratory performance. These measurements may be based on the skills listed below, on data obtained through quality assurance and quality control measures, or some combination of the two. It is the responsibility of each laboratory to develop performance standards and document that they are being monitored and enforced. Helpful suggestions for content and format of quality assurance reports can be found in publications such as the *Surgical Pathology/ Cytopathology Quality Assurance Manual* published by the CAP.

METHODS FOR MEASURING PRODUCTIVITY

Laboratory managers may need methods to measure the productivity of the individuals within their laboratory or of the laboratory itself. The number of full-time positions required is not always directly related to the case volume of the laboratory. Additional duties or special handling procedures required of the staff or even the complexity of the cases themselves can impact on the number of cases that can be processed from day to day. The work load limits (slides per day) established at state and federal levels are intended to represent the maximum number of slides screened by an individual per day or 24-hour period and are not to be construed as the minimum performance level expected for each individual in the laboratory. A laboratory manager must take a more comprehensive view of laboratory functioning.

One method for measuring productivity that had achieved widespread usage was the CAP Workload Recording Method. This system was based on work units established through time studies of procedures performed in the laboratory and was used with some degree of success in numerous laboratories throughout the country. However, CAP abandoned this method in 1992 because generic time studies done from a sampling of laboratories were not always appropriate for larger or smaller laboratories with different staffing, a greater mix of specimen types, or unique processing methods. In addition, values often had to be created by individual laboratories to account for specific work situations or administrative functions.

CAP has replaced the Workload Recording Method with the Laboratory Management Index Program (LMIP). LMIP is a comprehensive and systematic program for assessing laboratory operating performance. For clinical laboratories, 33 operating ratios based on individual laboratory statistics such as billable tests, number of individuals employed, worked laboratory hours, actual time spent on tests, consumable expenses, etc, have been established as a platform for comparison. For anatomic pathology laboratories, specific modules have been developed that recognize the distinct difference in management requirements for anatomic pathology compared with clinical pathology. Cytology laboratories will be required to submit information on the number of cases and slides for gynecologic, nongynecologic, and fine needle aspiration specimens, the number of cytotechnologists screening, the number of clerical staff, computerization of the laboratory, and total paid and worked hours. From the data collected from participating laboratories, CAP will establish a Laboratory Complexity Index (LCI) with which a laboratory will be able to compare its productivity, utilization, and cost-effectiveness with laboratories that have similar functions and testing complexity.

This will result in a more valid peer comparison than was possible with the Workload Recording Method. The laboratory manager will be able to identify areas that need improvement or demonstrate that the laboratory operates within reasonable parameters for its unique makeup. In addition, trend information from previous quarters will be provided to the participants and will help identify areas of stability or areas of change within the laboratory.

ASSESSING THE QUALITY OF THE WORK PERFORMED

There are many skills to be considered in the assessment of a cytotechnologist's or cytology student's ability to evaluate a cell sample. Qualitative and quantitative performance skills to be analyzed include those of detection, diagnosis, decision-making, recording, and communication. An objective evaluation mechanism for these skills should be designed to identify both strengths and weaknesses of the cytotechnologist or cytology student being evaluated.

The following are intended to suggest some of the criteria that may be used in the laboratory. Each cytopathology laboratory can adapt these measures to its own needs.

Detection Skills

1. Matching correctly the slide number with the appropriate requisition form
2. Identification of microbiologic findings that require the attention of the clinician
3. Identification of cellular changes that place patients in a high-risk group
4. Identification of ancillary findings, such as tumor diathesis, asbestos bodies, and carbon histiocytes
5. Identification and marking of atypical cells for further review

Diagnostic Skills

1. Correct cellular assessment of the type of lesion or entity represented in the cell sample
2. Correct prediction, by means of the cell sample, of the expected histologic or clinical diagnosis
3. Correct evaluation of the hormonal status of the patient and whether that status is compatible or incompatible with the patient's clinical history and age

Decision-Making Skills

1. Recognition of the inadequacy of a cell sample
2. Recognition of proper processing and staining of cell samples
3. Assessment of the disease process represented in the cell sample for the proper follow-up recommendations
4. Reliable recognition of what represents a clearly negative cell sample since, in most instances, clearly negative gynecologic cases will be reported to the clinician without further review by a pathologist
5. Recognition of cell findings that may require a search of the literature or require consultation; in other words, deciding what one does not know and when one should seek the aid of a more experienced cytologist

Recording Skills

1. Recording cell findings legibly for follow-up review and evaluation by the supervisor and/or pathologist
2. Recording cell findings accurately and precisely for the report to the clinician
3. Recording cell findings accurately for the data entry personnel
4. Recording cell findings for possible future research studies or teaching sets

Communication Skills

1. Ability to make clear verbal presentations to the cytopathologist regarding cell findings
2. Ability to present the final report to the clinician, if required, and to answer any questions that might be asked
3. Ability to explain the cell findings and demonstrate them in the microscope to the clinician who wishes to see the cell sample

The performance of an individual should be measured against a standard of performance decided on, in advance, by the laboratory director and senior staff members. Quality control and quality assurance requirements contained in federal and state regulations can serve as a basis for these and other laboratory measurements of performance.

REVIEW QUESTIONS

1. The CAP Laboratory Management Index Program is a
   a) procedure to ensure accurate screening of cytologic smears.
   b) means of measuring productivity in the laboratory.
   c) system for reporting diagnostic results.
   d) statistical record of specimen types received in the laboratory.

2. Carpal tunnel syndrome results from
   a) performing repetitive wrist movements.
   b) stretching the neck to reach the microscope eyepieces.
   c) being exposed to noxious fumes in the laboratory.
   d) using poorly designed chairs or poor posture while sitting at the microscope.

3. Specific guidelines for writing a laboratory procedure manual can be found in the
   a) College of American Pathologists Manual for Workload Recording.
   b) regulations implementing CLIA '88.
   c) publications by the National Committee for Clinical Laboratory Standards.
   d) standards for Medicare and Medicaid accreditation.

4. An initial overview or quick scan should be performed on each slide to
   a) detect the areas with abnormal cells.
   b) document presence of microbiologic elements.
   c) determine if the slide is clean enough for quick screening.
   d) obtain an initial impression of pertinent features and cellularity.

SELECTED READINGS

Bender JL, Bettner B, Blank CH, et al. *Clinical Laboratory Procedure Manuals.* Villanova, Pa: National Committee for Clinical Laboratory Standards; 1984;4(2).

Bogdanich W. Lax laboratories: the Pap test misses much cervical cancer through labs' errors. *Wall Street Journal.* November 2, 1987:1.

Browell B. Examining the cellular sample. In: Keebler CM, Reagan JW, eds. *A Manual of Cytotechnology.* 6th ed. Chicago, Ill: ASCP Press; 1983:38-44.

Deppisch H, ed. *Surgical Pathology/Cytopathology Quality Assurance Manual.* Skokie, Ill: College of American Pathologists; 1988.

Gill G. Practical considerations in microscopy. *The Cytotechnologist's Bulletin.* 1987;24:1-71,74-75.

Gill G. Practical considerations in microscopy: part II. *The Cytotechnologist's Bulletin.* 1988;25:19-21,25-26.

Karp R. Laboratory ergonomics. *The Cytotechnologist's Bulletin.* 1984;21:37-38.

Laboratory Management Index Program (LMIP). Northfield, Ill: College of American Pathologists; 1992.

Newton L. Carpal tunnel syndrome. *ASCT News.* 1986;7:73-77.

Smith V. The scoop on scopes. *ASCT News.* 1990;11:21-24.

Triol JH, ed. *ASCT Cytopathology Quality Assurance Guide, I.* Raleigh, NC: American Society for Cytotechnology; 1992.

Walensky G. Medicare, Medicaid and CLIA programs: regulations implementing the Clinical Laboratory Improvement Amendments of 1988 (CLIA '88). *Federal Register.* February 28, 1992;57:7002-7243.

Yokota S. Ergonomics and the laboratory. *ASCT News.* 1985;6:83-87.

CHAPTER 30

Management

GERALDINE O'NEILL HORAK,
MS, EMBA, SCT(ASCP), CFIAC

CONTENTS

The cytopathology laboratory in most private and hospital settings is managed as a separate entity or in conjunction with the pathology laboratory. The type of evaluative work required on the part of the cytotechnologist and the trust that develops between the cytotechnologist and cytopathologist is different from many other clinical laboratory personnel due to the interaction between the cytopathologist and cytotechnologist in the daily diagnosis of cellular samples.

Management of the cytopathology facility requires optimal use of the laboratory's resources to reach a final diagnostic assessment that results in quality patient care. In addition to being responsible for the day-to-day laboratory and hospital quality assurance program, managers must be cognizant of legal implications (related to patients and personnel), accreditation requirements (private, state, and federal), environmental regulations, safety precautions (especially those related to infectious diseases), and budgetary limitations and planning. The main components of managerial functions include:

1. Adherence and agreement with the written laboratory policy
2. Organization of people and tasks to be performed
3. Guidance and evaluation of personnel to match their written job descriptions and expected performance goals, especially those goals that pertain to quality work and participation in the laboratory's quality control program
4. Planning and adherence to the annual budget
5. Development of a continuing education program for all personnel
6. Allocation of funds for capital equipment
7. Development of quality controls to assure quality patient care within personnel and time constraints
8. Ability to handle public relations challenges: external (the media) and internal (administrators)
9. Knowledge of the market value for personnel and the cost of the cytologic sample
10. Working knowledge of all laboratory functions from cytopreparation, data entry, and computerized systems, through the final diagnostic assessment and report
11. Planning space for workstations
12. Knowledge of safety measures for personnel

This chapter covers some budgetary considerations for the cytopathology laboratory and methods to determine the cost of each procedure offered by the laboratory. In addition, personnel issues such as selection of personnel, orientation, job description, and performance appraisals will be briefly discussed.

THE BUDGET PROCESS

Each laboratory or institution has budgetary considerations. The following are some basic items with which a laboratory manager must be familiar to begin the budget process.

1. Direct costs: personnel, supplies, rental fees, maintenance contracts for computer and photocopying equipment and preventative maintenance of microscopes, average monthly charges such as telephones and beepers, paper, etc
2. Indirect costs, which in a hospital setting would include housekeeping, plant department, administrators, assessed overhead for electricity, heat, and air conditioning, room rental fees, telephone system, etc
3. Volume (real or estimated) and type of specimens
4. Capital equipment justification if equipment needs to be replaced or new equipment is needed; depreciation considerations depending on institution policy
5. Equipment inventory
6. Knowledge of union contractual agreements vs planned increases of nonunion personnel
7. Monies allotted for participation in continuing education programs
8. Inflation rate increases from suppliers
9. The cost of each test performed by the laboratory

Cost Analysis

The example below can be used to assess the actual cost of performing a cytologic evaluation of cerebrospinal fluid by two methods of preparation using the College of American Pathologists (CAP) *Manual for Laboratory Workload Recording Method* allotment of time for each portion of a task. Although CAP has recently converted to a new system for determining work load productivity (Chapter 29), laboratories can modify the CAP work load standards to their needs by performing time studies in their specific operation.

CSF Cytocentrifugation Procedure	Time Allowed, min
Specimen identification	5.0 per case
Matching slide to history	
Data entry of sample/patient information	
Gross description of sample	
Obtaining previous history/File search	2.0 per case
Centrifugation	2.0 per case
Cytospin preparation: 2 slides	4.0 (2.0 per slide)
Papanicolaou-stained sample: 1 slide	2.0 per slide
Diff-Quik–stained sample: 1 slide	2.0 per slide
(Includes preparation time, staining, coverslipping)	
Evaluation of samples by cytotechnologist	5.0 (2.5 per cytocentrifuge slide)*
Data entry/reporting	2.0 per case
Total unit value	24.0 per case

*The minutes allotted for interpretation of nongynecologic specimens depend on the type of cytopreparation performed on each type of specimen. For example, interpretation of membrane filter preparation is 5 minutes; interpretation of smear covering 50% or less of the glass slide is 2.5 minutes; interpretation of a cell block preparation is 2.5 minutes per slide; and so on. Time allotted to interpretation of negative gynecologic smear is 5 minutes, while 6.5 minutes has been assigned to interpretation of abnormal gynecologic smear (any slide that requires the review of a pathologist).

CSF Millipore Filter Procedure	**Time Allowed, min**
Specimen identification	5.0 per case
Matching slide to history	
Data entry of sample/ patient information	
Gross description of sample	
Obtaining previous history/ File search	2.0 per case
Centrifugation	2.0 per case
Cytospin preparation: 1 slide	2.0 per slide
Millipore filtration preparation: 1 slide	5.0 per slide
Papanicolaou stain/coverslip/labeling	
Cytocent sample: 1 slide	2.0 per slide
Millipore sample: 1 slide	4.0 per slide
Evaluation of samples by cytotechnologist	2.5 per cytocent slide 5.0 per filter
Data entry/reporting	2.0 per case
Total unit value	31.5 per case

Personnel Costs

Time of cytopreparatory personnel at $10.00/hour*
Time of data entry clerk at $12.00/hour*
Time of cytotechnologist at $20.00/hour*
Time of secretary at $14.00/hour*

*Salary estimations are based on present market conditions. Salaries vary depending on geographic region and what the marketplace will demand in that location. In addition to salary, employee benefits must be factored in. Employee benefit packages may be as high as 35% to 40% or as low as 25% of annual salary, depending on what is included in the package or how it is defined.

Equipment Costs

2 glass slides
1 centrifuge tube
1 Millipore filter
1/2 cytocentrifuge filter
Staining supplies
Mounting media
Applicator stick
2 coverslips
Requisition form and/or case work sheet
Specimen container
Final report paper (computer or manual generated)
Gloves, gowns, and face shield/mask/goggles worn during cytopreparation
Decontamination solution
Disposable wipes

1. All items supplied to clinical offices/physicians are counted into the cost of equipment, including slides, fixative, specimen containers, and requisitions.
2. The cost of the 10% rescreen on gynecologic samples is factored into the cost of a gynecologic Pap smear.
3. Waste may be factored in as a small percentage.
4. Equipment depreciation can be factored into the budget, depending on the institution's policy.
5. Cost of any special equipment, such as disposable cytospin equipment for handling of infectious material, should be considered.

The following is a sample worksheet to calculate costs for the cytocentrifuge of a cerebrospinal fluid sample.

	Cost/Unit	**x Units Used**	**Test Cost**
Supplies			
Slides	.06	2	.12
Coverslips	.035	2	.07
Labels	.01	2	.02
Cyto Filter	.07	2	.14
Gloves	.05	2	.10
Misc/gown			.18
Report paper	.05	2	.10
Waste factor			.05
Cost/test			.78
Reagents			
Stains	.06	2	.12
Alcohols	.06	2	.12
Mounting	.01	2	.02
Cost/test			.26

	Job Rate/Minute	**x CAP WLU***	**Test Cost**
Personnel/Labor			
Cytotechnologist	.33	5	1.65
Preparatory	.17	10	1.70
Secretary	.23	2	.46
Clerk	.20	7	1.40
Cost/test			5.21†

*WLU indicates Workload Unit expressed in minutes.
†It is necessary to factor in benefits—including vacation, holidays, health care, FICA, unemployment compensation, workers compensation, insurance, tuition reimbursement, and other items—on top of the base salary. The factor is set by the accounting department in each institution and is usually between 35% and 40% of the hourly base salary. For discussion purposes here, the factor will be set at 30%, thus 5.21 is multiplied by 1.30; thus the cost per test plus benefits is 6.78.

The personnel costs for each test vary depending on the laboratory operation. For example, cytotechnologists may routinely perform cytopreparatory and miscellaneous clerical operations in addition to microscopy, which increase costs since these tasks are done at a higher base salary.

CSF Cost Analysis

Supplies	.78
Reagents	.26
Personnel	6.78
Total direct costs	7.82

There are indirect costs, which are included as a predetermined factor established by the accounting department in each institution—sometimes as a set percent, or at times, an established dollar amount. It is usually around 80% of direct costs.

Total indirect cost 6.26 (80% of 7.82)

There is also a professional charge included, which is a predetermined factor established by the laboratory director or department chairman for physician services. It may be a set fee or a percentage of the total fee. The charge below is used for illustration purposes only.

Total professional charge	25.00
Total test cost	39.08

The following is a sample worksheet to calculate costs for Millipore filter preparation for a cerebrospinal fluid sample.

Direct Costs

	Cost/Unit	x Units Used	Test Cost
Supplies			
Slides	.06	2	.12
Coverslips	.035	2	.07
Labels	.01	2	.02
Cyto filter	.07	1	.07
Millipore	.35	1	.35
Gloves	.05	2	.10
Misc/gown			.18
Report paper	.05	2	.10
Waste factor			.05
Cost/test			1.14
Reagents			
Stains	.06	2	.12
Alcohols	.06	2	.12
Mounting	.01	2	.02
Cost/test			.26

	Job Rate/min	x CAP WLU	Test Cost
Personnel			
Cytotechnologist	.33	13.5	4.46
Preparatory	.17	9	1.53
Secretary	.23	9	2.07
Cost/test			8.06
(Benefit factor x 1.30)			
Cost/test			10.51

Personnel costs are increased in this sample because the cytotechnologist stained the slides and the secretary was used for all data entry tasks.

CSF Millipore Cost Analysis

Supplies	1.14
Reagents	.26
Personnel	10.51
Total direct cost	11.01
(Indirect costs x 80%)	
Total indirect cost	8.59
Total professional charge	25.00
Total test cost	46.44

Periodically, test costs need to be reevaluated and adjusted accordingly. As you can see from the test costing figures, the cytology laboratory is a labor-intense profession.

The Budget

The annual budget is a vital and necessary management tool used to project and match expenses with revenues as well as a control mechanism for sound, reliable, and accurate business decisions. Ideally, the supervisor, manager, and laboratory director will develop specific cost figures to use as guidelines to accomplish specific goals within the stated cost expenditures. The planned budget highlights where money can be saved by forecasting expected test volume, work load demands, and resources needed for the next budget period. Routinely throughout the year, budgeted expenses are monitored and tracked so the resulting information can be used by management to exercise greater control over costs and to use resources efficiently.

Some important questions are asked during the budget process:

1. Has there been a change in the volume and/or diversity of tests performed in the laboratory?
2. Has there been a steady increase/decrease in volume over the last 5 years?
3. Is a trend in test volume or work load demand developing?
4. Is there a new project planned, such as the introduction of new technology (eg, automation), that could substantially increase the volume of work?
5. Is a new test being marketed to meet the needs, wants, and desires of customers that will increase the volume of work?
6. What is the expected number of billable procedures for the upcoming year?

Caseload information and estimated annual volume help determine the number of employees needed to perform effectively in all aspects of the laboratory operation. Federal and state governments and accrediting agencies have set work load ratios for cytotechnologists. Each institution may use these guidelines to determine the number of cytotechnologists needed for operation. In addition, there should be enough properly trained support personnel, including technicians, clerks, and secretaries, to handle the size of the operation.

Position Vacancy

When a vacant position occurs, an assessment of that position should be done based on productivity data, scheduling needs including overtime, desired personnel qualifications, and full-time vs part-time options. Is there a work load fluctuation within a shift that needs to be assessed? For maximizing productivity, some areas may need staggered hours, flexible time shifts, split shifts, or even a decrease in staff size.

Salary Considerations

Salary surveys need to be performed regularly for all laboratory positions. The human resources department can survey similar hospitals and/or laboratories in a geographic region and/or national market in which it competes. It is important, therefore, for the human resources personnel to be familiar with laboratories performing at a similar level and with similar quality and quantity levels.

Salary data from the survey are collected and analyzed. This information provides clear market data indicating competitive rates for each position. More accurate information can be gained if the cytology manager participates in the survey, since awareness of comparative salaries at comparative positions is not always clear to administrators in human resources management. Based on the salary survey data, a salary range is established with a minimum, midpoint, and maximum salary for each job. The difference between the minimum and maximum of the salary range allows for salary differences based on experience and recognition of different levels of performance. Salary range adjustments are made annually based on the salary survey analysis, the institution's financial ability to increase it, and the competitive market demands. Salary increases are based on how well employees perform the duties of their job over a specified time. Each institution has its own performance review program with various performance rating levels.

At times, the laboratory manager must write a proposal to defend a salary increase or change. The proposal should address the need for a salary change, state the goals and objectives of the change, and estimate the cost. The proposal should be supported with information regarding impact on the annual budget and should offer alternative solutions. If a temporary position is needed during a crisis, a similar document may be necessary. The hourly salary rate for a temporary position is higher than that for full-time employees. This is primarily due to the fact that the cost of benefits is factored into (added to) the hourly pay rate of a temporary position while the hourly salary rate for full-time employees excludes the cost of benefits, which can cost the employer as much as one fourth to one third of the entire payroll. Questions that need to be asked at budget time are: Are cytotechnologists' salaries increasing regionally or nationally? If yes, by what percent or lump sum will the salary need to be increased to be competitive for the area? What are the conditions of the union contractual agreements, if any? What is the estimated annual percent increase of all the laboratory employees?

Laboratory Supplies

Laboratory supplies depend on work load needs. An accumulation of inventory and an inadequate turnover rate tie up laboratory funds. The stock and supplies should be rotated to avoid outdating. Contract bids may be obtained for common supplies. Some institutions have primary vendors that give substantial discounts on supplies. Standing orders on the largest volume of reagents and supplies usually assure that delivery is on time and alleviate the cumbersome paperwork and costs of the weekly/monthly orders. Standing orders, however, require close monitoring of supply delivery and billing to assure that orders are received and payments are made only for supplies actually delivered.

Cooperative purchasing with other laboratories within a section can yield bulk discounts. For example, cytology and histology laboratories could jointly purchase alcohols/stains and slides/coverglass, which could result in lower supply prices. Solutions and stains need to be dated and initialed when received and dated when opened. Vendors identify reagents/stains and their concentration, as well as their expiration date.

Equipment Purchases

Maintenance or service contracts offer warranties on equipment, parts, and labor. Know the effective date of the warranty. Does the warranty begin the day the instrument was installed or does the purchase order date trigger the warranty? Know what is covered and what the extra charges include. Some institutions have in-house clinical engineering departments able to service the instruments, thus saving expenditures. Check with in-house departments to see if they are willing to and comfortable with repairing the various instruments.

As instruments age, it is necessary to budget for repairs or maintain the service contract. Contingency plans need to be in place for instrument breakdown. If the instrument has to be sent to the manufacturer, what are the costs, how long will it take for repairs, and is there a loaner available to use during this downtime? If the vendor repairs the instrument on-site, what are the costs for the vendor repair personnel, such as travel time costs, hourly personnel rates, and parts prices?

Equipment preventative maintenance manuals often have space to document problems and resolution of these problems. Record potential or recurring problems. If the instrument is constantly under repair and it is documented in the preventative maintenance manual, it may be necessary to put a new instrument into the budget or capital equipment expenditure. A refresher course in instrument usage may be needed, especially if there has been employee turnover. Vendors usually are willing to hold refresher sessions for use of their instruments.

Continuing Education

Continuing education is mandated by some accrediting agencies and should be included in the budget. There should be an in-house continuing education program in place. Utilization of the pathology staff as well as staff from allied departments for an in-house continuing education program is a good cost-effective measure. Lectures, slide sets, glass slide teaching/examination sets, and teleconferences are excellent education tools. Cytotechnologists, residents, and pathologists can share with other personnel what they have learned at workshops, seminars, and national and regional meetings.

There are educational programs that can be purchased from various professional societies and can be included in the budget, eg, the American Society of Cytology's (ASC) Cytoteleconferencing series; the American Society of Clinical Pathologist's (ASCP) Check Sample, CheckPath, and Tech Sample self-study series; and CAP's Interlaboratory Comparison Program in Cervicalvaginal Cytology.

The educational needs of each individual in the laboratory should be determined. Goals should be established and programs put in place. With mandatory federal and state regulations governing cytology proficiency testing, each laboratory has to assess employees' needs for remedial work should they fail a test.

Capital Equipment Considerations

Capital equipment is long-term planning for the evaluation and selection of equipment and/or remodeling expenditures within the department usually in excess of $500. A typical formal proposal includes:

1. Type of equipment: lab equipment, word processing/office equipment, furniture and furnishings, and miscellaneous equipment
2. Reason for the request: replacement, increased demand, new staff, new technology/service
3. Cost
4. Suggested vendor and model number
5. Estimated date of purchase
6. Whether remodeling and/or utility changes are needed to install equipment; if so, who will make the installation
7. Whether additional employees are needed to operate this equipment
8. Priority of the equipment

Capital equipment is a multiple-step process involving a proposal, review and analysis, decision-making, implementing, and follow-up.

Remodeling of a laboratory area or building a new facility needs major consideration as to the design and execution of the physical facilities. All work areas must be designed to minimize problems with the work flow throughout the laboratory. Microscopy and administrative areas are separated from the cytopreparatory area. Environmental considerations—eg, proper ventilation, lighting, utility outlets—are needed. The workstations are arranged to be conducive to high-quality performance. Attention to safety and hazardous chemical precautions involve fireproof cabinets in a well-vented area. All equipment, new or used, must be in good working condition.

Simple and complex statistical analysis is performed monthly and year-to-date on operational and revenue reports for each cost center within the laboratory budget and for capital equipment acquisitions. Managers utilize this information to evaluate, compare, and control costs.

PERSONNEL ISSUES

Laboratories and institutions have established personnel practices. Employee records should include employee's education, experience, certification, records of illnesses and accidents occurring at work, job description, performance reviews, and miscellaneous items such as general accomplishments throughout employment.

The staffing of the laboratory involves obtaining and developing qualified individuals through recruitment, selection, orientation, and training. Managers do not usually have the primary responsibility for staffing but are often involved in manpower planning and determining compensation and promotions.

Job requirements for current and newly created jobs must be defined as precisely and completely as possible. The job description includes basic job function, minimum qualifications, on-the-job training, occupational exposure, and a detailed description of work or specific duties. A job description examines the job and its requirements, not the person in it.

Performance expectations need to be in place for each job description and must be discussed with each employee during orientation (or reiterated if discussed during the initial interview). A laboratory error policy guideline for each position defined as part of the quality control procedures serves to underscore the importance of accuracy and good judgment when dealing with patient confidential information and specimens. The policy emphasizes the possible consequences to the patient when a mistake occurs. This policy is not intended to intimidate employees or suggest that perfection is expected.

Error Policy

Laboratories should have well-defined error policies for all personnel, including cytotechnologists, cytopreparatory technologists, and clerical and secretarial staff, in order to maintain excellence in the delivery of health care through the recognition, timely correction, and prevention of errors. Utilizing team management, laboratory personnel should define the error policy for each laboratory section and the appropriate action to be taken. Internal quality control measures should be established to prevent errors. A suggested laboratory policy could be set up to define primary, secondary, and obscure errors. For example, an error policy for cytotechnologists could be set up as follows.

Primary Error

A cytotechnologist primary error could be defined as an error that originated with the cytotechnologist—such as missing an obvious malignancy or other benign condition on a case—that could have significant consequences for the patient. The error, when detected, would be noted in the supervisor's file with an anecdotal note. Should a second primary error occur within 1 month of the first error, it could be considered cause for the first step in the corrective action policy. A record would be placed in the permanent employee file in the human resources department. A third primary error within 1 year of the last disciplinary action could be considered cause for the second step in the correction action policy. A fourth primary error within 1 year of the last disciplinary action could be considered cause for suspension for 3 days without pay. A fifth primary error within 1 year of the last disciplinary action could be considered cause for termination.

Secondary Error

A secondary error could be defined as an error that should have been detected and corrected, but did not originate with the cytotechnologist, and may have significant consequences for the patient. For example, a cytotechnologist does not recognize a sample for what it is. The laboratory work sheet states that the specimen is a sputum; however, in screening the case the cytotechnologist should have recognized that the specimen was a bronchial brushing by virtue of the cells seen on the sample. The original error came from the attending physician's office, as noted on the incoming requisition. Two secondary errors within 1 month could be considered cause for an anecdotal note in the supervisor's file. This might not be placed in the institution's permanent record. This policy could be defined further by laboratory personnel, leading eventually to cause for termination.

Obscure Error

An obscure error could be defined as one that has significant consequences for the patient, but the origin of the error cannot be determined with certainty. For example, an obscure error would be an incorrect final diagnosis on a report that has gone to the patient's chart. Determining who entered the final diagnosis into the computer is obscure; it could have been the cytotechnologist who screened the case, the cytotechnologist who was helping in the clerical area on that particular day, or the clerical help. Errors could be recorded for those personnel who have handled the specimen, but no formal action is taken until three obscure errors for an individual employee have occurred within a 3-month period.

Productivity Issues

Standards of excellence in performance are found in all areas of the laboratory operation. They are defined in the quality control section of the laboratory procedural manual, which lists expected performance in a specific, observable, and measurable way. The quality control section also includes the following:

I. Cytotechnologist work load. Every 6 months, the technical supervisor (pathologist) establishes the work load for each cytotechnologist. General guidelines for daily work load considerations include
   A. Years of continued work experience in cytology
      1. Recent graduate of a cytotechnology program—maximum of 40 slides in an 8-hour period
      2. One to two years of continued work experience—minimum of 40 slides in an 8-hour period, not to exceed 100 slides
   B. Years of cytology employment at the present institution
   C. Participation in in-house continuing education programs should be at least 2 hours per month (by accrediting agencies' regulation) and may include
      1. Glass slide unknown cases
      2. Teleconferences
      3. ASCP Check Samples, CheckPath, and Tech Sample
      4. CAP Cervicalvaginal Cytology program
      5. Lectures by interdepartmental and intradepartmental staff, residents, cytotechnologists, and visitors
      6. American Medical Association and American Hospital Association programs
      7. Book or journal review conferences
   D. Amount of time allotted to screening excluding miscellaneous duties such as cytopreparatory and clerical assignments, travel time for fine-needle aspiration procedures, and special projects
   E. Each cytotechnologist's ability to accurately evaluate cases
   F. The laboratory's caseload variation such as gynecologic vs nongynecologic cases
   G. The laboratory's overall operation and environment

II. Tally of daily work load. Cytotechnologists document their daily work load by tallying total cases reviewed and calculating the number of slides screened each day [see **F**30.1-**F**30.3 at the end of the chapter] to assure that their performance is within the Health Care Financing Administration's and accrediting agencies' guidelines. The supervisor/technical director reviews this daily document as well as the monthly totals to assure that the cytotechnologists are not screening more than their established quotas, and to make daily work load adjustments as needed. A quality control log book is initialed by the supervisor/technical director after review of these documents.

    In addition to the tallying of the number of cases/slides, each cytotechnologist must keep a record/log book of each case screened, indicating patient/case number and case diagnosis.

III. Ten percent random rescreen of gynecologic cases. Ten percent of negative gynecologic cases evaluated by the cytotechnologists are randomly pulled, either by a preset computer program or manually, to be reviewed by the supervisor or pathologist for internal quality control rescreen prior to the issuance of a final report. These negative cases are selected from the total caseload and from patients that are identified as having high probability of developing cervical cancer based on available patient information. Each case is then documented either in the computer or manually. In the event of a discrepancy, the case is reviewed with the initial cytotechnologist, documented in a log book, and a corrected report is issued.

IV. During the cytopathologist daily sign-out of prescreened gynecologic work, disagreements in cellular study interpretations between the cytotechnologist and cytopathologist will be considered a discrepancy if it is either plus or minus two grades of severity, eg, negative findings vs a low-grade squamous intraepithelial lesion. The discrepancy will be discussed with the cytotechnologist, noted in a record book what adjustments or actions are taken, and initialed by the cytopathologist.

Selection of Personnel

To make employees aware of job vacancies, job posting is performed in central locations throughout the institution. Interested employees contact the personnel department, who initially screen the applicants and forward them to the manager. In unionized organizations and large institutions, specific job bidding and job posting procedures are normally spelled out.

Various employee recruitment methods include advertising in the "Help Wanted" section of newspapers, professional journals, and publications; announcements at professional meetings; recruitment letters to schools of cytotechnology and to individual cytotechnologists from lists or mailing labels purchased from professional societies; employee referrals; employment agencies; and personal contact.

The human resources department may perform the initial screening of applicants and does the background and reference checks. Interviews are set up with the laboratory director, staff pathologists, manager, supervisor, and other interested individuals. The interview is used to fully explain the job and its requirements, answer any questions that the applicant may have about the job, and eliminate unsuitable or unqualified applicants. The interview team determines which applicant is best suited and qualified for the laboratory and its current and future needs.

Interviewing techniques usually are of two types. (1) A structured interview is one in which the interviewer knows in advance what questions are going to be asked, asks the questions, and records the results. This type of interview has the advantage of providing the same information on all applicants, ensuring that all questions are covered with all applicants, and minimizing the personal biases of the interviewer. (2) An unstructured interview is one in which there is no definite checklist of questions. There is no planned strategy. Questions are open-ended, eg, "Tell me about your previous job."

Employment interviews are subject to legal considerations, and each institution has written interview guidelines and gives workshops defining lawful information that can be used to disqualify candidates. Considerations center around questions concerning age, arrest record, conviction record, credit rating, education, handicaps, marital and family status, military record, name, national origin, race/color, religion, sex, and work experience.

Not only in recruitment and selection of new employees but throughout the tenure of employment, one must abide by the established nondiscriminatory personnel policies that comply with state and federal law. These policies affect the whole employment process, from recruitment and selection to retention activities such as seniority systems, promotion and transfer, compensation, and layoffs. Equal employment opportunity was legalized in Title VII of the Civil Rights Act of 1964. Other legislation includes the Fair Labor Standards Act of 1963, the Age Discrimination in Employment Act of 1968, and the Rehabilitation Act of 1973. The purpose of all these laws and the many subsequent court interpretations of these laws is to ensure that the decisions to hire or not to hire an individual, to promote or transfer, and the compensation policies are all job-related.

Orientation of New Employees

The orientation program in large organizations is shared by both the human resources department and the laboratory manager to introduce the new employee to the organization and the job. An informational checklist of items to be covered in the orientation should include (1) job-related information: job description, duties, standards, and expectations; compensation; attendance, work hours, overtime, call-in policy, and vacation; patient awareness opportunities; (2) department related information: tour of department/introduction to coworkers and staff; location of time clock, rest rooms, supplies, bulletin board; (3) safety: fire alarm system and evacuation, laboratory safety and exposure control plan, chemical hygiene plan, accident report procedure; (4) institutional policies: objectives and philosophy of organization, brief history of organization, organizational chart, and operations related to laboratory.

A comprehensive cytopathology laboratory procedural manual serves as a good source and informational training manual for new employees. Also it serves as established, approved, measurable standards of performance for the competent practice of cytology, and a source document for inspection by regulatory and accrediting agencies. All the laboratory methods and procedures are outlined in detail, which promotes clarity, consistency, and continuity of performance and management decisions. It lists objectives, purposes, policies, procedures, methods, and rules. It clarifies management directives, reduces uncertainties, and saves time and energy. The new employee may even find that a change in laboratory procedure was overlooked and should be documented and dated in the manual.

The training of new employees involves the acquisition of skills, concepts, rules, or attitudes to increase their performance. On-the-job training is usually given by the supervisor or senior employee. For example, rescreening of slides by a supervisor from the newly hired cytotechnologist correlates the laboratory's diagnostic philosophy and expectations with the new hiree's diagnostic ability and provides positive reinforcing feedback along the way.

Performance Standards

Work expectations for new employees should be set at a reasonable level; demonstrate and define the proper way for the work to be done, let the trainee perform the work, and put the trainee on his or her own gradually. Supervisors should be available to answer questions and give positive encouragement.

The principle purposes of performance appraisal are to improve employee performance in the present job, to provide a record of employee performance that can be used as a basis for management decisions, and to prepare employees for future opportunities that may arise in the organization. Organizations use performance appraisals for wage and salary administration, promotions or demotions, transfers, layoffs, counseling employees, and human resources planning.

There are many types of performance appraisal methods used today, including graphic rating scale, critical-incident appraisals, work standards approach, ranking methods, and management by objectives. The human resources department or upper management decides which type of performance appraisal system the organization will use, and refinements are constantly made. The standards of performance should be specific, observable, and measurable. It is necessary that the employee be evaluated accurately and fairly. Considerable time and thought should be given to completing the performance appraisal form. The employee should be given at least 1 week's notice of the upcoming appraisal. The appraisal should be conducted in a private room or office without interruptions, and the confidential nature of this information should be explained to the employee. There should be ongoing, honest, and positive feedback to the employee. Some questions a supervisor should consider prior to the performance appraisal interview are: What are the specific good points on which you will compliment the employee? What are the specific negative points that you intend to discuss? What reactions do you anticipate? Can you support your performance appraisal with adequate facts? What specific help or corrective action do you anticipate offering? What follow-up action do you have in mind?

QUALITY MANAGEMENT

Patients and legislators demand quality health and customer satisfaction at a minimal cost. The Joint Commission on Accreditation of Healthcare Organizations, CAP, and ASC all define cytology quality control practices in their accreditation policies.

All laboratory procedural manuals have a section on quality assurance practices and quality control procedures. Quality is and must be built in at every stage in the laboratory process: specimen receipt, record-keeping and accessioning, processing, staining, microscopy, specimen-reporting, billing, and quality assurance procedures. There must be an ongoing assessment and revision of these simple and complex sequences of laboratory operations to strive toward excellence. The work flow, technology, and methodology should get the job done right the first time. Waste, repeated work, complexity, and error in the laboratory's daily life need to be eliminated. Through continuous daily improvement, the cytology laboratory will lower costs, improve efficiency, and achieve greater effectiveness. The bottom line is achieving what the customer wants when the customer wants it.

CRISES IN CYTOLOGY

Health care and the cytopathology laboratory are confronted with challenges from Medicare rules and third-party payers, corporate restructuring, uncertainties related to CLIA '88 and Occupational Safety and Health Administration regulations, and technological advances. External factors, such as the aging population, liability issues, escalation of medical costs, development of new technologies outside of medicine, constituent forces, economic issues, availability of health care insurance to the working poor, and the increasing incidence of human papilloma virus, impact cytology both directly and indirectly.

We now face automation of cytology screening and advances in computer image analysis and in molecular biology that pose both a challenge to cytology and a golden opportunity for change. Laboratory managers are being faced with new rules, demanding constituents, constraints, conflict, greater accountability, and an ever-changing internal and external environment. Planning that considers the past, present, and future will ensure a smooth transition into the next century.

CYTOLOGY LABORATORY MONTHLY WORK LOAD

Name: ______________________ Date: ______________________

Hours Worked: ______________________ Hours Screened: ______________________

Caseload:

Gynecologic Slides: ______________________ Gynecologic Cases: ______________________

Nongynecologic Slides: ______________________ Nongynecologic Cases: ______________________

CC/T-P Slides*: ______________________ CC/T-P Cases*: ______________________

Total Slides: __________

Total Cases: __________

Miscellaneous Daily Activities: ____

____

____

____

____

____

____

*Cytocentrifuge slides/Thin-Prep dispersion over one half or less of the slide counts as 1/2 slide.

F *30.1*

Example of daily work load form.

CYTOLOGY LABORATORY MONTHLY WORK LOAD

Name ______________________ Month ______________

ID# ______________________ Year __________

Day	Hours Worked	Hours Screened	Gynecologic Slides 1	Gynecologic Slides 2	Gyn Cases	QC* Slide /Cases	Nongyn Slides	CC/TP† Slides	Nongyn Cases	Total Slides	Total Cases
1											
2											
3											
4											
5											
6											
7											
8											
9											
10											
11											
12											
13											
14											
15											
16											
17											
18											
19											
20											
21											
22											
23											
24											
25											
26											
27											
28											
29											
30											
31											

* QC, quality control. † CC/TP, Cytocentrifuge slides/Thin-Prep or any dispersion over one half or less of the slide counts as 1/2 slide.

PLEASE LIST MISCELLANEOUS DAILY ACTIVITIES ON REVERSE SIDE

❑ I have not interpreted cytologic samples at any other site this month.

❑ I have interpreted cytologic samples at other sites this month, working within CLIA '88 guidelines.

Date Signature

F *30.2*

Example of monthly work load form.

WORK LOAD REVIEW

Cytotechnologist ______________________________

Work Load Limit ______________________________

Criteria ____

____

Month Year	#Cases/#Slides Reviewed		#QC Discrepancies*	#Sign-Out Cases	#Sign-Out Discrepancies†	Adjustments/Action Taken	Reviewed By
Jan							
Feb							
Mar							
Apr							
May							
June							
July							
Aug							
Sep							
Oct							
Nov							
Dec							

* A quality control (QC) discrepancy occurs when a cytotechnologist's interpretation of a cellular study is inconsistent with the interpretation of the QC reviewer.

† A sign-out discrepancy occurs when a cytotechnologist's interpretation of a cellular study is inconsistent with the pathologist's diagnosis by +/− 2 grades of severity (ie, negative findings vs a mild dysplasia).

F *30.3*

Example of work load review form.

REVIEW EXERCISES

1. Name at least six functions of management.

2. Briefly describe how you would determine the cost of a cerebrospinal fluid specimen.

3. Describe the major cost components of a test analysis.

4. Briefly describe some budget considerations of the following: work load, salary, supplies, equipment, and continuing education.

5. Briefly describe the recruitment, interview, and performance appraisal process.

SELECTED READINGS

Berman HJ, Weeks LE, Kukla SF. *The Financial Management of Hospitals.* 7th ed. Ann Arbor, Mich: Health Administration Press; 1990.

Department of Health and Human Services, Health Care Financing Administration. Medicare, Medicaid and CLIA Programs: Revision of Laboratory Regulations: final rule with request for comments (42 CFR Part 74, et al). *Federal Register.* March 14, 1990:9538-9610.

Department of Health and Human Services, Health Care Financing Administration, Public Health Service. Clinical Laboratory Improvement Amendments of 1988: final rule (42 CFR Part 405, et al). *Federal Register.* February 28, 1992:7002-7186.

Department of Health and Human Services, Health Care Financing Administration, Public Health Service. Clinical Laboratory Improvement Amendments of 1988: final rule (42 CFR Part 493). *Federal Register.* February 28, 1992:7188-7288.

Department of Labor, Occupational Safety and Health Administration. Occupational exposure to bloodborne pathogens: final rule (29 CFR 1910.1030). *Federal Register.* December 6, 1991:64004-64182.

Drucker PF. *Managing the Nonprofit Organization: Principles and Practices.* New York, NY: Harper Collins Publishers; 1990.

Drucker PF. *Managing for the Future: the 1990's and Beyond.* New York, NY: Truman M Talley; 1992.

Gitman LJ. *Principles of Managerial Finance.* 5th ed. New York, NY: Harper & Row, Publishers Inc; 1988.

Kovner AR, Neuhauser D. *Health Services Management: Reading and Commentary.* 4th ed. Ann Arbor, Mich: Health Administration Press; 1990.

Leeabov W, Scott G. *Health Care Managers in Transition: Shifting Roles and Changing Organizations.* San Francisco, Calif: Jossey-Bass Inc Publishers; 1990.

Lindorff D. *Marketplace Medicine: The Rise of the For-Profit Hospital Chains.* New York, NY: Bantam Books; 1992.

Marszalek-Gaucher E, Coggey RJ. *Transforming Healthcare Organizations: How to Achieve and Sustain Organizational Excellence.* San Francisco, Calif: Jossey-Bass Inc Publishers; 1990.

Medical Laboratory Observer. Montvale, NJ: Medical Economics Publishing. All issues.

Metzger N. *Handbook of Health Care Human Resources Management.* 2nd ed. Rockville, Md: Aspen Publishers Inc; 1990.

Omachanu VK. *Total Quality and Productivity Management in Health Care Organizations.* Norcross, Ga: Industrial Engineering and Management Press; 1991.

Schutz R, Johnson A. *Management of Hospitals and Health Services: Strategic Issues and Performance.* 3rd ed. St Louis, Mo: CV Mosby Co; 1990.

Shortell SM, Morrison EM, Friedman B. *Strategic Choices for America's Hospitals: Managing Change in Turbulent Times.* San Francisco, Calif: Jossey-Bass Inc Publishers; 1990.

Stevens GH. *The Strategic Health Manager: Mastering Essential Leadership Skills.* San Francisco, Calif: Jossey-Bass Inc Publishers; 1991.

Walton M. *The Deming Management Method.* New York, NY: The Putnam Berkley Group Inc; 1986.

CHAPTER 31

Safety

PEGGY PRINZ LUEBBERT, MS,
MT(ASCP) SC, CIC

CONTENTS

Laboratory personnel work with a variety of occupational health hazards on a daily basis. To ensure a safe workplace, cytotechnologists should be aware of potential hazards and should fully understand safety and infection control protocols.

A substantial set of safety regulations and standards have been developed by government agencies and professional organizations. This chapter can serve as a resource for safety and infection control information; however, an institution's specific policies and protocols should always be consulted.

CHEMICAL SAFETY

In 1988, the Occupation Safety and Health Administration (OSHA) introduced the Hazard Communication Standard, which was implemented to reduce the incidence of chemically related work illnesses and states that employees have the "right to know" about all chemical hazards with which they may have contact. In January 1990, OSHA released "Occupational Exposure to Hazardous Chemicals in Laboratories," known as the "Lab Standard." This standard went into effect January 31, 1991 and has the force of law.

OSHA recognized that laboratories differ from industrial operations in their use and handling of hazardous chemicals and promulgated a rule specific for clinical laboratories. This rule requires a facility to have a written program that includes warning labels on containers of hazardous chemicals, a material safety data sheet for each hazardous chemical and mixture in the workplace, and an employee information and training program.

Hazardous chemicals often found in a cytopathology laboratory include methanol, ethanol, xylene, chloroform, glacial acetic acid, hydrochloric acid, ammonium hydroxide, and bleach. If histologic preparations are made, toluene, formaldehyde, and picric acid may be present.

Product Warning Labels

All hazardous chemicals contain warning labels on the product that include the chemical and common names, warnings about physical and health hazards, and name and address of manufacturer. The label may also contain signs, symbols, or pictures depicting this information. When chemicals are transferred from large to small containers for ongoing use, the small containers must be labeled. However, a portable container (flask, cuvette) intended only for immediate use does not need to be labeled. Labels must not be removed or defaced; if one is damaged, it must be replaced immediately with a new and proper label.

Material Safety Data Sheets

Material safety data sheets, developed for each chemical by the manufacturer, should be readily available. Each sheet contains the following information:

1. Product or chemical identity used on the label
2. Name, address, and phone number for hazard and emergency information
3. Date the material safety data sheet was prepared
4. Chemical and common names of hazardous ingredients found in the product
5. Permissible exposure limits
6. Physical and chemical characteristics of the product, such as appearance, odor, boiling point, and vapor pressure
7. Physical hazards, including the potential for fire, explosion, and reactivity, and the proper extinguishing media
8. Primary routes of entry into the body (ingestion, inhalation, and skin absorption)
9. Acute and chronic health hazards, including symptoms of exposure, and medical condition aggravated by exposure
10. Carcinogenic hazard characteristics
11. Emergency and first aid procedures
12. Safe handling procedures, including work practice, spill or leak cleanup, storage and transport precautions
13. Appropriate waste disposal methods
14. Exposure control methods, including engineering controls

Cytotechnologists should know where the material safety data sheets are kept, read the material safety data sheets of all products, and follow the appropriate precautions in handling and disposal. Note that these data sheets do not all look alike; however, they must all contain the same type of information. Some laboratories provide a chart that contains the required information in a format that is easier to read and quickly accessible in case of an emergency.

Proper Handling and Disposal of Hazardous Chemicals

All chemicals should be treated as potential hazards. For proper handling and disposal of each chemical, follow the recommendations described on the material safety data sheets. General instructions to follow:

1. Discard all unlabeled bottles.
2. Clearly label all containers with the names of the chemicals and the hazards involved in their use.

3. Read all labels before using a chemical.
4. Avoid direct contact with chemicals.
5. Wear appropriate protective equipment (gloves, aprons, goggles) as necessary. This apparel should not be worn outside the laboratory.
6. Disposable gloves should be discarded after each use.
7. Handle one bottle at a time.
8. Use heavy duty "bottle carriers" for bottles larger than 500 mL.
9. Always add reagents slowly, pouring concentrated solutions into less concentrated solutions while stirring.
10. Pour acid into water, never water into acid.
11. Fill reagent bottles to within one fourth of their capacity. This will permit for heat expansion.
12. Do not use more of a chemical than directed and remove only approximately what is needed. Never return excess of a chemical to its original container.
13. Keep all chemical containers tightly stoppered.
14. Store flammable chemical in labeled explosive-proof refrigerators and cabinets.
15. Wash hands after completing any procedure.

Chemical Spills

When a hazardous chemical spill occurs, all persons in the immediate area of the spill should be alerted and evacuated if necessary. Report the incident to your supervisor and follow these general guidelines:

1. Review the material safety data sheet for appropriate ventilation, containment, and disposal instructions. Follow posted instructions if available.
2. A "spill kit" for the cleanup of chemicals may be available. It should contain spill pillows, silicon-based absorbent, dustpan, broom, plastic bags, waste labels, rubber gloves, rubber boots, and chemical splash goggles.
3. Small spills (<100 mL) can be absorbed by sand, paper towels, and neutralizers.
4. Solid spills may be brushed onto a dustpan by a person wearing gloves.
5. Take care to avoid reactive combinations of chemicals.
6. Dilute acids and alkalis before discarding down sinks and follow with copious amounts of water.

When a chemical is spilled on the skin, recommendations described on the appropriate material safety data sheet should be followed. General instructions include the following:

1. Remove all contaminated clothing as quickly as possible.
2. Flush the area of the body continuously for 15 minutes under a safety shower, faucet, or eye wash.
3. Wash the chemical off with soap and water. Do not use neutralizing agents, creams, lotions, or salves on the skin.
4. Obtain immediate medical attention.

FIRE PREVENTION

Explosions and fires can be encountered anywhere in the cytopathology laboratory. The most frequent causes of laboratory fires are carelessness, inattention, lack of knowledge, unattended equipment, and faulty electrical wiring and equipment. To prevent fires, your institution should have a fire safety program that includes training in safe work practices and use of fire extinguishers and blankets, fire drills, and evacuation procedures.

Fire Safety Precautions

1. Have an evacuation plan and know where the nearest exits are located.
2. Recognize the location and use of the fire extinguisher, blanket, and fire alarm.
3. Maintain marked, unobstructed exits.
4. Keep chemical inventory current and storage areas uncluttered.
5. Store incompatible chemicals separately.
6. Use safety cans instead of glass bottles to store flammable chemicals.
7. Store flammables in explosion-proof cabinets, refrigerators, or freezers.
8. Keep motors, switches, open flames, and other possible sources of ignition away from vapor or other flammable sources.
9. Limit chemicals on workbench to daily needs.
10. Use only equipment approved by Underwriters Laboratories (UL).
11. Avoid using extension cords. All equipment should go directly to socket. If an extension cord must be used as a temporary measure, it should be UL approved.
12. Keep safety storage cabinets and fire doors closed.

During a fire in your laboratory or on a fire drill act quickly and do the following:

1. Pull the fire alarm and alert personnel in immediate area.
2. If necessary, telephone the switchboard, identify yourself, and tell the operator the location of the fire. The operator may then announce the location of the fire over the paging system in code.
3. Remove visitors from immediate danger.
4. Contain the fire if you can with the appropriate fire extinguisher or blanket.

5. If someone's clothing catches on fire, wrap the person in a fire blanket or drench under the emergency shower.
6. Close doors and windows.
7. Disconnect electrical equipment.
8. Remove flammable liquid from the area.
9. If the fire cannot be contained, evacuate according to posted procedure.

If the fire is in another area of the institution, do the following:

1. Close doors and windows.
2. Clear exits and hallways.
3. Calm visitors; ask them to remain in the laboratory.
4. Remain in your department unless notified to assist elsewhere or to evacuate.
5. Wait for the "all clear" or evacuation procedures.

Fire Extinguishers

Portable fire extinguishers are classified by their ability to handle specific classes and sizes of fires. For burning combustible materials, such as wood, paper, clothing, and trash, use an extinguisher identified by a green triangle containing the letter "A." This type of extinguisher employs water or an all-purpose dry chemical. For burning liquids, use an extinguisher identified by a red square containing the letter "B." This type of extinguisher employs a foam, dry chemical, or carbon dioxide. For electrical fires, use an extinguisher identified by a blue circle containing the letter "C." This type of extinguisher employs nonconducting extinguishing agents, such as carbon dioxide or a dry chemical.

Multipurpose extinguishers recommended for all types of fires are the most common extinguishers found in clinical laboratories.

BIOSAFETY HAZARDS

The cytopathology laboratory environment poses special infectious disease risks to workers or visitors. Cytotechnologists should be aware of the identified risks and adhere to recommended policies and procedures to protect themselves and their coworkers.

Most infectious agents found in the cytopathology laboratory are spread by direct contact or respiratory exposure. Good hand washing and adherence to universal blood and body fluid precautions, as described below, helps break the chain of transmission and produce a safe work environment.

Hand Washing

Hands come in contact with many organisms and can therefore transmit infections. Frequent hand washing is essential for protection of both workers and patients. Hands should be washed

1. when visibly contaminated with blood, body fluids, or tissues.
2. after removal of gloves and other protective wear or equipment.
3. before leaving the clinical work areas.
4. before eating, drinking, smoking, applying makeup, or changing contact lenses outside of the laboratory, and after using the lavatory.
5. before all other activities that entail hand contact with mucous membrane or a break in the skin.
6. periodically during the day when routinely handling body fluids.

The wearing of rings and bracelets should be avoided because they might interfere with thorough hand washing (they also make it more difficult to don gloves). The following is proper hand washing procedure:

1. Wet hands and apply a small amount of an antiseptic soap.
2. Vigorously lather hands and rub together for at least 15 seconds.
3. Wash well between fingers and up the wrists.
4. Rinse well with a moderate stream of water in a downward motion.
5. Dry with a paper towel and use the towel to turn off the faucet. Dry skin adequately to avoid dermatitis.

Frequent hand washing can be very damaging to the skin's normal protective mechanisms by damaging or cracking skin, altering its pH, or changing its normal bacterial flora. Recent studies suggest that frequent application of hand lotion may reduce this damage. Laboratory personnel, therefore, are now encouraged to use it. This may be difficult, however, as one should avoid applying hand lotion immediately after washing or right before handling of sensitive instruments or equipment. Lotions might interfere with the residual action of the antimicrobial hand washing products.

Universal Precautions

Since medical history and examination cannot reliably identify the infectivity of all patients' blood and body fluids, universal precautions were first introduced in 1987 by the Centers for Disease Control to decrease the occupational risks of blood-borne diseases, such as the acquired immunodeficiency syndrome and hepatitis B, to health care workers. All body fluids should be handled with the same precautions as blood; this is known as body substance isolation.

In 1992, OSHA mandated the use of universal precautions with a new rule known as the Blood Borne Standard. This rule requires medical facilities to protect and educate personnel, and to monitor the use of universal precautions. The precautions specific for cytopathology laboratories include the following:

1. Use barrier protection routinely to prevent skin and mucous membrane contamination with blood or other body fluids.
2. Wear gloves when preparing nongynecologic samples or handling any body fluids or containers contaminated with body fluids. Always wear gloves when cuts, scratches, or other breaks in skin are present.
3. Change gloves when visibly contaminated with body fluids.
4. Wear a mask, eye glasses, goggles, or face shield during procedures that are likely to generate droplets of body fluids to prevent exposure of the mucous membranes of the mouth, nose, and eyes.
5. Wear a fluid-resistant gown, apron, or other covering when there is a potential for splashing or spraying of body fluids onto the body. Use disposable gowns when handling known infected material.
6. Wash hands or other skin surfaces thoroughly and immediately if contaminated with body fluids.
7. Wash hands immediately after gloves have been removed, even when no external contamination has occurred. Organisms on the hands multiply rapidly in the warm moist environment within the glove.
8. Handle laboratory instruments, especially needles, blades, and knives, with extreme caution.
9. Place used sharp items into a puncture-resistant biohazard container for disposal. The container should be located as close as possible to the work area.
10. Needles should not be recapped, purposely bent, cut, broken, or removed from disposable syringes otherwise manipulated by hand. If recapping is unavoidable, do it with one hand and use great caution.
11. Place large-bore reusable needles (bone marrow biopsy needles, etc) and other reusable sharp objects into a puncture-resistant container for transport to the reprocessing area.
12. All specimens should be put in well-constructed containers with secure lids to prevent leaking during transport. Care should be taken when collecting each specimen to avoid contaminating the outside of the container and the laboratory form accompanying the specimen.
13. Use biologic safety hoods (class 1 or 2) for processing all nongynecologic cell samples. Handle all samples as if infectious.
14. Decontaminate all laboratory work areas with an appropriate chemical germicide after a spill of blood or other body fluids and when work activities are completed. Laboratory countertops should be disinfected at least once per shift.
15. Rinse off all body fluids from reusable contaminated equipment prior to reprocessing, according to your institution's policies.
16. Clean and decontaminate scientific equipment that has been contaminated with body fluids before being repaired in the laboratory or transported to the manufacturer. Always follow manufacturer's recommendations.
17. Pregnant cytotechnologists are not thought to be at greater risk of infection than others in the laboratory. However, if an infection does develop during pregnancy or the mother is a carrier prior to the pregnancy, the infant is at risk of infection by perinatal transmission. Therefore, pregnant laboratory workers should be especially aware of universal precautions.

APPENDIX

The following list details incompatible chemicals:

Acetic acid: with chromic acid, nitric acid, hydroxyl-containing compounds, ethylene glycol, perchloric acid, peroxides, and permanganates

Acetone: with concentrated sulfuric and nitric acid mixtures

Ammonia, anhydrous: with mercury, halogens, calcium hypochlorite, hydrogen fluoride

Chlorine: with ammonia, acetylene, butadiene, benzine, and other petroleum fractions, hydrogen, sodium carbide, turpentine and finely divided powdered metals

Flammable liquids: with ammonium nitrate, chromic acid, hydrogen peroxide, nitric acid, sodium peroxide, halogens

The following chemicals should be stored and handled so they cannot accidentally contact each other:

Acetic acid, hydrogen sulfide, aniline, hydrocarbons, sulfuric acid, or any flammable liquid: with oxidizing agents such as chromic acid, nitric acid, peroxides, and permanganates

Halogens—fluorine, chlorine, bromine, iodine: with ammonia, acetylene, hydrocarbons

CHAPTER

32

Information Systems

Michael D. Glant, MD

CONTENTS

The need to collect, store, compile, and report laboratory data continues to increase and is paralleled by the growth of laboratory computerization. Over the last several decades the high volume of testing, widespread automation, and predominantly numerical data in areas of "clinical pathology" have made computerization a natural extension of those laboratory functions. The "anatomic pathology" components of the laboratory have different data manipulation and storage needs [**T**32.1]. Only more recently have hardware and software advances allowed the emergence of acceptable computerization for cytology, surgical pathology, autopsy pathology, and other areas of anatomic pathology. The recent mandates by the Clinical Laboratory Improvement Act of 1988 (CLIA '88) for documented quality assurance and quality control in cytology have forced most laboratories to seriously consider the cost-effectiveness of a computer system.

Laboratory personnel involvement is the key to successful computerization. The process of laboratory computerization in cytology needs to involve surgical pathology in addition to all aspects of cytology laboratory operations. A comprehensive review of the process is beyond the scope of this chapter. However, an overview of the process and reference to some further literature is recommended for anyone considering laboratory computerization. Most laboratories vastly underestimate the resources (mainly commitment of personnel) required to research, plan, and implement a computer system. It is a very expensive and "disruptive" process, with the potential for great benefit or even greater disappointment. The critical factors for success are the user's (laboratory's) commitment or involvement, the quality of the software and its vendor, and the complexity of the laboratory's needs. You do not always "get what you pay for," and a lack of involvement is one sure way to insure dissatisfaction. Expectations of computerization can be inappropriate and must be tempered by a knowledgeable user and vendor. This chapter discusses a variety of issues in cytology (and related anatomic pathology) computerization, provides a basic outline for computerization, and hopefully prepares the cytotechnologist or pathologist for the more extensive self-education needed for a successful computerization effort.

All laboratory computerizations need to proceed through a series of steps, which include (1) needs assessment, (2) organizing for computerization, (3) feasibility study, (4) system design/system selection, (5) implementation, and (6) maintenance and future planning. The majority of the computerization effort (about 80%) occurs before the system is implemented. If that degree of effort is not provided before implementation, numerous problems and additional expenses may occur.

NEEDS ASSESSMENT

Needs assessment evaluates whether a computer system is cost-effective. This is determined by the laboratory specimen volume and mix, the data management needs, the laboratory's financial resources, and the availability of a system to satisfy the laboratory's needs. Because of CLIA '88, nearly all laboratories with more than one cytotechnologist will find an appropriate computer system cost-effective. Manual record-keeping for all CLIA '88 quality assurance and quality control is very burdensome and erodes into valuable (and expensive) cytotechnologists' time. Based on present cytotechnologists' salaries and shortage of qualified personnel, a computer system payback in increased productivity is likely within a 2- to 3-year period.

ORGANIZING FOR COMPUTERIZATION

Organizing for computerization has three basic components: (1) forming a computerization project team, (2)

Need	Anatomic	Clinical
Dominant data type	Text	Numeric
Specimen volume	Small numbers	Large numbers
Data input	Multistep, transcription, or keyboard	Directly on-line by instrument interface
Specimen reports	Extensive text	Limited characters
Report retrieval	Long-term/on-line	Short-term/on-line
Diagnosis	Essential	Ancillary
Data management motivation	Archival and correlative	Immediate patient management
Turnaround	Days*	Minutes*
How long significant	Years	Hours, days
Work load	Per slide/block	Per test

* Excludes reference laboratory work, cytology rapid analysis, and frozen section diagnosis.

T *32.1*
Data Processing Needs: Clinical vs Anatomic Pathology

educating the project team, and (3) studying the laboratory's needs and desires.

This organization requires true commitment of several of the laboratory's key personnel to the project. For success, the laboratory will need to have a knowledgeable contingent to interface between the laboratory, the potential vendors, and all the clients and administration related to the laboratory. This project team needs to have representation from the following areas: the laboratory director, laboratory manager, quality assurance coordinator, data processing coordinator, and hospital administrator (if applicable).

The project team needs a leader. This person should have organizational skills, be interested in the computer, and have intimate knowledge of the day-to-day workings of the laboratory. In a larger laboratory this team may be a committee directed by a managing cytotechnologist or pathologist. The amount of work involved in the computerization process makes it very difficult for one person to do all of the work needed.

The project team needs to thoroughly study and document the present data processing and management system used by the laboratory. The team needs to form a concept of how they would like to see the computer used in the laboratory. This should focus on the integration of the present system's data management with the physical attributes of the laboratory. It needs to systematically contact vendors of computer hardware and software to gather information on the systems available. Site visits to active facilities with systems are very helpful to see how the hardware and software are used. Demonstration software can be purchased to closely review some vendors' offerings. Some basic reading about computerization is important. This early work by the team should concentrate on information gathering and getting an overview of the computerization process. Intensive vendor involvement should be discouraged until the team feels comfortable with discussing all of the issues pertinent to the laboratory's needs and resources.

The team needs to compose a questionnaire and hold meetings to get input from all personnel about the pros and cons of the present data management system. Additionally, the needs of client medical staff and related departments (such as accounting, billing, communications, or legal council) should be reviewed. This project team will need several months or more of concentrated effort to get a true picture of the laboratory's present data management approach and what needs to be improved. A flow chart of the work flow is helpful in the design and implementation of a new system.

FEASIBILITY STUDY

With the knowledge gained in the organizational phase, the project team can determine what is realistic in terms of how the laboratory will be computerized. This begins with the development of a prioritized list of goals for the system, including definite needs and less essential components. The organizational phase should have allowed for an estimate of personnel time and costs of the present system. A list of benefits expected from computerization should be made to serve as a guide when reviewing available systems. If possible, a basic estimate of cost for the most complete system should be prepared. This cost can be used to see what the laboratory's resources will allow.

This step is completed with the formal discussion of the laboratory's computerization project with a "decision maker" in the administration to establish how much money is available for computerization and to get administrative approval to continue the process. It is critical to get an administrative commitment to complete this process before a system is chosen. It is unfair both to the laboratory and to computer vendors to proceed with discussions before the decision maker has committed to completing computerization. Subsequent steps involve significant commitment by vendors and laboratory personnel, including visits to the laboratory by vendors and visits to review systems in outside sites by the laboratory's computerization team.

SYSTEM DESIGN AND SELECTION

This is the first step of the computerization process where detailed review and discussions with vendors of hardware and software should begin. The data gathered in the initial steps by the team should be well documented to provide vendors with an understanding of the laboratory's physical characteristics, data management, and resources (financial and personnel). A computer system is a complex mix of hardware and software. The variety of choices, their advantages and disadvantages, and the rapid emergence of new technologies make decisions complex. The choices made must be based on an understanding of the laboratory's "prioritized needs" and resources. For financial and planning reasons most laboratories can assume that a computer system will have the capacity to serve them for at least 5 years.

A detailed discussion about hardware and software cannot be addressed in this chapter; however, some basic definitions would be useful. Hardware is the electronic equipment in any system. For proper planning it is critical to understand how and where data input will be accomplished in a particular laboratory. Terminals (typically a screen and keyboard) need to be placed in areas where personnel can easily input data, and enough terminals must be available to avoid "logjams." Computer memory and processing speed need to be adequate to support all the data input and output devices without aggravating delay. Archival memory should allow on-line storage of patients' files for 5 to 10 years (or more if desired). The system needs a high capacity data backup system (usually tape). Output devices include printers, the terminals, and floppy disks. In addition modems, fax systems, and other communication hardware are often desired.

Hardware can be configured in three basic ways. A stand-alone "single user" computer is unlikely to be sufficient for a sizable laboratory but may serve a very small one. In most situations, either a "network" of personal computers (PCs) or a true multiuser computer system (minicomputer to mainframe) is the best choice. The highly competitive hardware market and the very strong "network" software make a PC-based network very economical, easily expandable, and powerful. The power of these networks has forced true minicomputer multiuser system prices down to a competitive level. Hardware choices may be mandated by a vendor's software; however, it is best if the software is "portable" to a variety of hardware configurations. This will allow transfer to different hardware if dictated by future needs.

Software is the information used by a computer system to operate. There are multiple "layers" of software. A good analogy is the laboratory/office setting in a manual system. Software is knowledge, organizational information, and "skills" that are usable by the computer hardware. In a manually run office, human knowledge and skills are similar to software. The lowest level of software is machine language. This is electrical charges, positive or negative, that form binary code. In humans this would be like the nervous system's nerve transmissions in the brain and peripheral nerves that direct the body: they are not realized by us at a conscious level. Low-level computer languages are the next layer and were used with machine language to write the early versions of essential computer software, including the types called "operating systems." The operating system is the computer's instructions to organize the input terminals, central processing unit (the brain of the computer), internal memory (random access memory [RAM] and read only memory [ROM]), archival memory (hard disks, magnetic tape, floppy disks), input/output devices (printers, keyboard, screens), and any other connection points that are attached to the system. This level of software is similar to reflex responses, involuntary muscular control, and other patterned responses that take little or no conscious thought to elicit. A variety of software packages are made to further direct the actions of the computer. These software packages are often called applications software and can be written in a host of languages, just like human beings can communicate with each other in a variety of languages and dialects.

Applications software provide instructions that impart specific "skills" to the computer. The ability to type, format, and organize papers and text while checking for spelling errors would be a skill of a secretary; software that imparts this to a computer is a "word processor." The ability to organize, file, retrieve, and sort complex data or records would be a skill of a clerical/demographics specialist; software that imparts this to a computer is a "data base manager." "Spread sheet" software programs organize data into columns and rows and allow rapid calculations "down and across" to further analyze data, particularly for comparisons as individual data points are altered. "Communications" software allows the computer to use phone lines or other transmission systems to communicate with other computers or devices.

In the computer, memory is available to store data, just as file cabinets are available in an office and the minds of the personnel contain information. RAM is the memory the computer stores electronically as it is "thinking." RAM is lost if the power switch is turned off (just like a person's knowledge is lost when brain function is lost). Archival memory is more static and permanent, like paperwork in a file cabinet. Software designs vary as to how they use the computer's resources. Some software is written in a language that is "older" and less refined than more recently developed languages.

Some languages were made for special purposes, eg, financial work, engineering, and basic teaching. Programming languages are placed in two basic groups. Lower-level languages are ones that are usually older and require more lines of instruction to get the computer to perform a function. They often are more machine specific (that is, they run on a limited or specific type of computer and are not "portable" to another system). More recently higher-level languages have been developed. They may have a specific targeted use as in many low-level languages, but they are usually easier to read because they are written similar to English text. Normally, a limited amount of instruction can accomplish many more functions with high-level language and the software is portable to more computer types. The highest-level languages of this type are called "fourth level" development languages. In choosing a system, the software types, languages used, and their portability should be considered. Programs written in lower-level languages are generally more expensive to develop, alter, and maintain. They are often hardware-specific and may limit future changes.

The basis of almost all anatomic pathology software is a data base management system and a word processor. The word processor is not likely to be difficult to choose. In fact many laboratories have replaced typewriters with PC-based word processors. If a laboratory is happy with a word processor it already uses, maintaining the same software may be sensible and cost-effective. The data base management system is another story. This has to be specifically designed to meet the needs of all aspects of data arrangement, including all quality control and quality assurance functions. Most vendors have only begun to approach this problem, and the CLIA '88 regulations will require that they make significant new development efforts. "Older" systems written in low-level languages will likely be expensive and slow to test and "debug" (the process of correcting software errors).

The most significant problem in any software development is the programmers' understanding of the field or application for which they are programming. The optimal situation would be one in which a programmer would have intimate knowledge and extensive experience in the area that is being programmed. If a pathologist or cytopathologist was an experienced programmer, then the software developed would likely be optimal. Unfortunately, this is rarely the case. Development of software is a series of explanations to a programmer by experienced persons in the field. Programs go through hundreds to thousands of revisions in an attempt to reach what is desired. The first commercial versions of any software are often crude and may be very confusing to the user, but seem fine to the programmer. Any laboratory that has developed its own software understands the long, painful, and expensive process of development. Also realize that just about anything can and will be promised by a computer vendor. Unfortunately, laboratories are not likely to realize how expensive extra development and programming will cost.

The above information helps form a basis for understanding some suggestions about system design and selection. The physical design of a system is dependent on (1) the laboratory's physical characteristics and personnel's functions, (2) the laboratory's work load, work flow, and specimen mix, (3) the laboratory's need to electronically communicate with clients via a modem, fax or hospital information system, and (4) the characteristics of the software/hardware chosen.

Whenever a system is designed, it has to comply with the vendor's requirements as well as the laboratory's. The vendor should be able to offer options for hardware to fit a range of budgets. The laboratory should not expect that a vendor will have all that is "wished" for by the laboratory, especially if a budget is limited. If options allow growth of a system at a reasonable cost it is often best to add hardware as needed and initially invest in more complete software.

Selecting a system from a vendor can be approached in two basic ways: by request for information or by request for proposal. Request for information is submission of the basic laboratory's needs with a series of questions to be answered by the vendor and is more commonly used in a smaller less complex situation. Request for proposal is a very detailed proposal submitted to a vendor that requires a complete and detailed response. Request for proposal is used more for complex situations where extensive development or customization is needed. As better systems become available with features desired by most laboratories, request for information will most likely be the most common approach.

The question of an integrated pathology system for clinical and anatomic pathology vs two separate systems frequently arises. Although "theoretically" integration seems best, in reality it is usually difficult to achieve, is much more costly, limits the choices of software, and functionally may be cumbersome. An integrated package, if the anatomic component is poor, is likely to be much less efficient than separate systems of good quality. "Interfacing" (developing communication links between software using different languages) is becoming increasingly more efficient and simple, but some vendors make it very difficult to accomplish. This may be a self-serving attitude to limit or block competition with their own software, particularly if they have good clinical pathology software and poor anatomic pathology software. Beware of a contract with a system vendor that blocks an interface (at a reasonable price) or prohibits the concurrent use of any software other than that which is installed.

There is often little advantage to integration particularly if an inexpensive interface is feasible. Even if an interface is not immediately available, a single clinical pathology system terminal in the anatomic pathology area is nearly as efficient. Separate terminals may require an occasional need to transpose clinical pathology data (usually some limited hematology results) into the anatomic system. In reality this is very inexpensive and requires little personnel time. An expensive interface to perform such a limited function may not be justified either in personnel cost or convenience. Technology does exist at limited cost to provide "terminal emulators" to easily and inexpensively provide interfaces with most systems, if vendors allow. Additionally, anatomic pathology and clinical pathology aspects of computerization are different enough or competitive enough when integrated to further justify separate hardware/software systems. The two areas often grow at different rates, have different maintenance needs, and have peak system demand times that conflict. In an integrated approach, when the system is down, the entire laboratory is at a standstill. With two systems, this is avoided. Nothing is more aggravating to anatomic pathology personnel than slow response times and limited archival memory due to the "priority" of clinical pathology functions on an integrated system. A hospital-wide computer system that includes the laboratory is even more likely to have very weak or nonexistent software for a laboratory's (particularly cytology's) special needs. The scenario of a hospital administrator forcing a system on a laboratory because a hospital-wide system is "best" is common in the small hospital setting.

Use caution when accepting a vendor's proposal to "develop" a system on-site. This will be a long and painful process during which the laboratory will invest many hours teaching programmers what is needed (so they can sell it somewhere else). Debugging such systems is very expensive and time-consuming. Also, care should be taken when investing in very expensive "unique" hardware or software systems that only provide a very limited application. Do not expect that a system will be easily customized. A good system for any laboratory is one that appears to need very little alteration.

It is very unlikely that a computer will immediately create "free time" for laboratory personnel. Such promises should be viewed with suspicion. More realistically, the system will initially require more personnel time for data input and training. Once implemented, a well-designed computer system will produce a highly organized data management system with uniformity and efficient output of reports—benefits not easily realized in a manual system.

Laboratory data management software should have a system for security of data access, data integrity, and patient confidentiality. Data access is often secured by providing passwords for entry into the system. Many operating systems can provide initial entry security. At times a laboratory may wish to limit access to particular programs within a system. A hierarchy of passwords is available in many systems. A program that requires a password to access a choice from a menu could also satisfy this function. Data integrity can be maintained in a number of ways. Integrity basically reflects the control over data alteration and the identification of any person responsible for data input or alteration. A system should be in place to identify personnel that input data. Once data are entered, the system should provide checks to avoid a report being generated without all pertinent data being present and verify that the report is appropriate for the diagnosis rendered. The file should be "locked" once the report is issued. When a report is amended it should be clearly identified and the original report must be documented for retrieval. Electronic signatures are very convenient but require a password system to guard against unauthorized report completion. Patient confidentiality is best guarded by overall system or menu level security.

A system should be menu driven, that is a series of screens with designated choices should lead the user to the functions available. A computer system that seems very logical and easy to follow is often call "user friendly." User friendly systems have the following characteristics: (1) easy to understand menu or navigational system, (2) uniform terminology, (3) uniform keyboard function with special function keys to expedite commonly desired operations, and (4) menus and programs that complement work flow.

Data input by keyboard entry is unavoidable in most technical uses for a computer, particularly when free text and other language-oriented data are used. The use of a "mouse" (a small device that rolls on a desktop to direct an arrow on the terminal screen) has become popular to make first time computer users very comfortable. By using menus or "windows" the user can navigate throughout the programs in a more visual way. Windows programs employ symbolic diagrams (icons) on the terminal screen that activate a computer program when a mouse is used. Laboratory software will likely evolve into the use of windows; however, presently most is more "user obvious" than user friendly.

Specific software programs needed for cytology are important to do all the documentation required by regulations. The following should be available in a system:

1. Report generator in Bethesda format*
2. Quality control case indication
   a) High-risk history indicators*
   b) Abnormal case reviews*
   c) Unsatisfactory case reviews*
3. Quality control data entry and reports (laboratory and individual)
   a) Statistics for cytotechnologist*
   b) Work load adjustment based on quality control*
   c) Laboratory's quality control statistics*
4. Quality assurance data entry and retrieval
   a) Prior abnormal case review with screening*
   b) Retrospective negative case review for abnormal findings*
   c) Case completion requirements and turnaround time*
5. Quality assurance reports
   a) Specimen quality reports for clinicians*
   b) Abnormal cases' summary for clinicians*
   c) Abnormal cases' follow-up letters for clinicians*
   d) Laboratory yearly statistics*
   e) Cytology/histology correlation with diagnostic accuracy statistics*
   f) Work load statistics (cytotechnologists)*
6. Electronic signature
7. Ad hoc report generator

*Indicate CLIA '88 requirements that in a manual system pose a tremendous clerical burden on laboratory personnel, especially cytotechnologists.

Specific information to request from a vendor [**T***32.2*] and attributes seen in high-quality software [**T***32.3*] are shown.

IMPLEMENTATION

Once a system is chosen, implementation begins. This step consists of three aspects: preparations for implementation, implementation in parallel, and full system dependence. Implementation is about 20% of the overall computerization effort. If you reach this point and do not have a clear idea of what you have purchased and how it will be installed, you are likely to have many problems with implementation.

Preparation for implementation has two aspects: preparation of the laboratory and preparation of the software. Laboratory preparation consists of training personnel and modifying facilities. Personnel will need orientation to the software and hardware. The use of a demonstration package with realistic data can be helpful. You must always assume that personnel have little or no computer experience. The computerization team should take the lead in educating key personnel about the computer's features. A visit to a laboratory with the system in active use is helpful. Always train personnel just before actual implementation. Facility preparation consists of hardware installation. The placement of equipment and wiring may require additional furniture or even environ-

Demonstration of all aspects of the system
Source code in escrow
Programming language
List of hardware compatibility (portability)
List of active users (best if on-site visit of a user with similar volume and laboratory setting can be arranged)
Vendor support
Option of local hardware support
Program to train staff members
Information on downtime of other users on system
Programs to satisfy regulations
Cost breakdown including customization and maintenance

T *32.2*
What to Request From Vendors

Users learn rapidly with fast input/output time
Provides the type of reports needed as well as ad hoc reports
Uniform in its approach throughout the system
Provides sophistication with less effort
Allows customization, but little appears needed

T *32.3*
Keys to Recognizing Software Quality

mental changes (air conditioning, temperature and humidity control).

Software preparation consists of the customization of any programs (if needed) and installation of institution-specific files or dictionaries. Customization may be the modification of present programs or the generation of new ones. Both typically will cause additional expenses and delay. If possible, avoid any nonessential customization and development. All software must evolve and be updated to meet the changing needs of regulations and other factors, but customization purely for "esthetics" or "to match past formats" should be avoided. Such changes may even hamper the maintenance and updating of a system by rendering it nonstandard. Again, the key is finding a package that meets your needs and has a format similar to what you would create if you had to develop it yourself.

Installation of laboratory-specific files or dictionaries includes an editing of any vendor-supplied diagnostic files (eg, systematized nomenclature of medicine files) to modify entries to match the institution's nomenclature. In addition, a variety of files (such as referring doctors, personnel names, and other standard data) used in a relational data base are built by the laboratory. This may be achieved on an individual PC on-site prior to the full system installation.

Once the laboratory's system is physically installed and tested, the actual implementation in parallel can be scheduled. This "live" use of the computer is done simultaneously with the prior data management system. It is important to initiate a system in parallel, since unexpected equipment failure or software problems are possible and backup is needed. In addition, personnel will understand the computer's strengths and weaknesses when the two approaches are compared in parallel. This is obviously a stressful process since it increases work load by doubling the data processing and generating questions about equipment and software. This step may last a few days to weeks. If a laboratory is poorly prepared then this step is likely to be prolonged or may need to be aborted.

If implementation is successful in parallel, then the laboratory will be able to go to full dependence on the computer. A manual system is then retained only as a backup for unexpected equipment failures. Once this is achieved, the project team will immediately turn to monitoring the system, planning maintenance, and predicting growth needs.

MAINTAINING THE COMPUTERIZED LABORATORY

Any computerized laboratory will need a method for monitoring the system. A variety of ideas will surface to further enhance the efficiency of the system's function and software, and bugs or software flaws will inevitably surface. All of these need to be discussed, documented, and communicated to the vendor. This information will help correct problems and allow the development of better software in updated versions.

Typically, a computer system will need software and hardware support by a maintenance contract. Separate contracts for software and hardware may be better. Most vendors for specialized laboratory software are unlikely to be local. Usually a hardware maintenance firm is local. Since hardware repairs require a physical presence, a local hardware support firm is more likely to respond rapidly to a need.

Software maintenance at a distance is not difficult with the technology of modems and communications software. Fees for hardware maintenance vary with the equipment type. The annual fee for software maintenance is generally about 10% of the software cost. This is usually a fair fee and should be a good investment. Often routine software updates are included in this charge. If a laboratory does not buy a software maintenance contract, desirable updates may be very expensive and implementation may be delayed.

Any laboratory should closely watch its growth to predict future needs. In the computer system, the need for more hardware (both input/output devices and memory) may grow faster than a "case load" would indicate. It is likely that an active laboratory will outgrow a system within 5 to 6 years.

CONCLUSION

Laboratory computerization is a very complex and comprehensive process that integrates an "electronic" data manager into all levels of function. For optimal results the laboratory personnel must become intimately involved in planning and implementation. In most laboratories the process will take as long as 1 to 2 years (each step above will last 1 to 3 months) to fully accomplish. A dedicated team needs to direct the project and commit substantial time to self-education in addition to the orientation of other personnel. Successful implementation has tremendous benefits in the quality and efficiency of the laboratory service.

REVIEW EXERCISES

1. What are the basic steps in laboratory computerization?
2. Who should comprise the computerization project team?
3. What are some of the features of "quality software"?
4. What are the three basic hardware system configurations?
5. What are the two main types of software used in anatomic pathology?
6. When implementation begins, about how much of the computerization effort should be finished?

SELECTED READINGS

Aller RD. Computers in anatomic pathology. *Clin Lab Med.* 1983;3:133-147.

Aller RD, French R, Mitchell S, et al. Computerized reporting and follow-up of gynecologic cytology. *Acta Cytol.* 1991;35:15-24.

Aller RD, Robboy SJ, Poitras JW, et al. Computer-assisted pathology encoding and reporting system (CAPER). *Am J Clin Pathol.* 1977;68:715-720.

Elevitch FR, Aller RD. *The ABC's of LIS: Computerizing Your Laboratory Information System.* ASCP Press; 1989.

McNeely MDD. *Microcomputer Applications in the Clinical Laboratory.* ASCP Press; 1987.

Weilert M, Aller RD, Pasia OG. System selection lessons learned the hard way. *CAP Today.* March 1991.

CHAPTER

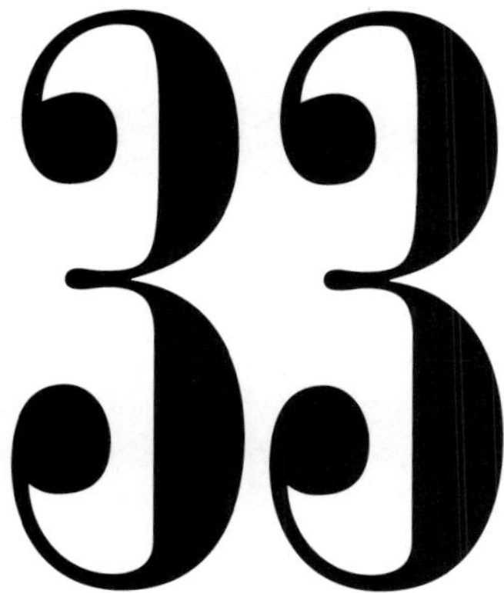

Quantitative, Analytic, and Automated Cytology Techniques

George L. Wied, MD, FIAC

CONTENTS

INTRODUCTION AND HISTORIC REVIEW

In 1924, Feulgen and Rossenbeck described their stain, which subsequently proved to be specific for double-stranded DNA. In the 1940s, Caspersson and Santesson measured fluorescence intensity and distribution of DNA, RNA, and proteins in individual cells and documented some fundamental differences between benign and malignant cells. In the 1950s, Mellors et al at the Sloan Kettering Institute applied the quantitative concept to the study of exfoliated human cells, using the fluorochrome berberin sulfate, and observed measurable differences of fluorescence between benign cells and cancer cells. Reagan et al and Patten introduced the concept of determining planimetric and cellular shape analyses into objectivation of cytologic diagnoses. Atkin was the initiator of studies using cytophotometry on tumors of the female genital tract and of breast.

Modern instruments use either static image analysis systems to measure cell components in smears or flow cytometry systems that use a suspension of single cells or cell nuclei. Analytic and quantitative cytology has two fundamental purposes: (1) to gather information of prognostic and therapeutic value, and (2) the construction of systems or machines that will complement the human eye in the performance of tedious and not easily reproducible tasks, such as the screening of cervical smears.

Flow cytometry for the determination of DNA content provides useful information only when very rigid criteria for the performance and interpretation are maintained. A cooperative study by five experienced laboratories demonstrated that this is not a trivial task. Since flow cytometric material always contains normal and tumor cells in practically all tumor cell suspensions, problems are encountered in detection of tetraploid tumors in lesions of the breast, the ovaries, and the colon. The methodologic difficulties in detecting tetraploidy by flow cytometry may be responsible for the controversy concerning the prognosis of tetraploid lesions.

When Hedley et al presented a technique to use paraffin-embedded material for flow cytometry, it seemed that this initiated a new vista for flow cytometry. However, in the meantime investigations by several authors, among them Berlinger et al, Cornelisse and Van Driel-Kulker, Frierson, and Jacobson et al, demonstrated that flow cytometric results differ when they are performed on fresh as compared with paraffin-embedded material. Additionally, rather high coefficients of variation were shown on paraffin-embedded material by de Vere et al, Cornelisse and Van Driel-Kulker, Quirke et al, and Wils et al. Tumors with near diploid stemlines may be classified as diploid because of the low resolution. This may be of critical prognostic importance, since Iversen showed on ovarian lesions that some of these near diploid tumors have the same poor prognosis as aneuploid tumors.

Image cytometry and flow cytometry each offer certain advantages and disadvantages. For many objectives the simultaneous use of both methods is proposed. A comparison between the two techniques is shown [**T** *33.1*].

Most of the information gathered on human cancer is retrospective, based on an analysis of archived material, be it aspiration smears or tissue blocks. Based on DNA measurements, human cancer can be divided into three groups. One group consists of a group of tumors wherein the DNA measurements appear to be of clinical value. A good example is the epithelial tumors of the bladder, wherein the diploid pattern corresponds to low-grade papillary tumors and the aneuploid DNA pattern to high-grade tumors and flat carcinoma in situ, a lesion that is the source of most invasive bladder cancers. The DNA measurements are of help in discriminating between bladder tumors of intermediate grade, which are about equally divided into diploid and aneuploid groups, with some evidence, mainly provided by Tribukait, that DNA patterns may be translated into behavioral differences. Another example is carcinoma of the prostate, wherein Koss et al showed in prospective and retrospective studies that tumors in the diploid range of DNA are much less likely to be aggressive than aneuploid tumors. The correlation between ploidy and histologic or cytologic patterns in the prostate is poor. DNA measurements are therefore of benefit in this case. Keep in mind that even in this group of tumors there are exceptions to the rule.

In the second group of human cancers, the value of DNA measurements is contradictory and must be considered unproved as an independent criterion. Carcinomas of breast, colon, kidney, endometrium, and other common cancers belong here, and long-term prospective studies are still needed to shed some light on the clinical usefulness of DNA measurements in tumors derived from these sites.

Finally, there is a group of human cancers wherein the DNA measurements are not of prognostic value, chief among them the tumors of the thyroid gland.

While theoretically DNA ploidy of human cancers should fall into two distinct categories, diploid and aneuploid, in reality there are many problems of histogram interpretation. These became apparent in a large prospective study of benign colonic mucosa as a baseline study of colonic cancer performed by Weresto et al. While 75% of the histograms disclosed an approximately diploid pattern, corresponding to normal lymphocytes, 25% of the histograms displayed significant variations in the position of the diploid peak. High-resolution cell image analysis can be effectively used in the quantitation of estrogen and progestogen receptors.

AUTOMATED SCREENING

The examination of cells is a subjective procedure dependent on the skill and expertise of the observer as well

	Low Resolution Flow Cytometry	High Resolution Cell Image Analysis
Personnel requirements	Special training required	Standard cytotechnology training
Sample preparation	Specially prepared complex single cell suspension	Existing, routine smear
Staining	Specific fluorochromes	Routine (Pap) or stoichiometric
Number of cells required	Tens of thousands, minimum	A few hundred, minimum
Cytometric features		
DNA Content	Yes	Yes
Size	Yes	Yes
Shape	No	Yes, with appropriate instruments
Texture	No	Yes, with appropriate instruments
Color	No	Yes, with appropriate instruments
Principal single parameter	Histograms of fluorescence (DNA content)	Histograms of digitized images based on light absorption or emission (DNA, steroid receptors)
Two or more parameter measurements	Limited to two (DNA vs oncogenes)	Synchronous or sequential
Visual control during measurement	None	Yes
Sorting	With sophisticated sorter only (after measurement)	Electronic sorting or selective scanning (selective enrichment)
Reexamination by reviewer of archived material	Impossible	Simple
Specimen retention as permanent record	Impossible	Simple
Comparisons of 2 reactions on the same cell	Impossible	Simple with motorized stage
Usefulness for histologic samples	Limited	Yes

* Modified from Koss LG. *Diagnostic Cytology and Its Histopathologic Bases.* 4th ed. Philadelphia, Pa: JB Lippincott Co; 1992:1616.

T*33.1*
*Comparison of Flow Cytometry and Image Cytometry Techniques**

as the time devoted to reviewing the slide. As such, it is fallible. No accurate, cost-effective automated system exists or is in commercial production at this time that would provide an objective analysis of the sample analogous to that available from the clinical hematology laboratory.

Historically, the attempt to automate cytologic screening used two major approaches: (1) high-resolution cell image analysis (cytoanalyzer) and (2) flow through cell analysis (Kamentsky et al). Flow cytometry as a screening technique for the early detection of ectocervical, endocervical, and intrauterine lesions is undoubtedly an inefficient, uneconomical experiment on the wrong anatomic site. It was a failure when it was conceived by Kamentsky et al, as shown by Koenig et al, and continues to be a dismal failure ever since. If fully automated or interactive diagnostic computerization is ever used and practically applied to the cytomorphologic screening for uterine lesions, it will be by high-resolution cell image analysis.

Prewitt and Mendelsohn used the modified cytoanalyzer, then called CYDAC, for an image analysis system for the classification of leukocytes. Subsequently, we developed TICAS (taxonomic intracellular analytic system) for the analysis of cells in cervical smears. Among the important design goals of TICAS was the establishment of standardized visible and subvisual diagnostic cell features. The introduction of computerized cell image analysis of the vaginal/cervical cell sample by the TICAS method was followed by many more or less futile attempts to introduce full automation of the gynecologic cell evaluation in Germany, England, Holland, Japan, Sweden, and the United States.

Many millions of dollars were spent in research and development funds in an attempt to fully automate the cytologic screening of the vaginal/cervical specimen. The idea was to automate a rather tedious screening job by a device that would not only be more accurate than cytotechnologists, but fully screen the entire slide, provide reproducible results, and do this quickly and in an economic fashion.

Why then are we not developing a fully automated high-resolution scanning system for gynecologic material? Why did so many attempts fail? The answers are relatively unsophisticated:

1. A fully automated device that reads the entire cell population of a given sample requires a monolayer of cells, which means that the material has to be put first in suspension and then placed with a rather sophisticated system on a glass slide. This is time-consuming for the clinician and the laboratory. Such a complex front-end system existed—probably the only one in actual operation in the 1980s—for the CYBEST System of Toshiba. Toshiba discontinued their entire automation effort in 1986.
   Automated systems that use the routinely prepared cell sample rather than a monolayer of cells will by necessity operate only on those cells that are "machine-readable," ie, on less than the entire specimen or on selected areas only.
2. The clinician expects a cytologic screening to provide information regarding vaginal microbiology, degree and type of infection (eg, human papilloma virus, trichomoniasis, herpes, etc), site of infection, hormonal classification, and identification of precursors of squamous and glandular cell lesions. The clinician expects definitely more than only "squamous cancer present" or "no squamous tumor cells found." The computerized image recognition of an actual malignant squamous tumor cell is a trivial computer identification routine. This has lead some bioengineers to believe that the entire task of fully automating diagnostic cytology is that simple. In fact, no automated system was or is being programmed to discern microbiologic entities and effects of human papilloma virus infection, to distinguish parabasal cells due to metaplasia from those due to epithelial atrophy, to clearly identify present well-differentiated adenocarcinoma cells, or to classify precursors. However, it is not the main goal of a screening system to identify the frank malignant tumor cells, but the precursor conditions and the clinically important alterations in nonmalignant cells and their "background."
3. The sample's quality has to be classified as "adequate," "inadequate," or "readable, but less than optimal, due to...." This is sometimes overlooked by instrument developers. In fact, in 1968, the Vickers Company in England announced with great pride, at a cytology conference in Cardiff, Wales, the completion of an automated screening instrument that was so poorly conceived that it could not even tell if there were or were not cells in the sample. It was thus an utter medicolegal monstrosity. The human observer can readily distinguish a well-fixed or well-stained sample from a poorly fixed or badly stained specimen, or an adequate sample from an inadequate or just barely readable sample. However, for a fully automated system, this is a very computer-intensive and time-consuming decision to make. On the other hand, if one has to place the slide under a microscope so that a human observer may scan the smear for sample adequacy, one can read it fully while one determines the quality and may not need an automated system, unless the automated system is significantly superior to human interpretation.
4. Any automated biologic device must, by necessity, set a threshold beyond which a sample is either classified "positive" vs "negative," or "alarm" vs "no alarm." It is medicolegally and ethically inconceivable that a machine would be intentionally set at a threshold to miss malignant tumor cell populations. However, if the threshold of an automated device is set such that it will never miss any tumor cell population, there will be a relatively large number of "false alarms." False alarms cost computing time and human reexamination time. This increases the actual cost of operation.
5. Some designers of automated systems state that their system is "as good as an average cytotechnologist," citing statistics in the literature and reports about the occasionally poor performance of cytotechnologists and/or cytopathologists. By saying this, these developers forget that none of us want or plan to make diagnostic mistakes, even if occasionally we do. As a matter of fact, we are very unhappy with ourselves or with one of our associates when such errors occur. However, by saying "statistically cytotechnologists miss one out of 20 cancers or worse, therefore, I can set my machine to miss that many cancers also," one is intentionally designing an ethically and medicolegally unacceptable, automated malpractice system.
6. Finally, a fully automated diagnostic system may bring about medicolegal problems for the producer of the system and the laboratory that uses it, if it were to operate as an unsupervised diagnostic system that would thus be liable for diagnostic errors.

The Committee on Cytology Automation of the International Academy of Cytology (IAC) published guidelines for designers of automated systems. The standards are divided into two major groups: (I) Mandatory Conditions and (II) Highly Desirable Features:

I. Mandatory Conditions (*Conditiones sine quae non*)
   I.1. The system shall not be designed or constructed as to pass as negative any sample that contains malignant tumor cells;
   I.2. The system shall not flag more "false alarms" on normal cells than could be readily handled by visual manual review;

- I.3. The system shall not use up the entire sample or render the sample unusable for classical microscopic review; the pathologist must be able to examine the sample after routine staining;
- I.4. The system shall yield reproducible results on repeated scannings of the same sample (within appropriate confidence limits);
- I.5. The system shall have an internal calibration standard for quality control; and
- I.6. The system shall identify the inadequate (or empty) slide.

II. Highly Desirable Features (required for clinical application)

- II.1. The system should be able to demonstrate clearly the item that led to an "alarm" for subsequent review by a human observer;
- II.2. The system should include dysplastic cells in the alarm group and should not restrict itself to the identification of frankly malignant tumor cells;
- II.3. The system should detect and identify contamination and artifacts as such to avoid unnecessary human review;
- II.4. The preprocessing of the sample required to a given system should be convenient and inexpensive for the clinician and laboratory (worst case: a system requiring specific preprocessing that is more expensive than the entire routine classical work-up and evaluation while not offering improved diagnostic quality);
- II.5. Infectious organisms, such as trichomonads and fungi, as well as "footprints," as in herpes inclusions and koilocytosis, should be identified; and
- II.6. The system should operate cost-effectively.

To my knowledge, no fully automated system has been designed or developed that meets these criteria, and it is highly doubtful that a commercial system satisfying them will be operational in the foreseeable future. However, it is quite conceivable that an *interactive* system can be successfully developed that leaves diagnostic judgment largely to the professional and medical personnel. Such interactive systems, on the least sophisticated level, may simply be high-resolution cell image scanners that identify "alarms" in the smears, mark their coordinates on the slide electronically, and then replay these cells or artifacts to a human observer for visual reassessment and diagnostic judgment.

We designed such a prescreening alarm identification module that was used to scan the slide in relatively low resolution for alarms while it recognized and "discarded" erythrocytes, leukocytes, and normal squamous epithelial cells. Later, a high-resolution program using the same microscope reevaluated the "alarm," discarded artifacts, and attempted to classify the remaining cells. This system worked as far as the software and hardware were concerned, but did not comply fully to the above IAC standards and did not operate in an economic fashion.

DIAGNOSTIC CONSULTANTS: EXPERT SYSTEMS AND ARTIFICIAL NEURAL NETWORKS

The use of expert systems and artificial neural networks represents new approaches to the design of medical consultants. Both of these techniques fall into the domain of artificial intelligence: expert systems are knowledge-based programs designed to solve "expert" problems, while artificial neural networks are computational analogue to biologic neural systems that have the ability to "learn" by example. See the selected readings for recent publications that describe these two approaches in detail.

Years ago, expert systems had to be developed with major programming efforts and expenditure of huge sums of money, since most were developed from "scratch" using artificial intelligence languages such as LISP or PROLOG, and there were few commercially available "shells" available on anything less than a mainframe computer. This is no longer true; one can find suitable software packages that provide the novice a sufficiently structured system to enter the facts and rules necessary to specify appropriate action in appropriate cases. Much time is often wasted evaluating the expert system tools or shells. There are usually only minor differences between them. It is much more effective to select an expert system tool useful for the problem and do something with it, even on a limited scale.

Most expert system application domains involve uncertainty. Rule-based expert systems require a mechanism for managing and reasoning with uncertain knowledge. These mechanisms are usually referred to as uncertainty management systems. Many uncertainty management systems have been proposed; four of the most well-known are bayesian inference, the MYCIN certainty factors, the Dempster-Shafer evidential reasoning, and fuzzy logic. These four systems are commercially available in expert system tools and it is up to the user to select the appropriate system for the specific problem at hand.

Practically all knowledge outside of pure mathematics involves some degree or level of uncertainty. Uncertainty arises from limited measurement accuracy, fuzziness, deficient knowledge or lack of knowledge, or observability or sensitivity to initial conditions. The type of uncertainty most often experienced in applications exists when measurement devices with limited accuracy are used to observe quantitative parameters. Since these devices have limited accuracy and resolution, some degree of uncertainty is inherent in these measurements. Consider the display of measurements of DNA content in nuclei with a histogram showing four bins between 4N and 8N. Although, at least in our microTICAS system, the individual nuclear measurements are stored accurately, the observer of the histogram sees only bins of 4N, 5N, 6N, etc. Uncertainty due to real or perceived limited measurement accuracy is generally modeled as a random error.

Another important type of uncertainty is fuzziness. Fuzziness relates to the inherent vagueness of specific classifications or descriptors. Most knowledge obtained from human experts is fuzzy. Fuzziness may appear similar to randomness, but it differs significantly. Fuzzy uncertainty is not necessarily created by any random process. In this case the uncertainty arises from the fuzziness of the knowledge itself. Consider the concept of normal ("benign") and abnormal ("malignant") nuclear/cytoplasmic ratios. Evidently, a squamous epithelial cell with a nuclear/cytoplasmic ratio of 1:30 is a normal mature cell, and a squamous cell with a nuclear/cytoplasmic ratio of 1:1 is abnormal, not even considering other parameters. However, many if not most cells fall somewhere in between these extremes. Ignorance of one or more cellular parameters often causes uncertainty in other parameters. Uncertainty arises in practically all domains that apply to artificial intelligence technology. In cytopathologic and histopathologic diagnoses and prognoses, the expert system developer must deal with randomness, fuzziness, limited measurement accuracy, ignorance, and deficient or lacking observability.

An uncertainty management system is a set of mathematical algorithms or software shells for the management of uncertain knowledge. The system provides the ability to store, generate, and reason with uncertain knowledge. Since each system is based on different mathematical formalism and each assumes a dissimilar model of uncertainty, the selection of the appropriate one for developing applications in cytopathology and histopathology is often key to a project's success. Using the wrong uncertainty management system may compromise the system's performance, potency, robustness, and reliability. A system that ignores basic uncertainties may erroneously provide completely "certain" definitions and recommendations that may have very fragile performance. Space does not permit describing the various uncertainty management systems in detail; see the appropriate monographs and publications on the subject.

Expert systems assist in many levels of diagnostic cytology and histopathology, especially in an automated approach. These expert systems provide consultations much as a human expert would, and can be restricted to rather brief answers, actions, or recommendations. We are using expert systems of various levels of sophistication in a variety of applications:

1. Cytologic and histologic samples from a given patient are compared cytometrically, and the expert system decides for the purpose of quality assurance if the biopsy is representative of the cytologic sample.
2. Previously stored cytometric, histometric, and clinical data from patients are searched for patterns similar to that from a new patient. When such patterns are identified in the data base, the biologic behavior of similar previous lesions is checked, along with therapeutic history, and the clinician is provided with a comparative assessment for the recommendation of therapy and/or probable prognosis.
3. DNA ploidy measurements are assessed by the expert system, taking into account body site and type of material submitted for DNA analysis. The expert system sets prognostic criteria dependent on this information (as entered by the microscopist); eg, the system will react to hyperdiploidy differently if it occurs on material from the hematopoietic system as compared with squamous epithelium. It will also check the available data base for examples of this type of lesion and provide prognostic probabilities.
4. The cytologic sample of a gynecologic patient with an intraepithelial squamous lesion of the ectocervix is cytometrically evaluated and the data entered into a data base. When and if the patient is treated by laser or cryosurgery, the postoperative sample is rescanned 4 to 6 weeks after therapy and the original scannings are compared with the postoperative scannings. The expert system then compares the preoperative and postoperative cytometric findings and evaluates whether the therapy was successful in returning the ploidy pattern to normal. Future reexaminations are treated in the same manner, so that the expert system provides a mechanism for ongoing quality control and improved likelihood of success of the therapy.
5. The expert system may also be used to assess anamnestic data and compare these data in conjunction with cytometric data to alert the clinician about possible differential diagnoses. Meta-rules of the expert system may also be constructed to have a different set of rules invoked for a different set of input data; eg, if the anamnesis shows that the patient was born in England and now lives in Brisbane, Australia and exhibits dark nevi, the system flags the greater possibility of the presence of melanotic cells and consults accordingly. Or if a 65-year-old patient is obese, diabetic, and a nullipara, then rules are invoked to consider small squamous parabasal cells as "normally expected" and to be more alert to glandular cells from the endometrium.
6. Expert systems can also be used to evaluate subjectively obtained criteria on cytologic and/or histologic samples, such as the descriptive histometric clues a pathologist may use in diagnosis of a tissue specimen. Probabilities of various diagnoses for a given specimen may then be evaluated based on previous cases, together with an explanation as to why the expert system recommended a particular diagnosis.
7. In cytometry, expert systems are being used for scene segmentation (ie, delineation of nuclei and cytoplasm), for automated focus of the microscope, and for recommendations regarding optimal staining and fixation for a given case and the selection of appropriate filters if fluorochromes are used.

These are only a few of our applications of expert systems that are operational or in development. While expert systems are essentially based on rules comprised of "if" and "then" clauses by means of which the user can always trace how the system arrived at a given answer or recommendation, neural networks are nonalgorithmic and acquire knowledge by learning, essentially like how an infant learns to walk. Artificial neural networks are based rather loosely on the underlying mathematics of the processing in biologic neural systems, and are comprised of a great many very basic processing elements roughly corresponding to neurons. They are being used extensively in military reconnaissance to discern man-made objects and identify their possible military intention. They are also being used for voice and handwriting recognition. We have developed hybrid systems incorporating frame-based and rule-based expert systems integrated with artificial neural networks often operating as intelligent front-end processors to such systems. The use of artificial neural networks to interpret DNA ploidy spectra, essentially as sophisticated pattern recognition software, is one such example. Using trained artificial neural networks to analyze several hundred ploidy spectra from cervical neoplasias, we were able to obtain 20% better diagnostic separation between various classes compared with that obtained using a discriminant function classifier.

The usefulness of embedded artificial intelligence systems such as these will become increasingly evident in the near future, as more research centers enter this important field and as expert system shells and neural network software and hardware become available on inexpensive general purpose microcomputers. Their application will not lead to the replacement of cytotechnologists or pathologists, but will increase the objectivity, reproducibility, and accuracy of their work.

EXPECTATIONS AND THOUGHTS FOR THE FUTURE

What can be done using quantitative cytologic techniques to improve a potentially superior diagnostic technique and to assure that the quality of cytology stays at the cutting edge of modern development?

The expectation, which prevailed for about two decades, that monoclonal antibodies of diagnostic value can be found has not been verified with any existing substance, and there is not a single antibody known to date that would selectively react with cancer cells to the exclusion of all other cells.

Chromatinic surface texture criteria can be identified by computerized cell image analysis, but the clinical utility and reliability of these "markers" depends largely on the optical resolution of the scanning system and the experience of the investigators. Extensive research is required to determine the occurrence of cell texture changes relative to the distance from the lesion, therapy for the condition, and which diagnostic specificity and sensitivity the changes may have in a possible screening environment.

Quantitative cytology provides the eventual success in objectifying our cellular evaluations. DNA measurements are an important parameter, although not the only useful one in this endeavor. In addition to visual so-called global descriptors, such as cell size, shape, color, nuclear size, shape, density, etc, there are significant subvisual features. In the near future, a multitude of unresolved fundamental problems will have to be addressed. There need to be agreements on standards for sample preparation, fixation, and staining, including purity of dyes, nature of solvents, the pH, temperature of staining baths, image recording, microphotometric quality, data collection and representation, scene segmentation of the cell images, type and numbers of reference cells, and the hydrolysis procedure, if any.

The International Academy of Science has established a Task Force on Quantitation and Standardization that attempts to arrive at internationally acceptable standards on many of these fundamental problems. Assuming that such controls can be accomplished, quantitative and analytical cytology may eventually represent the technique at arriving at a reproducible and reliable diagnostic interpretation, and finally at the "biologic or diagnostic truth."

Automated screening for gynecologic cancer was the daydream of the 1950s and 1960s. No fully automated system worked economically and sufficiently accurately in a clinically useful operation. None of the systems evaluate the microbiologic, cytophysiologic changes (hormonal classification) and detailed information on inflammatory changes, although these are important data that should be obtained from the cellular samples. From the sublime (Toshiba system) to the ridiculous (Vickers system), several fully automated instruments were proposed, supported, and finally discontinued.

If automation has a place in screening cytologic samples, it will be in an interactive mode where the system scans the sample and shows so-called "alarms" to a human observer for final analysis. The accelerated scanning by modern parallel processing computers and the decrease of the prices of the processors may make an economical, interactive system a reality.

Some of us mistakenly expect artificial intelligence systems to produce miraculous results that could not be achieved by the best human brain. Probably only those expert systems with limited size and clearly delineated purpose will have clinical utility in the foreseeable future.

It may be assumed that many diagnostic operations, such as data handling, microscope control, and quality assurance projects, will have some or more artificial intelligence rules added, and in years to come expert systems will be part of many laboratory mechanisms without the user necessarily being aware that there is an artificial intelligence component present.

SELECTED READINGS

Armitage NC, Robins RA, Evans DF, et al. The influence of tumour cell DNA abnormalities on survival in colorectal cancer. *Br J Surg.* 1985;72:828-830.

Atkin NB. Modal DNA-value and survival in carcinoma of the breast. *Br Med J.* 1972;86:271-272.

Atkin NB. Prognostic significance of modal DNA value and other factors in malignant tumors based on 1465 cases. *Br J Cancer.* 1979;40:210-221.

Atkin NB, Richards BM. Clinical significance of ploidy in carcinoma of cervix: its relation to prognosis. *Br Med J.* 1962;2:1445-1446.

Bacus S, Flowers JL, Press MJ, et al. The evaluation of estrogen receptor in primary breast carcinoma by computer-assisted image analysis. *Am J Clin Pathol.* 1988;90:233-239.

Bahr GF. Frontiers of quantitative cytochemistry: a review of recent developments and potentials. *Anal Quant Cytol.* 1979;1:1-19.

Bahr GF, Bartels PH, Wied GL, et al. Automated cytology. In: Koss LG, ed. *Diagnostic Cytology and Its Histopathologic Bases.* 3rd ed. Philadelphia, Pa: JB Lippincott Co; 1979:1123-1186.

Bahr GF, Bibbo M, Oehme M, et al. An automated device for the production of cell preparations suitable for automatic assessment. *Acta Cytol.* 1978;22:243-249.

Baildam AD, Zaloudik J, Howell A, et al. DNA analysis by flow cytometry, response to endocrine treatment and prognosis in advanced carcinoma of the breast. *Br J Cancer.* 1987;55:553-559.

Bartels PH, Abmayr W, Bibbo M, et al. Computer recognition of ectocervical cells: image features. *Anal Quant Cytol.* 1981;3:157-164.

Bartels PH, Bahr GF, Wied GL. Information theoretic approach to cell identification by computer. In: Wied GL, Bahr GF, eds. *Automated Cell Identification and Cell Sorting.* New York, NY: Academic Press; 1970:361-384.

Bartels PH, Graham A, Kuhn W, et al. Knowledge engineering in quantitative histopathology. *Appl Optics.* 1987;26:3330-3337.

Bartels PH, Koss LG, Wied GL. Automated cell diagnosis in clinical cytology. In: Koss LG, Coleman D, eds. *Developments in Clinical Cytology.* London, England: Butterworths Co; 1980:314-342.

Bartels PH, Wied GL. Performance testing for automated prescreening devices in cervical cytology. *J Histochem Cytochem.* 1974;22:660-662.

Bartels PH, Wied GL. Automated image analysis in clinical pathology. *Am J Clin Pathol.* 1981;75:489-493.

Berlinger NT, Malone BN, Kay NE. A comparison of flow cytometric DNA analyses of fresh and fixed squamous cell carcinomas. *Arch Otolaryngol Head Neck Surg.* 1987;113:1301-1306.

Bibbo M, Bartels PH, Dytch HE, et al. High-resolution color video cytophotometry. *Cell Biophys.* 1983;5:61-70.

Bibbo M, Bartels PH, Dytch HE, et al. Ploidy measurements by high-resolution cytometry. *Anal Quant Cytol Histol.* 1985;7:81-88.

Bibbo M, Bartels PH, Dytch HE, et al. Rapid cytophotometry and its application to diagnostic pathology. *Appl Pathol.* 1987;5:33-46.

Bur M, Bibbo M, Dytch HE, et al. Computerized image analysis of estrogen receptor quantitation in FNA of breast cancer: a preliminary report. *Lab Invest.* 1987;56:9A.

Burger G, Ploem JS, Goerttler K, eds. *Clinical Cytometry and Histometry.* London, England: Academic Press; 1987.

Caspersson T, Santesson L. Studies on protein metabolism in the cells of epithelial tumors. *Acta Radiol.* 1942;46(suppl):1-105.

Coon JS, et al. Interinstitutional variability in DNA flow cytometric analysis of tumors: the National Cancer Institute's Flow Cytometry Network experience. *Cancer.* 1988;61:128.

Cornelisse CJ, van de Velde CJH, Caspers RJC, et al. DNA ploidy and survival in breast cancer patients. *Cytometry.* 1987;8:225-234.

deLaplace PS. Concerning probability. In: Newman JR, ed. *World of Mathematics.* New York, NY: Simon & Schuster; 1956.

de Vere White RW, Deitch AD, West B, et al. The predictive value of flow cytometric information in the clinical management of state 0 (Ta) bladder cancer. *J Clin Pathol.* 1988;139:279-282.

Dytch HE, Bartels PH, Bibbo M, et al. Computer graphics in cytodiagnosis. *Anal Quant Cytol.* 1982;4:263-268.

Dytch HE, Bibbo M, Bartels PH, et al. Computer graphics in cytologic and pathologic microscopy: tools for the clinician and researcher. *Anal Quant Cytol Histol.* 1986;8:81-88.

Dytch HE, Bibbo M, Puls JH, et al. Software design for an inexpensive, practical, microcomputer-based DNA cytometry system. *Anal Quant Cytol Histol.* 1986;8:8-18.

Dytch HE, Bibbo M, Puls JH, et al. A PC-based system for the objective analysis of histologic specimens through quantitative contextual karyometry. *Appl Optics.* 1987;26:3270-3279.

Feulgen R, Rossenbeck H. Mikroskopisch-chemischer Nachweis einer Nukleinsaure vom Typus der Thymonukleinsaure Praeparaten. *Hoppe-Seylers Z Phys Chem.* 1924;135:203-248.

Franklin WA, Bibbo M, Doria MI, et al. Quantitation of estrogen receptor and Ki-67 in breast carcinoma by the microTICAS image analysis system. *Anal Quant Cytol Histol.* 1987;9:279-286.

Friedlander ML, Hedley DW, Swanson C, et al. Prediction of long-term survival by flow cytometric analysis of cellular DNA content in patients with advanced ovarian cancer. *J Clin Oncol.* 1988;6:282-290.

Frierson H. Flow cytometric analysis of ploidy in solid neoplasms: comparison of fresh tissues with formalin-fixed paraffin-embedded specimens. *Hum Pathol.* 1988;19:290-294.

Galera-Davidson H, Bibbo M, Bartels PH, et al. Differential diagnosis between follicular adenoma and follicular carcinoma of the thyroid by marker features. *Anal Quant Cytol Histol.* 1986;8:195-200.

Greenebaum E, Koss LG, Elequin F, et al. The diagnostic value of flow cytometric DNA measurements in follicular tumors of the thyroid gland. *Cancer.* 1985;56:2011-2018.

Hecht-Nielsen R. Neural analog processing. *Proceedings of SPIE-International Society of Optical Engineering.* 1982;360:180-189.

Hedley DW, Friedlander ML, Taylor IW, et al. Method for analysis of cellular DNA content of paraffin-embedded pathologic material using flow cytometry. *J Histochem Cytochem.* 1983;31:1333-1335.

Iversen OE. Flow cytometric deoxyribonucleic acid index: a prognostic factor in endometrial carcinoma. *Am J Obstet Gynecol.* 1986;155:770-776.

Iversen OE. Prognostic value of the flow cytometric DNA index in human ovarian carcinoma. *Cancer.* 1988;61:334-339.

Jacobsen AB, Thorund E, Fossa SD, et al. DNA flow cytometry in metastases and a recurrency of malignant melanomas: a comparison of results from fresh and paraffin embedded material. *Virchows Arch B.* 1988;54:273-277.

Kamentsky LA, Melamed MR, Derman H. Spectrophotometer: new instrument for ultrarapid cell analysis. *Science.* 1965;150:630-631.

Koenig SH, Brown RD, Kamentsky LA, et al. Efficiency of a rapid cell spectrophotometer in screening for cervical cancer. *Cancer.* 1968;21:1019-1026.

Koss LG. Automated cytology and histology: a historical perspective. *Anal Quant Cytol.* 1987;9:369-374.

Koss LG. *Diagnostic Cytology and Its Histopathologic Bases.* 4th ed. Philadelphia, JB Lippincott Co; 1992:1613-1641.

Koss LG, Czerniak B, Herz F, et al. Flow cytometric measurements of DNA and other cell components in human tumors: a critical appraisal. *Hum Pathol.* 1989;20:528-548.

Koss LG, Greenebaum E. Measuring DNA in human cancer. *JAMA.* 1986;255:3158-3159.

Mellors RC, Keane JF, Papanicolaou GN. Nucleic acid content of the squamous cancer cell. *Science.* 1952;116:264-269.

Mellors RC, Kupfer A, Hollender A. Quantitative cytology and cytopathology. *Cancer.* 1953;6:372-384.

Ng ABP, Atkin NB. Histological cell type and DNA value in the prognosis of squamous cell cancer of uterine cervix. *Br J Cancer.* 1973;28:322-333.

Patten SF Jr. Sensitivity and specificity of routine diagnostic cytology. In: Wied GL, Bahr GF, Bartels PH, eds. *The Automation of Uterine Cancer Cytology.* Chicago, Ill: Tutorials of Cytology; 1976:406-415.

Patten SF Jr. *Diagnostic Cytopathology of the Uterine Cervix.* 2nd ed. Basel, Switzerland: S Karger; 1978. Monographs in Clinical Cytology, vol 3.

Pressman NJ, Wied GL, eds. *The Automation of Cancer Cytology and Cell Image Analysis.* Chicago, Ill: International Academy of Cytology; 1979.

Puls JH, Bibbo M, Dytch HE, et al. microTICAS: the design of an inexpensive video-microphotometer computer system for DNA ploidy studies. *Anal Quant Cytol Histol.* 1986;8:1-7.

Quirke P, Dixon MF, Clayden AD, et al. Prognostic significance of DNA aneuploidy and cell proliferation in rectal adenocarcinomas. *J Pathol.* 1987;151:285-291.

Reagan JW. The nature of the cells originating in so-called "precancerous" lesions of the uterine cervix. *Obstet Gynecol Surv.* 1958;13:157-179.

Reagan JW. Recent advances in the use of the cytological studies in the diagnosis of cancer of the uterus. *Acad Med N J Bull.* 1962;8:210-217.

Reagan JW. Presidential address. *Acta Cytol.* 1965;9:265-267.

Reagan JW, Bell BA, Neuman JL, et al. Dysplasia in the uterine cervix during pregnancy: an analytical study of the cells. *Acta Cytol.* 1961;5:17-29.

Reagan JW, Hamonic MJ, Wentz WB. Analytical study of the cells in cervical squamous-cell cancer. *Lab Invest.* 1957;6:241-250.

Reagan JW, Moore RD. Morphology of the malignant squamous cell: a study of six thousand cells derived from squamous cell carcinoma of the uterine cervix. *Am J Pathol.* 1952;27:105-127.

Reagan JW, Patten SF. Analytic study of cellular changes in carcinoma in situ, squamous-cell cancer, and adenocarcinoma of uterine cervix. *Clin Obstet Gynecol.* 1961;4:1097-1125.

Reagan JW, Scott RB. The detection of cancer of the uterine cervix by cytological study. *Am J Obstet Gynecol.* 1951;62:1347-1352.

Reagan JW, Seidemann IL, Patten SF. Developmental stages of in situ carcinoma in uterine cervix: an analytical study of the cells. *Acta Cytol.* 1962;6:538-546.

Tanaka N, Ikeda H, Ueno T, et al. Fundamental study for approaching the automation of cytological diagnosis of cancer and a new automated apparatus CYBEST [in Japanese]. *Jpn J Clin Pathol.* 1973;22:757-768.

Tanaka N, Ikeda H, Ueno T, et al. Fundamental study of automated cytoscreening for uterine cancer: new system for automated apparatus (CYBEST) utilizing pattern recognition method. *Acta Cytol.* 1977;21:85-89.

Tolles WE. The cytoanalyzer: an example of physics in medical research. *Trans N Y Acad Sci.* 1955;17:250-256.

Tribukait B. Flow cytometry in surgical pathology and cytology of tumors of the genito-urinary tract. In: Koss LG, Coleman DV, eds. *Advances in Clinical Cytology.* New York, NY: Masson Publishing; 1984;2:163-189.

Tribukait B. Flow cytometry in assessing the clinical aggressiveness of genito-urinary neoplasms. *World J Urol.* 1987;5:108-122.

Weresto RP, Greenebaum E, Deitch D, et al. Deoxyribonucleic acid ploidy and cell cycle events in benign colonic epithelium peripheral to carcinoma. *Lab Invest.* 1988;58:218-225.

Wied GL. Automated cell screening: a practical reality or a daydream? In: Evans DMD, ed. *Automated Cytology.* London, England:E & S Livingstone Ltd; 1970:43-47.

Wied GL. *History of Clinical Cytology.* 7th ed. Chicago, Ill: Tutorials of Cytology; 1992:1-36. Compendium on Clinical Cytology.

Wied GL, Bahr GF, eds. *Automated Cell Identification and Cell Sorting.* New York, NY: Academic Press; 1970.

Wied GL, Bahr GF, eds. *Introduction to Quantitative Cytochemistry II.* New York, NY: Academic Press; 1970.

Wied GL, Bahr GF, Bartels PH. Automated analysis of cell images by TICAS. In: Wied GL, Bahr GF, eds. *Automated Cell Identification and Cell Sorting.* New York, NY: Academic Press; 1970:195-360.

Wied GL, Bahr GF, Bartels PH. The taxonomic intra-cellular analytic system (TICAS) for cell diagnosis. In: Evans DMD, ed. *Automated Cytology.* London, England: E & S Livingstone Ltd; 1970:252-259.

Wied GL, Bahr GF, Bibbo M, et al. The TICAS-RTCIP real time cell identification processor. *Acta Cytol.* 1975;19:286-288.

Wied GL, Bartels PH, Bahr GF, et al. Taxonomic intracellular analytic system (TICAS) for cell identification. *Acta Cytol.* 1968;12:180-204.

Wied GL, Bartels PH, Bibbo M, et al. Computer recognition of ectocervical cells: classification of the efficacy of contour and textural features. *Acta Cytol.* 1977;21:753-764.

Wied GL, Bartels PH, Bibbo M, et al. Image analysis in quantitative cytopathology and histopathology. *Hum Pathol.* 1989;20:549-571.

Wied GL, Bartels PH, Dytch HE, et al. Rapid high-resolution cytometry. *Anal Quant Cytol.* 1982;4:257-262.

Wied GL, Bartels PH, Dytch HE, et al. Rapid DNA evaluation in clinical diagnosis. *Acta Cytol.* 1983;1:33-37.

Wied GL, Bartels PH, Weber J, et al. Expert systems design under uncertainty of human diagnosticians. IEEE Proceedings. 8th Annual Conference on Engineering in Medicine and Biology, 1986. CH 2368-9, Vol 25:757-760.

Wied GL, Bibbo M, Bartels PH. Computer analysis of microscopic images: application in cytopathology. *Pathol Annu.* 1981;16:367-409.

Wied GL, Messina A, Meier P, et al. DNA-assessment on Feulgen-stained endometrial cells and comparison with fluorometric values. *Lab Invest.* 1965;14:1494-1499.

Wied GL, Messina A, Rosenthal E. Comparative DNA-measurements on Feulgen-stained cervical epithelial cells. *Acta Cytol.* 1966;10:31-37.

Wied GL, Weber JE, Dytch HE, et al. TICAS-STRATEX: an expert diagnostic system for stratified cervical epithelium. IEEE Proceedings, EMBS-EMSA, Boston, Mass, November 1987.

Wils J, van Geuns H, Baak J. Proposal for therapeutic approach based on prognostic factors including morphometric and flow cytometric features in stage III-IV ovarian cancer. *Cancer.* 1988;61:1920-1925.

Zadeh Laffi A. Fuzzy sets. *Information & Control.* 1965;8.

CHAPTER 34

The Light Optical Microscope

Peter H. Bartels, PhD, FIAC(hon)

CONTENTS

Diagnostic clinical cytology is based on the microscopic assessment of cellular material. The light optical microscope is, therefore, the single most important instrument for the cytologist. Effective use of the microscope is not difficult to learn; the principles involved are simple. This chapter discusses the design and function of the light optical microscope; its component parts, alignment, and proper use; and procedures to follow when images lack clarity. To understand how to attain optimum performance and best use of the microscope's capabilities one has to know something about diffraction. A discussion of principles of image formation and diffraction is therefore provided. A brief survey of various optical methods in light optical microscopy concludes the chapter.

THE MICROSCOPE AND ITS COMPONENTS

The microscope shown [**F***34.1*] is typical of the many designs commercially available. While there are variations, all microscopes have the following components in common. The microscope stand (18) houses in its base the light source (1). A collector lens (2) sends a beam of light forward. A mirror (3) in the microscope base, often protected by a glass dust cover (5), sends this illuminating beam upward toward the substage condenser (6). Also mounted in the microscope base, somewhere between the collector lens and the glass dust cover, is a field iris diaphragm (4). Here, it is shown just below the dust cover.

The substage condenser can be focused up and down by means of a rack and pinion (9). The condenser is equipped with an iris diaphragm, the so-called aperture stop (7). The condenser usually contains two optical lens systems. The top element can, in some microscopes, be swung out of the way to allow the illumination of a very wide field of view under low power. As a rule though, the top element is in the optical beam path. With the top element in place, the condenser focus actually involves only very small adjustments. Under normal conditions the surface of the condenser's top element is almost flush with the microscope stage (10). The condenser can be centered by means of two centering screws (8). The stage can be moved in x and y directions by control knobs (11). In some microscopes the specimen is moved in x and y directions by means of a "mechanical stage" attached to a fixed microscope stage.

The slide with the object under a coverslip (14) rests on the microscope stage. The objective (15) is mounted in a revolving nosepiece (16), supported by the arm of the microscope stand (18). Built into the nosepiece, or immediately above it into the arm of the microscope stand, one often finds a tube lens (17). The nosepiece may allow the mounting of three to five objectives. Such a set of objectives usually includes a scanning lens of very low magnification, such as 3.2:1, a low-power objective of 10:1, a "high

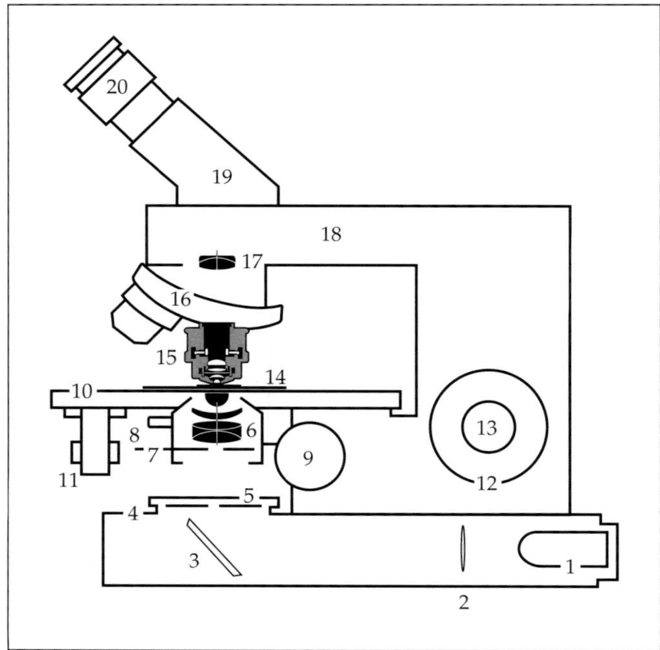

F*34.1*

Components of the light optical microscope.

dry" objective of 40:1, and an oil immersion objective of 100:1 magnification.

Focusing of the microscope is done by means of a coarse adjustment (12) and a fine adjustment (13). These two independent controls may be separated altogether, they may have two control knobs mounted coaxially, or they may be actuated by the same knob. In some microscopes focusing moves the microscope arm portion of the stand up and down. In other designs it is the stage that is moved; note that the substage condenser as a whole then moves with the stage. Recent designs move only the nosepiece with the attached objectives.

The microscope tube (19) attaches to the microscope stand above the nosepiece. It may be a binocular tube or a trinocular tube (which allows mounting of a camera or a video system). A slider with a reflecting prism then directs the light either into the binocular observation tubes or to the camera. In the binocular tube the beam is split by a prism system. The oculars (20) are merely inserted into the observation tubes, for ease of exchange.

For comfortable viewing it is important that the two oculars in their tubes are set to correspond to the interpupillary distance of an individual observer's eyes. This may vary from 55 to 75 mm. The adjustment is effected either by a control knob between the two tubes, a small lever , or simply by pulling the two tubes apart laterally. One of the two observation tubes may allow a small adjustment in tube length, to allow for the interpupillary distance adjustment. Oculars sometimes have focusable eye lenses; these may be focused sharply on a set of cross hairs or micrometer plates inserted into the ocular.

WORKING PRINCIPLES

As an object is viewed, its "apparent size" changes with the distance from which it is observed. From afar, an object may appear small; at closer view, the same object appears much larger. The "actual size" or the physical dimensions of the object have not changed, only the apparent size changes.

The lens in the observer's eye projects an image of the object onto a light-sensitive layer in the back of the eye. This layer is called the retina. The closer the object is to the observer and the larger the viewing angle, the larger is the area that the projected image covers on the retina. This is shown for two objects viewed under different viewing angles [**F***34.2*]. The retina holds individual light-sensitive cells called cones and rods. They are spaced with variable density; the closest spacing occurs in the foveal area, where there is most acute vision.

The average distance between light-sensitive cells is approximately 5 µm. Let it be assumed that the retinal image of an observed object covers an area containing, eg, 400 light-sensitive cells. Each of these cells contributes a signal adding to perception of the object. In effect, the object is represented by an array of 400 sampling points. These 400 points may well be sufficient to show the object with all the detail necessary for its identification. However, there may be occasions when finer detail is desired. This requires a "closer look," which is accomplished by simply getting closer to the object. It then appears under a larger viewing angle and its retinal image may now cover as many as 1500 points.

There is a limit, however, to the fineness of detail for perception with the unaided eye. When an object is brought too close to the eye, the eye lens can no longer focus its image onto the retina. The increase in viewing angle and of the retinal image are worthless; the retinal image becomes blurred.

How small an object can be seen with the unaided eye from a normal viewing distance? This is best answered by schematic drawing [**F***34.3*]. On the left is an object. Assume that two very small holes were punched, close together, into the object and held up against the light. The eye lens projects the two bright spots onto separate retinal cells. They are perceived as two tiny bright spots separated by a narrow dark space. The object is "resolved"—there are two spots and we see two spots. As the holes are punched closer together, they are projected onto two adjacent sensory cells or even onto the same retinal cell. Eventually, the holes are perceived as a single, oblong spot, or simply as a single bright spot. While the object would have been visible, it would not have been resolved in its true structure.

The smallest object structures that can be resolved with the unaided eye, from a normal viewing distance of 250 mm, are approximately 100 µm in size. To see finer detail, optical instruments must be used to increase the viewing angle. In the simplest case an enlarged image of the object may be projected and viewed from a convenient normal viewing distance. Home movies are an example of this principle. An object is projected onto a screen by a lens [**F***34.4*]. On the screen appears a "real image": it is actually present at the location of the screen. This image is viewed under a viewing angle that is much larger than that attained by just looking at the object itself from a normal viewing distance. The lens projecting the image faces the object and is, therefore, called the "objective." The objective is schematically indicated by a single lens [**F***34.4*]; however, actual objectives are often complex optical systems that, in the case of oil immersion systems for microscopes, may contain as many as 16 lens elements. Such objectives produce images of very fine detail and of structures that, even in the enlarged image, have not yet reached a dimension of 100 µm. This means that the image may contain

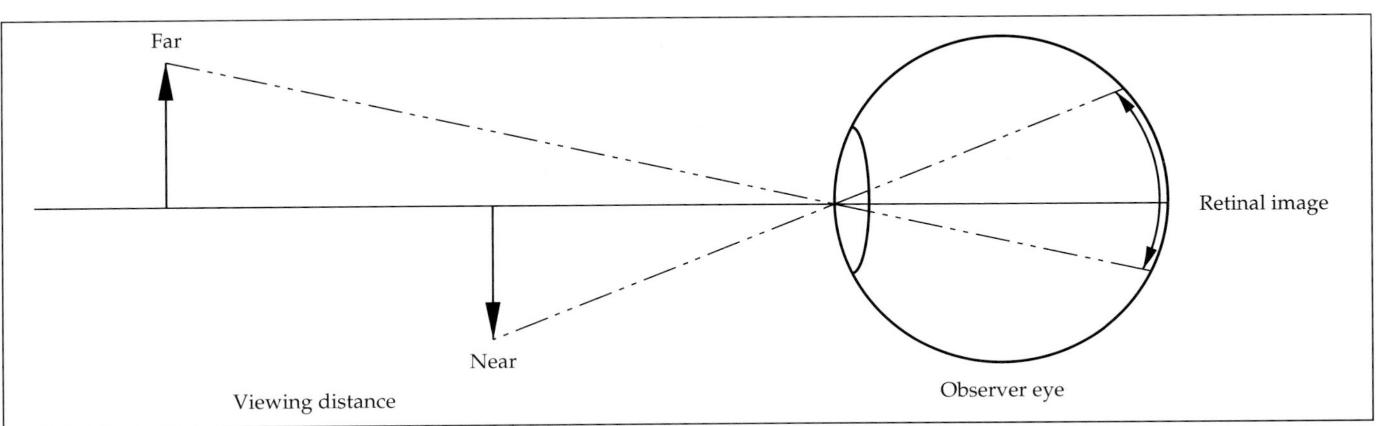

F*34.2*
Viewing distance and its relation to the size of the image on the retina.

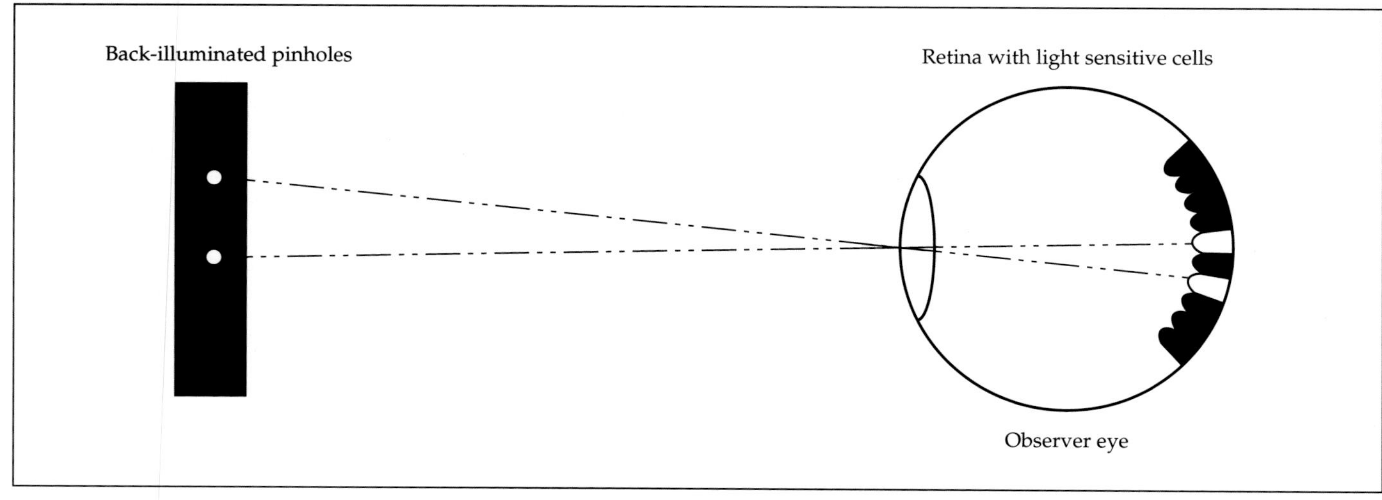

F34.3
Schematic representation of "resolution" in the retinal image.

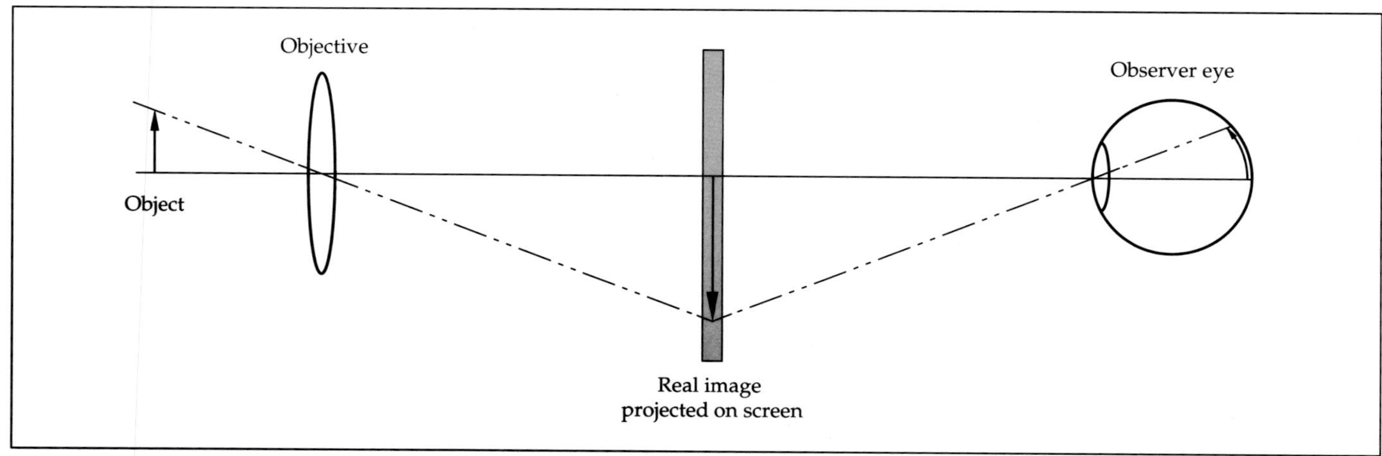

F34.4
Increase of viewing angle by employing an objective lens.

more detail than the eye can see. This problem is remedied by the use of an additional magnifier.

Magnifiers let a light ray in under a large viewing angle. The observer sees a greatly enlarged image of the viewed object [**F***34.5*]. The image seen through a magnifier is not really present where it appears to be. This is why such images are called " virtual images."

The magnifier used to look at the image projected by a microscope objective is called an "ocular," since it faces the observer's eye. The final magnification of the light optical microscope is thus reached in two stages. The objective projects an enlarged image, the "primary" or "intermediary" image. This is viewed through an ocular, which further increases the viewing angle. Systems of this kind are called "compound microscopes" [**F***34.6*].

It is important to realize that the resolution of the microscopic image is determined by the objective. Detail not imaged into the primary image plane by the objective is not presented in the final image: the ocular is merely a magnifier.

The intermediary image produced by the objective is a real image. It could be seen on a screen. The image seen through the ocular is a virtual image [**F***34.6*]. The objective contains several lens elements. The intermediary image is slightly reduced before it is formed. This reduction is introduced by the "field lens" located at the bottom of the ocular. The reduction makes it possible to accommodate slightly larger field sizes. The eye lens of the ocular projects the image out to infinity. For the observer it seems to come from far away, and one can make observations for hours without strain and with a relaxed, "infinity-adapted" eye.

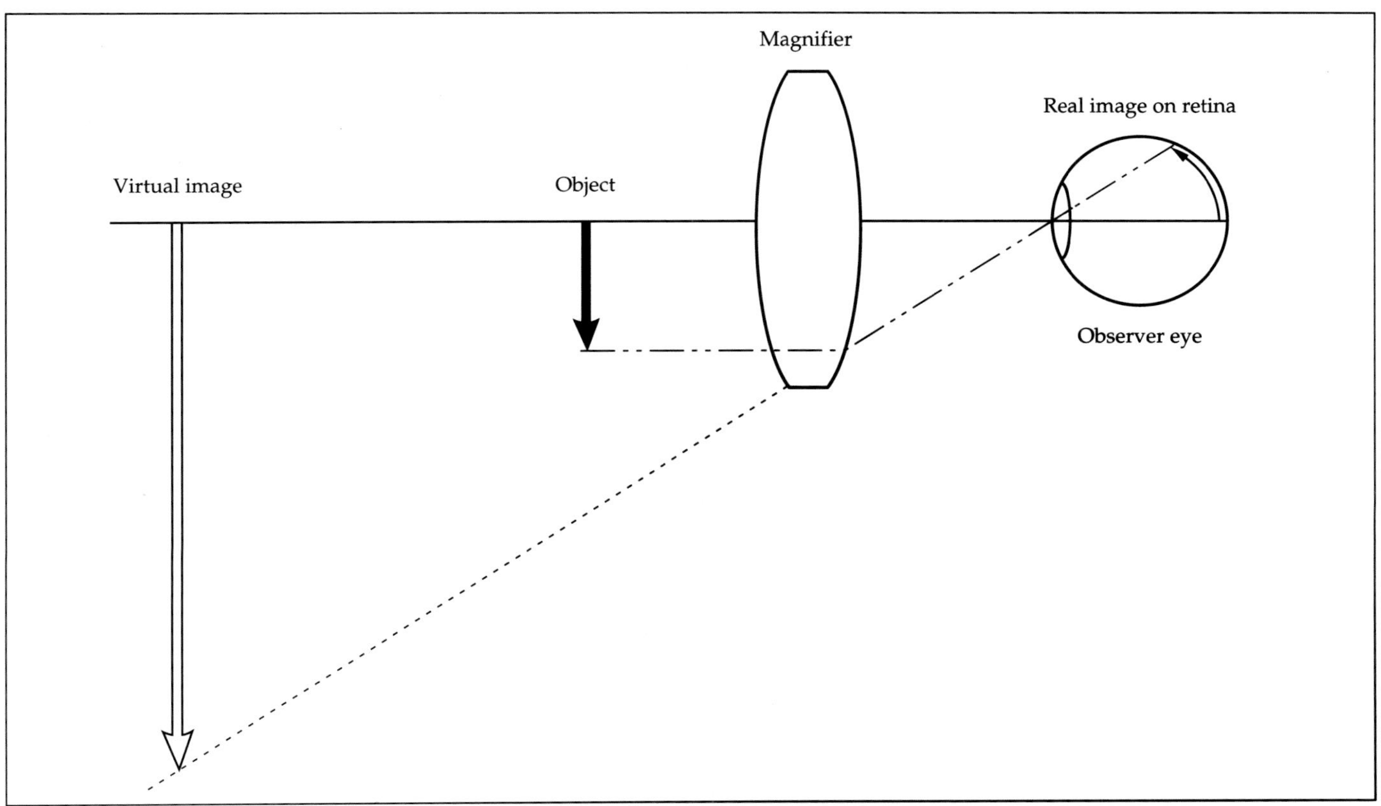

F34.5
Principle of a magnifier.

The microscopic specimen must be illuminated. This is done by means of a lens system mounted below the stage of the microscope, the substage condenser (or simply condenser), and a light source. The light source is usually mounted somewhere in the rear of the microscope so that its heat causes no problem. To gather its light more effectively, it is equipped with a collector lens.

All research microscopes and most of the better laboratory microscopes are equipped with two iris diaphragms. One is mounted in the substage condenser and is called the "aperture stop." The other is mounted below the condenser, usually close to the collector lens, and is called the "field stop." The function of the field stop is to reduce stray light, which interferes with image brilliance and contrast. When we use objectives with increasing magnification, we see a smaller and smaller area of the microscopic specimen. Yet, the condenser illuminates the entire specimen from below. Stray light originating in portions of the specimen that may not even be in the field of view may reduce the brilliance of the image. This is especially important in photomicrography. By closing the field stop to where it just encloses the object area seen by the objective the amount of stray light can be reduced significantly. The function of the aperture stop is to regulate image contrast. It thus has a direct effect on the attainable resolution. The **aperture stop is the most important control on a light optical microscope. It should never be used to regulate image brightness. To understand the working principle of the aperture stop it is necessary to briefly discuss image formation and light diffraction.**

Koehler Illumination

In a light optical microscope two distinct beam paths exist: the beam path of the transilluminating light [**F**34.7, left] and the beam path of the image-forming light [**F**34.7, right]. The direct light provides the uniform bright background; its beam path begins at the light source. The source's collector lens images the light source into the plane of the aperture stop of the condenser, which, in effect, becomes the source. The aperture stop is located in the front focal plane of the condenser, ie, the condenser sends a parallel beam through the object. This transilluminating, parallel beam enters the objective. It is focused by the objective in its back focal plane, another plane that is equivalent ("conjugate") to the light source. Finally, the direct beam comes to a focus again at the exit pupil of the microscope—at the "eye point" approximately 1 cm above the ocular. The exit pupil of the microscope is the plane where the

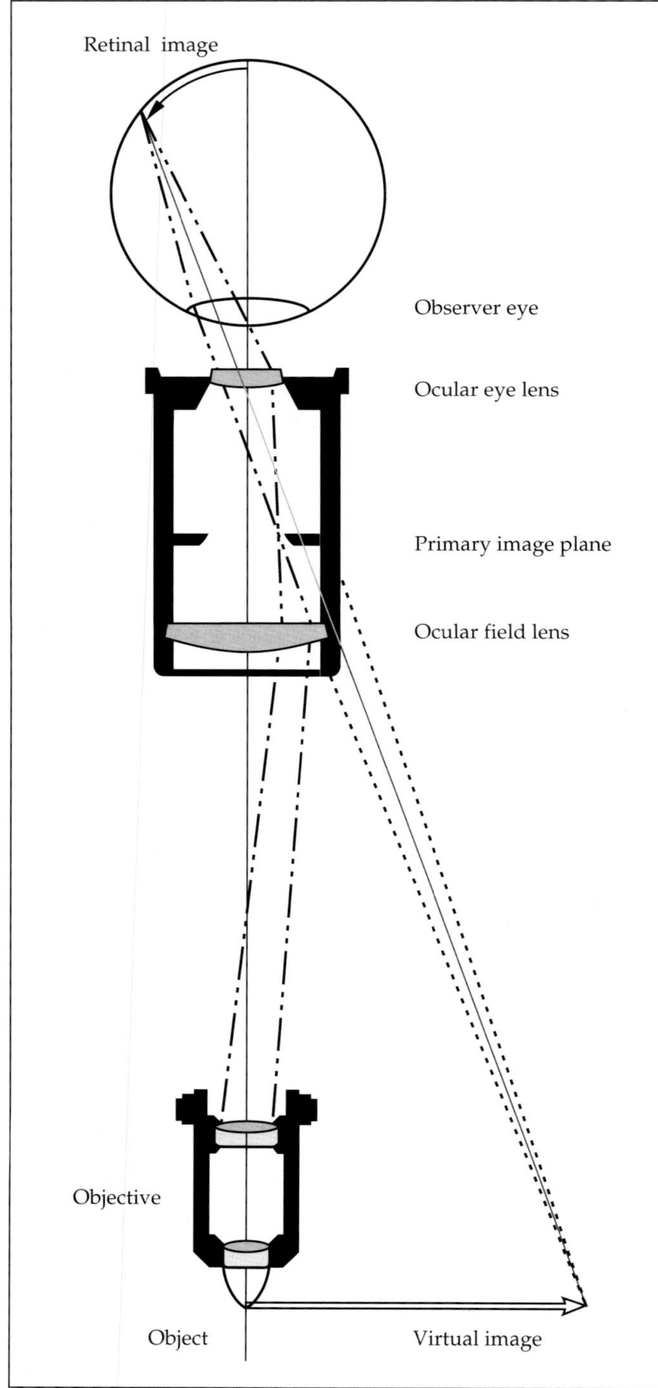

F34.6

Compound microscope.

pupil of the observer's eye should be positioned, so that there is a match between the exit pupil of the microscope and the entrance pupil of the eye. There are thus four conjugated planes in the direct beam path in simultaneous focus: light source, aperture stop, objective back focal plane, and microscope exit pupil.

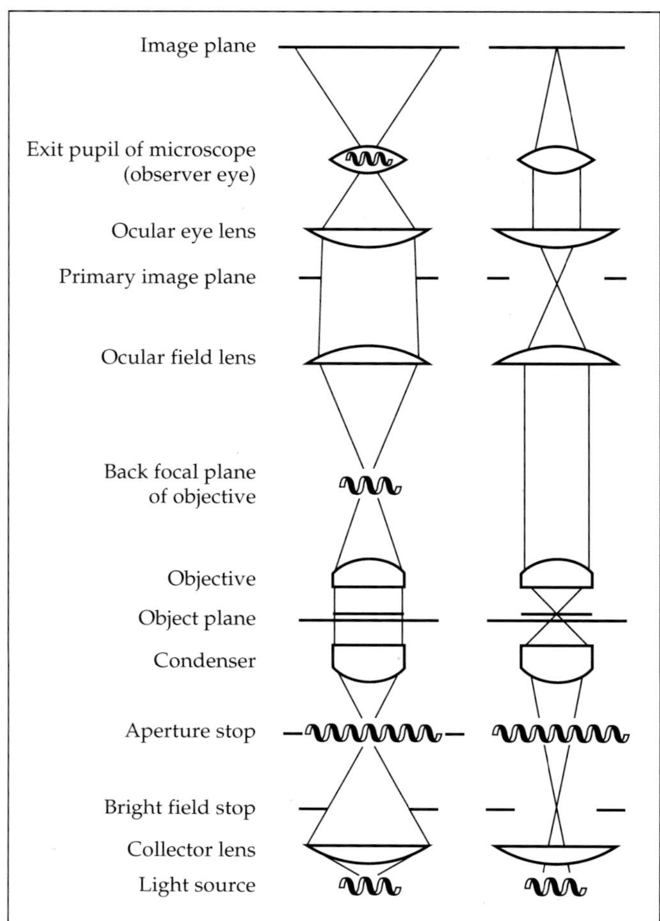

F34.7

Beam paths in Koehler illumination (left, transilluminating light; right, image-forming light).

The beam path for the direct light is shown for an on-axis beam [**F**34.7]; an off-axis beam transilluminating the specimen is also shown [**F**34.8]. It originates off center, at the source filament, and comes to a focus at the edge of the aperture stop, in the front focal plane of the condenser. It also passes through the specimen as a parallel beam—under an angle determined by how far the aperture iris had been opened. It is a parallel beam nevertheless. The steeper the angle of the light transilluminating the specimen, or "the higher the aperture of the illumination," the farther towards the periphery it will be focused in the back focal plane of the objective.

In the image-forming beam path there are also four conjugated planes. The first is the plane of the field stop. The field stop is imaged sharply into the object plane by the condenser. The object plane is the second conjugated plane. It is imaged by the objective into the primary image plane, inside the ocular. The ocular projects the image to infinity, and the observer's eye lens finally focuses the microscopic image onto the retina.

A light microscope set up so that these two beam paths coexist is an example of "Koehler illumination," named

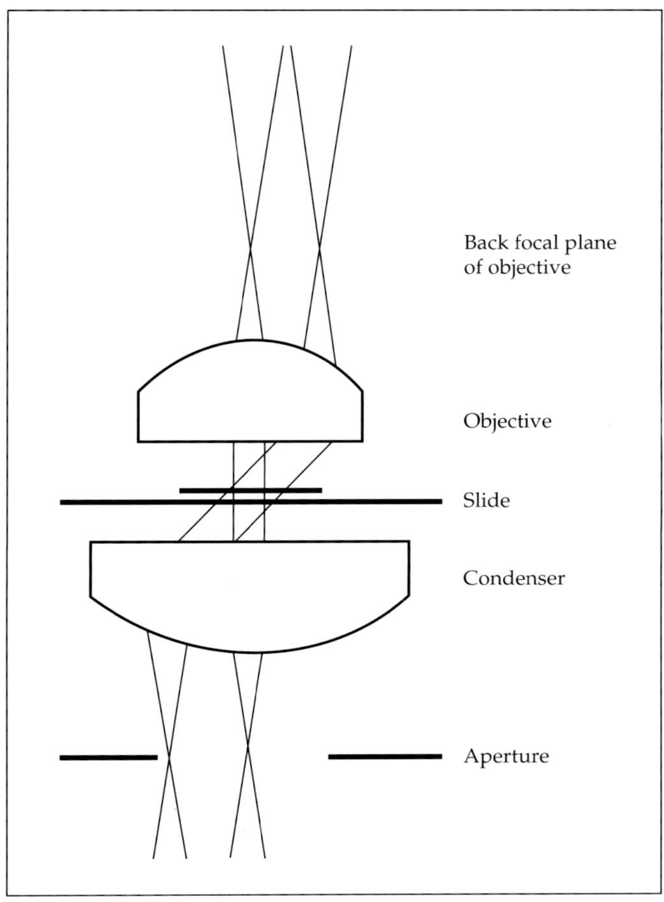

F34.8
Transillumination of object by parallel beams.

after Dr August Koehler, of Carl Zeiss, Jena, Germany (1866-1948). Koehler illumination provides uniformity of illumination and conditions for which image formation is theoretically well understood.

Image Formation in Light Optical Microscopy

The propagation of light through an optical system is commonly illustrated by "geometric optics": light beams are shown in their extension and direction by drawing straight lines, so-called "rays of light." Geometric optics are an eminently useful method to design optical systems, to show how beams of light diverge or converge. Rays are shown as they bend sharply at precise angles when refracted by an optical element, or reflected at a surface. Geometric optics shows rays intersecting to form a mathematically fine focal point.

Geometric optics are, however, a simplified abstraction that provides valid predictions only under conditions where light interacts with relatively large objects, such as lenses, prisms, and mirrors. Geometric optics ignores the wave

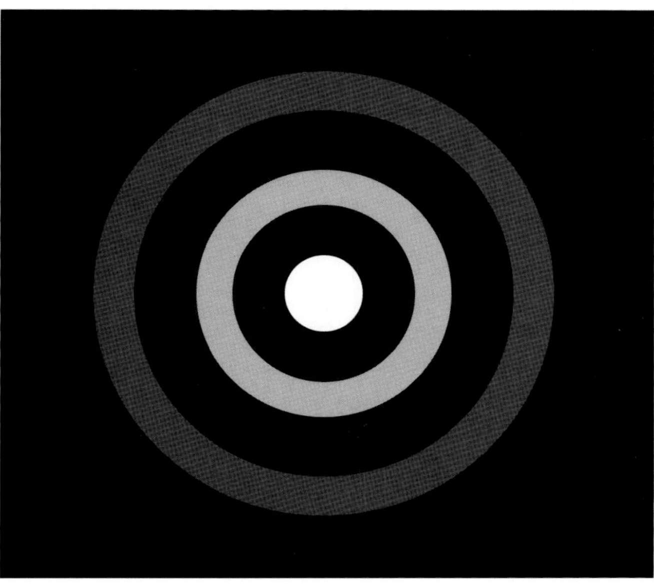

F34.9
Schematic representation of the diffraction pattern for a high-aperture objective.

nature of light. Geometric optics, therefore, implies infinitely fine resolution. In reality, light propagates as electromagnetic waves. The wave field has a distinct structure: there is the amplitude of the electromagnetic field, the frequency of the radiation, and the divergence of the wave fronts. The imaging of an object point into an image point, realistically, has to be represented by the process where focus is the point of greatest constriction of the wave field. Geometric optics with its rays and mathematically sharp image points assumes the wavelength to be zero. Under this assumption all objects are large compared with this inherent structure of the wave field. "Resolution" is infinite in geometric optics. In the real world, waves interact with objects. When the objects or their structures are comparable in size to the wavelength of light, one has to consider diffraction theory. Most certainly this applies when one discusses the limit of resolution of the light optical microscope.

The image of a small, back-illuminated pinhole is not simply a sharply delineated small round spot. Rather, the object is imaged as a "diffraction pattern." A central bright maximum is surrounded by a series of dark and bright rings, decreasing rapidly in brightness [**F**34.9]. The diameter of the central maximum is determined by the numerical aperture of the objective and by the wavelength of light. It is independent of how small the pinhole in the object plane actually is: it is as small a point as the particular objective is able to image. The diffraction pattern is characterized by the "point spread function" of the objective. The higher the numerical aperture of the objective, the smaller is the half-intensity diameter of the point spread function [**F**34.10]. When the point spread function is as sharply defined as the objective's design specifications

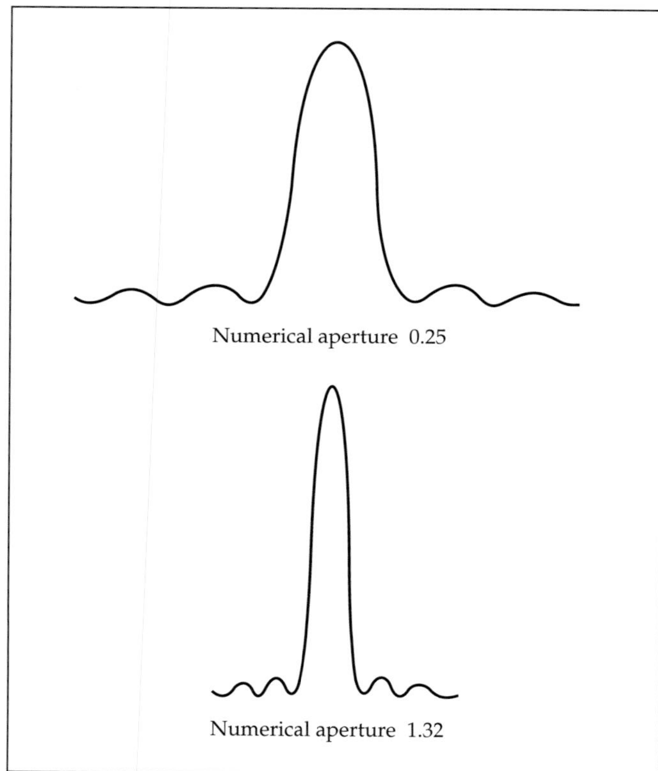

F34.10
Point spread function: width of the diffraction pattern of an objective; role of numerical aperture.

allow and not broadened by optical system aberrations, this is considered diffraction-limited imaging.

The point spread function limits how closely two points may be spaced in the object plane and still be discerned as two separate points. Convention has defined this limit of resolution as equal to the distance from the maximum of the point spread function to the location of the first dark ring. If the maximum of one point's diffraction pattern is not closer than this distance to the maximum of the diffraction pattern of another point, the dip in image intensity is considered to offer sufficient contrast for the human eye to discern two points. This limit is also known as the Rayleigh limit. It is calculated as

d = (1.2 x wavelength)/(2 x numerical aperture)[**F**34.11]

For example, an objective of numerical aperture 1.3 and illuminating green light of wavelength 540 nm would lead to a Rayleigh limit of (1.2 x 0.54 μm)/(2 x 1.3) = 0.25 μm = d.

To develop an understanding of the factors ultimately limiting performance in diffraction-limited imaging, idealized "model objects" are used. For the imaging of an object point into an image point, consider a very small round, back-illuminated object, such as a tiny pinhole in a metallized slide. For the discussion of image resolution and diffraction-limited imaging, consider such model objects as gratings, ie, arrays of parallel, opaque, and fully transparent stripes, each grating with a different spacing of the stripes.

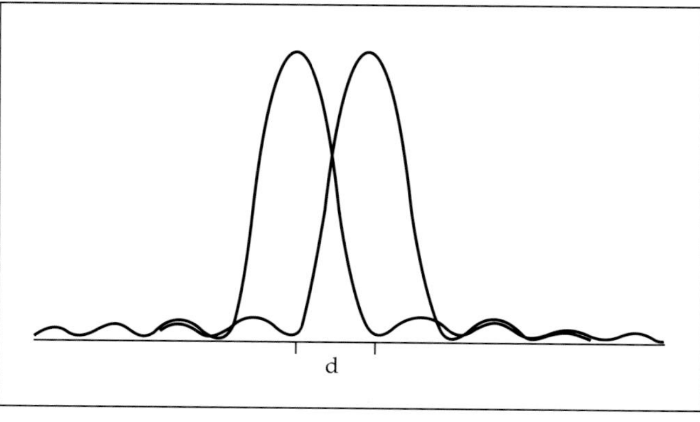

F34.11
Resolution of two diffraction patterns.

Applied to the resolution of such a set of alternating opaque and transparent stripes, the distance translates into line pairs/mm, or spatial frequency. To sample the image information fully, the so-called Nyquist theorem requires that sample spacing provides at least two sampling points for the highest spatial frequency, hence the line pair. The spatial frequency at which contrast has decreased so much that the line structure can no longer be seen and the area simply appears uniformly gray is called the spatial cutoff frequency of the objective. For the objective in the above example this would be at 4000 line pairs/mm.

The ability of the objective to transfer object contrast to the image, as a function of spatial frequency, is defined by the contrast transfer function. When the opaque and transparent stripes are wide and the number of line pairs/mm is modest, at low spatial frequencies, contrast may be fully preserved in the image. As the spatial frequency of the grating increases and there are more lines/mm, image contrast decreases gradually. At the Rayleigh limit, the human eye can just barely discern stripes [**F**34.12].

Gratings of different spatial frequencies are the model underlying the mathematical considerations that enter into an analysis of diffraction-limited imaging in light optical microscopy. Objects in general, whether a cell or tissue section, contain structural details falling into a wide range of spatial frequencies (as discussed in more detail below). Objects diffract light. This may be modeled as a superposition of diffraction gratings from the full range of spatial frequencies. The smallest detail that a microscope objective can "resolve" or the highest spatial frequency for which the image still offers acceptable contrast is defined by the numerical aperture of the objective and the wavelength of light. How they affect the image resolution requires some understanding of the role of diffraction.

How direct light encounters a very small object is depicted [**F**34.13]. The parallel wave fronts of the illumi-

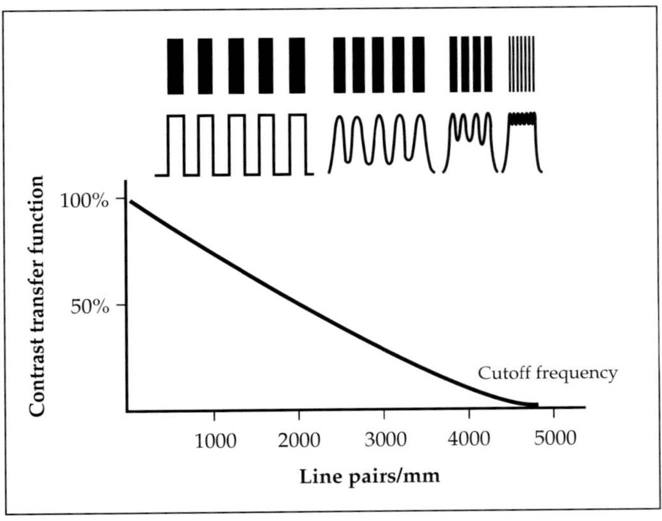

F*34.12*

Contrast transfer function and cutoff frequency.

nating light interact with the object structure. The structure disturbs the plane wave front, and as a result a wavelet of light is generated, called an "object wave" or elementary wavelet. Its point of origin is the object structure and from there it spreads forward with a spherical, diverging wave front. If another tiny object is close by, its interaction with the same wave front also produces an elementary wavelet. The two object waves are generated by the same wave front. Consequently, they retain a fixed mutual relationship. They are "in phase" and coherent. Therefore, their electromagnetic wave fields can interact. This interaction takes the form of "interference." The strength or the amplitude of the two wave fields may at a given point add up, leading to constructive interference. Under slightly different conditions the two wave fields may counteract each other and cancel out, in a process called destructive interference.

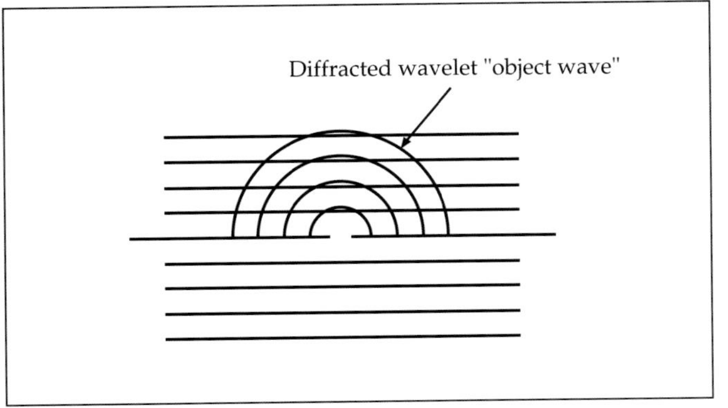

F*34.13*

Interaction of illuminating wave front with an object structure; origin of an object wavelet.

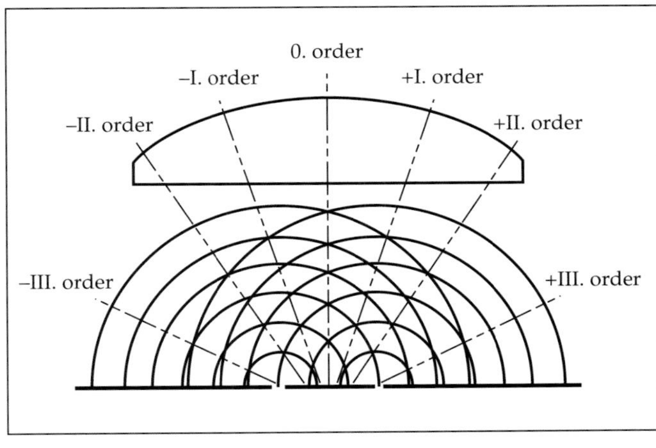

F*34.14*

Orders of diffraction.

Two object points giving rise to diffraction are shown [**F***34.14*]. They are separated from each other by a distance that is of the order of magnitude of the wavelength. The spherical wave fronts of the two object waves shall be assumed drawn on the wave crests, ie, at the point of greatest amplitude of the wave field. Where wave crest from one wave field falls on wave crest of the other, constructive interference can occur. The two wave fields will reinforce each other. As can be seen, such reinforcement occurs in certain directions only [**F***34.14*].

Conditions for constructive interference exist in direction of propagation of the original illuminating wave front. This is called the zero order of diffraction. There are higher orders. The first order appears under an angle and closest to the zero order. There is a symmetry about the direction of the original illuminating wave front. There is a +1 order and a –1 order. At higher angles one can observe a +2 order and a –2 order, a +3 order and a –3 order, and so forth. In these directions the interfering elementary wavelets combine to form parallel beams [**F***34.15*].

Without an object structure there is no diffracted light, and no structure in the uniformly illuminated image plane. The information about the object is, so to speak, entrusted to the diffracted wavelets to carry forward and form an image. To do so, the diffracted light must enter the objective, which explains the role of the numerical aperture of the objective. The numerical aperture expresses the largest angle of acceptance for light. As depicted the two first orders just enter the aperture of the objective [**F***34.15*]. Light diffracted under a very high angle, eg, some of the higher orders, at an angle beyond the angle of acceptance of the objective, never enters the aperture. It simply cannot contribute to the formation of the image: it is lost, and with it the information it carries. Fortunately, while contribution of light of the higher orders to the formation of the image is helpful, it has been established that sufficient information to image an object is retained if at least light diffracted into the first order enters the objective.

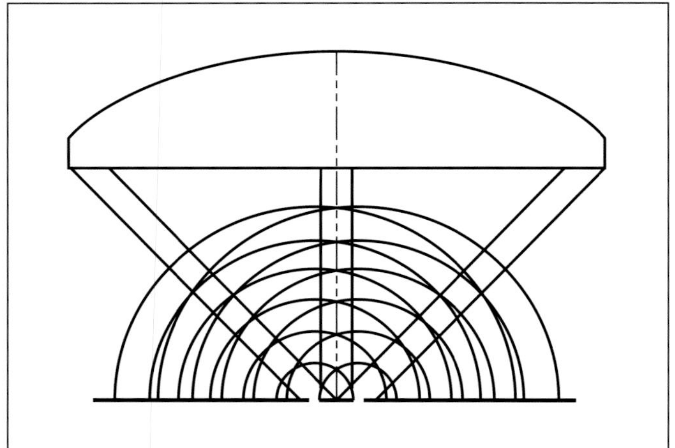

F34.15

Diffraction by a structure of higher spatial frequency than F34.14. The first orders are barely entering the objective aperture: their angle here just corresponds to the acceptance angle (numerical aperture) of the objective.

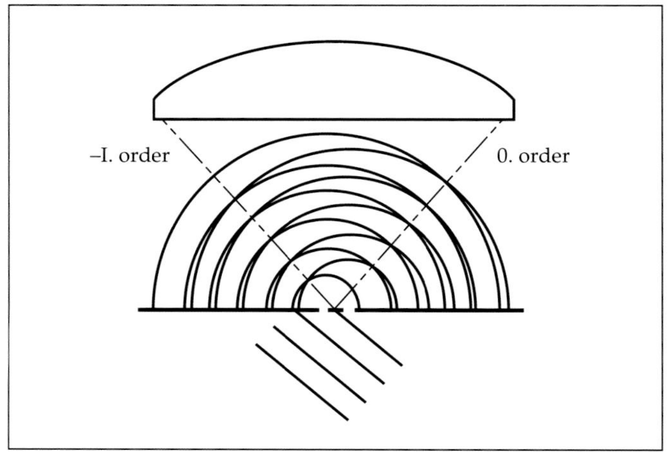

F34.16

Gain in cutoff frequency by using high aperture of illumination.

The relationship between numerical aperture, the diffraction of light by object structures, and the attainable resolution can be considered further [**F**34.15]. In this figure the same situation as shown above [**F**34.14] is depicted; however, the two diffracting object points are much closer together. The directions under which conditions for constructive interference occur now appear under a much greater angle. The first order of diffracted light just barely enters the objective aperture. The dimension of the object structure is still below the spatial cutoff frequency of the objective. For two object points any closer the angle of diffraction for the first order would be so high that the diffracted light would bypass the objective aperture. The limit of resolution has been reached.

Actually, it has been shown that it is not necessary to have diffracted light from both the –1 order and the +1 order to image an object. A contribution from one of the two is sufficient. Thus, if an object is illuminated with a plane wave under a high angle to begin with, so that the zero order barely enters the aperture on one side, the full angle of the objective aperture is open to accept the first order of light diffracted by object points twice as closely spaced [**F**34.16] as those shown above [**F**34.15]. This explains why the objective and condenser aperture should match and the aperture stop should be fully opened for the objective to attain maximum resolution. Only when this is achieved can the object be illuminated with parallel light under such a high angle of incidence.

To show the role of the wavelength of the illuminating light on resolution, a drawing with the wave fronts spaced to scale of two diffracting object points is helpful [**F**34.17]. The top portion shows the object with a fine structure such that the first order of diffraction appears under an angle that just misses the aperture of the objective for red light of 650-nm wavelength. In the bottom portion, the same object is illuminated with blue light of 400-nm wavelength. Blue light is diffracted at a lesser angle than red light. Therefore, for the small structures where the first order of diffraction for red light already misses the aperture of the objective, the first order of diffraction for blue light still contributes to the image. Blue light can therefore resolve finer detail. The point spread function is smaller. The spatial cutoff frequency for shorter wavelengths is higher.

The interaction of the illuminating light with the object structure, the generation of diffracted object wavelets (their

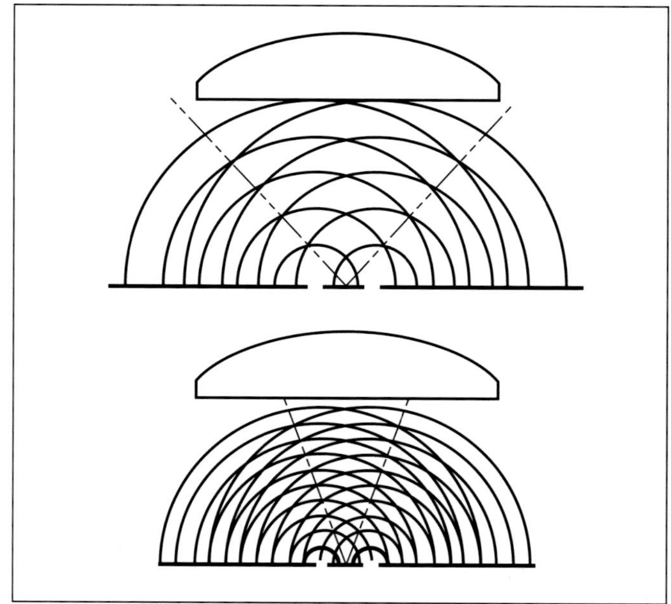

F34.17

Top, Object of such high spatial frequency that the first orders of red light no longer enter the objective. Red light will not resolve this structure. Bottom, Blue light of shorter wavelength still resolves the structure.

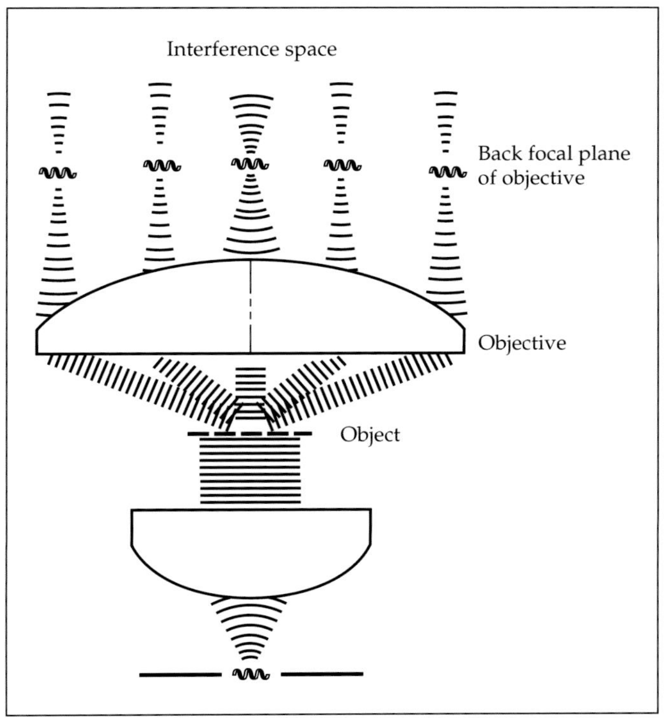

F34.18
Image formation in a light optical microscope. Processes giving rise to the events in the interference space are schematically represented.

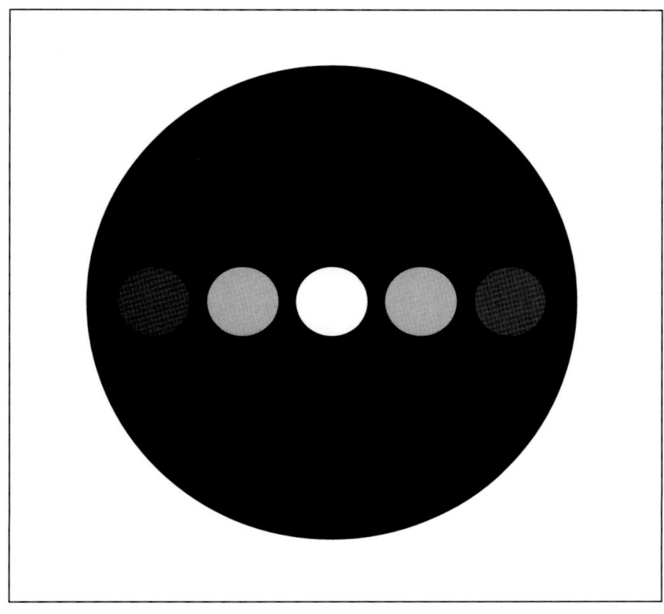

F34.19
Appearance of the back focal plane of the objective when a grating is used as a test object. The aperture stop is closed to demonstrate the processes shown in F34.18. The bright first order image of the aperture stop is seen at the center. The higher diffracted orders are arranged in direction of the grating, with diminishing intensities towards the periphery of the back focal plane.

interaction resulting in interference), and the propagation of diffracted light only in certain directions have been described. The roles of the numerical aperture of the objective and of the wavelength of light are understood. Thus, the processes involved in the formation of an image can now be discussed.

A model object will be used to discuss the underlying processes: a grating with opaque and transparent parallel stripes of a spatial frequency such that even some of the higher orders of diffraction enter the aperture of the objective. For purposes of discussion, assume that the aperture stop has been almost completely closed [**F**34.18]. Light diffracted by the specimen, light of the zero order, and direct light enter the objective. Since the superposition and constructive interference of the diverging wave fronts of the object wavelets lead to the formation of parallel wave fronts in direction of the different orders, this light, as it enters the objective, is focused in the back focal plane of the objective. There, a small image of the source and of the almost completely closed aperture stop is formed on axis by the zero order, flanked by fainter images of the –1 and +1 order and the higher orders of diffracted light. Since the test object was a grating, the images of the aperture stop all lie on one diameter of the back focal plane of the objective, spread out in the direction of the grating [**F**34.19].

Wave fronts propagating in the space between object and objective, under different angles to the optic axis, come to focus in the objective's back focal plane in different locations. The greater the angle to the optic axis, the more towards the periphery of the back focal plane they come to focus. Since, as we have seen, structures of higher spatial frequencies give rise to diffracted light whose first orders form a large angle with the optic axis, the high-frequency information about the object, ie, the information about the finest detail, appears at the periphery of the back focal plane of the objective.

The higher the numerical aperture of the objective, the more the high spatial frequency detail of the object can contribute to the image. If one closes the aperture stop in the condenser—which is in a plane conjugated to the back focal plane of the objective—diffraction from some of the higher spatial frequency components in the object never even enters the objective. From the back focal plane the light from all of these source images spreads out into the space behind the back focal plane, with all of the wave fields permeating each other. Remember that the diffracted light and the direct light are coherent and can interfere. This is precisely what happens throughout this space, which therefore is also referred to as the "interference space." The interference leads to a distinctive distribution of brightness and darkness throughout the interference space. However, we are interested only in the distribution of brightness and darkness—and of color—in a very specific plane in that space, at right angles to the optic axis. It is the plane where all the rays as traced by geometric optics, from the object and through the objective, come to a sharp focus. It is the primary image plane, the image of the object plane projected by the objective. The distribution of brightness and darkness and of color is the result of multitudinous interference processes between the direct and the diffracted light. It is hoped that the image reflects, in its visual appearance, its morphometric properties and photometric values, the physical characteristics of the object.

ALIGNMENT AND SETUP

There is some variation in microscope design, but the sequence of steps to align or set up an instrument is generally the same. A typical sequence of steps follows:

1. Turn on the light source.
2. Open the field stop.
3. Observe whether the light beam falls fully on the mirror in the base of the microscope. In instruments where the source is mounted in a separate housing, position the source until it is approximately centered and its beam fills the mirror fully. In instruments with a built-in light source you can see whether the light beam is centered or not by observing it as it passes through the glass dust cover plate in the front base of the microscope. Place a piece of thin paper on this dust cover and adjust the position of the bulb until the beam is centered. As a rule, the socket of the bulb can be centered by means of centering screws, accessible on the outside of the lamp housing.
4. Use the coarse adjustment to move the stage away from the objective.
5. Swing a 10:1 objective into position.
6. Put a slide onto the stage, with coverslipped side up, and position it with the mechanical stage so that the specimen can be expected to lie approximately under the objective.
7. Swing the condenser top element into place. The top element is often mounted so that a lever can flip it into place or out of the way, but the latter should be done only for observation under very low power.
8. Move the condenser all the way up by means of the control knob next to the substage. This control knob operates a rack and pinion, which is simply a gear arrangement that allows a precise positioning, up and down, of the condenser. The top element of the condenser should be approximately flush with the stage surface; it should never lift the slide.
9. Look into the oculars. If the field looks entirely dark, the condenser may be very far off center, or it may not have been moved up by the rack and pinion control. Some microscopes have not only the two oculars for binocular observation, but a third tube straight up, to accept a camera. Such trinocular tubes often have a built-in prism that sends the light either to the visual, binocular tube, or lets the light pass straight up into the tube for the camera. These prisms are frequently mounted on a slider. If the field looks entirely dark there is a good chance that this prism is not set for binocular visual observation. Slide the prism over to send the light into the binocular tube. If the condenser is approximately centered and the light source not entirely misaligned, one should at this point be able to see at least part of the field illuminated and be able to focus. This is done by very slowly turning the coarse adjustment until one can make out the specimen. If the specimen has very low contrast the proper object plane is easier to find if one moves the specimen back and forth with the mechanical stage. The eye picks up motion quite readily and helps to find the object and correct plane of focus. Once the specimen is in approximate focus, use the fine adjustment to correct the focus. It is most likely that at this point the field is still unevenly illuminated and the image may be poor, but one can fine-focus the specimen, which is sufficient at this point.
10. Open the aperture stop fully.
11. Slowly close the field stop. As it is being closed, the field may become completely dark; this means that the condenser is grossly decentered. Open the field stop again and keep recentering the condenser as you close it gradually, so that it always stays in the center of the field of view.
12. Focus the condenser until the edges of the field stop appear in sharp focus with the specimen. Do not touch the fine adjustment for the objective at this time, unless the specimen is no longer in sharp focus. In that case, refocus the objective, then refocus the condenser.
13. Give the condenser a final centration so that the image of the closed field stop appears at the exact center of the field of view.
14. Open the field stop until its edges just disappear symmetrically around the field's periphery.
15. The aperture stop has already been fully opened. It should now be closed very slowly while observing the image. At a given setting the image will undergo a rather sudden change. Contrast increases sharply and bright fringes (so-called diffraction seams) surround small detail and appear along sharp edges in the specimen. The aperture stop has been closed too far and, while for the beginner the gain in contrast looks desirable, the image has in fact seriously deteriorated and resolution is greatly impaired. It is helpful to take this point in the setting of the aperture stop as a starting point from where one opens the aperture stop again, watching for loss of contrast, and specifically for the appearance of milky haze in the image. The image should be clear, brilliant, and free from haze and milkiness. In a well-prepared preparation,

stained to high contrast, the aperture stop can be opened all the way. Imperfections in specimen preparation usually require that one backs up from a fully opened position of the aperture stop, particularly when high dry objectives are used.

16. As a final check, remove one ocular and look down into the tube. The back focal plane of the objective will be seen. It should be uniformly illuminated and the light distribution should be centric. When the collector lens in front of the light source is focused, the illumination in the back focal plane of the objective should "breathe," ie, it should expand and contract in a concentric manner. No crescent-shaped darker areas should appear on the sides. Should this occur, the light source requires recentering. It is always possible to tell whether the source or the condenser is off center. When the aperture stop is opened, its edges should disappear symmetrically all around the edges of the back focal plane. If they do, the condenser is centered. Replace the ocular.
17. Binocular microscopes permit an adjustment of the spacing between the tubes to match the interpupillary distance of an observer's eyes. In some instruments this adjustment includes an automatic compensation for the change in distance from the object to the primary image plane. In other instruments the tubes can be individually adjusted after the interpupillary distance has been found. Focusable eye lenses in oculars should be set so that a reticle is seen sharply in focus. The microscope is then focused so that the image is also in focus with the lines of a reticle.

IMAGE PROBLEMS AND SOLUTIONS

A very common condition is a hazy or milky image. Although in focus, the specimen appears to be washed out, even in the center of the field. This condition occurs particularly under high dry observation—the same specimen may look fine under low-power objectives and even under an oil immersion.

Milky images result from spherical aberration. There are several possible causes for this. The coverglass on the specimen is too thick or too thin, or there is no coverglass. The layer of mounting medium is too thick. The optics and the microscope stand were made by different manufacturers and the mechanical tube lengths do not match. Objectives and oculars were made by different manufacturers. The plane in which the ocular has its sharp round stop—where the primary image is expected to be (the ocular adjustment length)—and the plane onto which the objective projects the primary image do not match. The objectives are corrected for infinity tube length (see below), but the microscope tube lens is for a finite tube length.

When photomicrographs show image haze, especially under a high dry objective, a 35-mm camera has often been mounted by a mechanical adapter without proper optical consideration. To get the image into focus the objective has to be moved from its designed working distance, which introduces spherical aberration. Some of the very highly corrected flat field optics and oil immersion objectives require that the manufacturer's immersion oil be used. Also, some of these systems are sensitive to plastic coverslips and some synthetic mounting media, which have a dispersion very different from glass.

When a lack of image definition exists, even under low-power observation, check the following possibilities. There is an oil film or fingerprint on the front lens of the objective. Some flat field optics have a concave front lens, where such films are hard to see. There are fingerprints on surfaces inside the microscope, very often on the tube lens. The oculars are smudged; the eye lenses in particular are often filmed with remnants of eye makeup. To remove such films or prints from hard-coated surfaces, it is best to use polystyrene pellets ("peanuts") from packing material. A pellet is broken to provide an absolutely clean and fresh surface and a soft cleaning tool. Some lens cleaner is placed on the fresh surface and the pellet is pressed slightly against the surface to be cleaned. This is better than lens paper, which often accumulates gritty dust particles that scratch the optical coatings. One should not use alcohol as solvent, as it will attack lens cements. Interior surfaces, such as prism surfaces, are soft coated and scratch even at a slight touch.

If the image of the field stop is not sharp even when it should be in focus, and at times appears smeared in streaks in one direction, this is caused by an oil smudge on the bottom of the slide or the surface of the condenser top element. In the first instance the streak would move with the slide, in the second it would move when the condenser centering is used. Such smears are caused by immersion oil spilled onto the microscope stage and transferred to the condenser and bottom surface of a slide.

Dust particles may appear either sharply outlined or diffused. To locate them the following measures are helpful. Rotate the oculars in the tubes. If the dust particles rotate with them, they are on an ocular. Lower the condenser. If the particles go out of focus they are somewhere below the microscope stage. Small fibers or particles that appear at the same location on every photomicrograph are usually on the camera attachment's projective lens.

Dust particles or fibers on internal optical surfaces are best removed by a short burst from a compressed air can sold for the purpose. One may also glue a very small piece of chamois leather to a thin wood rod and very carefully pick up particles from interior surfaces. The microscope mirror may be cleaned by rinsing with water to which some detergent has been added, and swabbed with cotton while there is a fluid film on the mirror.

When the image looks sharp and crisp at the center of the field of view but out of focus around the periphery of high dry and oil immersion objectives, it is caused by curvature of field, an optical systems aberration that cannot be eliminated. Flat field objectives have been corrected for this and are preferable for photomicrography. However, apparent curvature of field may also result from a serious mismatch of objective and ocular, such as when they are of different manufacture.

Optical Correction

The design of high-performance optics involves many trade-offs and compromises. Microscope objectives may contain from 4 to 16 optical elements. To attain very high precision and achieve cost-efficient manufacture, the surfaces of these elements are ground to spherical shapes. The trade-off is that diffraction-limited, aberration-free imaging is possible only under specific, rather precise conditions.

Spherical aberration causes hazy, milky images over the entire field of view. It occurs when a coverglass of incorrect thickness is used, or if too heavy a layer of mounting medium is present. It may also occur when optics from different manufacturers are combined on the same microscope, and when a camera or video system is improperly mounted. In most of these instances, to get the image into focus, one has to move the objective from its designed working distance, which causes spherical aberration. Low-power systems are not sensitive to this and neither are oil immersion objectives—a slight change in working distance merely means a different thickness of oil, which is not that different from glass. High dry systems are very sensitive: with their high aperture and short working distance any deviation from the design working distance causes severe spherical aberration.

Chromatic Aberration

Uncorrected optical systems have different focal lengths for light of different wavelengths. In microscope objectives even the least corrected systems are chromatically corrected. In condensers, however, one frequently sees strongly colored fields when the focus of the condenser is changed slightly, the sign of a chromatically poorly corrected system. So-called "aspheric" condensers usually have no chromatic correction; they should not be used for color photomicrography. A laboratory microscope should have at least an achromatic condenser, and for photomicrography or video recording an aplanatic/achromatic system.

Microscope objectives are offered in three grades of correction: achromats, fluorite objectives, and apochromats. Achromats are corrected spherically for one wavelength and chromatically for two wavelengths; fluorite objectives are corrected spherically for two wavelengths and chromatically for two wavelengths; apochromatic objectives have a spherical correction for two wavelengths and chromatic correction for three. Curvature of field correction, ie, flat field optics, are offered in each of these grades. Generally, fluorite objectives tend to render the crispest, high-contrast images. Apochromats produce very finely resolved images of generally fainter contrast; they demand a carefully stained specimen.

Curvature of Field

One optical correction that leads to severe image degradation is astigmatism. It can be corrected in an objective; however, historically one then had to accept that the microscopic image was no longer flat but had a curvature. By introducing so-called "meniscus lenses," curvature of field can today be completely controlled in flat field optics. Meniscus lenses have concave surfaces. In medium and high dry objectives the best design often puts the concave surface on the front lens of the objective, and particular care in cleaning is required because the concave front surface of these objectives tends to accumulate dirt and oil films. Use of polystyrene pellets with lens cleaning fluid is the best cleaning method.

Depth of Field and Focus

Total depth of field comprises two components: the "wave optical depth of field" and the "geometric optical depth of field." The image of a sharp bright point in the object is, even in an ideally corrected system, imaged into a diffraction pattern. Its lateral extension in the image plane is described by the point spread function. However, the diffraction pattern also has an extension in direction of the optic axis as the wave fronts converge to the plane of focus. The image thus is not formed as a two-dimensional surface but as a three-dimensional layer. It is not very meaningful to define—within the diffraction-limited range along the optic axis—where exact focus is. The wave optical component of the total depth of field thus is due to diffraction effects.

Detectors such as the human eye, photographic film, or a video tube have limited resolving power. As long as some image detail is smaller than this limit, the detector records it as a sharp point. The detector has no way to decide whether the detail is in sharp focus or not. There is a range of focus then where details, whether slightly below or slightly above geometric focus, appear to be in perfect focus. This range is called the geometric optical depth of field.

There is a distinction between depth of field and depth of focus. Depth of field refers to a range in the object space. Depth of focus is the corresponding range in the image plane. The wave optical depth of field is proportional to the wavelength and inversely proportional to the square of the numerical aperture of the objective. The geometric optical depth of field is inversely proportional to the magnification and the numerical aperture.

In low-power objectives almost all of the total depth of field is due to geometric optical depth of field. In a high numerical aperture system, such as an oil immersion objective, the two components contribute approximately the same to the total depth of field.

Chromatic Magnification Difference

It is possible to get the images for different wavelengths to come to the same focus and even to be free from spherical aberration over a given wavelength range. However, one has to accept as a compromise that the red and the blue images may have slightly different magnifications at focus in the primary image. This is not a serious defect: one simply never sees the effect—the design of the oculars compensates for the difference. However, different manufacturers use different amounts of chromatic magnification difference, which is another reason why optics from different manufacturers should not be mixed.

FIELD OF VIEW DIAMETER

It is useful to compute the diameter of the field of view in a microscope. It is determined by the magnification of the objective and that of the tube factor, but not by that of the ocular. For the ocular the so-called field of view number is important to know; it is provided by the manufacturer. For a typical wide-field ocular the field of view number is 18 mm. To compute the field of view diameter, divide the field of view number of the ocular by the magnification of the objective times that of the tube factor. One obtains the field of view diameter in millimeters. For example:

$M_{objective} = 40:1$, $M_{tube\ factor} = 1.25$, field of view number = 18 mm; thus, $18/(40 \times 1.25) = 0.360$ mm = 360-μm diameter

INFINITY-CORRECTED OPTICS

Historically, microscope objectives were designed to project the primary image to a plane somewhat below the upper edge of the tube, the plane where the fixed round stop in the ocular provides a sharp edge for the field of view. This design did not allow changing of the relative position of objective and ocular, which is desirable when one wants to achieve fine focusing by moving the nosepiece only; also it is difficult to insert beam splitters or prisms into this space without providing for proper optical correction.

Infinity-corrected optics give the designer such freedom. The objective is designed to have the object at its front focal plane, which projects the primary image to infinity. A tube lens above the nosepiece is used to bring the image in and focus it into the appropriate primary image plane. The beam path between objective and tube lens now is telecentric, and its length is no longer critical.

IMAGING MODALITIES

Light optical microscopy offers a multitude of different imaging modalities. Each is designed to bring out particular optical properties of microscopic objects or to allow observation of particular processes. In clinical cytology, transmitted light microscopy (bright field microscopy) is the standard modality. The specimen is transilluminated with white light and appears in good contrast, stained to bring out cellular or tissue detail in various colors. Some stains, such as the Feulgen reaction, selectively show specific cytochemical cell constituents.

In darkfield microscopy, the specimen is illuminated with a hollow cone of light of such high aperture that all of the direct light (the zero order) bypasses the objective. Only scattered and diffracted light enters the objective aperture. The specimen thus appears on a completely dark background, with its edges and other structural details brilliantly outlined by the scattered light. The condenser aperture has to be larger than the aperture of the objective. Darkfield microscopy was the standard modality to observe spirochetes; it is very useful in revealing the chitin structure of protozoa or to see cilia.

Increasingly important is fluorescence microscopy. The specimen is stained with a fluorochrome, a dye that gives off fluorescence when illuminated with short wavelength light. In a fluorescence microscope the specimen is illuminated with blue or ultraviolet light, also called the "exciting light." The object shines in brilliantly luminous fluorescence and high contrast against a dark background. Fluorescence microscopy offers extreme sensitivity of detection; combined, as a label, with immunologically selective and specific markers, it has become a very valuable and clinically useful methodology.

In phase-contrast microscopy contrast is generated optically. Unstained, live cells can be observed in high contrast. Most clinical materials are almost pure phase objects, ie, they do not exhibit natural contrast. Their structure is expressed only in differences in refractive index and does not lead to visible differences in image brightness. Phase objects are like a piece of clear glass in water. Phase contrast makes phase structures appear as if they did absorb light. Phase contrast requires a special condenser and special objectives.

Interference-contrast microscopy also images phase objects in high contrast; interference optics offer a variety of modalities. There is differential interference contrast, where the specimen is shown in sharp relief, as if embossed. Other interference schemes show the specimen in luminous colors, with color hues indicating differently refracting cellular or tissue components.

Microscopy under polarized light is used to show and identify crystalline objects, and to analyze their internal microscopic and submicroscopic structure. The method requires, at the simplest level, two polarizing filters; analytical polarizing microscopy is done on highly specialized instruments.

Confocal microscopy permits the imaging of very sharply defined optical sections. It is valuable for observing details in thick, highly scattering objects so that the image-degrading effects of the overlaying tissue are minimized. Confocal microscopy allows fine depth discrimination.

Video-enhanced contrast microscopy uses optical and video-electronic means to generate and enhance contrast, to show objects or cellular processes where extremely small phase differences are involved.

In digital microscopy the optical image is converted to a numeric/digital representation, processed, stored, redisplayed, archived, and quantitatively analyzed. Such analysis may involve micromorphometric as well as microphotometric methods. Quantitative DNA measurement to establish a ploidy distribution for a clinical specimen is an example of such a microphotometric method.

Many of the mentioned modalities are applied primarily in research; however, there is an increasing tendency to transfer research methods to the examination of clinical specimens.

REVIEW EXERCISES

1. Why will the correct setting of the bright field stop reduce stray light?

2. Why is the aperture stop not used to regulate image brightness?

3. Which iris appears in sharp focus together with the specimen in Koehler illumination?

4. Which image will show more detail—an image projected by an objective 25:1, numerical aperture 0.65, and viewed with an ocular x12.5; or an image projected with an objective 40:1, numerical aperture 0.95, and viewed with an ocular x8?

5. You want to have a field of view diameter of 600 μm, and you have a wide-field ocular with a field of view number of 24; the tube factor of the microscope is x1. What is the highest power objective you could use?

6. Does the finer structural detail in an image correspond to the higher spatial frequencies?

7. Do the higher spatial frequencies in the object give rise to light diffracted under large angles?

8. Why will blue light illumination render higher resolution than red light illumination?

9. Which objective will allow a larger depth of field: 40:1, numerical aperture 0.95; or 40:1, numerical aperture 0.65?

10. Why would an oil immersion objective be less sensitive to cover glasses of incorrect thickness than a high dry objective?

11. Does a flat field objective have a shallower depth of field than a corresponding traditional objective?

12. Explain the difference between visibility of some small object, and resolution in its image.

SELECTED READINGS

Baak JPA, Oort J. *Morphometry in Diagnostic Pathology.* Berlin, Germany: Springer Verlag; 1983.

Bennet AHB, Jupnik H, Osterberg H, Richards OW. *Phase Microscopy.* New York, NY: John Wiley & Sons; 1951.

Bennett HS. The microscopical investigation of biologic materials with polarized light. In: McClung CE, ed. *Handbook of Microscopical Technique.* New York, NY: Harper & Row; 1950.

Determan H, Lepusch F. *The Microscope and Its Application.* Wetzlar, Germany: E. Leitz Optical Company; 1974.

Inoue S. *Videomicroscopy.* New York, NY: Plenum Press; 1986.

Moellring FK. *Microscopy From the Very Beginning.* Oberkochen, Germany: Carl Zeiss; 1968

Pawley J. *Handbook of Biological Confocal Microscopy.* Madison, Wis: IMR Press; 1989.

Ploem JS , Tanke HJ. *Introduction to Fluorescence Microscopy.* Oxford, England: Oxford University Press; 1987.

CHAPTER

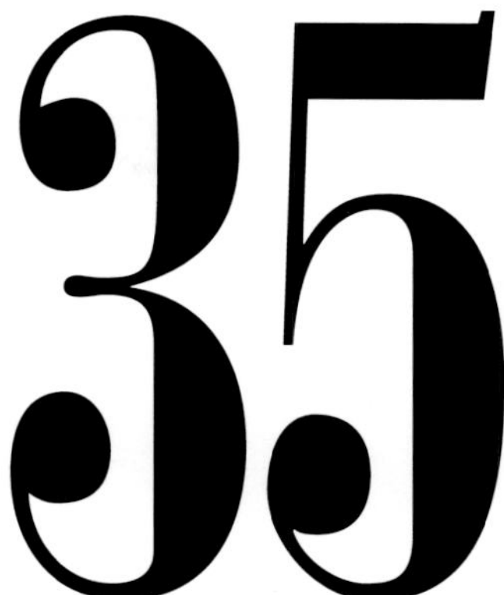

Cytopreparatory Techniques

MARION D. HOLMQUIST, CT(ASCP)

CATHERINE M. KEEBLER, CT(ASCP), CFIAC, SCD(HON)

CONTENTS

Because cytopreparatory techniques vary from laboratory to laboratory, it is not possible to include in any one book all the procedures currently used for processing cytologic specimens. Thus, general techniques will be described that illustrate basic principles of cytopreparation. An understanding of these principles and procedures will enable the student to prepare good cytologic preparations.

FIXATION

Immediate and proper fixation of cellular material is essential for accurate cytologic interpretation. Knowledge of different fixatives and their effects on cells and tissue is a prerequisite of cell preparation.

A fixative is defined as an agent used to maintain the existing form and structure of constituent elements in a cytologic or histologic specimen. The fixative specifically recommended for cytologic preparations is alcohol, which has a characteristic effect on the nuclear content of the cell. Alcohol, a dehydrating agent, causes cells to shrink as it removes or replaces water, an essential ingredient in protein structure. In this process, cellular structures are coarsened and nuclear detail is sharpened, resulting in the nuclear chromatinic patterns seen in cytologic cell preparations. Because of its essential contribution to final cell preparations, alcohol fixation is the first step in the Papanicolaou staining procedure.

Wet Fixation

Originally, a solution of equal parts of diethylether (ether) and 95% ethanol was the fixative recommended for cytologic preparations. However, because of the safety hazards of ether, this compound is not used today. Now, most cytopathology laboratories in the United States use 95% ethanol, or an acceptable substitute.

Ethanol is readily available to most hospital laboratories at a concentration of 95%. Absolute (100%) ethanol is more expensive and has not proved to be a superior cytologic fixative. Ethanol is subject to federal taxation unless a license to purchase it is obtained. Most hospitals and large laboratories have this license. For those laboratories unable to purchase ethanol, substitutes are methanol, isopropanol or *n*-propanol, and denatured alcohol. These are purchased at 100% concentration, but by knowing the effect of these alcohols on cells, proper concentrations can be determined, resulting in a fixative similar to ethanol.

Methanol produces less cell shrinkage than ethanol. Therefore, 100% methanol has an effect on cells comparable with that of 95% ethanol. Methanol is the preferred fixative for processing chromosomes for cytogenetics because it preserves delicate detail.

Isopropanol causes slightly greater cell shrinkage than methanol and ethanol. A recommended substitute for 95% ethanol is 80% isopropanol. The increased amount of water counteracts the shrinkage effect of the alcohol. *n*-Propanol is similar to isopropanol in effect.

Denatured alcohol is ethanol that has been changed by the addition of additives to render it unfit for human consumption. Specially denatured alcohol is a commercial form of industrial ethanol. There are many different formulas for denatured alcohol, but all of them contain ethanol as the main ingredient. Therefore, this alcohol should be used as a cytologic fixative at a concentration of 95% or 100%. One formula for denatured alcohol is 90 parts ethanol (95%), five parts methanol (100%), and five parts isopropanol (100%).

The alcohols described should be applied as wet fixation, which is the immediate submersion of freshly obtained cells in a fixative. A slide should remain in the fixative a minimum of 15 to 30 minutes. Because it is difficult to transport bottles containing liquid and against postal regulations to mail alcohol, it is not always possible to keep slides immersed in solution. After slides have been wet-fixed for 15 to 30 minutes, remove them from the fixative, place them in a container, and mail or carry them to the laboratory. These slides should be reimmersed in 95% ethanol or its equivalent prior to staining.

Coating Fixatives

Coating fixatives, a combination of an alcohol that fixes the cells and a wax-like substance that forms a thin, protective coating over the cells, are used increasingly in both hospital and nonhospital settings. Once a coating fixative has been applied over the cells the slides can then be mailed or carried to the laboratory.

Coating fixatives can be nonaerosal solutions that are applied by spraying the cell sample or by dropping a liquid solution onto the slide. These fixatives may be purchased under many brand names from pharmaceutical supply houses. The alcohol base for these fixatives is not ethanol but one of its substitutes. It is important to determine the proper equivalent concentration. When using spray fixatives, the distance to be held from the slide should follow the manufacturer's recommendation.

An excellent liquid fixative that can be prepared in the laboratory and used to coat the slide is a polyethylene glycol and alcohol solution (see "Formulas" section). Slides fixed in coating fixatives must be immersed in 95% ethanol or its equivalent (several rinses) to dissolve the wax coating prior to staining. Hair sprays are not recommended as coating fixatives because the formulas may change without notice to consumers, and substitute chemicals in the sprays may be detrimental to cell preservation.

Air-drying

Air-drying is not acceptable for samples to be stained by the Papanicolaou method or one of its modifications.

Air-drying causes nuclear swelling and distortion and loss of chromatin detail; the nuclear size may be four to six times the size of a fixed nucleus. The cytoplasm in air-dried samples appears less dense and cannot be colored properly by the EA polychrome stain. Therefore it is important for air-dried slides to be differentiated from those that are wet-fixed or spray-fixed by careful labeling so that proper staining methods are utilized for each specimen.

Air-dried samples collected in conjunction with fixed samples are the choice of many cytopathologists for the evaluation of fine needle aspirates. The air-dried sample can be stained with one of a number of hematologic staining methods, including the Diff-Quik method, which is easy and quick. As stated above it is important that the clinician label the specimens properly so that the samples can be stained correctly.

Cell Samples Fixed in the Laboratory

The fixatives discussed in the preceding sections are used by clinicians or technologists to fix cell samples capable of adhering to glass slides throughout the staining procedure. Cell samples in a fluid medium, especially cerebrospinal fluid, should be brought to the laboratory without delay. If some delay is unavoidable (12-24 hours), body fluids may be refrigerated. For sputum samples, a solution of 50% to 70% ethanol with or without the addition of polyethylene glycol is suggested for collection of the sample or can be added to the specimen when received in the laboratory.

Cytopathologists sometimes recommend that fluid specimens be brought to the laboratory fresh—without the addition of a fixative or heparin—for the following reasons:

1. The body fluid acts like a tissue culture medium and protects cells for a limited time, especially when kept below body temperature.
2. Unfixed body fluids contain soluble proteins, which pass more readily through membrane filters. Alcohol coagulates protein and causes clogging of the filter, which is already filled with small quantities of filtrate.
3. Coagulated proteins retain much of the stain, interfere with visibility of cells and prevent adherence of cells to the glass slide. It is therefore necessary to pretreat the surface of the slide with a substance such as albumin to make the cells adhere to the glass surface.
4. Prefixed specimens can restrict the utilization of additional staining procedures that may support the cytologic diagnosis.
5. Immunocytochemical studies or estrogen and progesterone receptor determinations may require individual fixation and preparation.

If a long delay is expected prior to processing a body fluid, a 1:1 solution of specimen and 50% ethanol may be used.

Fixatives for Mucoid or Viscous Cell Samples

A fixative that combines 50% ethanol and a 2% polyglycol solution may be used to collect sputum and tracheal samples and some bronchial samples. More information is contained in the section on respiratory tract sample preparation.

Lysing Fixatives

There are times when the cell sample may be grossly obscured with blood and when a fixative and lysing solution may be required to produce a microscopically better image. Some formulas for lysing solutions are shown in the "Formulas" section.

Fixatives for Cell Block Preparation

The cytotechnologist may be required to prepare a cell sample for a cell block. In selected cases, immunohistochemical staining procedures, hybridization techniques, and special stains of histologic sections prepared from cell blocks can provide useful diagnostic information to the cytopathologist.

The fixatives described above contain concentrations of alcohol that are excellent for preserving cytologic samples but detrimental for preserving tissue samples. Preserving whole tissue or cells packed tightly by centrifugation for embedding and sectioning requires a different type of fixation. Since tissue must be soft enough not to crumble when cut with a microtome, alcohol is not recommended for histologic fixation because alcohol hardens the tissue. A good fixative for tissue contains a high concentration of water.

The most widely used fixative is a saturated solution of formaldehyde gas in water (37% by weight or 40% by volume). Such solutions are commonly called formalin or formol. One part 40% formaldehyde with nine parts water is designated as 10% formalin.

To be most effective, formalin needs to be maintained at a pH of 7, ie, near neutrality. This near neutrality is best preserved by adding phosphate buffer (0.067 mol/L) to the solution of 10% formalin, which compensates for the slowly progressing production of formic acid. Formic acid results from oxidation of formaldehyde, promoted by the action of light. To avoid this, formalin should be kept in a dark bottle. The water in 10% buffered formalin causes edema of the cells, resulting in swollen amorphous nuclear content. However, this does not interfere with the histologic diagnosis. Fixation by formalin improves considerably if after 6 to 12 hours the old fixative is poured off and replaced by a fresh formalin solution. Buffered 10% formalin is a good preservative for lipids, carbohydrates, and mucin. Substitution of alcohol for formalin fixation results in faster fixation, increased hardening, better preservation of glycogen, and loss of fats and lipids.

Bouin's fixative solution provides a balance between those ingredients that cause shrinkage (picric acid) and those that cause swelling (glacial acetic acid).

PAPANICOLAOU STAINING METHOD

The Papanicolaou method is a polychrome staining reaction designed to display the many variations of cellular morphology showing degrees of cellular maturity and metabolic activity. In his study to detect the action of ovarian hormones on the vaginal epithelium, Papanicolaou modified the conventional hematoxylin-eosin (H&E) stain to be more specific for cytoplasmic changes. To do this, he incorporated the features of Shorr's staining technique, a single differential stain with an alcoholic base, to provide sharp cytoplasmic contrast between cells of the vaginal epithelium. Because intact cells overlap and some appear in three-dimensional configurations, the greatest value of the Papanicolaou staining method is the resultant cell transparency. By using solutions of high alcoholic content, the counterstains provide clear visualization through areas of overlapping cells, mucus, and debris.

Papanicolaou also changed the fixative for slides from an aqueous to an alcoholic solution, resulting in a nuclear stain that demonstrates unique chromatinic patterns found in normal and abnormal cells. The combination of the modified H&E and Shorr's staining procedures produced the Papanicolaou staining method for the visualization of benign and malignant cells. The main advantages of this stain are (1) definition of nuclear detail, (2) cytoplasmic transparency, and (3) cell differentiation.

This section provides a general overview of the Papanicolaou staining method, including the various modifications, stains, and procedures. A diagram of the progressive and regressive methods is shown [**F**35.1]. The four main steps are (1) fixation (discussed above), (2) nuclear staining with hematoxylin, (3) cytoplasmic staining with counterstains orange G and EA, and (4) clearing and mounting.

The four main steps are interspersed with steps to add solutions that hydrate, dehydrate, and rinse cells. Hydration may begin with a high concentration of alcohol; gradually, the alcohol content of each hydrating solution is lowered until the cellular material is immersed in water ($95\% \rightarrow 80\% \rightarrow 70\% \rightarrow 50\% \rightarrow H_2O$). Hydration may also be abrupt by immediate immersion of the cellular material from a high concentration of alcohol directly into water ($95\% \rightarrow H_2O$).

After some minutes in hematoxylin, the cells are dehydrated gradually ($H_2O \rightarrow 50\% \rightarrow 70\% \rightarrow 80\% \rightarrow 95\%$) or abruptly ($H_2O \rightarrow 95\%$) prior to immersion in the alcoholic counterstains orange G and EA. The gradual displacement of alcohol by water and water by alcohol is thought to minimize cell distortion and to reduce cell loss from the glass slide caused by convection currents of the solutions. Gill disputes this and has eliminated the graduated alcohols, using a one-step hydration and dehydration method.

Rinses following staining must be done in the solvent of the stain. Following aqueous hematoxylin, the slides are rinsed in water; following orange G and EA the slides are rinsed in alcohol.

Because there is variability, both with fixation and the pH of the cell sample itself, the Papanicolaou method should be thought of as an aid, but not the final answer, in differentiating one cell type from another. Knowledge of normal variations in color for a specific cell type will help the cytotechnologist check a particular batch of stained slides. The staining reaction can be monitored and adjusted by microscopic checks.

Nuclear Stain

The nuclear stain used in the Papanicolaou staining method is hematoxylin, one of the few natural stains in laboratory use. Used for over 100 years in histology, it has an affinity for chromatin. The precise chemical formula is known but synthesis is not practical, and for this reason bottles of hematoxylin powder vary. The formulas for four different types of hematoxylin are shown [**T**35.1].

There are two ways to stain nuclei. One is to stain for the desired color intensity, which eliminates decolorizing with hydrochloric acid and the subsequent running-water bath. This is the progressive method of staining [**F**35.1]. The second is to overstain with an unacidified hematoxylin, then remove the excess stain with dilute hydrochloric acid. This is the regressive method of staining [**F**35.1]. Because nongynecologic cell samples do not adhere to slides as well as those from the female reproductive tract, the progressive method of staining (without a running-water bath) is recommended.

Even though alum hematoxylin acts like a basic stain (ie, appears to have an affinity for basic nucleoproteins), the pH of the solution is only 2.95, even without the addition of glacial acetic acid. With 2% acetic acid added, its pH is 2.34. To cause the color of the stain to change from red to the desired blue, it is necessary to raise the pH to over 8.0, ie, to make it alkaline. This can be accomplished by rinsing with tap water if the pH of the water is over 8.0, or the slides may be "blued" with dilute solutions of ammonium hydroxide (NH_4OH, pH 8.0-8.5), lithium carbonate (Li_2CO_3, pH 8.0-8.5) or Scott's tap water substitute (pH 8.2). If the blueing agent is not removed by water its action continues. The action of the hydrochloric acid also continues if it is not removed thoroughly by rinsing gently in lukewarm tap water.

Once the nuclei have been stained, the stain is usually "set." The stain can be removed by chlorinated tap water but not by the alcohol rinses in subsequent solutions. Tap water may contain chlorine in varying amounts. If there is a high amount of chlorine in the water used, fading of cell samples may be experienced. Therefore, both chlorine and pH levels of the water should be tested.

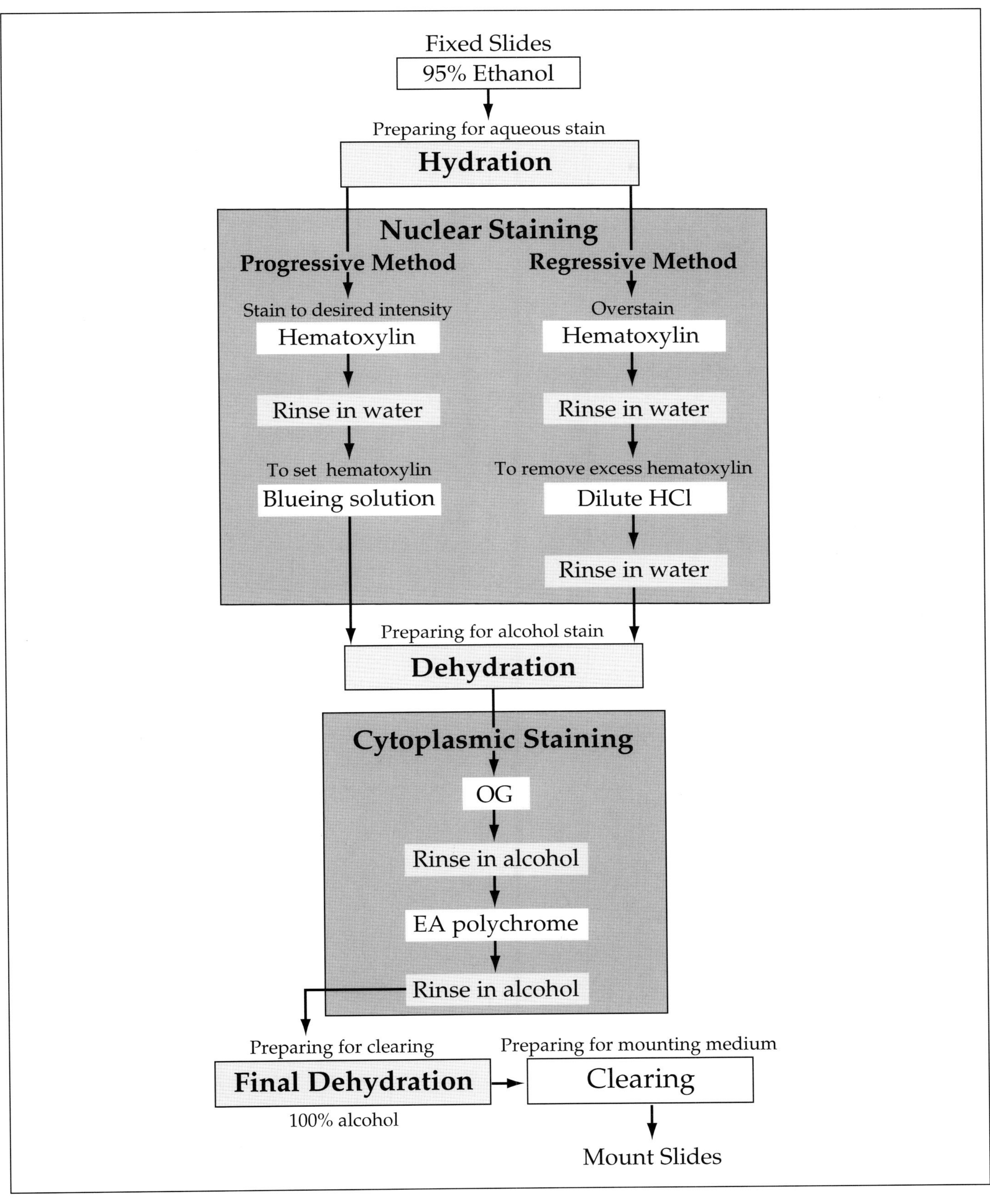

F *35.1*

Principles of the Papanicolaou staining procedure.

Ingredients	Harris (1900)	Mayer (1904)	Lillie-Mayer (1941)	Gill Half-Oxidized Hematoxylin (1973)
Hematoxylin	5 g	1 g	5 g	2 g anhydrous or 2.36 g crystalline
Ammonium aluminum sulfate (ammonium alum)	100 g	50 g	50 g	17.6 g aluminum sulfate or 23.5 g aluminum ammonium sulfate
90% ethanol or absolute ethanol (if hematoxylin dated after 1973)	50 mL	—	—	—
Glycerol or ethylene glycol	—	—	300 mL glycerol	250 mL ethylene glycol
Distilled water	1000 mL	1000 mL	700 mL	730 mL
Chemical ripening agent	2.5 g mercuric oxide	0.2 g sodium iodate	0.2-0.4 g sodium iodate	0.2 g sodium iodate
Temperature and time	100°C, a few minutes	15°C, instantly	25°C, instantly	25°C, instantly
Added acid				
Normal	None	None	20 mL glacial acetic*	20 mL glacial acetic
Variant	40 mL glacial acetic	20 mL glacial acetic	—	1 g citric acid
Stated life	Months to years	2-3 months	Months to years	Over 1 year

* Saccomanno technique substitutes 20 mL normal acetic acid for 20 mL glacial acetic acid.

T35.1
Formulas for 1 L of Alum Hematoxylin

To have consistently stained cells day after day, it is important to make checks with the microscope after critical steps in the procedure, eg, after the progressive blueing and water rinses and after the regressive hydrochloric acid plus running tap water rinses. As recommended by Gill, the dyes should be changed after a specific number of slides have been stained or a specific time has elapsed. In daily practice it is recommended that the dyes be changed after 2000 slides or 6 to 8 weeks, whichever comes first.

Cytoplasmic Stains

The next steps in staining involve the cytoplasmic stains (counterstains). These are synthetic dyes, derivatives of coal tar products, whose chemical formulas have been standardized, so there should be no variation in bottles of these synthetic dye powders.

Orange G (Papanicolaou formula OG-6) is a monochromatic stain that colors keratin a brilliant orange. Because this stain has relatively small molecules, it rapidly penetrates the cytoplasm. Keratin, not normally present in vaginal and cervical epithelium, is found in keratinizing carcinomas, and therefore the presence of bright orangeophilic cytoplasm is significant. Some authors believe the orange G dye can be eliminated. Some laboratories delete the OG stain when staining cerebrospinal fluids, since the presence of squamous epithelial cells can be determined by their morphology and their coloration with EA. EA is a polychrome stain composed of eosin, light green, and, in the original formula, Bismarck brown. Eosin stains the cytoplasm of mature squamous cells, nucleoli, and cilia. Light green stains the cells that are metabolically active, such as parabasal and intermediate squamous cells and columnar cells. Bismarck brown does not add a characteristic color to the cytoplasm. Its reason for inclusion in the original formula is uncertain and it has been eliminated from many formulas.

Superficial cells stain pink with eosin; hence they are described as eosinophilic. Parabasal and intermediate cells stain green, blue-green, or blue, depending on time in the EA stain, and are referred to as cyanophilic.

The formula for the original stain developed by Papanicolaou for staining vaginal smears is designated by a code number, EA-36. A commercial preparation, EA-50, is made from a similar formula except for the solvent; since commercial preparations cannot be made with ethanol, usually methanol is used. EA-36 made in the laboratory and EA-50 purchased from a pharmaceutical supply house are interchangeable. EA-65 is a third formula, which contains half the amount of light green of EA-36 and of EA-50, while the eosin and Bismarck brown remain the same. This reduced amount of light green is sometimes preferred for nongynecologic preparations, particularly if they are thick and absorb too much of the green color. EA-65 also has been recommended for specimens from the female reproductive tract to help differentiate adenocarcinomas of the endocervix from those of the endometrium. Any of the EA stains may be used, however, for all specimen types.

Counterstains are removed from the cells if slides are allowed to remain in the alcohol rinses for an extended length of time.

Clearing

The final step in the Papanicolaou staining method is clearing, which results in cellular transparency. This is the step between dehydration and mounting. The solution used for dehydration is replaced by a substance that is miscible with both alcohol and mounting media. This substance transmits light rays from the microscope illumination in the same manner as the cell itself, thereby making the cells transparent. Xylene at one time was the most commonly used clearing solution. It is colorless and chemically nonreactive, and has a refractive index of 1.494 (approximately that of glass, 1.515). There are substitutes for xylene on the market that have yet to be fully tested. The substitutes may have a greasy feel or a citrus odor, and require alteration of the clearing and coverslipping steps. There is a clearing agent in current use, Clearium, that allows the slide to be taken directly from the last alcohol rinse to the coverslipping medium, eliminating the need for xylene. Until clearing solutions are proven environmentally safe, it is recommended that one work with them under a fume hood.

Procedures and Troubleshooting

Various modifications of the Papanicolaou staining method are presented in the "Procedures" section. The Papanicolaou staining method can be relied on to yield consistently good results provided a few simple guidelines are followed. If problems arise, refer to the appendix of troubleshooting guidelines in this chapter. A more in-depth explanation of cytologic staining mechanisms may be found in "Fundamental Mechanisms of Cytological Staining" by R. W. Horobin (see "Selected Readings").

FILTERING STAINING SOLUTIONS

The purpose of filtering staining solutions is to remove any cellular material that has fallen from the slides. Filtration depends on two elements: the ability of the filter paper to retain particulate matter, and the speed of the filtration process. The correct grade of paper filters rapidly yet retains most microscopic particles, giving a clear filtrate.

Unlike membrane filters, filter papers are not sold by pore size but by numbers indicating retention power. A list of filter paper grades from one company to demonstrate their power of retention and speed is shown [**T**35.2]. Note the shortest time (3 seconds) will not filter out most epithelial cells. With the separatory filter system introduced by Gill, cross-contamination was apparently reduced to zero.

Type of Filter Paper	Retention, 95% Efficient, μm	Filtration Speed, sec
1	11	40
2	8	55
3	5	90
4	20-25	12
5	2-3	250
6	3	175
7	16	30
90	30+	3

* Reprinted with permission from Whatman Catalogue, Clifton, NJ.

T35.2
*Properties of Various Types of Filter Paper**

MOUNTING THE CELL SAMPLE

A mounting medium is a substance that acts as a permanent bond between the slide and the coverslip. It protects the cellular material from air-drying and shrinkage, and acts as an effective seal against oxygen to prevent fading of the stain. It must be miscible with the clearing agent, and must have a refractive index that closely matches the specimen and the glass slide, yielding the best possible transparent image.

Use the smallest amount of liquid mounting medium that will completely cover the area under a coverslip without evaporating after drying. This is best determined by experience. Too rapid evaporation of the solvent causes air bubbles to appear in the mounting medium as it dries. Xylene evaporates more slowly than toluene. A mounting medium with a xylene solvent is particularly recommended for cellulose ester membrane filters. The pH of the mounting medium should be as neutral as possible to inhibit the fading of stains. Regular balsam and even "neutral" Canada balsam are slightly acidic. A list of mounting media solvents and their refractive indices is shown [**T**35.3].

Product Name	Solvent	Refractive Index Liquid
Clearium	NA	1.4998
Clearslip	NA	1.5
Eukitt	Xylene	1.4948
Harleco, HSR	Xylene	1.5202
Histoclad	Toluene	1.586
Permount	Toluene	1.5144
Pro-Texx	Toluene	1.4950

NA, not applicable.

* Companies' names and locations follow: Surgipath Medical Industries Inc, Grayslake, Ill (Clearium); IMEB, San Diego, Calif (Clearslip); Calibrated Instruments, Ardsley, NY (Eukitt); Curtin Matheson Scientific Inc, Houston, Tex (Harleco, HSR); Clay Adams Co, Parsippany, NJ (Histoclad); Fisher Scientific Co, Pittsburgh, Pa (Permount); and Lerner Laboratories, Stamford, Conn (Pro-Texx).

T *35.3*

*Solvents and Refractive Indices for Mounting Media**

There are quick-drying mounting media such as Clearslip (IMEB, San Diego, Calif) and Clearium (Surgipath Medical Industries Inc, Grayslake, Ill) that do not require the use of a solvent.

Refractive Index

The velocity of light in air is a constant. When light passes through any other medium, it is slowed down. The net effect of this is a bending (refraction) of the light ray. The amount of bending that occurs depends on the particular solution through which it passes. A relative fraction, called the refractive index, is the ratio of the speed of light in air to the speed of light in a medium.

$$\text{Refractive index} = \frac{\text{speed of light in air}}{\text{speed of light in a medium}}$$

Note: The refractive index of light in air is given the value of 1.

The refractive index is a useful value in cytology because the closer the refractive index of the mounting medium is to the refractive index of the specimen on the slide, the more transparent the specimen becomes. This is particularly important in mounting membrane filters [**T** *35.4*]. Eukitt (1.4948) and Pro-Texx (1.495) have the lowest refractive indices and are recommended for cellulose filters. Histoclad (1.586) is recommended for polycarbonate filters because its higher refractive index approaches that of the filter. Before using a new mounting medium, it is advisable to check the refractive index to obtain as clear an image as possible. An alternative solution may be to mount a polycarbonate filter on a specifically made slide (Poretics Corporation, Livermore, Calif) that according to the manufacturer, "virtually eliminates distracting pore outlines in polycarbonate filters."

Material	Refractive Index
Membrane filters	
Millipore (cellulose)	1.49
Nuclepore (polycarbonate)	1.62
Poretics Corp (polycarbonate)	1.584
Birefringent	1.625
Glass slide	1.51
Coverslip†	1.52

* Companies' names and locations follow: Millipore Corp, Bedford, Mass (Millipore); Nuclepore Corp, Pleasanton, Calif (Nuclepore); and Poretics Corp, Livermore, Calif (Cyto-Clear).

† No. 1 thinness, 0.96-1.06 mm.

T *35.4*

*Refractive Indices**

Glass Slides and Coverslips

The glass slide beneath the specimen and the coverslip above it also have refractive power. A refractive index for each that is as close as possible to the tissue and the mounting medium produces the optimal visual image [**T** *35.4*].

The thinnest slides are desirable for use in exfoliative cytology, because thick glass slides have a tendency to be uneven and to lead the light from the condenser in an unfavorable way. Slides with a thickness of 0.96 to 1.06 mm are preferable. Coverslips that cover all the cellular material contained on a slide (24 x 50-60 mm) are recommended for cytology to avoid the possibility of losing cells only microscopically visible.

For highest resolution, ie, when oil immersion objectives are used, but also when photomicrographs are to be made using a x40 to x45 objective (high dry), only coverslips of specified thickness should be used because microscope objectives are corrected for this thickness. American- and British-made microscope objectives are corrected for use with 0.18-mm-thick coverslips. German- and Japanese-made objectives are corrected for use with 0.17-mm-thick coverslips. These figures assume that tissue sections are being examined; a No. $1^1/_2$ coverslip would correspond well with these measurements. Since cell samples are usually much thicker in cytology, and a thinner coverslip would compensate for the difference in the specimen, a No. 1 coverslip is recommended for cytologic use.

How to Coverslip Slides

The method of coverslipping a slide, while not difficult, requires practice to achieve speed and dexterity. Coverslipping should be performed only in a well-ventilated space, preferably with the fumes drawn away from the person who is coverslipping. A good light very close to the work area is necessary. One slide at a time should be removed with forceps from the final clearing solution, and the underside quickly wiped dry with cotton gauze. A drop or two of mounting medium is placed on the coverslip, which is then inverted and lowered onto the slide. A dropper may be used to drop mounting medium to the cells on the slide if care is taken to prevent the dropper from touching the surface cells.

All implements used to process specimens should be thoroughly cleaned or discarded after each use. Cross-contamination can occur during coverslipping if the glass rod, dropper, or pipette used for applying the mounting medium touches one cell sample and then another. Also, all instruments used to position the coverslip onto the slide should touch only the outer surface of the coverslip and never the cellular surface of the slide.

A common problem with mounting media is evaporation of the solvent, which causes thickening of the medium, making it difficult to apply. The problem can be eliminated if the viscosity of the fluid is tested weekly. A determination of the normal flow rate of newly opened mounting medium is necessary to establish a standard. This is accomplished by filling a pipette with the fresh medium, taking care to wipe off any excess on the outside of the pipette, and counting the drops that fall in 5 seconds. This number may be used to monitor viscosity of the same medium each week. If the number of drops decreases, add enough solvent to return the flow to the established standard.

Mounting slides with a coverslip and mounting medium are achieved with practice. A No. 1 coverslip that covers the entire cell sample is preferred. Some of the problems that may occur related to coverslipping are shown in the appendix of troubleshooting guidelines at the end of this chapter.

Mounting Cellulose Filters

Proper mounting of filters is not easily achieved. The procedure itself must be followed with attention to detail. It is best to practice on blank filters first. One must avoid the "hills and valleys" only apparent when screening the sample, especially under x40 magnification, and drying out of the filter, which can occur if excess xylene is not removed from the filter during the mounting process.

To avoid the hills and valleys when screening filters, the entire filter must lie flat on the glass slide surface. The flattening is aided by expansion of the filter, which is done before processing the cell sample, when using vacuum pressure to place the filter on the grid, and finally, and perhaps more importantly, when mounting filter preparations. To avoid the appearance of hills and valleys and to avoid evaporation of mounting medium in filter preparations, follow the procedures on page 438.

Mounting Polycarbonate Filters

The same procedure as coverslipping cellulose filters is used. Note that the polycarbonate filter should not be left in the final xylene clearing solutions or the filter will curl at the periphery and be unwieldy to coverslip.

DESTAINING THE CELL SAMPLE

To destain slides the following steps are taken:

1. Removal of the coverslip is accomplished by one of several methods: (1) soaking the slide in xylene until the coverslip falls off, (2) placing the slide in a freezer up to 1 hour (not for newly stained and coverslipped slides; see "Procedures" section), or (3) placing the slide on a warming plate at 60°C for 3 to 4 hours.
2. Once the coverslip is off, put slide through two changes of xylene or xylene substitute to remove all traces of mounting medium. The time it takes to remove the old mounting medium varies with the mounting medium used, how long ago the slide was stained and coverslipped, the thickness of the cell sample, and the thickness of the mounting medium originally used. The time necessary may vary from a few hours to overnight. Then proceed backwards through the staining procedure omitting the stains themselves. By carrying the slide through the alcohols to water, the counterstains will be removed. Gentle dipping for 1 minute in each solution is usually sufficient; however, destaining process times are not critical. In fact, it is better not to rush this process and be sure all the original stain is removed.
3. To remove nuclear stain, soak the slide in dilute hydrochloric acid. This is usually an aqueous solution, but an acid alcohol can also be used. After soaking in dilute hydrochloric acid for 5 to 10 minutes, remove the slide and quickly look at it under the microscope to determine how much nuclear stain is still present. Return it to the acid if the nuclear stain is still apparent. The slide may remain in the acid as long as 1 hour without ill effect.

After the nuclear stain is removed, eliminate the acid by placing the slide in a 10- to 15-minute bath of running water or rinse well in several washes of water. Finally, to remove the acid completely (including the acid counterstains), place the slide in a blueing solution such as Scott's tap water substitute (pH approximately 8.02). After this solution has been rinsed off in two changes of tap water, the slide is ready for restaining and may be placed directly into hematoxylin. Filtering solutions after restaining samples is especially important since cells in specimens being restained may more readily float into the staining solutions than those in freshly fixed cell samples.

RESTAINING THE CELL SAMPLE

In the restaining procedure it has been noted by one of the authors (Keebler) that the cells appear to be more sensitive in their uptake of hematoxylin. It is important, therefore, that one slide be tested prior to restaining a group of slides so the time spent in the hematoxylin does not exceed the time necessary to stain the nucleus. The type of fixation originally used to fix the cells may affect the destaining and restaining procedures and in most cases is an unknown parameter.

PROCESSING FLUID CELL SAMPLES

Macroscopic Observation of Fluids

Macroscopic observations of fluid samples should be recorded prior to processing and before the final diagnostic assessment is made. These notes should include the specimen type, ie, the precise site of anatomic origin must be carefully recorded and clearly designated on the acquisition form. A list of macroscopic descriptions and their possible significance is shown [**T***35.5*].

Because each cell sample is different and thus must be handled individually, there is no single way to assess the presence or absence of malignant tumor cells in a particular cell sample. Not all bloody fluids contain malignant tumor cells, and not all clear fluids are devoid of malignant tumor cells. The technique selected to process a given specimen depends on its volume and consistency. A cloudy fluid often yields a sediment after centrifugation from which direct cell spreads can be made. A small amount of clear fluid such as a cerebrospinal fluid can be filtered through a membrane filter or cells can be concentrated onto a glass slide by means of a cytocentrifuge. Emphasis in the cytopreparatory laboratory should be on individual preparation of each specimen. Small fluid samples can be prepared in their entirety, while 50-mL aliquots of larger samples may be prepared for microscopic examination as long as the sample is either well mixed and equal aliquots are sampled or the natural forming sediment is used to prepare the sample.

Gross Appearance	Possible Disease Process
White, milky (emulsified lipid) chylous	Malignancy, lymph retention, diffuse scleroderma, tuberculosis, filariasis, trauma to thoracic duct
Whitish "woolly" (supernatant has appearance of pineapple juice)	Rheumatoid arthritis
Chylous-like opalescent (fat-free)	Unknown origin
Yellow, milky "gold paint" appearance	Cholesterol crystals
Yellowish white	Collagen disease
Pale yellow, mucoid or jelly-like consistency	Pseudomyxoma peritonei
Yellowish green with odor	High bacterial count If peritoneal fluid, might indicate presence of intestinal bacteria If pleural fluid, might indicate pneumonococcal or streptococcal pneumonia or a lung abscess
Honey-like consistency	Mesothelioma, possible presence of hyaluronic acid
Pale brown	Old hemorrhage
Dark brown (clear yellow supernatant)	Melanoma
Brownish-orange or brownish-green (color remains in centrifugate)	Jaundice
Watery, clear	Transudate
Watery, brownish	Transudate bilirubin

T*35.5*

Descriptive Terminology for Body Cavity Fluids and Their Possible Significance

Sediment may occur in some body fluids if the fluid is allowed to stand for a time. The upper portion contains serum and may ultimately be discarded, while the bottom portion contains the majority of valuable cells that are then used for centrifugation. Some laboratories use this natural sedimentation to their advantage, especially in the preparation of urinary tract samples. Other fluids can be gently rotated in their containers, and the fluid for centrifugation is obtained from a sampling of the entire specimen.

Transudates and Exudates

There are two types of fluid samples: transudates and exudates. Transudates are usually caused by infiltration of blood serum through the intact vascular wall into the pleural or peritoneal cavity. Transudates have a low protein content and a lower specific gravity than exudates. Exudates result from an active accumulation of fluid within a body cavity, apparently associated with damage to the capillary walls. Exudates are usually rich in fibrin and protein and may coagulate on standing.

Knowing whether a fluid is a transudate or an exudate is not only clinically significant but also aids in the correct processing of a specimen. The cells from an exudate usually adhere better to a slide than cells from a transudate. If the fluid contains abundant protein, some of the proteinaceous material can be removed from the cells by centrifugation, discarding the supernatant fluid, and rinsing the cells. Subsequently, interference with the staining reaction is avoided.

A method for handling smaller clotted material is to twist the clotted or fibrin-like material with tissue forceps. Epithelial cells including tumor cells may be trapped within the clotted material. By strenuously wringing out the clot, the cells will be released into the remaining fluid, and the cell sample can then be processed. The remaining portion of the clot can be processed as a cell block or discarded. To prevent clotting, heparin can be added to the collecting container. A clotted specimen can be processed and should not be discarded. Clotting of the cell sample reflects a high protein content. A large clot can be transferred to a beaker twice the size of the clot; by exerting pressure on the clot, the cells trapped within it will be exuded as a fluid sample. The fluid can then be processed like any other fluid sample.

Clinical Information

The patient's clinical history must be checked. The clinician may request special staining procedures on the cytologic sample, or in cases of suspected malignant lymphoma, additional air-dried samples for Wright-Giemsa stain could be made that may be helpful to the cytopathologist in the evaluation of the cell sample. Stains for fat may be of value for a patient suspected of having lipid pneumonia: alcohol fixation of the cell spreads would yield unsatisfactory samples for detection of lipid and formalin vapor fixation would be required. The cytotechnologist should be aware of various disease processes, staining procedures, and requirements for processing samples for immunologic study, and of staining procedures other than the Papanicolaou method that will provide helpful information to the cytopathologist.

Safety of Laboratory Personnel

Clinical information regarding the presence of infectious disease should be obtained by the clinician, but there are instances when this information is not provided to the laboratory or when patient confidentiality conflicts with information given to laboratory personnel. Laboratory personnel should therefore handle every cell sample as one deriving from a patient with an infectious condition, thus protecting themselves and their colleagues from potential danger.

All specimens processed in the cytopathology laboratory must be handled as if they are infectious in order to reduce the risk of transmission of hepatitis, human immunodeficiency virus (HIV), or other infectious conditions to cytopathology personnel. *Universal precautions* is the term used for such protocols that must be utilized when processing biologic specimens, including blood, body fluids and body secretions, according to the Blood Borne Standard issued by the Occupational Safety and Health Administration (OSHA). Precautions to be taken in the cytopathology laboratory have been discussed in Chapter 31, "Safety." However, due to the importance of maintaining a clean environment and minimizing the risk of infections to cytopathology personnel, several points are reiterated in this section.

Handling cell samples from patients with acquired immunodeficiency syndrome (AIDS), hepatitis, and other infectious disease requires special attention, but since we often do not know this information prior to handling a specimen it cannot be emphasized enough that all cell samples should be handled as though infectious. Laboratory personnel must be informed when a cell sample derives from a patient with Creutzfeldt-Jakob disease, especially when handling neurologic material. The mode of transmission of this disease is not known. All cell samples and all equipment used in the preparation of the cell samples must be destroyed, including the actual glass slide material once the diagnostic assessment has been made.

Many hospitals have an Infection Control Committee, a multidisciplinary committee that is responsible for the prevention, control, and investigation of infections within the hospital as well as establishing and monitoring pertinent environmental policies. It is important to have a cytotechnologist involved with this committee to help assess clinical practices regarding handling specimens. An annual review of handling specimens is necessary to maintain the standard of each institution.

Personal hygiene is particularly important. Handwashing is required when handling infectious material and prior to leaving the laboratory. The key to good handwashing is vigorous rubbing. Vigorously rub hands together after lathering with soap and warm water for at least 15 to 30 seconds. Rinse hands well under a stream of water. Use a paper towel to dry hands and use a clean paper towel to turn off the faucet.

Eating and drinking are expressly prohibited in the cytopathology laboratory. Food must not be placed in a refrigerator used for specimens or reagents. Personal items such as purses, books, and glasses should be kept out of the cytopreparatory work area.

Clothing and other apparel worn in the cytopathology laboratory when processing specimens (laboratory coats, paper gowns, masks, goggles, and gloves) should remain in the laboratory. A "clean" laboratory coat should be kept outside the cytopathology area for use when one leaves. Paper gowns, shoe covers, and masks should be discarded after each use in a designated biohazard bag. Gloves are worn to handle all specimens. To avoid contamination, gloves should be removed and discarded when answering the telephone, opening a door, turning on/off switches and using a typewriter, bar coder, computer keyboard, and/or writing implements. Note: Wearing gloves does not eliminate the need for proper hand-washing.

Specimens should be individually placed in self-sealing plastic bags for transport. The requisition is attached to the bag without puncturing a hole in the bag, this prevents contamination of the requisition if the specimen container leaks. Plastic bags or requisitions contaminated by blood should not be accepted by the laboratory.

Specimens collected in syringes should have the needle removed before submitting the specimen to the laboratory. The syringe cap should be used to seal the syringe. In some institutions a specimen sent to the laboratory with the needle attached is not processed until the physician responsible is notified to come to the laboratory to replace the needle with the syringe cap.

Universal precautions are practiced in laboratories because many times accurate clinical information is missing or unknown when the specimen is sent to the laboratory. A biologic safety cabinet/hood should be used when processing specimens that are blended or vigorously mixed to minimize risk of contamination by aerosolization of the specimen. Even with the use of a hood it is recommended to allow the specimen to settle before opening the container cover.

All pipetting of specimens should be done manually. Mouth pipetting is prohibited. Disposable pipettes are preferred and should be disposed of in biohazard containers.

Specimens to be centrifuged are placed in disposable sealed tubes. The amount of specimen should be below the brim to prevent spillage of the contents. The centrifuge cover is kept closed until the centrifuge comes to a complete stop. The cytocentrifuge, used to process small amounts of specimen, is operated with the same precautions as other centrifuges. The main difference is the cytocentrifuge uses chambers and filter paper that directly affix the specimen onto the slide. The cytocentrifuge filter papers are discarded in a biohazard bag. The chambers are soaked in a disinfectant and scrubbed with a small brush to prevent cross-contamination of specimens. Disposable cytocentrifuge chambers are available. Some cytocentrifuges are self-decontaminating; however, in the event of gross contamination the head of the cytocentrifuge may be autoclaved.

Specimens are kept in a refrigerator until all laboratory studies have been completed. Biohazardous waste is any waste that potentially could cause infection, including fluids, blood, body tissue, secretions or excretions, and disposable items used to collect and/or process specimens such as tubes, filter paper, pipettes, and syringes. A sink should be designated for the disposal of urine; any sink reserved for such use should not be used for hand-washing. When pouring specimens, care should be taken not to splatter. The sink should be flushed with water. All other specimens are discarded in double-lined biohazard bags. All disposable items used in the laboratory are discarded in biohazard bags. Sharp items such as glass and needles are disposed of in rigid labeled containers, which are carefully sealed.

All reusable equipment such as blender cups, glassware, centrifuge containers, and cytocentrifuge chambers should be placed in an iodophor solution containing 70% isopropanol, 80 ppm free iodine, or other Environmental Protection Agency (EPA)-approved disinfectant before routine cleaning. Generally, equipment and instruments should be maintained and cleaned according to manufacturer's specifications.

Work surfaces, including countertops, instrument surfaces, and trash lids, are to be cleaned by laboratory personnel at the end of the day or immediately if biohazardous spillage occurs, using 70% isopropanol, 5% sodium hypochlorite, or an iodophor solution containing 80 ppm free iodine.

Genitourinary Tract Samples

Processing urine samples may pose different problems for the cytotechnologist. Fresh urine samples are recommended for cytologic evaluation. Cool or cold urine samples may cause clogging of cellular filters because of the formation of salt crystals in the urine sample [**T**_35.6_]. If the sample is collected in alcohol it is either difficult to attach the cells to the surface of a glass slide or proteinaceous material may adhere to the cells. In the first instance the cells tend to harden and round up, requiring the addition of a cohesive agent on the glass slide, which may interfere with staining the specimen. In the second instance the stain will also not be optimal because of the proteinaceous material. The optimal cell sample, ie, the sample that contains well-preserved and well-stained cells and minimal cell loss, is the freshly collected sample that is prepared immediately on a polycarbonate filter.

Cerebrospinal Fluids

It is recommended that equipment used in the preparation of cerebrospinal fluids be kept separate from other equipment. It is also recommended that a separate staining setup be maintained for cerebrospinal fluids. These two measures will avoid the possibility of floaters from other fluids appearing in cell samples from cerebrospinal fluids.

Substance	Description	Solubility Characteristics	Line Drawing
Acid Urine			
Urates	Calcium, magnesium, and potassium: mostly amorphous	In alkali; at 60°C	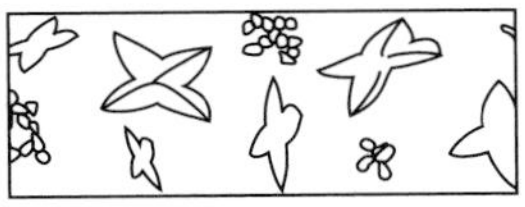
	Ammonium: thorn apple	At 60°C with acetic acid	
	Potassium: small, spherical	Strong alkali	
	Sodium acid urate: needles or amorphous	At 60°C	
Uric acid	Large variety of crystals: rhombic, 4-sided plates, or rosettes; polarizes	In alkali	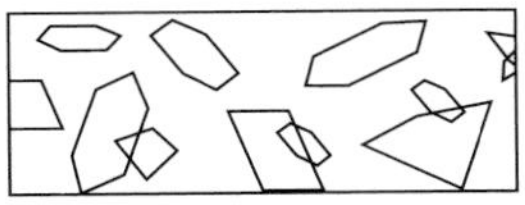
Calcium oxalate	Small octahedron common; dumbbell, ring form	In dilute HCl	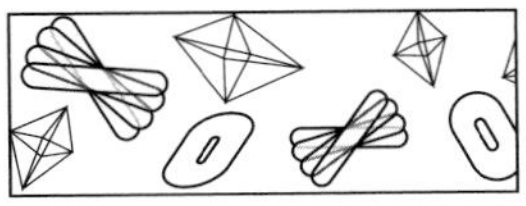
Alkaline Urine			
Triple phosphate	3- to 6-sided prisms, "coffin lid"; sometimes fern leaf	In dilute acetic acid	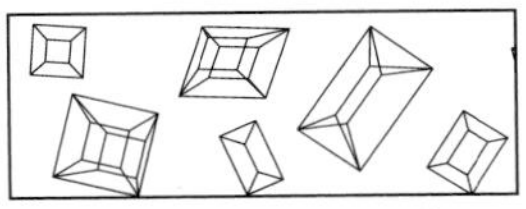
Calcium carbonate	Small dumbbells or spheres; rarely needles	In acetic acid with effervescence	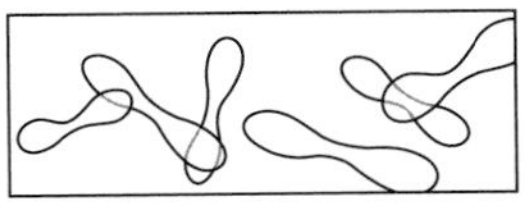
Calcium phosphate	Star-shaped or long, thin prisms; needles or occasional plates	In dilute acetic acid	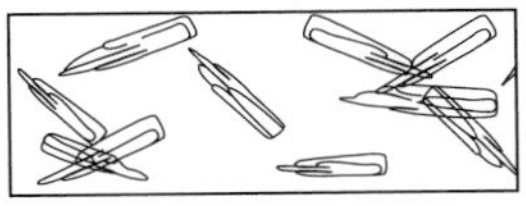
Abnormal Urine			
Cystine	Hexagonal, flat; may be confused with uric acid; does not polarize	In alkali, especially ammonia and dilute hydrochloric acid	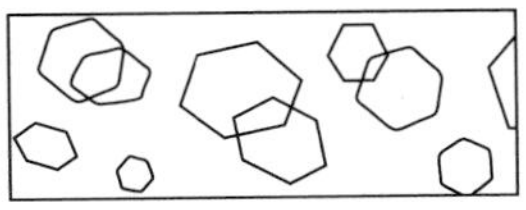
Tyrosine	Fine, silky needles in sheaves or rosettes	In alkali, dilute mineral acid, relatively heat soluble	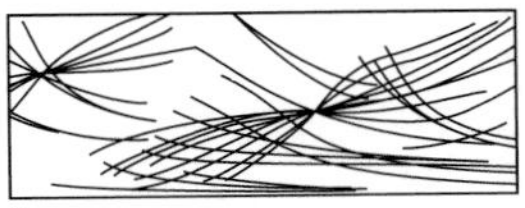
Sulfonamides (eg, sulfadiazine)	Striated sheaves, eccentric binding	In acetone	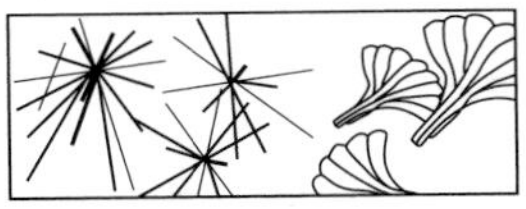
Renografin™, radiographic media	Thin, rhombic, source with notch; easily polarized	In 10% NaOH	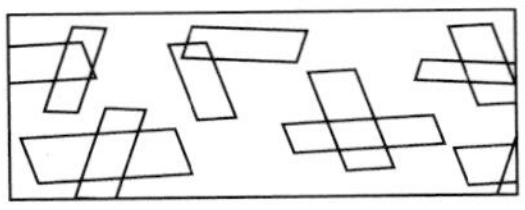
Ampicillin	Long, fine crystals		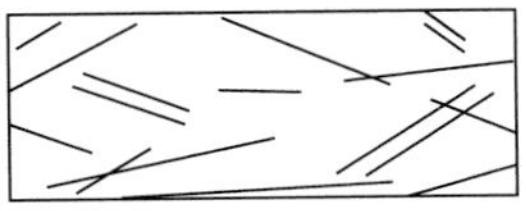
Cholesterol	Flat plates with corner notch	In chloroform, ether, hot alcohol	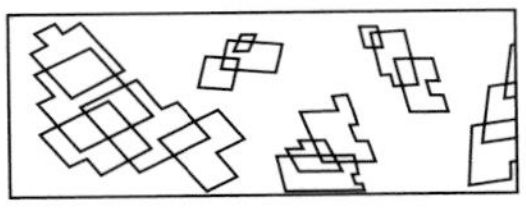

T35.6

Characteristics of Some Crystals and Amorphous Material in Urinary Sediments

The staining procedure can be shortened and OG may be omitted from the procedure without adverse effect.

Preparing Fluid Specimens

The following steps are to be performed prior to processing fluid samples to ensure safe conditions in the cytopreparatory work area, which should be separate from the microscopic evaluation area.

The germ-free hood should be turned on at least one half-hour before processing begins. If filters are to be prepared this is a good time to check the pressure gauge and oil level of the vacuum pump. After donning gown and gloves the specimens are prepared for processing. If refrigerated, the specimens should be removed from the cold and wiped clean with 70% isopropanol. If the hospital does not have double-bag collection containers the requisition forms also need to be wiped clean with 70% isopropanol.

Specimens are matched to the requisition forms. Any discrepancies found should be discussed with the clinician requesting the test. It is at this time that a search by computer or manually is done to see if the patient has had previous cytologic or histologic testing performed. A laboratory acquisition is given to each case and a gross description is written on the requisition form. Slides are numbered, as well as test tubes, specimen containers, and Petri dishes (for filter preparations). Type of sample and patient identification are included on the slides. Filters are numbered with a permanent marking pen and are placed in 95% ethanol for expansion(cellulose filters) or a physiologic solution(polycarbonate filters).

Fluid samples may be divided into equal portions and placed in plastic test tubes for centrifugation. Plastic containers are recommended since they are less likely to break than glass test tubes. To determine the proper centrifugal speed, see the "Technical Section." After initial centrifugation, several processing methods are available. If the specimen is clear and contains few cells, a filter preparation may be the method of choice. If the specimen has a cell button after centrifugation and tests cellular with toluidine blue, direct smears or filters can be made, or cytocentrifugation can be used. If the specimen is bloody, the saponin method can be used, especially when a button cannot be seen after centrifugation. Direct smears or a filter and/or cytocentrifugation may also be tried. If a sample is viscous or mucoid, direct smears or the Saccomanno technique is utilized. For specific details for processing fluid samples, see the "Procedures" section.

Centrifugation

Centrifugation is used to separate cells from the fluid. This processing method may be used for all body cavity fluids, urine samples, and gastric and bronchial washings, or for any specimen where the volume of fluid is large enough or the cellular content sufficient enough to produce a tangible pellet or sediment during centrifugation. Mucoid specimens do not lend themselves to centrifugation unless pretreated or blended prior to centrifugation

Fluid samples may be divided into equal portions and placed in plastic test tubes for centrifugation. Plastic containers are recommended since they are less likely to break than glass test tubes. Additionally, fewer cells adhere to plastic surfaces than to glass. Procedures vary from laboratory to laboratory regarding the recommended time and speed a specimen should be centrifuged. Experiments in cell fractionation show that whole cells sediment optimally at a relative centrifugal force of 600*g* in 10 minutes. To determine what speed will produce 600*g* for a centrifuge, see the "Technical Section."

Once the size of the centrifuge has been determined, the speed to operate it should remain constant, assuming that the liquid media are constant. The speed should be raised only if the specimen is mucoid and very thick. As the head rotates, cells are forced outward and collected in the bottom of the centrifuge tube, forming a button or pellet. The remaining clear liquid is called the supernatant fluid.

Solid particles sediment at different rates; this is true of liquids allowed to stand as well as centrifuged liquids. Specifically, sedimentation depends on the density difference between particle and medium, the size of the particle, and the viscosity of the suspending medium. The suspended matter settles in order of weight and size, the heaviest and largest elements settling first.

The centrifuge should be considered a contaminated area and should be thoroughly cleaned after each use. Prior to centrifugation, examine each plastic test tube for cracks. However, careless balancing of the tubes is a more common cause of breakage than defective test tubes. If breakage does occur, use a germicidal solution to carefully clean out the entire apparatus. A germicidal solution added between the test tube and the centrifuge chamber helps keep the centrifuge chamber uncontaminated and easier to clean in case of breakage. Safety shields or safety trunion cups should be used. Disposable centrifuge tubes should have a screw top to avoid aerosol sprays from the cell sample. Gloves and a mask should be worn when handling cell samples during centrifugation and handling. The cell sample should be permitted to settle prior to removal of the centrifuge cap. Some cytocentrifuges have built in self-decontamination mechanisms. Bench-type centrifuges without a self-decontamination mechanism should be placed in biologic safety cabinets when in use.

Slide Preparation After Centrifugation

After centrifugation, the supernatant fluid is poured off and discarded. The sediment is removed from the test tube by a disposable pipette or a thin cotton-tipped applicator (premoistened by the supernatant fluid).

Most exudates adhere well to plain glass slides. Urine samples, cerebrospinal fluids, and watery samples may not adhere. The following methods may help prevent this problem:

1. Polylysine-coated slides can be used. A solution of polylysine (Polysciences Inc, Warrington, Pa) is spread evenly over a glass slide or the slide may be dipped into the solution.
2. Frosted slides are sometimes used to aid cellular adherence to glass surfaces. Force should not be used to apply the cell material to the frosted slide or cell distortion will result. A light, gentle touch and even spreading of the cell material across the surface of the rough glass slide is best.
3. Albuminized slides can be used. Apply a minimum amount of albumin to glass slides and spread evenly across the entire slide surface. This should be done well in advance to allow the slides to become "tacky," thereby increasing adherence of the cell material to the glass surface. If used too soon, the entire albumin layer and cell sample may slough off during fixation and staining. Albuminized slides may be prepared weeks in advance and kept in a closed container. One disadvantage of this method is that albumin tends to pick up a blue color in staining.
4. The cell sample itself can be albuminized. Add two to three drops of albumin to the cell sample before the material is centrifuged.

When fixing fresh cellular material, especially transudates, allow the sample to dry slightly at the periphery of the cell material prior to placing it in the fixative solution. This will result in better adherence of the cells to the slide. Practice is required, as overdrying may leave the specimen unsatisfactory for cytologic diagnosis.

Lysing Fixatives for Bloody Cell Samples

Too much blood on a slide obscures cellular elements. Fortunately there are ways to remove excess blood from a slide, which should be done before the specimen is stained. Methods to hemolyze and fix bloody cell samples are described below:

1. Place slide in 50% or 70% ethanol, then dehydrate by transferring slide to 95% ethanol.
2. Place slide in modified Carnoy's fixative for 3 to 5 minutes, then place in 95% ethanol. Note: If this lysing fixative is used the staining procedure is altered. The time in the hematoxylin and EA must be reduced since this fixative causes considerable shrinkage of cells and may result in an overstained sample if stained with other samples fixed by different methods.
3. Place slide in 95% ethanol for 5 minutes, then in urea solution (120 g powdered urea dissolved in 1 L distilled water) for 20 to 30 minutes. Then place in 95% ethanol to halt hemolysis.
4. Place slide in solution of one drop of concentrated hydrochloric acid in 500 mL of 95% ethanol for 3 to 5 minutes, then place in 95% ethanol.
5. For handling fluids that are extremely bloody, see the saponin procedure (page 441). A good ventilation system is needed if one works with saponin because it is considered to be a carcinogenic.

Lysing Bloody Air-Dried Samples

Excessive blood can be removed from specimens if the material has been air-dried on a glass slide using a simple but effective procedure (see page 441).

Membrane Filters

Filtration of a specimen through a membrane filter, first applied to routine cytologic examination of urine, can be used for all types of fluid specimens. With this method, a higher rate of cell recovery is often possible than by spreading cells on a glass slide. Commercially prepared cellulose or polycarbonate membrane filters are available and effective in collecting cells for cytologic examination. A list of solutions that have a deleterious effect on filters is shown [**T***35.7*].

Cellulose membrane filters are opaque in appearance until cleared in the staining procedure and covered with a mounting medium with a similar refractive index. Filters must be placed in 95% ethanol a few seconds before use to expand them, otherwise a "hill and valley" effect will interfere with screening. These filters require a modification of the Papanicolaou staining procedure. Once the filter has been moistened it should not be permitted to dry or it will flake, crack, and crumble.

Polycarbonate filters are very thin (10 µm) plastic films. The pores are uniform in diameter and randomly spaced in a straight path through the thin plastic. The total area covered by the pores occupies no more than 2% of the surface area. Because they are initially transparent, Nuclepore filters are not affected by background staining. Expansion in 95% ethanol is not necessary but moistening in physiologic solution is suggested. If left too long in the final xylene or clearing solution the filter tends to curl up. Unlike the pores of other cellulose membrane filters, polycarbonate filter pores remain visible in the finished specimen if standard mounting medium and coverslipping procedures are used. If this is objectionable to the viewer, special steps may be taken to eliminate them (see next paragraph).

Solvent	Cellulose Filter Millipore	Polycarbonate Filters Nuclepore	Poretics
Ethanol, 95%	Swells	None	None
Ethanol, 100%	Softens, deforms, and dissolves	Softens, deforms, and dissolves	None
Methanol	Dissolves*	None	None
Chloroform	None	Dissolves	Not recommended
Ammonium hydroxide, 3 N, 6 N	None	Dissolves in 6 N	Not recommended
Acetone	Dissolves	Bleaches	Limited

* The Gill EA stain contains 250 mL in a 1000-mL solution. This amount does not appear to damage filters.

T35.7
Effect of Solvents on Filters

Dissolving the Polycarbonate Filter

To eliminate the pores in the polycarbonate filter that remain visible, chloroform can be used to dissolve the filter, leaving only the cells visible. This can be performed before or after the staining procedure (see page 441).

Solutions Used in the Preparation of Membrane Filters

The following solutions have little or no effect on filters: *n*-propanol (1-propanol), isopropanol (2-propanol), ethylene glycol, propylene glycol, glacial acetic acid (10%), hydrochloric acid (3 N), formaldehyde, formalin, xylene, and ammonium hydroxide (weak solutions).

To wash cytologic preparations with an isotonic solution, one that will neither shrink nor swell cells, it is necessary to maintain an osmolality of sodium chloride (NaCl), ie, the same as the osmolality of serum and tissue fluid. The formula that achieves this is 8.5 g of NaCl per liter of water (isotonic saline). This solution so nearly approaches the osmolality of fluid from living human beings that it has acquired the appellation "normal." This is an unfortunate word choice that has created confusion because in chemistry the term "normal" describes solutions of higher concentration than that of isotonic saline.

In chemistry, two terms describe concentration: molarity and normality. A one molar solution (1 mol/L) contains one gram molecular weight of a substance per liter of solution (mole = the weight of a substance equal numerically to its molecular weight). A one normal solution (1 N) contains one gram equivalent weight of substance per liter of solution (a gram equivalent weight is the weight of the substance that reacts with one mole of hydroxide ions). For NaCl, the one molar solution and the one normal solution contain the same amount of NaCl, 58.5 g per liter of water. As can be readily seen, the 1 N NaCl (58.5 g/L) is much more concentrated than the isotonic NaCl (8.5 g/L). The 1 N NaCl solution is hypertonic to cells rather than isotonic.

Physiologic saline is another saline solution, and is isotonic to cells and contains ingredients in addition to NaCl, such as trace elements necessary for nourishing cells. Hank's balanced salt solution is an example of a physiologic saline solution. The ingredients in the various types of saline solutions are compared [**T**35.8]. Hank's solution may be preferred over saline solutions in the preparation of fresh body fluids because it is physiologic. The procedure to prepare an inexpensive solution is shown [**T**35.9].

Wet Preparations

A temporary, rapid examination is possible on any nonfixed cellular fluid. After the specimen is centrifuged, a drop of sediment is mixed with an aqueous toluidine blue stain and examined with the microscope. This technique may be used for determining the cellularity of a specimen or for a preliminary search for abnormal cells. This quality control measure will help select those samples that have a potential of floating tumor cells onto other samples if stained together.

The stain is impressive. The cells appear three-dimensional and are much larger than cells that have been fixed in alcohol. In urine samples casts and crystals can be seen, which will dissolve out in the Papanicolaou staining procedure. More cells are seen on the wet preparation than on the smear fixed in 95% ethanol. Since the cells appear larger

Solution	Sodium Chloride (NaCl) g/L H_2O
Isotonic saline (normal)	8.5
1 N NaCl (normal)	58.5
1 mol/L NaCl (molar)	58.5

T35.8
Comparison of Saline Solutions

than those seen on the fixed sample, some individuals may take awhile to adjust to these alterations in appearance of the cells. This procedure is shown on page 438 .

Solute	g/L H_2O
Sodium chloride	8.0
Potassium chloride	0.4
Calcium chloride	0.14
Magnesium chloride·$6H_2O$	0.1
Magnesium sulfate·$7H_2O$	0.1
Disodium phosphate·$2H_2O$	0.06
Monopotassium phosphate	0.06
Sodium bicarbonate	0.35
Dextrose	1.0

T35.9
Hank's Balanced Salt Solution (Physiologic)

PROCESSING RESPIRATORY TRACT SAMPLES

Mucoid samples such as sputum specimens lend themselves to direct spreading of the fresh sample onto the glass slide after careful selection of bloody and white flecks within the sample. However, the preferred method for sputum sample processing is the technique recommended by Saccomanno because of its ability to sample the entire cell sample, not only an arbitrary sample selected by an individual who may or may not be experienced in the handling of mucoid samples or for those individuals who cannot deal with such samples. This technique for handling respiratory material is presented below.

The following information relating to respiratory tract cell samples was contributed by Fern Miller, CT(ASCP).

Fresh (Unfixed) Specimens

Aerosol-induced specimens and an occasional specimen from hospitalized patients may come to the laboratory without preservative. These unfixed specimens are prepared without delay to prevent degeneration of cells, or a polyethylene glycol/alcohol fixative may be added to the sample on arrival in the laboratory. In the latter instance, the Saccomanno technique (page 441) can be used for further processing.

The fresh specimen must be carefully sampled. Transfer multiple discolored portions of specimen (blood-tinged area, blood flecks, etc) to slides by means of forceps or applicator sticks.

Gently crush specimens between two slides until large lumps disappear. Separate slides and, with an applicator stick, tease out material to form a uniform smear over the surface of the slide. Avoid leaving rough or raised areas that may create coverslipping problems. Drop immediately into 95% ethanol. Do not allow material to dry during smearing procedures. A few drops of isotonic saline may be added to soften the material and keep it moist during the process.

Prefixed Specimens

Specimens are collected in 70% ethanol. Excessive hardening of the specimen (coagulation of mucoproteins) is encountered when 95% ethanol is used.

Sample material carefully, selecting discolored areas if present. Place multiple small samples of these areas on a slide thinly coated with commercial egg albumin. Using a second albuminized slide, break up the material with a firm rotating motion. If the specimen has become hard or rubbery, a drop of tap or distilled water on the slide will soften it adequately. Continue to crush the specimen between two slides with alternate rotating and up-and-down motion until there is a thin, evenly distributed film on each slide. Do not allow the material to dry on the slides during smearing; keep wet with drops of water or isotonic saline solution.

If in doubt as to how well the material will adhere to the slides through rehydration and staining, test before dropping into 95% ethanol fixative by pulling slides apart. Well-smeared slides should come apart cleanly. If material from one slide comes off on the other, continue working with rotating and up-and-down movement until test is successful. Drop immediately into 95% ethanol.

Allow slides to remain in fixative for a minimum of 30 minutes. Longer periods of fixation are not harmful to cells. Remove slides from fixative and immerse in distilled or tap water for 15 to 20 seconds. Drain well. Slides may be stained immediately or allowed to air-dry, thus reducing the risk of cell loss.

The technique of smearing sputum specimens is easily learned, but practice with various types of material is necessary to make cell spreads that are diagnostically acceptable. Extremely thin smears do not provide sufficient cells for fair assessment, and a thick smear is microscopically unsatisfactory. The goal is to obtain a thin, uniformly distributed layer of cells over each side.

Cells prefixed in a polyethylene and alcohol solution lend themselves to processing with the Saccomanno technique (page 441). Grossly, the technique used to make cell spreads, with practice, will yield a finely granular, uniform appearance. Microscopically, an even distribution of cells is revealed. The background is relatively free of mucus, the bulk of this having been suspended and discarded in the supernatant fluid.

With the Saccomanno technique, some cell-group fragmentation has been noted in tumor cells deriving from adenocarcinomas. In addition, tumor cells from small cell carcinoma tend to be more widely dispersed and thus the microscopic appearance may differ considerably from the prominent clusters and/or streaks seen with the conventional sampling method. If small cell carcinoma is suspected on a given specimen, blending at a slower rate and for a lesser time may be advantageous.

Occasionally a specimen is difficult to prepare. Extremely degenerated, purulent material is hard to process, as is firm rubbery mucus that may be a secretion from the nasopharynx. For these specimens, proceed in the manner described above. Purulent specimens are most satisfactory if very thinly smeared. There is no best way to handle the mucoid material that may originate in the nasopharynx.

Bronchial Secretions and Washings

For processing of these samples, see page 441.

Pneumocystis carinii

Detection of *Pneumocystis carinii* in bronchial wash samples stained with the Diff-Quik method is fairly reliable and rapid, and has a reported sensitivity of 76%. The routine Papanicolaou staining method may be less sensitive for the washings but improves in bronchoalveolar lavage specimens. Sensitivity is increased with the use of Grocott-Gomori methenamine-silver stain and cresyl echt (fast violet), in addition to the Diff-Quik stain. The Gram-Weigert stain is also good.

Bronchial Brushing Technique

Brushings from the bronchial tree are prepared in the bronchoscopic examining room. Operating room personnel are instructed in preparation of slides. The material from the brush should be confined to an area on the slide approximately the size of a nickel. The slides are placed immediately into 95% ethanol and sent to the cytology laboratory. Brushings smeared in too thin a fashion over the surface of the slide tend to dry rapidly before immersion in the fixative, thus distorting the cells and making microscopic assessment difficult.

TECHNICAL SECTION

Laboratory Measurements

Volume

The basic unit of volume measurement in the metric system is the liter. One liter is approximately equivalent to one quart (1 L = 1.0567 qt). Volume is also frequently expressed in terms of cubic measurement of length. The cubic centimeter (cu, cc, cm^3) is probably the most commonly encountered, but the trend is to use the milliliter (0.001 L), especially for volume of liquids. The difference in the two measurements is very small (1 mL = 1.000027 cc), and a liter is now defined so that 1 mL exactly equals 1 cc.

To measure the volume of liquids in the laboratory, graduated cylinders of various sizes, burets, and pipettes are generally used. Because they have a larger diameter than pipettes, graduated cylinders are less accurate than pipettes. In reading any of these, the container is held so that the liquid surface is level with the eye; the volume is read to correspond with the bottom (concave) surface of the meniscus of transparent liquid or the top (convex) surface of opaque liquids.

Weight

The basic unit of weight is the gram. One gram is approximately 1/30 of an ounce. One kilogram (1000 g) is about 2.2 lb.

Size

The term micrometer (μm) was adopted in 1967 by the Thirteenth General Conference of Weights and Measures as the official designation for 10^{-6} meters. It has replaced the micron (μ).

Solutions

The amount of a substance (solute) that will dissolve in a solution (solvent) is not fixed. Different concentrations can be produced. There is an upper limit, however, to the amount of solute that can be dissolved in a solvent. A solution containing the limiting amount is called a saturated solution. Any additional solute will settle to the bottom of the container and will not dissolve. One way of guaranteeing a saturated solution is to keep adding solute until there is an excess.

The three most common percentage solutions used in the laboratory are (1) grams of solute in 100 mL of solution (wt/vol, ie, weight per volume), (2) grams of solute in 100 g of solution (wt/wt, ie, weight per weight), and (3) milliliters of liquid in 100 mL of solution (vol/vol, ie, volume per volume).

In most laboratories the weight per volume solutions are used because the solvent is merely the vehicle for the solute. The preparation of a 5% solution of sodium chloride, for example, on a weight per volume basis, would consist of dissolving 5 g of sodium chloride in water and then diluting the solution to a final volume of 100 mL. The preparation of a 1% weight per volume concentration of 2,6-di-tert-butyl-*p*-cresol in a mounting medium would consist of dissolving 1 g of the antioxidant in 100 mL of the mounting medium.

A one normal solution is abbreviated 1 N solution; sometimes the "1" is eliminated and just implied [**T**35.10].

Concentration of HCl, %	Amount of HCl, mL
36	86.0
37	83.3
38	80.8
39	78.4
40	76.2

T35.10
Amount of Hydrochloric Acid Needed to Make 1 L of a 1 N Solution

Specific Gravity

The specific gravity of a solid or a liquid is a number that expresses the ratio of the weight of the solid or liquid to the weight of an equal volume of water at 4°C used as a standard.

$$\text{Specific gravity} = \frac{\text{weight of solid or liquid}}{\text{weight of an equal volume of water at 4°C}}$$

The density of water changes very little between 4°C and 30°C; therefore, the value of 1 g/mL may be used as a standard for specific gravity measurements at ordinary laboratory temperatures. The specific gravity of a solid or liquid is the same when any system of units is used because it expresses the ratio of the weight of the solid or liquid to the weight of an equal volume of water. Specific gravity values are therefore expressed as a number without any units. The measurement of the specific gravity of urine is a standard component in routine urinalysis. It is a screening test that provides information about the concentrating and diluting ability of the renal tubules. It reflects the concentration of dissolved substances; the normal range is 1.008 to 1.030.

Transfer of Materials

To transfer solids into wide-mouth containers, such as beakers or dishes, or onto paper sheets, tilt the bottle containing the solid and rotate it. Do not shake the bottle as you pour and do not insert any object into the bottle. (It may be advantageous to shake the bottle before opening it to loosen the contents.)

To transfer liquids, place a stirring rod against the lip of the bottle or other container from which the liquid is to be removed. Tilt the bottle so that the liquid flows down the rod into the receiving container.

When using pipettes, medicine droppers, or aspirators, first pour a small quantity of the solution from the reagent bottle into a beaker; do not put the dropper into the reagent bottle. Draw a small quantity of the solution from the beaker into the dropper and, without inverting the dropper, place its tip against the inside upper edge of the receiving container and squeeze the bulb to force the liquid without splashing.

Centrifugal Speed

Procedures vary from laboratory to laboratory regarding the recommended time and speed a specimen should be centrifuged. To determine the centrifugal speed that will produce 600*g* speed, measure the radius of the rotating head of the centrifuge (from the center to the bottom of the test tube holder) in centimeters [**F**35.2] and apply this measurement to the chart shown [**F**35.3]. This chart relates relative centrifugal force (expressed in gravities) to revolutions per minute (rpm) and the radius of the centrifuge head (expressed in centimeters). Place a line on the chart that will intercept 600*g* and the known radius of the centrifuge. The recommended speed (rpm) will be evident where the line intercepts the column on the right. For example, if the radius of the centrifuge from the center of the rotating head to the bottom of the test tube holder is 20 cm, then fluid specimens are centrifuged at 1200 rpm for 10 minutes.

This chart can also be used to determine the relative centrifugal bar force when the rpm is given and the radius is known. Intercept these two points, and the line will cross the middle column at the centrifugal force this combination will produce.

Once the size of the centrifuge has been determined, the speed to operate it should remain constant, assuming that the liquid media are constant. The speed should be raised only if the specimen is mucoid and very thick.

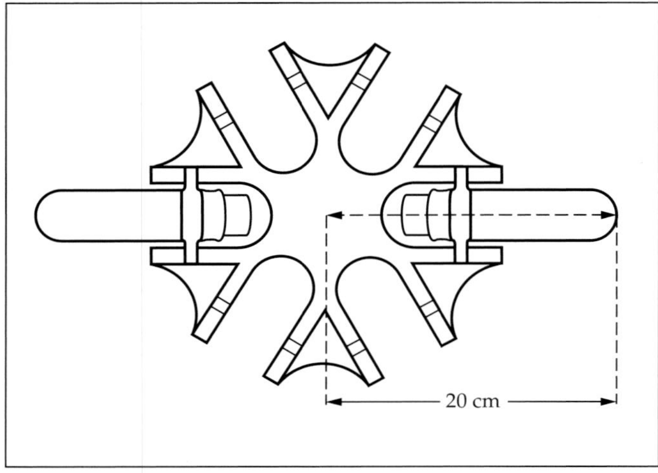

F35.2

*Determining rotating speed of centrifuge (rpm): (1) Measure radius of centrifuge in centimeters. (2) Using the chart [**F**35.3], draw a line from the determined radius in the first column through 600g in the second column, which can be considered a constant for sedimenting whole, intact cells. The projected line will intercept the last column at the recommended rate of speed to be used for 10 minutes.*

Rotating Radius, cm: 20, 19, 18, 17, 16, 15, 14, 13, 12, 11, 10, 9, 8

Relative Centrifugal Force (600*g*): 2,000, 1,000, 1,000, 800, 700, 600, 500, 400, 300, 200, 150, 100

rpm: 3,000, 2,500, 2,000, 1,500, 1,400, 1,300, 1,200

F35.3

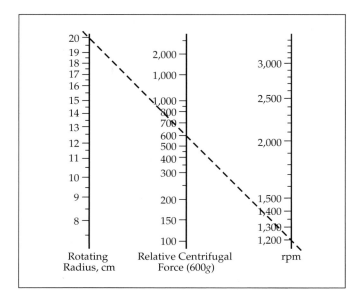

Determination of recommended speed for centrifuge.

FORMULAS

Cytologic Use

Equivalent concentrations of alcohols for cytologic fixation:

100% Methanol
95% Ethanol
95% Denatured alcohol
80% Propanol
80% Isopropanol

Commercially available spray fixatives for cytologic use

Coating fixative (prepared in the laboratory):

Polyethylene (Carbowax 3350 Flake; Union Carbide Chemicals, New York, NY)	*50 g*
95% ethanol or equivalent	*950 mL*

Combine and shake vigorously until dissolved. The bottle may be placed in warm water to hasten the process. This fixative must be removed before staining by soaking in 95% ethanol or equivalent for 15 to 30 minutes.

Lysing Fixatives for Bloody Cell Samples

Urea, 2 mol/L solution:

Powdered urea	*120 g*
Distilled water	*1 L*

Modified Carnoy's fixative:

95% ethanol	*7 parts*
Glacial acetic acid	*0.5 parts*

Hydrochloride lysing fixative:

95% ethanol	*500 mL*
Hydrochloric acid, concentrated	*1 drop*

Histologic Use

Neutral-buffered formalin, 10% (pH, 7.0):

Concentrated formaldehyde solution (37%-40%)	*100 mL*
Water	*900 mL*
Acid sodium phosphate, monohydrate	*4 g*
Anhydrous disodium phosphate	*6.5 g*

Bouin's fluid:

1.2% aqueous picric acid solution	*75 mL*
10% formalin	*25 mL*
Glacial acetic acid	*5 mL*

Stains Used in the Papanicolaou Staining Method

Half-Oxidized Hematoxylin (Gill)

The following chemicals are combined in the order given, stirring for 1 hour on a magnetic mixer at room temperature:

Distilled water	*730 mL*
Ethylene glycol	*250 mL*
Hematoxylin, anhydrous (color index [CI] No. 75290, certified)	*2.0 g*
Sodium iodate	*0.2 g*
Aluminum sulfate, $Al_2(SO_4)_3 \cdot 18H_2O$	*17.6 g*
Glacial acetic acid	*20 mL*

1. CI No. 75290 includes crystalline hematoxylin ($C_{16}H_{14}\cdot 3H_2O$, molecular weight 356.336) and powdered anhydrous hematoxylin ($C_{16}H_{14}O_6$, molecular weight 302.288). Catalogs do not always describe which form is available. The laboratory worker must distinguish between them simply by inspecting the hematoxylin sample. To equal 2.0 g of anhydrous hematoxylin, 2.36 g of crystalline hematoxylin must be used.
2. The amount of sodium iodate must be weighed accurately to ±0.01 g.
3. Use of other aluminum sulfate formulas requires amounts other than 17.6 g to provide the same number of aluminum ions.
4. One gram of citric acid can be substituted for 20 mL of glacial acetic acid.
5. The chemicals are of reagent quality.

The stain can be used immediately but may require 3 to 4 minutes to achieve the intensity attained routinely in 2 minutes by hematoxylin that has remained covered for 1 week at room temperature or in a 37°C incubator.

Although no visible precipitate is recovered, it is good practice to filter the stain through medium grade filter paper before using it for the first time.

Harris Hematoxylin (Stock Solution)

Hematoxylin (CI No. 75290, certified)	*5 g*
95% ethanol	*50 mL*
Aluminum ammonium sulfate	*100 g*
Distilled water	*1000 mL*
Mercuric oxide (red or yellow)	*2.5 g*

Dissolve the hematoxylin in alcohol. Dissolve the aluminum ammonium sulfate in water and bring to a boil. Add the hematoxylin solution, and again bring to a boil. Remove from heat and add mercuric oxide immediately. Stir until the solution assumes a dark purple color, and then plunge the flask into a cool water bath. When the solution has cooled, filter it into a dark bottle.

Harris Hematoxylin (Working Solutions)

Technique 1: Dilute a sufficient amount of the stock solution with an equal volume of distilled water. Keep in a well-stoppered, dark bottle when not in use. Filter each time before using.

Technique 2: Add glacial acetic acid to 4% (vol/vol) concentration and use acetified Harris hematoxylin full strength. Keep in a well-stoppered, dark bottle when not in use. Filter before each use.

Hematoxylin

Hematoxylin is a yellow or red crystalline compound, the coloring principle of logwood, oxidized in solution to form hematein, the active dye.

The nuclear stain is hematoxylin and is extracted from the inner parts of the stem of the logwood tree found in Central America. Today most of the extract or wood comes from Brazil. Supplies in the United States and other parts of the world are dependent on local conditions of production and shipment. Hematoxylin is a colorless compound, easily oxidized to hematein, an orange to reddish compound (not to be confused with hematin, a constituent of hemoglobin). The brownish powder used to make up the dye solution is a varying mixture of hematoxylin and hematein. Hematein is not an efficient colorant of tissue by itself and would be easily removed by solvents were it not for its ability to link up with the metal salts of alums in forming what is called a dye lake. Alums are double sulfates of two- and three-valent metals or other cations such as ammonia. Hematein binds firmly to the aluminum alum of the hematoxylin staining solution and changes its color in the process to a deep blue (lake). It is the trivalent metal from the alum that binds to tissue (and is therefore called the mordant). It in turn has the dye attached to it. Once a lake is bound to tissue it is not easily removed by neutral fluids and is therefore ideal with respect to counterstains.

Many of the manipulations associated with the hematoxylin stain of cytology and histology are to accomplish adequate concentration of oxidized hematoxylin (hematein), to prevent excessive oxidation, and to eliminate eventually from the tissue all compounds other than the blue hematein-alum lake. Staining by other constituents of the hematoxylin mixture occurs occasionally and is usually reddish. The hematein lake is assumed to bind to the phosphate groups of DNA and RNA. Some arguments against this concept of exclusive binding to nucleic acids have, however, been raised. It is likely that nuclear proteins also participate to a certain extent in stain uptake. Extensive discussions of this interesting and crucial dye can be found in a book by Baker and in an article by Gill et al (see "Selected Readings").

OG-6 Counterstain

The OG-6 staining solution is 0.5% (wt/vol) orange G in 95% ethanol. Since the crystalline dye is not readily soluble in 95% alcohol, the following procedure should be used:

1. Prepare a 10% aqueous solution of orange G (CI No. 16230, certified), using distilled water. Allow to stand for several days.
2. Prepare the OG-6 staining solution (0.5%) as follows:

Orange G, 10% aqueous solution	*50 mL*
95% ethanol	*950 mL*
Phosphotungstic acid	*0.15 g*

Store in a well-stoppered, dark bottle and filter before using.

Modified Orange G

1. Prepare a 10% total dye content aqueous solution of orange G (CI No. 16230, certified) by dissolving a corrected weight of dye in 100 mL of distilled water at 70°C to 80°C. The corrected weight of dye is obtained by dividing 10 g by the percent dye content that is

printed on the label of bottles of synthetic dyes certified by the Biological Stain Commission. For example, 12.5 g of orange G must be weighed out for a lot that contains 80% dye (10 g + 0.80 = 12.5 g).

2. To prepare a working solution of modified orange G, combine the following ingredients:

Orange G, 10% (total dye content [TDC]) aqueous solution	*20 mL*
95% ethanol	*980 mL*
Phosphotungstic acid	*0.15 g*

No precipitate forms; the solution is ready for immediate use.

Orange G

Orange G is a strongly acidic dye. It stains keratin within the cytoplasm and reacts with the basic groups of protein. It is only slightly soluble in ethanol, and 50 times more soluble in water. In 95% ethanol, orange G stains cytologic material sufficiently lightly to maintain transparency of cytoplasm. Phosphotungstic acid was added by Papanicolaou as a substance to enhance the depth of color. It is known as a mordant and for its effects on metachromasia or chromotropism. Phosphotungstic acid strongly binds to proteins; in fact, it is one of the strongest protein precipitants. In turn, orange G appears to bind more strongly with tungstate-treated cytoplasm. No metachromasia is known or likely for orange G, and neither is the formation of a lake.

EA

EA is a polychromatic stain, whereas hematoxylin and orange G are monochromatic. EA is an unfortunate experimental label chosen by Papanicolaou to indicate a mixture of light green SF, eosin Y, and Bismarck brown Y. The numbers 36, 50, and 65 that usually follow the designation EA are laboratory codes and bear no direct relation to the composition of the mixture.

Light green SF carries the designation SF (Saurefarbstoff) because German chemists made it as an acid dye. It is a good stain for cytoplasm, as it binds well to basic protein side chains. It is the most light-sensitive of stains in the Papanicolaou series.

Eosin Y (yellowish) is tetrabromofluorescein. When all four bromine atoms are present, it is deepest red; at lower bromine content, eosin tends to stain more yellowish. Mixtures of various levels of bromination are sold commercially. Eosin is the most widely used stain for the cytoplasm, rendering strong tinctorial effects as an acid dye.

The significance of Bismarck brown Y in the Papanicolaou series is obscure. Baker identifies it as a basic dye convenient for coloring lipid cytoplasmic inclusions in living cells. Most of the Bismarck brown is precipitated out of the mixture by reacting with phosphotungstic acid. It has been eliminated from the Gill formula altogether.

EA-36

EA-36 was originally formulated for staining gynecologic smears but can be used for other types of body secretions and fluids. The original formula was modified slightly in 1954.

1. Prepare the following aqueous solutions, using distilled water: 2% light green SF yellowish (CI No. 42095, certified) and 10% Bismarck brown Y (CI No. 21000, certified). Allow to stand for several days.
2. Prepare alcoholic stock solutions:

0.1% light green	
2% aqueous light green	*50 mL*
95% ethanol	*950 mL*

0.5% Bismarck brown	
10% aqueous Bismarck brown	*5 mL*
95% ethanol	*95 mL*

0.5% eosin Y	
Eosin Y, water, and alcohol soluble (CI No. 45380, certified)	*5 g*
95% ethanol	*1000 mL*

3. Prepare EA-36 staining solution:

0.1% light green	*450 mL*
0.5% Bismarck brown	*100 mL*
0.5% eosin	*450 mL*
Phosphotungstic acid	*2 g*
Lithium carbonate, saturated (about 1.3% wt/vol) aqueous solution	*10 drops*

Mix well and store in a well-stoppered, dark bottle. Filter before using. Bismarck brown was included as a background stain, but it has no discernible color effect.

EA-65

EA-65 is a modification of EA-36 developed for staining thicker cell spreads of nongynecologic specimens. Use of either EA-36 or EA-65 for staining is a matter of personal preference.

1. Using 2% aqueous light green solution, prepare 0.05% light green in alcohol.

0.05% light green:	
2% aqueous light green SF yellowish	*25 mL*
95% ethanol	*975 mL*

2. Prepare EA-65 staining solution:

0.05% light green	*450 mL*
0.5% Bismarck brown	*100 mL*
0.5% eosin Y	*450 mL*
Phosphotungstic acid	*6 g*

EA-50

EA-50 is a ready-made solution prepared commercially by several manufacturers. It is supposed to be similar to EA-36 but its composition varies from one manufacturer to another. Variables include the type of solvent (by federal law it cannot be undenatured ethanol); the presence or absence of Bismarck brown, acetic acid, and lithium carbonate; and the amount of light green and eosin.

Modified EA

The formula for modified EA is the result of testing by Gill that has shown that Bismarck brown exerts no discernible color effect and can also form a precipitate with phosphotungstic acid. Therefore, it has been deleted from the original formula. Modified EA is used for gynecologic and nongynecologic cellular preparations.

1. Prepare two solutions: a 3% TDC aqueous solution of light green SF yellowish (CI No. 42095, certified) and a 20% TDC aqueous solution of eosin Y (CI No. 45380, certified) by dissolving separately corrected weights of each dye in separate amounts of up to 100 mL of 70°C to 80°C distilled water (see step No. 1 of directions for modified orange G for remarks regarding corrected weights).
2. To prepare a working modified EA staining solution, combine the following ingredients:

95% ethanol	*700 mL*
Absolute methanol	*250 mL*
Glacial acetic acid	*20 mL*
3% light green TDC aqueous solution	*10 mL*
20% eosin (TDC) aqueous solution	*20 mL*
Phosphotungstic acid	*2 g*

Stat OG/EA

The procedure (from the Johns Hopkins Cytopathology Laboratory, Baltimore, Md) requires the preparation of 1 L of stat OG/EA. Combine the following:

10% orange G, aqueous	*6 mL*
3% light green SF yellowish, aqueous	*20 mL*
20% eosin Y, aqueous	*20 mL*
95% ethanol	*680 mL*
absolute methanol	*250 mL*
Glacial acetic acid	*20 mL*
Phosphotungstic acid	*4 g*

Blueing Solutions

Blueing solutions differentiate and "blue" the nuclei in the progressive staining method of Papanicolaou.

1. Tap water alone, if pH is higher than 8.0.
2. Ammonium hydroxide (NH_4OH) in 70% ethanol (or water): Add 15 mL NH_4OH to 985 mL 70% ethanol (or water).
3. Lithium carbonate (Li_2CO_3): Mix 1.5 g Li2CO3 in 100 mL water. Add 1 mL of mixed solution to 99 mL water.
4. Scott's tap water substitute: Add 2 g sodium bicarbonate ($NaHCO_3$) and either 10 g magnesium sulfate anhydrous ($MgSO_4$) or 20 g magnesium sulfate ($MgSO_4{\cdot}7H_2O$), crystalline (Epsom salt) to 1000 mL water. The pH of Scott's tap water substitute is about 8.02. This blueing agent is replaced after every second rack of slides or filters is processed. Its pH plays an important role in determining the color of the nuclei. Suitable alternatives to this blueing agent are 0.5% sodium acetate (pH 7.13); 0.1% sodium bicarbonate (pH 8.05), and 1.0% potassium acetate (pH 7.45).

Destaining Solution

Acid alcohol solution:

Hydrochloric acid (5N) concentrate reagent grade	*10.0 mL*
70% ethanol	*1000 mL*

Note: Always add acid to alcohol.

Toluidine Blue

Formula 1 (McCormack et al modified by Naylor)
Stock solution of toluidine blue:

Toluidine blue	*0.5g*
95% ethanol	*20.0 mL*
Distilled water	*80.0 mL*

Dissolve toluidine blue in alcohol and then add distilled water, filter, and store in dark bottle. Store in refrigerator to prevent fungal growth.

Formula 2 (Holmquist)
Stock solution of toluidine blue:

Toluidine blue	*1 g*
Distilled water	*100 mL*

Working solution of toluidine blue:
1 part stock to 15 parts water

Thionin Blue

Thionin blue	*1.0 g*
25% ethanol	*100 mL*
Glacial Acetic Acid	*2 drops*

Dissolve the thionin blue in alcohol, add acetic acid, let stand for 30 minutes, filter, and store in a dark bottle. Frequent filtration is needed for this solution as it tends to form crystals. Thionin blue does not stain red blood cells. The Papanicolaou stain can be performed over the thionin blue stain.

Hydrochloric Acid Solution

A one normal solution is abbreviated 1 N solution; sometimes the "1" is eliminated and just implied. To make a 1 N hydrochloric acid (HCl) solution, follow this procedure:

1. Check the assay on the bottle of concentrated HCl to determine the percent of concentration.
2. Choose the appropriate amount of HCl based on the concentration of HCl [**T** *35.10*].
3. In a 1000-mL graduated cylinder place 700 mL of distilled water. Add appropriate amount of HCl. Cool. Add water to 1000 mL.

Solutions for Saponin Method for Bloody Fluid Samples

1% saponin solution (Fisher Scientific Co, Pittsburgh, PA) (prepare under a fume hood):

Saponin	*1 g*
0.2% stock solution of sodium p*-hydroxybenzoate*	*100 mL*

1. Mix thoroughly.
2. Filter through 8-µm membrane filter.
3. Refrigerate.

0.2% stock solution of sodium *p*-hydroxybenzoate (Eastman Kodak Co, Rochester, NY):

1. Dissolve 2 g sodium *p*-hydroxybenzoate in 1000 mL distilled water.
2. Refrigerate.

3% calcium gluconate solution:

1. Dissolve 3 g calcium gluconate in 100 mL 0.2% stock solution of sodium *p*-hydroxybenzoate.
2. Mix thoroughly.
3. Filter through 8-µm membrane filter.
4. Refrigerate.

Hank's Solution

The procedure for preparing 1 L of solution is as follows:

1. Gently stir the prepackaged powdered medium (Grand Biological Co, Grand Island, NY) into 950 mL of deionized distilled water at 15°C to 30°C (room temperature). Do not heat the water.
2. Rinse out inside of package to remove all traces of powder.
3. Add 0.35 g of $NaHCO_3$ per 1 L of medium.
4. Add 50 mL deionized distilled water to bring the volume to 1 L.
5. Adjust the pH of the medium to 0.2 to 0.3 below the desired final working pH (pH units will usually rise 0.1-0.3 with filtration). Use of 1 N NaOH is recommended; add slowly with stirring.

PROCEDURES

Papanicolaou Staining Procedure, Progressive Method

95% ethanol (fixative)	15 min
80% ethanol	6-8 dips
70% ethanol	6-8 dips
50% ethanol	6-8 dips
Water, distilled	6-8 dips until glossy look disappears
Harris hematoxylin,* undiluted	45 sec
Water, distilled	Rinse
Water, distilled	Rinse
Water, distilled	Rinse
50% ethanol	6-8 dips
Ammonium hydroxide NH_4OH (1.5% in 70% ethanol)	1 min
70% ethanol	6-8 dips
70% ethanol	6-8 dips
80% ethanol	6-8 dips
95% ethanol	6-8 dips
OG-6	1-1/4 min
95% ethanol	Rinse
95% ethanol	Rinse (do not allow slides to remain in alcohol)
EA-50 or -65	3 min
95% ethanol	Rinse gently
95% ethanol	Rinse gently
95% ethanol	Rinse gently
100% ethanol	6-8 dips
100% ethanol (if large volume)	6-8 dips
100% ethanol:xylene (1:1)	6-8 dips
Xylene	6-8 dips
Xylene	6-8 dips
Xylene	Until ready to mount

*Undiluted stock to which 4 mL glacial acetic acid per 100 mL of stain has been added.

Papanicolaou Staining Procedure, Regressive Method

95% ethanol (fixative)	15 -30 min
80% ethanol	6-8 dips
70% ethanol	6-8 dips
50% ethanol	6-8 dips
Water, distilled	15 sec-2 min until glossy look disappears
Harris hematoxylin: distilled (1:1) stock solution diluted with an equal volume of distilled water	6 min
Distilled water	Rinse to remove excess stain

Distilled water	Rinse
Aqueous hydrochloric acid solution HCl (0.25% aqueous)	6 dips
Gentle running tap water (lukewarm)	6 min
50% ethanol	6-8 dips
70% ethanol	6-8 dips
80% ethanol	6-8 dips
95% ethanol	6-8 dips
OG-6	$1^1/_2$ min
95% ethanol	Rinse off excess stain
95% ethanol	Rinse (do not allow slides to stand in the alcohol as it will decolorize them)
EA-36, -50, or -65	$1^1/_2$ min
95% ethanol	Rinse gently (do not leave slide in alcohol)
95% ethanol	Rinse gently (do not leave slide in alcohol)
95% ethanol	Rinse gently (do not leave slide in alcohol)
100% ethanol	6-8 dips
100% ethanol (if large volume)	6-8 dips
100% ethanol:xylene (1:1)	6-8 dips
Xylene	6-8 dips
Xylene	6-8 dips
Xylene	Until mounted

Gill Half-Oxidized Hematoxylin Staining Method

Solutions for slides and filters:	
Tap water	10 dips
Tap water	10 dips
Gill hematoxylin	2 min
Tap water	10 dips
Tap water	10 dips
0.05% hydrochloric acid (omit for slides) (color of filter should be very pale yellow)	Up to 30 dips in 1 min
Tap water	10 dips
Tap water	10 dips
Scott's tap water substitute	1 min
Tap water	10 dips
Tap water	10 dips
95% ethanol	10 dips
95% ethanol	10 dips
Slides and polycarbonate filters:	
Modified orange G	$1^1/_2$ min
95% ethanol	10 dips
95% ethanol	10 dips
95% ethanol	10 dips
Modified EA	10 min
95% ethanol	30 dips
95% ethanol	30 dips
95% ethanol	30 dips
Absolute ethanol	10 dips
Absolute ethanol	10 dips
Absolute ethanol	10 dips
Xylene	10 dips
Xylene	10 dips
Xylene	Until coverslipped
Cellulose filters:	
Modified orange G	2 min
95% ethanol	1 min
95% ethanol	1 min
95% ethanol	1 min
EA* for filters	8 min
95% ethanol	4 min (no dips)
95% ethanol	2 min (no dips)
95% ethanol	1 min (no dips)
Absolute isopropanol	1 min
Absolute isopropanol	1 min
Absolute isopropanol	1 min
Xylene	1 min
Xylene	1 min
Xylene	Until coverslipped

*Formula for EA for cellulose filters differs from that for slides and polycarbonate filters. See Gill and Miller in "Selected Readings."

A modified Papanicolaou procedure for samples from the female reproductive tract [**T***35.11*] and a Papanicolaou staining method for tissue sections [**T***35.12*] are shown.

Quick Papanicolaou Staining Procedure for Stat Specimens (Johns Hopkins Cytopathology Laboratory, Baltimore, Md)

Tap water	5-10 dips (until surface is smooth)
Gill's hematoxylin No. 2	1 min, including 10 initial dips
Tap water	5 dips
Scott's tap water substitute	15 sec
Tap water	5 dips
Stat OG/EA	1 min, including 10 initial dips
95% ethanol	5 dips
95% ethanol	5 dips
Absolute ethanol	10 dips
Absolute ethanol	10 dips
Xylene	5 dips
Xylene	5 dips
Coverslip	

Procedure	Time	Points of Emphasis
95% ethanol	30 min	Slides fixed with a Carbowax component (some spray fixatives) must be rinsed well in two separate solutions of 95% ethanol prior to staining the cells. These washes are designed to remove the waxy coating from the cells for a better uptake of the stains.
95% ethanol	30 min	These two alcohol solutions should be discarded after every second basket or filtered for reuse.
Tap water	Time varies	The glassy appearance of the water on the glass slide must disappear prior to placement in hematoxylin. This may take as long as 5 minutes, depending on the thickness of the cell sample. Drain the water thoroughly from the slides so as not to dilute hematoxylin. Discard the water after each use.
Half-oxidized hematoxylin	4-6 min	A microscopic check may be made after 2 minutes to determine the total time needed for adequate nuclear staining.
Running tap water	Time varies	Gently run tap water until all traces of hematoxylin are removed and the water runs clear.
Scott's tap water substitute	1 min	The Scott's solution must be removed from the slide. If not, a white filmy coating will appear on the slide.
Tap water	25 dips*	
95% ethanol	10 dips	The 95% ethanol solutions are rotated when the first ethanol is discolored by stain.
95% ethanol	10 dips	
Modified orange G	1 min	
95% ethanol	10 dips	Rotate ethanol solutions as each one becomes discolored by dye.
95% ethanol	10 dips	
95% ethanol	10 dips	
Modified EA	10 min	
95% ethanol	20 dips	Rotate ethanol solutions as each one becomes discolored by dye.
95% ethanol	20 dips	
95% ethanol	20 dips	
Absolute ethanol	10 dips	
Absolute ethanol	10 dips	
Absolute ethanol	10 dips	
Xylene or substitute	10 dips	It is recommended that all xylene be kept under a hood.
Xylene or substitute	10 dips	Coverslipping must be performed under a hood as must the filtering of all xylene.
Xylene or substitute	Until coverslipping	
Mounting medium		

* To avoid loss of cells due to mechanical agitation, slides should be dipped gently. A dip is the complete submersion of the slides in a solution and their complete removal from the solution in a continuous and somewhat quick fashion. The cell sample must never be allowed to air-dry between solutions.

T*35.11*

Modified Papanicolaou Staining Procedure for Samples From the Reproductive Tract (Chicago Lying-In Hospital, 1991)

Procedure	Time	Points of Emphasis
80°C oven	2 hours	Use to melt paraffin. Note: Oven time and staining time may vary with thickness of section.
Xylene	5 min	
Xylene	5 min	
Xylene	5 min	
100% ethanol	5 min	
95% ethanol	30 min	Slides fixed with a polyethylene glycol component such as hair spray must be rinsed well in two separate solutions of 95% ethanol prior to staining the cells. These washes are designed to remove the waxy coating from the cells for a better uptake of dye. These two solutions should be discarded after every second basket or filtered for reuse.
95% ethanol	10 min	
Tap water	Variable	The glassy appearance of the water on the glass slide must disappear prior to placement in hematoxylin. This may take as long as 5 minutes, depending on the thickness of the cell sample. Drain water thoroughly from slides so as not to dilute hematoxylin. Discard water after each use.
Half-oxidized hematoxylin	8 min	A microscopic check is made to assess time factor.
Tap water	Variable	Gently run tap water until all traces of hematoxylin are removed and the water runs clear.
Scott's solution	1 min	
Tap water	40-50 dips*	Scott's solution must be removed from the slide, otherwise a white filmy coating will appear on the slide. Discard water after each use.
95% ethanol	10 dips	
95% ethanol	10 dips	
Orange G	1 min	
95% ethanol	10 dips	Rotate ethanol solutions as each one becomes discolored by dye.
95% ethanol	10 dips	
95% ethanol	10 dips	
EA	10 min	
95% ethanol	20 dips	Rotate ethanol solutions as each one becomes discolored by dye.
95% ethanol	20 dips	
95% ethanol	20 dips	
Absolute ethanol	10 dips	
Absolute ethanol	10 dips	
Absolute ethanol	10 dips	
Xylene	10 dips	Xylene must be covered at all times and used under a hood.
Xylene	10 dips	
Xylene	Until cover-slipping	Coverslipping and filtering of xylene must be performed under a hood.
Mounting medium		

* To avoid loss of cells due to mechanical agitation, slides should be dipped gently. A dip is the complete submersion of the slides in a solution and their complete removal from the solution in a continuous and somewhat quick fashion. The cell sample must never be allowed to air-dry between solutions.

T *35.12*

Papanicolaou Staining Method for Tissue Sections (Chicago Lying-In Hospital, 1988)

Destaining and Restaining Procedures

Procedure 1(Chicago Lying-in Hospital):

1. Remove old mounting medium using xylene. The time needed is variable; it is necessary to check the slide at selected time intervals until one is certain that the old mounting medium has been removed.
2. Rinse in a clean xylene solution.
3. Rinse in absolute ethanol (10 dips).
4. Rinse in absolute ethanol (10 dips).
5. Rinse in absolute ethanol (10 dips).
6. Rinse in 95% ethanol (10 dips).
7. Rinse in 95% ethanol (10 dips).
8. Rinse in tap water (10 dips).
9. Place in acid-alcohol solution (see "Formulas" section). Time varies (3-5 minutes or until slide appear colorless).
10. Rinse in running tap water. The time needed varies (5 -10 minutes) to remove all traces of acid.
11. Restain with Gill half-oxidized staining method.

Procedure 2 (Case Western Reserve University, Cleveland, Ohio):

1. Remove old mounting medium using xylene. The time needed varies.
2. Rinse in absolute ethanol/xylene (1:1).
3. Rinse in absolute ethanol.
4. Rinse in absolute ethanol.
5. Rinse in 95% ethanol.
6. Rinse in 95% ethanol.
7. Rinse in 95% ethanol.
8. Rinse in 95% ethanol.
9. Rinse in 80% ethanol.
10. Rinse in 70% ethanol.
11. Rinse in 50% ethanol.
12. Rinse in distilled water.
13. Place slides in 1% HCl for 1 to 20 minutes to remove hematoxylin (hematein). The time will vary depending on the thickness of the material.
14. Wash slides under gently running tap water for 10 minutes to remove all traces of acid.
15. Restain the slides.

This procedure is also used to remove the golden brown artifact or "corn flakes."

Procedure 3 is used for cellulose filter preparations (Henry Ford Hospital, Detroit, Mich):

1. Hang filter on clip, as in staining procedure for cellulose filters.
2. Rinse in xylene (30 minutes minimum).
3. Rinse in absolute ethanol (1 minute).
4. Rinse in absolute ethanol (1 minute).
5. Rinse in 95% ethanol (20 dips).
6. Rinse in 95% ethanol (20 dips).
7. Rinse in 0.05% HCl (10-20 minutes or longer, depending on how long decolorization takes).
8. Rinse in running (distilled) water (2 minutes).
9. Stain beginning with Gill's hematoxylin No. 1.

Toluidine Blue Staining

1. Pour supernatant off specimen.
2. Place one drop of sediment on a slide with a disposable eye dropper.
3. Place one drop of stain near the cell sample on the slide with a second disposable eye dropper.
4. Mix the two drops together with the eye dropper.
5. Coverslip with small coverslip so cells and dye stay in a central location on the slide.
6. Let sit for a few seconds.
7. Examine cell sample under the microscope for the presence of malignant tumor cells and their cell type. This information will help determine the amount of sample to be used for a filter preparation and if the sample should be stained separately from other specimens.

This staining procedure may be used for the rapid evaluation of fine needle aspirates. Rapid Papanicolaou staining procedures and a thionin staining procedure are also in use in some laboratories.

Thionin Staining Method

Fixation in 99% isopropanol	$1^1/_2$ min
Tap water	5 dips
Thionin blue	5 dips and then sit for 1 to $1^1/_2$ min
Tap water	5-10 dips
99% isopropanol	Rinse
99% isopropanol	Rinse
Coverslip	

Diff-Quik Staining

The Diff-Quik staining procedure for air-dried smears is shown [**T***35.13*].

Mounting Filters

To avoid evaporation of mounting medium the following procedure should be followed:

1. Place a strip of mounting medium lengthwise on labeled glass slide.
2. Place cellulose filter, cell side up, on top of mounting medium.
3. Place clean applicator across middle of filter.
4. Roll applicator stick like a rolling pin toward one edge of filter. Flatten filter as you roll applicator stick. This flattening process avoids "hills and valleys" in the filter and places cells on the same focal plane. This step also avoids excessive evaporation of the clearing agent.

Procedure	Time	Points of Emphasis
Fixative (aqua solution)	25-30 dips	Before staining the sample it is advisable to immerse the slide in 95% methanol for 5-10 minutes or longer if sample is bloody.
Solution I* (orange solution)	25-30 dips	To enhance eosinophilia, increase the number of dips; for paler staining, decrease the number of dips (to no fewer than 3 dips).
Solution II* (purple solution)	25-30 dips	To enhance cyanophilia, increase the number of dips; for paler staining, decrease the number of dips (to no fewer than 3 dips).
Distilled water		May be examined wet or dry.
Allow to dry		
Xylene	Several seconds	
Coverslip		

* Solutions should be tightly capped when not in use and changed once a week.

T*35.13*
Diff-Quik Stain for Air-Dried Smears

5. Bring applicator stick to middle of filter again.
6. Roll applicator stick toward second edge of filter, flattening the filter with the applicator stick.
7. Discard applicator stick.
8. Place strip of mounting medium lengthwise across top of flattened filter.
9. Place coverslip on top of mounting medium on slide.
10. Press coverslip down with slight pressure to ensure mounting medium covers entire area of slide. No open areas should remain or evaporation of remaining clearing fluid will occur, resulting in an opaque, dried out filter. If air bubbles appear at periphery of slide between filter border and edge of slide it is possible to fill in gaps with the use of a disposable aspirator syringe containing mounting medium held alongside the edge of the slide next to the air bubble; osmotic action will help fill in the empty spaces.
11. Store the filter samples in a flat horizontal position for at least 3 months prior to storing in an upright position. This, as well as not wiping the excess mounting medium from the sides of the slide, will help prevent the filter from drying out.

Freezer Method to Remove Coverslip

1. Place slide flat in freezer compartment of refrigerator with coverslip side down. Freezer time varies from 10 minutes to 1 hour, depending on how long ago the slide was coverslipped. The more time that has elapsed the less time required in the freezer.
2. Remove slide from freezer. Area between coverslip and slide should appear frosty and there should be a separation of the coverslip from the slide along the periphery. If the slide does not appear frosty and there is no visible separation between slide and coverslip, go back to step 1.
3. Place a razor blade under the coverslip where separation already exists and move it along the outer edge of the slide. The coverslip should pop or fall away from the slide easily. Note: Protective gloves and goggles should be worn for this step.

Preparing a Cellulose Filter

1. General introductory steps are to be found on page 425.
2. If a cell button is apparent, pour off supernatant in disposable plastic container. If no cell button is apparent, proceed to step 11.
3. Carefully decant one test tube.
4. Save and refrigerate second test tube.
5. Resuspend button in 10 mL of Hank's balanced salt solution. To achieve a thorough mixing of the cell sample, use a vortex blender.
6. Mix one drop of resuspended specimen with one drop of toluidine blue with one drop of resuspended fluid on a glass slide.
7. Cover with No. 1 coverslip (24 x 24 mm).
8. Wait 1 minute.
9. Examine under x10 objective of microscope to determine how many drops of fluid should be added to filter.
10. Make a direct smear from sediment if air-dried sample deemed necessary.
11. Moisten grid of filter apparatus with isotonic solution.
12. Place moistened and expanded filter on grid.
13. Use vacuum to secure placement of filter on grid.

14. Place funnel over filter on grid. Be sure placement of filter is in correct position, then clamp the funnel to grid.
15. Allow the isotonic solution to pass through the clean filter. This will allow the filter to flatten out on the surface of the grid. Pleating or wrinkling of the filter is avoided. The filter is now ready for the cell sample.
16. Add 20 mL of Hank's or isotonic saline solution to the funnel. Note: When adding solutions to filter funnel, let fluid run along the side of the funnel.
17. Add 50 to 100 mL of Hank's or isotonic solution to funnel.
18. Add one or more drops of sediment with a disposable pipette (depending on cell number). Add the drops of sediment above and close to the filter in an even motion across the surface of the filter.
19. Slowly begin the vacuum.
20. Continue the vacuum until the Hank's solution is barely covering the filter. The filter must be covered with fluid at all times.
21. Add the isotonic solution from a rinse bottle along the sides of the reservoir to retrieve any cells clinging to the sides of the funnel. When the solution has almost disappeared, stop the vacuum.
22. Add 20 to 30 mL of 95% ethanol to the reservoir to fix the cells on the filter. Allow the fixative to remain on the filter for 1 minute, then begin the vacuum again and pull most of the fixative through the filter. A small amount of fixative should remain on top of the cells. Stop the vacuum. Pouring 95% ethanol onto the already present Hank's solution will result in a 50% alcohol solution, which in turn acts to lyse red blood cells in the cell sample. One can see the filter turn from red to white very quickly. If the 50% alcohol solution does not work, a second preparation may be required or the saponin technique should be tried.
23. Remove the clamp, lift the funnel, and transfer both to disinfectant solution.
24. Remove the filter from the grid with forceps and quickly place filter, cell side up, in a labeled Petri dish containing 95% ethanol.
25. Run disinfectant solution through the grid, followed by 95% ethanol, then transfer grid to disinfectant solution.

Cytocentrifugation Using Cytospin 2

Cytospin 2 procedure for samples with a cell button:

1. Place labeled slides, filter cards, and perspex chamber into slot at periphery of cytocentrifuge.
2. Balance chambers.
3. Add Saccomanno preservative for slides intended for Papanicolaou staining: four drops for body fluids and bronchial washings, two drops for urine samples, and four to six drops for patients with AIDS or with Creutzfeldt-Jakob disease when no filter will be made. In the latter case, disposable cytofunnel chambers should be used. If slides are to be air-dried for hematologic staining, no preservative is added.
4. Place specimen drops into the chamber with a disposable pipette, depending on the results of the toluidine blue procedure, or use number of specimen drops in step 3.
5. Balance remaining chambers with Hank's solution.
6. Centrifuge at 600 rpm for 4 minutes; if cerebrospinal fluid, centrifuge at 500 rpm for 5 minutes.
7. Turn timer to the "off" position.
8. Allow centrifuge to come to a stop. Do not brake mechanism.
9. Remove slide from each chamber with care. The cell sample should not be disturbed.
10. Immediately place slides for Papanicolaou staining into 95% ethanol.
11. Repeat steps 7 and 8 for the remaining slides.
12. Place slides to be air-dried in a staining holder.
13. If the sample is not considered infectious the perspex chambers are placed in a 10% bleach solution for one half-hour. If the specimen is considered contaminated the disposable chambers are placed directly into specially marked bags for contaminated material (red bags would help separate this material from less contaminated material and would alert disposal personnel to material to be handled as infectious).
14. Remove chambers from disinfectant after 15 to 20 minutes.
15. Rinse chambers with distilled water after removal from bleach solution and dry thoroughly.

Cytospin 2 procedure for samples with no cell button:

1. Remove test tubes from centrifuge.
2. Invert test tube to drain off supernatant.
3. Take sample from base of test tube and mix with Hank's solution.
4. Mix on vortex mixer to resuspend cells.
5. Add preservative to each cytocentrifuge chamber.
6. Add a few drops of resuspended specimen to chamber.
7. Spin specimen for 4 minutes at 600 rpm; if cerebrospinal fluid specimen, spin for 5 minutes at 500 rpm.
8. Remove slides with care.
9. Place filters and disposable cytofunnel chambers directly into red bag.
10. Place chambers and slide clips into disinfectant.
11. Place slides for Papanicolaou stain into 95% ethanol or fix with spray fixative. The latter may help cells adhere to glass slide surface.
12. Place air-dried sample in staining dish.
13. Remove chambers from disinfectant after 15 to 20 minutes.
14. Rinse chambers well with distilled water and dry thoroughly.

Saponin Method

The saponin method may be applied to all excessively bloody samples:

1. Centrifuge specimen at 3000 rpm for 10 minutes.
2. Discard supernatant.
3. Add 25 mL of Hank's or isotonic solution to cell button.
4. Mix well and add up to 45 mL of Hank's or isotonic solution.
5. Resuspend the cell concentrate by repeatedly inverting the centrifuge tube, or better, by agitation on a vortex mixer.
6. Add 2 mL of 1% saponin and mix by inversion. Note: Refrigerate solution when not in use, because at room temperature fungal growth occurs. Usefulness of the solution is determined solely by whether it continues to hemolyze erythrocytes. With refrigeration the solution may keep for one week or possibly longer.
7. After 1 minute, add 3 mL of 3% calcium gluconate and mix by inversion. Note: Refrigerate the solution when not in use. It may keep for 1 week or longer.
8. Centrifuge at 3000 rpm for 10 minutes. The supernatant is colored red; the cell concentrate, white. Unburdened of hemoglobin, the red blood cell ghosts remain suspended in the supernatant and cannot contaminate the cell concentrate. The increased number of nonerythrocytes available for microscopic examination is remarkable.
9. Prepare cell spreads or centrifuge sample when cell concentrate permits; otherwise, resuspend the cell sample in a small amount of Hank's or isotonic solution (depending on size of button) and prepare a cellulose filter.

Rehydration Method for Air-Dried Bloody Smears

Rehydration (Case Western Reserve University method) of air-dried smears with normal saline is used for bloody smears, ie, bronchial washings, fluids, and needle aspirates:

1. Spread material on clean glass slide.
2. Allow the slide to dry completely and quickly (air-dry for no longer than 30 minutes).
3. Place slide in normal saline for 30 seconds to rehydrate (to prevent cross-contamination, change saline after each specimen).
4. Transfer the wet slide to 95% ethanol for fixation.
5. Use Papanicolaou staining method.

Dissolving Polycarbonate Filters

Method before staining:

1. Remove the filter from fixative; cut and trim it if necessary. Do not let the filter dry. Reimmerse in fixative.
2. Place the filter cell side down on a plain slide that has been labeled with the specimen's accession number. Do this on a paper towel.
3. Working quickly, lay two pieces of medium-grade filter paper (or paper of similar absorbent texture) over the filter and either roll a tape roller over it or use finger pressure. Once over and back is sufficient; speed is important to avoid air-drying.
4. Remove the paper and make sure alcohol is under the filter to keep the cells wet. The filter must not look as it does when dry; if it does, the cells will take up stain poorly and be unsatisfactory to examine.
5. Still working quickly, take a Pasteur pipette already filled with chloroform and cover the filter with the solvent. This anchors the cells and filter to the slide.
6. Without waiting, put the slide (still covered with chloroform) in a Coplin jar of chloroform. Cap the jar.
7. After 30 minutes, transfer the wet slide to 95% ethanol. Dip it several times. If the slide remains clear, the polycarbonate filter has been dissolved completely. If a milky film appears on the slide, dissolving is incomplete. If incomplete, return the slide to chloroform for about 15 to 30 minutes or until it remains clear when placed in ethanol again.
8. Routinely stain and coverslip the slides.

Method after staining:

1. Remove filter from the last dish in staining procedure.
2. Remove the holding clips from the filter.
3. Remove filter from slide and dry slide completely on an absorbent paper towel.
4. Place filter on slide with cell side down (ie, cells against glass).
5. Blot filter dry with absorbent tissue, using either finger pressure or a glass rod. The filter will be slightly opaque when completely dry.
6. Place a 4 x 4-in gauze pad in a Petri dish, and place slide with filter on top if it.
7. With slide tilted and with chloroform in a pipette, flood chloroform evenly over entire filter surface. It is best to start at the center of the filter and work toward each end.
8. Immediately place slide on flat surface. The cover of the Petri dish should be inverted. If moisture in the air contacts the filter at this point, the filter will become cloudy. If the chloroform has been applied spottily, holes will appear in the filter.
9. Remove slide from Petri dish, dip in xylene, and mount.

Saccomanno Blending Technique

First, prepare a 2% polyethylene glycol solution as follows:

1. Add 2 mL of melted polyethylene glycol to 948 mL of 50% ethanol.

2. A supply of melted polyethylene glycol may be kept at 56°C for ready use. Glassware used to make the solution must be kept warm to prevent hardening of wax on the surface during preparation, which can cause inaccurate measurement.
3. Mix polyethylene glycol solution and ethanol on a magnetic stirrer for 30 minutes. Once in solution, polyethylene glycol does not coagulate.

Perform the Saccomanno blending technique as follows:

1. Collect sputum in 120-mL plastic containers half-filled with polyethylene glycol solution. The polyethylene glycol is essential to prevent shrinkage of the cells and to retain nuclear detail.
2. When a sputum specimen is received in the laboratory, shake the container vigorously to mix specimen thoroughly with preservative solution. Prepare slides with proper identification. Egg albumin is not necessary, as material adheres well to slides.
3. Pour into a 50-mL plastic centrifuge tube. If contents of collection bottle do not equal 50 mL, add 50% ethanol to bring to this level.
4. Pour contents of tube into a 250-mL Eberbach semimicrocontainer (Scientific Products, Minneapolis, Minn).
5. Homogenize specimen using a blender at high speed for 5 to 10 seconds or less. If flecks and fine threads are visible in the specimen, return to blender for an additional 10 to 15 seconds. Avoid excessive blending.
6. Return the specimen to the tube.
7. Centrifuge in plastic tubes for 10 minutes at 2100 rpm.
8. Decant supernatant fluid, leaving 1 or 2 mL to admix with sediment.
9. Agitate on electric mixer for 10 seconds.
10. Aspirate sediment into Pasteur pipette.
11. Place one or two drops of centrifugate, if thick, or two to four drops, if thin, on a slide.
12. Lay a second slide over the centrifugate and allow it to spread evenly between the two slides. If necessary, gentle manipulation of the two slides may be used to aid in dispersion of the sediment.
13. Pull slides apart with an easy, sliding motion.
14. Air-dry slides, leaving a thin coating of wax. Drying causes cells to become firmly adherent to slides, thus virtually eliminating the possibility of cell loss during rehydration and staining. Smears may be left in this condition for days or weeks without ill effect. As far as is known, the function of polyethylene glycol in solution is to prevent shrinkage of cells during air-drying. Since polyethylene glycol precipitates on the slides, it must be removed to allow full penetration of stains.
15. Remove polyethylene glycol from cell samples by immersion of slides in 95% ethanol for 10 to 15 minutes with occasional dipping.
16. Rinse slides in two stages of tap water of 10 seconds each.
17. Stain by Papanicolaou method.

APPENDIX: TROUBLESHOOTING GUIDELINES

Staining

General staining problems and their possible causes are shown [**T***35.14*].

Papanicolaou Staining Methods

1. Cover solutions when not in use.
2. Filter stains daily.
3. Staining dishes should be thoroughly cleaned of stain residue each day.
4. The level of all solutions should be checked prior to beginning the procedure.
5. Stains are added to the staining baskets from the working solutions as needed to maintain the appropriate level in the staining dishes.
6. When using the progressive method, it is necessary to maintain the alkaline pH of the blueing agent to "blue" the nuclei the same intensity every time. The pH can be checked with specifically graded litmus paper.
7. When using the regressive staining method, the percent and formula used for the hydrochloric acid solution varies greatly from laboratory to laboratory. It is therefore necessary to make this step as uniform as possible.

Stains

1. Stains are light sensitive and subject to oxidation. Oxidation may be slowed by keeping the stains in opaque dishes and covered as much as possible during staining and when not in use. Stains should be stored in dark opaque bottles.
2. The life expectancy of stains can be lengthened by filtering them at the end of each day and returning them to brown storage bottles. Gill suggests using separatory funnels for filtering and storing the stains. An 8.0-mm membrane filter is incorporated into the system to remove cellular material from the stains.
3. Stains should be filtered daily before use.
4. Most commercially sold hematoxylin stain today is more variable in quality than that sold prior to October 1, 1973, and requires 5 to 6 g of hematoxylin to equal the stain intensity that 1 to 2 g produced previously. The lot numbers given by the Biological Stain Commission are listed in their journal, *Stain Technology*, published bimonthly, and serve as a guideline for determining hematoxylin quality. If

Problem	Possible Reason
Dark nuclei	Sample was overstained in Harris hematoxylin. Excess stain was not removed by rinses following hematoxylin. There were too few dips in HCl, or the HCl concentration was less than recommended. The ammonium hydroxide solution was too strong. Note: An overly potent ammonium hydroxide solution may cause sedimentation to appear at the base of the staining dish and require frequent changes.
Pale nuclei	The polyethylene glycol coating was not removed from cells prior to hematoxylin. HCl was not removed in the tap water rinse. The concentration of HCl was greater than recommended or slides were dipped too many times in HCl. The ammonium hydroxide solution was too weak. Note: One can test this solution by waving one's hand across staining dish toward stainer. If odor is apparent, solution should be active; if not, discard. The percentage of this solution is difficult to control and variation of staining will most likely occur. The time in hematoxylin was inadequate. The time in chlorinated tap water was excessive. The pH of the tap water following hematoxylin was not sufficiently alkaline. The hematoxylin was diluted by water if water was not properly drained from the slides. Stains should be changed each 2000 slides or each 6 to 8 weeks, whichever comes first. Prior to placing slides in hematoxylin, the refractile "glassy" or "bubbly" appearance must be eliminated by increasing the time the slides are left in water. If this is not done, penetration of the dyes is impaired. This step usually takes longer than the time designated in most staining procedures [**F**35.4, **F**35.5].
Cytoplasmic color not consistent	Air-drying occurred prior to fixation. Solutions were not at proper level within dishes. Slides were left too long in alcohol rinses or clearing solutions following OG and EA. Polyethylene coating was not adequately removed from cells. The time in hematoxylin was too long, or hematoxylin was not removed prior to OG and EA dyes. Rinsing of slides between solutions was inadequate. Rinsing following staining solutions was insufficient. Improper draining of slides between rinses occurred. Various times and types of stains were inconsistent from day to day. pH of tap and distilled water was not sufficiently alkaline. pH of EA needs to be controlled (pH 4.5-5.0 achieves maximum results). pH of cell sample may vary from sample to sample (enzymes released by microorganisms may alter pH of cell sample). Water temperature may vary from season to season. Thickness of cell sample is variable; look to the periphery of cell groups to check color and consistency of staining results. Cell sample was left near heat during mailing process or during the time between obtaining the sample and staining. Slides were fixed in a variety of fixatives, each reacting differently to staining.
Intense green cytoplasm	Eosin in the EA stain has been overpowered by green dye. Time in EA may be reduced to achieve desired "greenness." Note: The greenness or blue-green color of the cytoplasm is a good way to determine if EA is functioning. Once the greenness of the cytoplasm disappears, the EA is exhausted and should be changed.
Macroscopically the slides or filters are pink, orange, or yellow	Oven temperature was too high; if so there is nothing that can be done to obtain a well-stained sample. To avoid this disaster the oven temperature should be checked and recorded each day.
Dull, grayish hazy appearance of cells	Water contamination of dehydrating and clearing solutions has occurred. Polyethylene glycol coating was not removed from cells prior to staining of filter.
Lack of contrasting cytoplasmic colors	Hematoxylin and EA dyes were exhausted.
Opaque white color on back of slide	Scott's tap water substitute was not rinsed from slides. Use two separate but thorough water rinses following Scott's tap water substitute.

T35.14

Staining Problems and Solutions

Gill's or Mayer's hematoxylin is used, there is little chance of overstaining.
5. Chlorinated tap water will bleach hematoxylin.
6. If hematoxylin is diluted with tap water, the water should be slightly alkaline.
7. The pH of the EA should be on the acidic side (4.5-5.0) to achieve optimal results.
8. If polyethylene glycol fixatives are used, the hematoxylin stain requires constant observation to avoid contamination by the coating substances. Frequent changes of hematoxylin may be required. As mentioned previously, prior to staining slides fixed with coating fixatives it is recommended that the slides be immersed in two separate rinses of 95% ethanol or 80% ethanol for at least 20 minutes each, depending on the thickness of the smears.
9. Staining times for the hematoxylin and counterstains are often a matter of personal choice and depend on the type of cell sample. Individual experimentation may be necessary.
10. If slides remain in alcohol or clearing solutions longer than the prescribed time, the stains will be removed from the cells, especially the EA.
11. The use of a separatory funnel permits solutions to be filtered cell-free and without loss of staining constituents. This is especially important to know if using Harris hematoxylin, for which other methods of filtration may result in a weaker staining solution.

Rinsing Slides

1. Prior to placing slides in hematoxylin, the refractile "glassy" or "bubbly" appearance (due to removing alcohol from cells and cell clumps) must be eliminated by increasing the time the slides are left in water. If this is not done, penetration of the dyes is impaired. This step usually takes longer than the time designated in most staining procedures [**F***35.4*, **F***35.5*].
2. Slides should be well drained between solutions, but should not be permitted to dry. Staining racks may be blotted with paper towels between solutions when using manual method.
3. If the tap water rinse following hematoxylin is not sufficiently alkaline (approximately pH 7.4) the staining results will differ from time to time.
4. Gentle dipping of slides may avoid cell loss and possible cross-contamination, especially for nongynecologic samples.
5. Equating one dip to 1 to 2 seconds is a way to stabilize staining, especially when more than one person is responsible for staining. A dip is defined as the act of first submerging a rack of slides in a solution (without touching the bottom of the dish) and then raising the rack completely from the solution. These motions may be synchronized so that each dip is completed within one to two seconds.
6. Water rinses following hematoxylin should be changed after each use. Effective rinsing is judged by the disappearance of the dye color in the dishes, usually after the first two rinses; the third dish should be practically colorless.
7. Discard alcohol rinses following stains if deeply colored with stain. Rotate alcohol rinses following stains so the cleanest or clearest one is nearest the stain.
8. Alcohol solutions used for hydration and dehydration need to be discarded periodically.
9. Remove Scott's tap water substitute from slides by two separate tap water rinses. Discard after each use.

Cross-Contamination

1. It is recommended that three separate staining setups be used: one for gynecologic samples, one for cerebrospinal fluids, and one for all other nongynecologic cell samples. All stains and solutions should be filtered frequently, and in the case of nongynecologic samples, after a known malignant case has been stained.
2. In the case of body fluids the performance of a wet film preparation reveals the sample containing malignant tumor cells. The sample can then be stained after all other slides have been routinely stained that day.
3. Gentle dipping of slides may help avoid cell loss.
4. Xylene can be kept free of water contamination by adding silicic acid pellets to the absolute alcohol in the final dehydration rinse or by filtering xylene or its substitute with medium-grade filter paper daily.
5. Stains are filtered daily and stored in dark bottles.
6. Cross-contamination is controlled more stringently with the separatory funnel system. Filters need replacement when filtration becomes labored after several filtrations. Filtration may be slow to start if the pores are wet. Wet pores may require substantial vacuum to break loose the liquid held in the pores. Once the pores are open again, filtration proceeds smoothly. In other words, slow-starting filtration may mimic an overloaded filter that needs replacement.
7. With the separatory filter system, cross-contamination at the Johns Hopkins cytology laboratory was reduced virtually to zero. Spills are also avoided since the stain is vacuumed into the storage unit. Soiled laboratory coats and hands can also be avoided if the tube for vacuuming up the solution is long enough to be placed into the base of the staining dish containing the dye.
8. Floaters:
   a) Use the separatory funnel as described above.
   b) Change alcohols twice daily.
   c) Discard water rinses after each usage.
   d) Replace blueing and differentiation solutions frequently during the day.
   e) Known positive cases can be stained separately in disposable tubes or Coplin jars, or stained last in the regular staining dishes, provided that the regular setup is then discarded or all solutions are filtered.

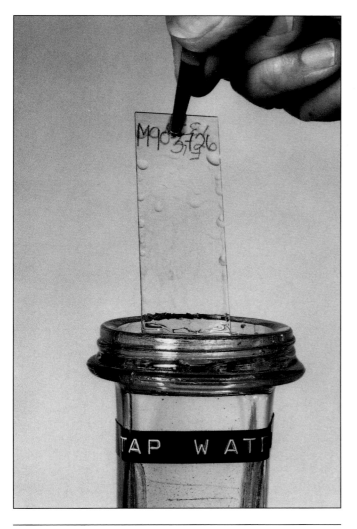

F35.4
"Glassy" or "bubbly" appearance of slides if not left long enough in water prior to placement in hematoxylin.

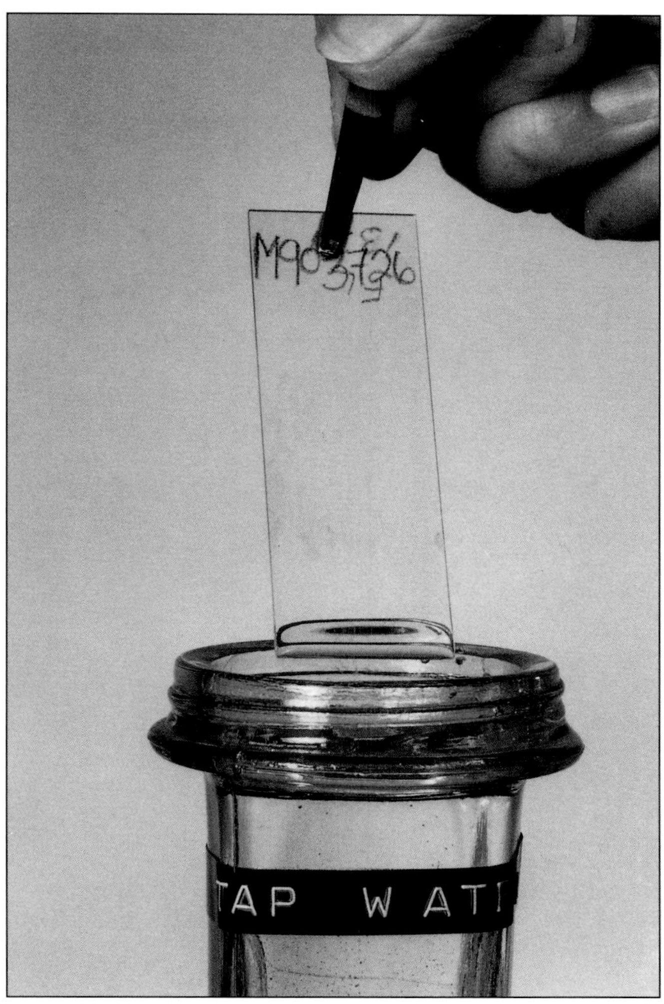

F35.5
Clear, nonbubbly appearance of slides when slides have been left in water for adequate length of time prior to placement in hematoxylin.

f) Use the toluidine blue technique to determine if a given fluid or specimen is positive.

Staining Cellulose Filters

Problem	*Possible Reasons*
Dull, grayish hazy appearance of cells	Mounting medium did not match refractive index of filter.
Unevenly stained	Rinsing in clearing solutions was inadequate.
	Filter may have adhered to another filter and solutions were not adequately circulated throughout filter.
Opaque white filter	Xylene was not adequately removed from cellulose filter prior to coverslipping.
	Mounting media was not put underneath and above cellulose filter.

Mounting Slides

Problem	*Possible Reasons*
Specimen wiped off because not on proper side of slide	When placed in staining rack, make sure cell surfaces are facing in same direction.
	If cell sample is thin or transparent, determination as to which side of the slide contains the sample may not be possible until specimen has been stained and coverslipped.
Rust-like coloration covering cells ("corn flakes")	Remove one slide at a time from final clearing solution; cover as fast as possible to prevent drying of cell surface.

Mounting Filters

Problem	*Possible Reasons*
Constant focusing of objective required to evaluate cells, especially under x40 magnification	Cellulose filter was not expanded in 95% ethanol prior to preparation as recommended in procedure. Prior to placing cells on the grid the filter may be flattened on the grid by pressure from a vacuum pump. Cellulose filter was not flattened on slide as described in mounting procedure.
Opaque, flat white filter noted after staining and drying	Filter was not properly mounted. Too much xylene or too little mounting medium was used in coverslipping procedure.

Cellulose Filter Preparation

Problem	*Possible Reasons*
Cell sample does not flow easily through cellulose filter	Sample was not centrifuged prior to the filtration procedure (necessary particularly for urine samples). Concentration of proteins and salts or crystals may clog filter. If urine sample is cold, allow it to reach room temperature before processing. Crystals may form when specimen is cold and disappear after specimen has returned to room temperature.
Cell loss in final preparation when abundance of cells are seen on toluidine blue cell film	Filter apparatus was improperly aligned. Filter was left too long in alcohol solution after preparation. Cells have floated away from filter surface or filter was allowed to sit overnight in final clearing solution. Space was inadequate between filters during staining procedure; cells attached themselves to back of another filter. If specimens are divided in two separate aliquots, a second filter may be prepared.

Contamination of Cell Sample

Problem	*Possible Reasons*
Fungal growth on all specimens (seasonal: higher in spring and fall)	Physiologic solutions grow fungi and should be discarded frequently. When not in use they should be refrigerated. If the saponin procedure is being used, the fresh solutions should be refrigerated when not in use. Specimen was left unrefrigerated after collection. Water supply may be contaminated. Periodic microbiologic analyses should be performed.
Water droplets on all specimens	When using staining machines, water droplets may appear at the bottom edge of stained slides. Water may collect in the bottom of staining dishes.

With manual staining, water droplets are likely to be spread across all areas of slide:

1. Discard final xylene clearing solutions. Water can usually be detected in xylene by the presence of a "wavy" look to solution instead of a "clear and clean" look. Xylene absorbs moisture from the air and water or may be carried over from the previous solutions.
2. Discard final clearing solutions of alcohol, because alcoholic solutions are prone to absorb water.
3. If water is still present, discard all alcohol and clearing solutions and filter stains.

   In general, xylene should be filtered through laboratory-grade filter paper daily.

   Gill recommends maintaining higher levels in the staining dishes of all solutions that follow the water baths.

Floaters

Problem	*Possible Reasons*
To detect floaters	Microscopic checks should be made of all samples stained together. If presence of atypical cells on a different focal plane is noted during microscopic examination of specimen, depress coverslip; floater will usually move or "float" away from view. One individual within the laboratory should check all fluid samples stained in 1 day to ascertain the possibility of floaters.

If floater detected	Make a second filter for samples, or prepare cell spreads on all samples to compare with filter preparations.
To avoid floaters	Perform toluidine blue procedure on all body fluids to determine if malignant tumor cells are present. If present, specimen should be stained after negative samples have been processed. Change all solutions completely after staining a known positive sample. Filter stains daily (separatory funnel apparatus is more effective than other methods). Stain nongynecologic samples separate from cerebrospinal fluids. Stain cellulose filters separately. Stain gynecologic samples separate from all other samples. Discard water rinses after each usage. Replace blueing and differentiation solutions frequently during the day. Known positive cases can be stained separately in disposable tubes or Coplin jars, or stained last in the regular staining dishes, provided that the regular setup is then discarded or all solutions are filtered. Use separatory funnel system.

SELECTED READINGS

Baker JR. *Principles of Biologic Microtechnique.* New York, NY: John Wiley & Sons Inc; 1958.

Bales CE, Durfee GR. Cytologic techniques. In: Koss LG, ed. *Diagnostic Cytopathology and Its Histologic Bases.* 4th ed. Philadelphia, Pa: JB Lippincott Co; 1992:1451-1531.

Barrett DL. Sources of cell loss using membrane filter and cytocentrifuge preparatory techniques. *Cytotechnol Bull.* 1975;12:7-8.

Barrett DL. Cytocentrifuge technique. In: Keebler CM, Reagan JW, Wied GL, eds. *Compendium on Cytopreparatory Techniques.* 4th ed. Chicago, Ill: Tutorials of Cytology; 1976:80-83.

Barrett DL, King EB. Comparisons of cellular recovery rates and morphological detail using membrane filter and cytocentrifuge techniques. *Acta Cytol.* 1976;20:174-180.

Beyer-Boon ME, Voorn-Den Hollander MJA. Cell yield obtained with various cytopreparatory techniques for urinary cytology. *Acta Cytol.* 1978;22:589-594.

Bigner SH, Johnston WW. Cytopreparation. In: Johnston WW, ed. *Cytopathology of the Central Nervous System.* New York, NY: Masson Publishing USA Inc; 1983:5-15.

Bonfiglio TA. Cytopathologic interpretation of transthoracic biopsies. In: Johnston WW, ed. *Masson Monographs in Diagnostic Cytopathology.* New York, NY: Masson Publishing USA Inc; 1983:187-194.

Boon ME, Wickel AF, Davoren RAM. Role of the air bubble in increasing cell recovery using cytospin I and II. *Acta Cytol.* 1983;27:699-702.

Chan JKC, Kung ITM. Rehydration of air-dried smears with normal saline. *Am J Clin Pathol.* 1988;89:30-34.

Danos M. On understanding the Papanicolaou stain: an interview with Ralph D. Lillie. *Cytotechnol Bull.* 1970;7:1-2.

Danos M. Fixatives for cytologic use. In: Keebler CM, Reagan JW, Wied GL, eds. *Compendium on Cytopreparatory Techniques.* 4th ed. Chicago, Ill: Tutorials of Cytology; 1976:7-9.

Fawcett DW, Valee BL, Soule MF. Method for concentration and segregation of malignant cells from bloody, pleural, and peritoneal fluids. *Science.* 1950;111:34-36.

Gill G. Saponizing bloody cytologic specimens. In: *The Shandon Cytospin 2 in Diagnostic Cytology: Techniques, Tips and Troubleshooting.* Sewichley, Pa: Shandon Southern Instruments; 1982:44-46.

Gill GW. Controlling the Papanicolaou stain. *ASCP Cytotechnology Check Sample*, C-66. Chicago, Ill: American Society of Clinical Pathologists; 1979.

Gill GW, Frost JK, Miller KA. A new formula for half-oxidized hematoxylin solution that neither overstains nor requires differentiation. *Acta Cytol.* 1974;18:300-311.

Gill GW, Miller KA. *Laboratory Techniques for Specimen Preparation.* 5th ed. Baltimore, Md: The Johns Hopkins School of Medicine; 1973.

Harris MJ, Schwinn CP, Marrow JW, Gray RL, Browell BM. Exfoliative cytology of urinary bladder irrigation specimens. *Acta Cytol.* 1971;15:385-399.

Hickling RA. Vital staining of malignant cells in a peritoneal effusion. *Cancer.* 1931;34:789-791.

Hinds IL. A comparison of three xylene substitutes. *Lab Med.* 1986;17:752-755.

Holmquist MD. Detection of urinary tract cancer in urinalysis specimens in an outpatient population. *Am J Clin Pathol.* 1988;89:499-504.

Horobin RW. Fundamental mechanisms of cytological staining. In: Boon ME, Kok LP, eds. *Standardization and Quantitation of Diagnostic Staining in Cytology.* Leyden, the Netherlands: Couloml Press; 1986:9-14.

Horobin RW. An overview of the theory of staining. In: Bancroft JD, Stevens A, eds. *Theory and Practice of Histological Techniques.* 3rd ed. New York, NY: Churchill Livingstone Inc; 1990:93-108.

Husain OAN, Millett JA, Grainger JM. Use of polylysine-coated slides for preparation of cell samples for diagnostic cytology. *Technical Methods.* 1979:309-311.

Johnston WW, Frable WJ. *Diagnostic Respiratory Cytopathology.* New York, NY: Masson Publishing USA Inc; 1979:5-18.

Lillie RD. *Histopathologic Technic and Practical Histochemistry.* 3rd ed. New York, NY: McGraw-Hill Inc; 1965.

McNair J, Scott TF, Finland M. The cytology of pleural effusions in pneumonia studied with a supravital technique. *Am J Med Sci.* 1934;188:322-332.

Naylor B. Pleural, peritoneal and pericardial fluids. In: Bibbo M, ed. *Comprehensive Cytopathology.* Philadelphia, Pa: WB Saunders Co; 1991:541-614.

Papanicolaou GN. A new procedure for staining vaginal smears. *Science.* 1942;95:438-439.

Papanicolaou GN. *Atlas of Exfoliative Cytology.* Cambridge, Mass: Harvard University Press; 1954:3-12, suppl 2.

Pharr SL, Farber SM, King EB. Cellular concentration of sputum for cytologic examination. In: *Transactions of the Fifth Annual Meeting of the Inter-Society Cytology Council.* Philadelphia, Pa: 1957:65-68.

Precautions in taking care of patients with suspected Creutzfeldt-Jakob disease. In: *Nation Nosocomial Infections Study Report, Annual Summary 1979.* Atlanta, Ga: Centers for Disease Control; 1982.

Reynaud AM, King EB. A new filter for diagnostic cytology. *Acta Cytol.* 1967;11:289-294.

Saccomanno G, Saunders RP, Ellis H, Archer VE, Wood BG. Concentration of carcinoma or atypical cells in sputum. *Acta Cytol.* 1963;7:305-310.

Seal SH. A method for concentrating cancer cells suspended in large quantities of fluid. *Cancer.* 1956;9:866-868.

Smith MJ, Naylor B. *Techniques of Cytopathology: Laboratory Manual.* Ann Arbor, Mich: Department of Pathology, University of Michigan; 1970:8-10.

Smith MJ, Naylor B. A method for extracting ferruginous bodies from sputum and pulmonary tissue. *Am J Clin Pathol.* 1972;58:250-254.

Soost HJ, Falter EW, Otto K. Comparison of two Papanicolaou staining procedures for automated prescreening. *Anal Quant Cytol.* 1979;1:37-42.

Street CM. Papanicolaou techniques in exfoliative cytology. In: Cowdry EV, ed. *Laboratory Technique in Biology and Medicine.* 3rd ed. Baltimore, Md: Williams & Wilkins; 1952:253-259.

West PW. *Calculations of Quantitative Analysis.* New York, NY: Macmillan Publishing Co; 1947.

Index

Numbers in **boldface** refer to pages on which images, figures, and tables appear.

B

C

D

E

F

M

Q

R

S

T

U

V

W

Y